The Complete Cancer
Survival Guide

The Complete Cancer Survival Guide

■

**The Most Comprehensive, Up-to-Date Guide
for Patients and Their Families**

*With Advice from Dozens of Leading
Cancer Specialists at More than 30
Major Cancer Centers*

Peter Teeley and Philip Bashe

MAIN STREET BOOKS

DOUBLEDAY
New York   London   Toronto   Sydney   Auckland

A Main Street Book
PUBLISHED BY DOUBLEDAY
a division of Bantam Doubleday Dell Publishing Group, Inc.
1540 Broadway, New York, New York 10036

Main Street Books, Doubleday and the portrayal of a building with a
tree are trademarks of Doubleday, a division of Random House, Inc.

Chapter Seven's table of anticancer drugs and their potential side effects is
adapted from the *USP DI*, vol. 2, *Advice for the Patient, Drug Information
in Lay Language*, 18th ed., Copyright © 1998 by the USP Convention, Inc.
Permission granted.

All illustrations courtesy of the National Cancer Institute.

Book design by Richard Oriolo

Library of Congress Cataloging-in-Publication Data
Teeley, Peter.
The complete cancer survival guide / Peter Teeley and Philip Bashe.
p.   cm.
Includes index.
1. Cancer—Popular works.   I. Bashe, Philip.   II. Title.
RC263.T39   2000
616.99′4—dc21   98-28588
CIP

ISBN 0-385-48605-7

Printed in the United States of America

May 2000

FIRST EDITION

1   2   3   4   5   6   7   8   9   10

To my grandfather, Thomas Ambrose Cullen:
Though severely wounded and gassed twice in World War I,
he never lost his great spirit, Irish humor, and dashing self-confidence.

To my mother, Winifred Cullen Teeley, and my father, Francis Albert Teeley,
whose strength during World War II and courage and hard work as
immigrants made a better life for us in America.

To my daughters, Adrienne, Laura, Randall, and Susan,
who have filled me with love and joy for all their years.

—PETER B. TEELEY

Peter Teeley would like to acknowledge the following people:

I am alive today partly because of the efforts of my former wife Valerie Teeley, former President George Bush, and former First Lady Barbara Bush. I thank Valerie for her total dedication to my well-being, her vigilance and determination in assuring that my medical care was comprehensive, and for being my advocate. She was protective and supportive of me throughout an eight-month medical ordeal that was physically and emotionally debilitating.

I owe a great debt to Barbara Bush, who informed the president of my grave condition while I was in a coma following a second life-threatening surgery. He in turn dispatched White House physician Dr. Larry Mohr to oversee my medical care. Larry became both friend and adviser. He called Dr. Samuel Broder, then the head of the National Cancer Institute, to find out which hospitals were offering the most promising, cutting-edge clinical trials for stage III colon cancer. That call led to my successful treatment at Georgetown University's Lombardi Cancer Center.

There are many other people I would like to thank, beginning with Linda Hodgson. After hearing a doctor tell Valerie that I might die, Linda called the White House and conveyed to the Bushes the seriousness of my condition. The next morning, the president called Valerie, triggering events that helped me survive.

I am eternally grateful to my two primary physicians at Lombardi, Dr. Paul Woolley and Dr. John Marshall, for their honesty and directness, their tremendous knowledge of treating colon cancer, and their warm, reassuring natures.

Thanks also go to:

The other doctors and nurses who made up my medical team, particularly Dr. Chitra Rajagopal. All of them made me feel like the most important patient on earth, and I am indebted to them for their extraordinary attention and care.

My two intensive-care nurses at the community hospital, Beth Maday and Ann Saether. They bathed me, treated me, encouraged me, and were instrumental in my pulling through.

Mary Morgenstern, my former assistant and longtime friend, who maintained my business and performed countless personal and professional tasks for my family and me.

John White, the former chairman of the Democratic National Committee, and a very close friend who called every day to offer encouragement and provide humor. Our long political discussions helped to lift my spirits and keep my mind off my illness. John died a few years ago, and I regret that I was unable to help him as he had helped me.

Alixe Glen Mattingly, a miraculous cancer survivor at age sixteen, who was an inspiration during my illness and, as always, a caring friend.

I deeply appreciate the kindness extended to me and my family by members of the Bush cabinet and executive branch, especially Secretary of State James A. Baker III, Commerce Secretary Robert Mosbacher, and Margaret Tutwiler, former Assistant Secretary of State.

Many journalists displayed a deep caring by calling, writing, or just checking in to see how I was doing, but I'd especially like to thank Andy Rosenthal and Maureen Dowd of the *New York Times,* Michael Duffy of *Time* magazine, Al Hunt of the *Wall Street Journal,* John Mashek of the *Boston Globe,* Gene Gibbons of Reuters, and Ann Devroy of the *Washington Post.* Sadly, Ann later succumbed to cancer.

Finally, I want to express my deepest gratitude to Philip Bashe, my coauthor, who actually wrote this book, compiled the research, and turned what was originally my story into a much more important comprehensive cancer survival guide that will benefit many thousands of cancer patients, their families, and friends.

Philip Bashe would like to thank Robert and Rochelle Bashe, the late Evelyn Bashe, Justin Bashe, and, as always, Patty Bashe, for everything.

Together the authors would like to thank the following physicians, nurses, and other health-care professionals at Georgetown University Medical Center's Lombardi Cancer Center for kindly taking the time to speak with us: director Dr. Marc Lippman, Dr. John Marshall, Dr. Christine Berg, nurse Merilyn Francis, Leslie Freeman, Dr. Michael Hawkins, Dr. Jane Ingham, Dr. Kenneth Meehan, Dr. Marie F. Pennanen, Dr. Chitra Rajagopal, clinical social worker Dominica Roth, Dr. Julia Rowland, nursing coordinator Maureen Sawchuk, clinical dietitian Susan Sloan, Dr. Scott Spear, chaplain Christine Swift, and Dr. Rebecca Zuurbier.

We are grateful as well to these other cancer specialists and health-care professionals who consented to be interviewed. Alphabetically, they are: Dr. Jeffrey Abrams (National Cancer Institute), Dr. Rocco Addante (Norris Cotton Cancer Center, Dartmouth-Hitchcock Medical Center), Dr. Fred Appelbaum (Fred Hutchinson Cancer Research Center), Elizabeth Augustine (National Institutes of Health Clinical Center), Dr. Paul A. Bunn, Jr. (University of Colorado Cancer Center), Dr. John Butler (Chao Family Comprehensive Cancer Center, Unversity of California at Irvine), Dr. Paul Carbone (University of Wisconsin Comprehensive Cancer Center), Dr. Christine Cassel (Mount Sinai Medical Center), Dr. Visalam Chandrasekarian (Long Island Jewish Medical Center), Dr. Michael Cooper (Duke University Medical Center), Dr. Larry Copeland (Arthur G. James Cancer Hospital and Research Institute, Ohio State University), Dr. Vincent DeVita (Yale University Cancer Center), Dr. Michael Friedman (Food and Drug Administration), Dr. Charles Fuchs (Dana-Farber Cancer Institute), Dr. Harinder Garewal (Arizona Cancer Center, University of Arizona Health Sciences Center), Dr. T. S. Greaves (Kenneth Norris Jr. Comprehensive Cancer Center, University of Southern California), Dr. Michael Gruber (Kaplan Cancer Center, New York University Medical Center), Dr. William H. Hartmann (American Board of Pathology), Dr. Todd Heniford (Cleveland Clinic Foundation), Dr. Michael Hogan (Fox Chase Cancer Center), Dr. David Johnson (Vanderbilt Cancer Center, Vanderbilt University), Dr. Brian Kimes (National Cancer Institute), Dr. Barnett Kramer (National Cancer Institute), Dr. Jill Lacy (Yale University Cancer Center), Dr. Frederick Lang (University of Texas M. D. Anderson Cancer Center), Dr. Ted Lawrence (University of Michigan Comprehensive Cancer Center), Dr. Cathy L. Lazarus (Northwestern University Medical School), Matthew LoScalzo (Johns Hopkins Oncology Center), Dr. Jim Mohler (UNC Lineberger Comprehensive Cancer Center), Dr. Paul Moots (Vanderbilt Cancer Center, Vanderbilt University), Dr. Mitchell Morris (University of Texas M. D. Anderson Cancer Center), Dr. Edward Neuwelt (Oregon Cancer Center, Oregon Health Sciences University), Dr. Larry Norton (Memorial Sloan-Kettering Cancer Center), Dr. Allan Oseroff (Roswell Park Cancer Institute), Dr. Margaret Pratila (Memorial Sloan-Kettering Cancer Center), Dr. Bruce Redman (University of Michigan Comprehensive Cancer Center), Dr. Douglas Reintgen (H. Lee Moffitt Cancer Center and Research Institute at the University of South Florida), Dr. Fred Richards II (Comprehensive Cancer Center of Wake Forest University), Dr. Mary Ann Richardson (Center for Alternative Medicine in Cancer), Dr. William Richtsmeier (Duke Comprehensive Cancer Center, Duke University Medical Center), Dr. Nicholas Robert (Inova Fairfax Hospital), Dr. Peter Rosen (Jonsson Comprehensive Cancer Center, UCLA), Dr. Steven Rosen (Robert H. Lurie Comprehensive Cancer Center, Northwestern University), Dr. Mark Sherer (Mississippi Methodist Rehabilitation Center), George Silberman (U.S. General Accounting Office), Dr. Franklin Sim (Mayo Clinic Cancer Center), Dr. Colin Paul Spears (Eli Lilly and Company), Dr. Kasi Sridhar (Sylvester Comprehensive Cancer Center, University of Miami Medical School), Dr. Michael Sterchi (Baptist Hospital at the Bowman Gray School of Medicine of Wake Forest University), Dr. David Tubergen (University of Texas M. D. Anderson Cancer Center), Dr. Anil Tulpule (Kenneth Norris Jr. Comprehensive Cancer Center, University of Southern California), Dr. Rick Ungerleider (National Cancer Institute), Dr. Donald Urban (University of Alabama at Birmingham Comprehensive Cancer Center), Dr. Randal Weber (University of Pennsylvania Cancer Center), Dr. Larry White (Association of Community Cancer Centers), Dr. Paul Woolley (University of Pittsburgh Cancer Institute at University of Pittsburgh Medical Center Lee Regional, and formerly of the Lombardi Cancer Center), Dr. Kenneth Yaw (University of Pittsburgh Cancer Institute), and Dr. Charles J. Yeo (Johns Hopkins University School of Medicine).

Finally, very special thanks to our talented editors, Judy Kern and Rob Robertson, for their expert guidance, saintly *patience,* and support; Judy's assistant, Kendra Harpster; copy editor Bill Betts; designer Richard Oriolo; Gilbert G. Bashe, for bringing the two of us together; Maggie Bartlett of the National Cancer Institute's Office of Cancer Communications, Graphics and Audiovisual Section; Sue Lin Chong, the Lombardi Cancer Center's senior associate director of public relations, for effort above and beyond the call, fax, and e-mail of duty; everyone at James Levine Communications, Inc.; and especially our agent, Arielle Eckstut, for her guidance and advice, and for making the difficult process of getting a book published appear simple and orderly, a tribute to her impressive talents.

Normally I do not write Forewords, but in this case I am particularly pleased to write about *The Complete Cancer Survival Guide*. This is because of my respect for Peter Teeley, my press secretary for six years, former U.S. Ambassador to Canada, and my friend. Also, because he and coauthor Philip Bashe have written a book that will help a great many people with cancer, as well as their families.

Barbara and I know all too well the devastating impact this disease can have. In 1953, just a few weeks after the birth of our third child, Jeb, our three-year-old daughter was diagnosed with pediatric leukemia.

Robin was an adorable child, with golden curls and the sweetest smile you could imagine. That spring, however, she seemed unusually lethargic. At first Barbara wasn't overly concerned, but when the fatigue persisted, she brought Robin to our hometown pediatrician in Midland, Texas. Dr. Dorothy Wyvell took a blood sample and said she'd call us later that day, after the test results were in. She also suggested cryptically that Barbara have me meet her at the office.

Back then people didn't talk openly about cancer like they do today, undoubtedly because the prospects for survival were so slim. When Dr.

Wyvell informed us that Robin had leukemia, our faces registered little shock; we'd never heard of the disease and didn't understand the implications of the news she'd just delivered.

I vaguely remember asking the doctor what could be done to cure our daughter. In a compassionate voice, she explained that there *wasn't* any cure. Dr. Wyvell gently advised us to take Robin home, care for her and love her, and wait for the end, which would come swiftly—perhaps in a matter of weeks.

My uncle, Dr. John Walker, happened to be a surgeon at Memorial Hospital in Manhattan. Today it is known as Memorial Sloan-Kettering Cancer Center, one of the world's preeminent cancer research and treatment facilities. Uncle John concurred with our pediatrician's bleak prognosis. But he recommended that we bring Robin to Memorial for chemotherapy, a treatment that was then in its infancy. The best we could hope for was that the medication might extend our little girl's life long enough for a medical breakthrough to come along. We flew to New York the next day, determined to give our three-year-old every conceivable opportunity to live.

Based on the standards of fifty years ago, we succeeded. The leukemia went into remission, only to recur. Robin's condition seesawed back and forth like this several times over the next half a year. That summer she did get to visit her grandparents in Connecticut and spend time in Maine with her brothers Jeb and George, our oldest. We even took Robin home to Texas at one point. Despite the painful tests and blood transfusions and side effects from the chemotherapy, those last six months were a gift, both for her and for us. In October our darling daughter passed away peacefully in Memorial Hospital, with us at her bedside.

Soon after, we established a foundation to raise funds for leukemia research: the Bright Star Foundation. It was just one of many efforts under way at the time in search of a cure. All Americans should be grateful to the cancer research hospitals, the National Cancer Institute, pharmaceutical companies, and the thousands of medical professionals who have participated in developing and investigating new therapies. Thanks to them and to the patients who volunteered to enter these studies, remarkable strides have been made.

Today, about four in five boys and girls with Robin's disease live, as do three in four of all youngsters with cancer. For adults the overall cure rate has edged steadily upward. In 1995 it surpassed 66 percent, or two-thirds, for the first time. Many patients are now routinely offered choices of treatments where not all that long ago none may have existed.

When Pete was diagnosed with colon cancer in 1991, he wasn't satisfied with the limited treatment options available at one hospital outside of Washington. He discussed treatment options with my personal physician, who told him about a National Cancer Institute sponsored clinical trial being conducted at Georgetown University Medical Center's Lombardi Cancer Center. Pete credits the then investigational protocol of two chemotherapy drugs with possibly saving his life.

We still have a long way to go, however, which is why my wife and I remain involved in the cancer community. Barbara sits on the board of trustees at the Mayo Clinic, while I serve in a similar capacity at the M. D. Anderson Cancer Center in Houston. Together we cochair the National Dialogue on Cancer (NDC), comprised of an impressive array of cancer experts from around the country. One of the NDC's goals is to increase funding for research. Another is to educate cancer patients on how to advocate for themselves within the health-care system.

This book is part of that process. If *The Complete Cancer Survival Guide* merely recounted Pete's personal battle with the disease, it would be inspiring enough. But the authors have brought together the most up-to-date information on cancer, its diagnosis, and its treatment, and distilled it in a warm, authoritative style that will be readily understandable to people with cancer and the people who love them. Pete and Philip also weave in the perspectives of cancer specialists at more than three dozen state-of-the-art cancer centers in the United States.

Today's cancer patients have more choices than ever before; *The Complete Cancer Survival Guide* will help you to make sense of them and obtain the most appropriate medical care for your type of cancer.

—GEORGE BUSH,
Houston, Texas

Contents

As far as I knew, and as far as my doctors were concerned, I was scheduled to undergo a routine appendectomy. When I awoke from surgery the next morning, I found my wife, Valerie, sitting at the foot of my hospital bed, bearing devastating news: What had appeared on an MRI scan to be nothing more than an inflamed appendix was, in fact, cancer.

Shortly afterward the surgeon appeared. "You must feel like you've been run over by a Mack truck," he said. "You've had a tough night." I could only wince in agreement. The doctor proceeded to explain the diagnosis: A tumor in the large intestine had burrowed through the bowel wall and infiltrated the adjoining appendix as well as several nearby lymph nodes. This put the cancer at stage III on a scale of I to IV, with IV being the most life-threatening. He'd cut out the malignant portion of the colon, then rejoined the severed ends. Nearly two dozen nodes also had to be removed.

"What are my odds for beating this?" I asked.

"About fifty-fifty."

I was fifty-one years old. Two thoughts flashed through my mind. The first—*You may not have long to live*—was immediately replaced by images of my little girls, four-year-old Randall, and Adrienne, just eighteen months old, and my two grown daughters, Susan and Laura.

Standard treatment for stage III colon cancer calls for postoperative chemotherapy to eradicate any stray cancer cells that might be lurking in the body. But before I could begin the fight of and for my life, a new hurdle arose when the intestine twisted, blocking digested food from passing through.

"I'm afraid I have to open you up again," the surgeon informed me. For the second time in a week, a supposedly routine procedure proved anything but. A medical error led to my developing pneumonia and slipping into a coma. For the next week, I hovered between life and death, my breathing regulated by a mechanical respirator. One night Valerie asked a member of the medical team outright, "Is my husband going to die?" The doctor paused uncomfortably, then answered, "He might."

A few days later, while I was recovering, the surgeon ambled into my hospital room accompanied by two doctors, who pulled up chairs and introduced themselves as my oncologists. They outlined a treatment plan that consisted of the then-conventional regimen of cancer-fighting drugs. Both men were congenial and, I'm sure, highly capable. "I don't want to be disrespectful," I told them, "but I think I'm going to go somewhere else."

"Where?" they asked.

To be honest, I had no idea. Like most newly diagnosed patients, I knew little about the disease and less still about its treatment. What I did know was that I had scant confidence that this community hospital held my best hope for a cure. Before I made any decision, I wanted to learn what my options were—if I *had* any options. After finally leaving the hospital, I rested at home in Alexandria, Virginia, for a few days, mulling over what to do next.

Perhaps because I'd spent twenty years in politics as a press secretary—to Vice President George Bush, and before that to U.S. Senators Jacob Javits of New York and Robert Griffin of Michigan—networking for information came naturally. A doctor friend of mine referred me to Georgetown University's Lombardi Cancer Center in Washington, D.C., which offered an experimental treatment for stage III colon cancer as part of a large study funded by the National Cancer Institute, the federal government's main agency for cancer research. The purpose of this clinical trial was to evaluate the effectiveness of a new combination of drugs, though the two agents themselves had been used in cancer therapy for some time. Based on earlier studies, the doctors felt confident that the regimen would prove superior to the current standard chemotherapy, or would be at least as beneficial. I met the eligibility requirements and enrolled in the trial.

Today, more than eight years later, I can be said to be cured. There are 8 million other cancer survivors like me who have successfully completed the difficult journey that you are just starting.

Where to Seek Cancer Care: The Most Important Consumer Decision of Your Life

I went about lining up medical care much as I would any other service. The analogy isn't original, but if your car's engine needs repair, you probably call around for referrals and quiz the mechanic about his experience. Yet when faced with the most critical consumer decision of their lives, the majority of cancer patients accept without question the recommendation of the doctor who diagnosed the disease. Eighty-five percent of the time, that person is not an *oncologist,* a specialist in the detection and treatment of cancer.

These patients are putting themselves at risk. An alarming report issued by the National Cancer Policy Board in 1999 concluded that a considerable number of cancer patients were receiving substandard medical care. "Based on the best available evidence," wrote the authors, "some individuals with cancer do not receive care known to be effective for their condition. The magnitude of the problem is not known, but the National Cancer Policy Board believes it is substantial."

There are many reasons why cancer therapy can deviate from the optimal course. Some of them may surprise you; all of them should concern anyone faced with having to decide where to go for medical care.

• You risk receiving less than state-of-the-art care if your physician lacks experience in treating your form of cancer.
The word "cancer" actually refers to a constellation of many different diseases, most of them relatively rare. Only 30,200 new cases of leukemia are diagnosed annually. Kidney cancer: 30,000. Cervical cancer: 12,800. Testicular cancer: 7,400. (By contrast, consider that each year brings 400,000 new cases of heart failure, another 500,000 men

and women suffer strokes, and 1.5 million more are felled by heart attacks.) So it's highly conceivable that a general oncologist—one who treats a variety of cancers—sees but a few patients with your particular disease each year. Given the ever-evolving landscape of cancer therapy, you cannot presume that a physician has experience in, or even knowledge of, the latest developments just by virtue of being a "cancer doc."

"In a country this size, the dissemination of information is sometimes very slow," observes Dr. Vincent DeVita, director of the Yale University Cancer Center in New Haven, Connecticut. Even in the absence of an established treatment, it can take a long time for new techniques to trickle down through the ranks of physicians, especially those not associated with medical centers carrying out clinical research. Dr. DeVita, who directed the National Cancer Institute from 1980 to 1988, points to his own work in the 1970s, when he and other NCI oncologists specializing in cancer of the lymphatic system pioneered the first curative therapy for advanced Hodgkin's disease.

"The cure rate," he says, "went from zero percent to 70 percent. Yet it took *eleven years* for that to be fully integrated nationwide, despite the fact that no competing therapy existed and the treatment was widely accepted." Would you want to entrust your life to an oncologist whose information is limited, someone who might not be aware of or have the opportunity to implement today's treatment advances for another month, another year?

"Cancer is too complex and too curable to have someone 'catch up' at your expense," Dr. DeVita emphasizes. "There are some kinds of cancer treatments that simply are carried out better by people with experience."

Medical Terms You're Likely to Hear

Surgical oncologist: a surgeon who specializes in cancer surgery. He or she may further specialize in breast surgical oncology, gynecological surgical oncology, and so on.

Medical oncologist: a physician who specializes in treating cancer with chemical agents, or *chemotherapy.*

Radiation oncologist: a physician who specializes in treating cancer using high-energy X rays, or *radiation therapy;* also referred to as *radiotherapy.*

• **You risk receiving less than state-of-the-art care if your treatment isn't planned by a multidisciplinary oncology team.**

For many cancers, the most effective therapy often integrates two or more *disciplines,* or methods of treatment: perhaps surgery followed by chemotherapy, which is what I underwent; or chemo or radiation therapy up front, in the hopes of shrinking an otherwise inoperable tumor to an operable size. There are many other permutations, involving not only surgery, chemo, and radiation but hormone therapy, biological therapy, bone-marrow transplantation, and still other complementary therapies.

A multidisciplinary team brings together experts in the different disciplines to collaborate on a treatment strategy, or *protocol*—ideally, at the outset. "The idea," explains Dr. Marc Lippman, director of the Lombardi Cancer Center, "is that surgeons, medical oncologists, and radiation oncologists can make valuable contributions to the initial treatment planning for any kind of cancer. Oftentimes, better recommendations are made simply because other people with varying perspectives see the case. Heaven only knows that I've modified my views about certain patients' cases based on what colleagues had to suggest."

Although the multidisciplinary concept is gaining prominence at many medical centers, the reality is that most patients won't have a team behind them unless they expressly seek out a cancer facility where the multidisciplinary concept is practiced. Should they see only one doctor, it's possible they'll never be exposed to other approaches to treatment. Or they may trek from surgeon's office to chemotherapist's office to radiotherapist's office and wind up with three conflicting recommendations.

Based on the findings of three major studies, the National Cancer Institute in 1988 issued a rare "clinical alert" advising physicians of the striking benefits that *adjuvant* therapy demonstrated with early-stage breast tumors. "Adjuvant" refers to drug therapy administered after a patient recuperates from surgery, to patrol the circulation and kill any lingering malignant cells. But a decade later, only about one in two women with stage I or II breast cancer receive either postoperative chemotherapy or hormone therapy as recommended. One reason why, suggests Dr. DeVita, a cancer specialist since 1963, is that "there are plenty of surgeons who don't believe in adjuvant therapy for breast cancer at all. So they never refer their patients to a medical oncologist. After the operation, the woman is told, 'Don't worry, Mrs. Smith, I got everything.' That sounds like great news. But we've known for fifty years that when you think you've eliminated every last trace of cancer in the breast, most of the time it eventually comes back, spreads to other parts of the body, and the patient dies of her cancer."

• **You risk receiving less than state-of-the-art care if the medical facility treating you does not participate in a broad range of** *clinical trials*.

When you're contending with a disease that, despite strides in treatment, claims more than half a million lives each year, "in many cases," notes Dr. Lippman, "the best therapy is an experimental one."

The Lombardi Cancer Center, one of thirty-five facilities designated a "comprehensive cancer center" by the National Cancer Institute, attracts many patients seeking cutting-edge treatments. "That's the majority of the patients we see," says Dr. John Marshall. Dr. Marshall, a subspecialist in gastrointestinal cancers, was one of my two attending physicians. "Usually, they get their adjuvant therapy out in the community," meaning community hospitals not always affiliated with extensive research. "And when the community has nothing more to offer them, they come here."

Until recently, clinical trials were generally perceived as the last resort. But as my case illustrates, it is not uncommon nowadays for oncologists to propose an investigative protocol from the start. It is through such studies that new strategies find their way into the mainstream. Fluorouracil and leucovorin, the experimental drug combination that I received, is now regarded as standard treatment for stage III colon cancer, and an improvement over what I would have been given had I not actively sought out other options.

• **You risk receiving less than state-of-the-art care if the medical facility treating you is inadequately equipped to manage any serious side effects that may arise from treatment**.

Both chemotherapy and radiation therapy carry risks. No matter how precise the dosage, some degree of healthy cells inevitably are ravaged along with malignant cells. This is what causes adverse side effects, which range from disagreeable to fatal. In the most serious complication—immune suppression—the anticancer drugs destroy white blood cells, the body's foot soldiers against viruses, bacteria, and other infectious agents. Should the white-cell count drop below a certain level, patients can become dangerously susceptible to pneumonia and other life-threatening infections.

As a result, treatment may have to be suspended until the white count rebounds. If a patient's blood counts repeatedly take a battering, the drugs may have to be given at longer intervals or the dosage may need to be lowered. In either instance, the patient is deprived of the full benefit of therapy. A 1995 Gallup survey revealed that half of patients undergoing chemotherapy had their treatment delayed due to diminished white-cell counts.

According to Dr. DeVita, your chances of being able to stick to the original course are enhanced considerably if you receive outpatient treatment at a major medical center, "where we're surrounded by experts in infectious diseases, cardiology, and other fields of medicine, so that we can deal with unusual complications more readily." A major medical facility is also more likely to have access to any new drugs or techniques for controlling side effects. In the same 1995 Gallup poll, three in four chemotherapy recipients said they were never informed of, much less offered, a biological agent proven to stimulate the body's production of white cells, though the product has been available since 1991.

"Oncologists and radiotherapists in private practice are far more inclined to modify dosages in ways that can be harmful to the outcome," says Dr. DeVita, "because they're usually less equipped to handle the side effects that might occur."

• You risk receiving less than state-of-the-art care if your medical insurer denies payment for a doctor-recommended treatment on the grounds that it is experimental.

The growing practice among third-party payers of broadly defining "experimental" therapy might be the single greatest threat to the quality of cancer care. Examples of rejected claims range from debatable (treating women at heightened risk for a recurrence of breast cancer with bone-marrow transplantation, a costly and risky procedure that is still being studied to see if it indeed benefits those patients) to unconscionable (the absurd contention, made by a number of insurance carriers, that breast reconstruction following a mastectomy is "cosmetic" surgery and therefore not covered).

Perhaps most insidious are the reimbursement policies that restrict doctors from prescribing a chemotherapy drug "off-label": that is, to treat a form of cancer other than those spelled out in the drug's accompanying package insert. Prescribing off-label is a common practice in oncology, with more than half of all patients receiving at least one drug prescribed in this fashion. However, in a U.S. General Accounting Office study made public around the time my cancer was discovered, in September 1991, one in four oncologists surveyed admitted that they'd had to alter their optimal treatment plan and order less effective agents, because the preferred drugs would not be reimbursed by the patient's insurer.

At the time, one of the off-label applications most frequently turned down was the use of leucovorin in treating stage III colon cancer—the protocol that may have saved my life. "Until very recently," says Dr. Lippman, "fluorouracil was an approved treatment, whereas fluorouracil modulated by leucovorin was not. Yet it was known among experts and widely published that fluorouracil and leucovorin was superior." I was fortunate that my insurance company never questioned the claim, and I was able to complete the clinical trial. However, for other patients, particularly those on managed-care plans, "it was impossible," says Dr. Lippman, "to get payment for giving them the superior care."

Cancer Treatment Today: Cause for Optimism

There are still other factors that could compromise the quality of your cancer treatment, but let's stop here, before we give the impression that outstanding medical care isn't to be found. On the contrary, most cancer patients in this country receive appropriate, compassionate care from dedicated doctors, nurses, and other healthcare professionals.

In 1996—twenty-five years and $28 billion in research after President Richard Nixon signed the National Cancer Act, the opening salvo in the "war on cancer"—it was announced that for the first time, the overall cancer mortality rate (the number of cancer deaths per 100,000 people) had dipped slightly over the previous five years. From the mid-1970s to the mid-1990s, the survival rates for most cancers rose, in some cases dramatically.

This progress can be attributed partly to greater public awareness of preventive measures, but also to improved screening techniques for detecting cancer earlier, when it is generally more treatable, and to more effective therapies. In the mid-1950s, only about one in three people with the disease lived five years or longer. Today three in five reach that landmark, which for certain cancers signifies a cure.

While it is true that the 1990s brought incremental gains in treatment, there is still no so-called magic bullet. But then, this is a frustratingly complicated disease. "In terms of our overall ability to cure cancer, we've been on a plateau since the early 1980s," concedes Dr. DeVita. Significant headway has been made, however, in enhancing patients' quality of life, through such advances as the following:

Less invasive surgeries: for instance, a nerve-sparing approach to prostatectomy (removing the prostate gland) that better preserves the ability to achieve an erection, an all-too-frequent result of the conventional operation. Or laparoscopic colectomy for resecting some colon tumors. Instead of a large incision in the abdomen, the surgeon makes several small cuts, inserts a flexible viewing instrument, and performs the procedure through this scope, resulting in less scarring and a speedier recovery.

Combined treatments that spare patients disfiguring operations or allow them to forgo surgery altogether. Today most women with early-stage breast cancer can be offered the choice of a mastectomy or equally effective breast-conservation surgery, also known as a lumpectomy, followed by radiation. Likewise, laryngeal-cancer patients may be treated with chemotherapy and radiation therapy in lieu of a laryngectomy to excise the voice box.

More precisely targeted external-beam radiation therapy, which allows for higher dosages while safeguarding surrounding normal tissues, reducing side effects.

Greater use of screening procedures, tests that can detect certain cancers in their early stages, before symptoms arise. For instance, many of the growing number of people who survive colorectal cancer owe their lives to having had an endoscopic exam of the colon and rectum. Credit for the marked decline in deaths from cervical cancer belongs largely to the simple Pap smear, which enables gynecologists to catch incipient carcinoma of the cervix before it even becomes cancer.

Improved medications for controlling disease symptoms and treatment side effects like pain, nausea, diarrhea, constipation, and low blood counts.

At many cancer centers, a greater emphasis on offering patients and their families professional mental-health care, peer support groups, and social-work services, to better help them cope with the psychological and financial burdens cancer can impose.

Most people live within driving distance of excellent cancer care. But unless you take it upon yourself to become an educated medical consumer, how can you be sure if you are indeed receiving the most appropriate therapy for *your* cancer?

"If patients don't know what treatments are out there," cautions George Silberman, assistant director of the General Accounting Office, and an author of the GAO report on off-label usage of chemotherapy drugs, "they're going to get treated however the physician wants to treat them, and they won't ever know the difference." In the current uneasy climate surrounding health care in America, with more and more men and women being herded into health-maintenance organizations and entering the rolls of the ailing Medicare system, acting as your own consumer advocate has never been more important.

Consider *The Complete Cancer Survival Guide* your comprehensive consumer's manual to obtaining the best cancer care available. Drawing on advice from dozens of top cancer specialists at major cancer centers around the country, it maps out a practical game plan that you can put into action the day you're diagnosed or at any point along your journey. Rely on it not only to help you make sense of therapy choices that may seem at odds with one another, but to learn how to best care for yourself during this time—physically, emotionally, spiritually, financially— and how to navigate the health-care-system maze. When you've just been told you have cancer, and your life is on the line, this is precisely what you need. I know.

Your Game Plan

1. Learn about your disease and how it is diagnosed and treated. *See Chapters Two, Three, Four, and Six.*
2. Find out about any clinical trials that might be beneficial for your type and stage of cancer. *How can you do this in just a few phone calls? See Chapter Four.*
3. Arrange a consultation for an independent multidisciplinary second opinion. *Where should you seek a second opinion regarding treatment? See Chapter Five.*
4. Based on the treatment options presented to you, decide on the plan and where to have it carried out. *What should you look for in a cancer-treatment facility? See Chapter Five.*
5. Ask your oncologist to prescribe medications in advance for any anticipated symptoms and side effects. *What are the most effective*

remedies for pain, nausea, and other complications? See Chapter Eight.

6. Follow a diet high in protein and calories, and learn how good eating habits can help you avoid or alleviate nausea, diarrhea, constipation, and other gastrointestinal-related side effects. *How can you best maintain your weight and energy during treatment? See Chapter Eight.*

7. Don't neglect your emotional health! *How are stress, anxiety, and depression controlled? See Chapter Nine.*

8. Accept offers of help from family, friends, and neighbors, and utilize any services that may be available in your community: home-delivered meals, transportation to and from medical appointments, homemakers and home-health-care professionals, and so on. *How do you go about tracking down local services for patients and families? See Chapter Ten and the appendices.*

9. Learn how to make your medical insurance work effectively for you. *How do you contest a rejected insurance claim? If your oncologist recommends an experimental therapy, what steps can you take to help win approval from your insurer? See Chapter Ten.*

Make no mistake: Taking charge of your medical care—and, in effect, your destiny—is a daunting responsibility. At first you'll likely feel overwhelmed by the barrage of unfamiliar concepts and medical jargon. You might be intimidated by the medical establishment and the doctors themselves. That was true for me and is probably true for anyone else who's ever been told he or she has cancer.

"During that first visit, nobody hears anything after the word 'cancer,'" says Dr. John Marshall, who reckons he's delivered hundreds of cancer diagnoses over the years. "But eventually, most patients come to understand what they need to know about their disease, and they become quite savvy about their medical care and making decisions about treatment."

I can tell you from experience that all of this is far easier if you have the support of a loved one or trusted friend. I am convinced that I would never have survived my illness had it not been for Valerie. It was she who took notes at appointments, filled the doctors in on details about my condition that escaped my notice, and generally helped me to sort out my options and work in partnership with the medical team. With this in mind, *The Complete Cancer Survival Guide* is intended as much for concerned family members as it is for patients.

"I'll Do Anything to Get Better"

I often think back to something my other attending physician, Dr. Paul Woolley, said to me during the low point of my treatment. Following my second cycle of chemotherapy, I was racked with explosive diarrhea that left me weak and dehydrated, unable to eat. More serious, though, my level of white blood cells had plummeted to the extent that Dr. Woolley immediately admitted me to the hospital.

"You know," he remarked later that week as he perused my medical chart, "you're one of the best patients I've ever had."

"Why's that?" I asked.

"Because you'll do anything to get better."

And it's true. With the knowledge always in the back of your mind that nearly one in two people with cancer die of their disease, most of us would do virtually anything to give ourselves an edge, no matter how seemingly slight or statistically insignificant.

Certainly an element of luck, fate, providence—call it what you will—plays a part here. We all know that a patient can make all the "right" decisions about his health care and ultimately suffer the "wrong" outcome, for reasons that often defy medical explanation. But looking back, I firmly believe that participating actively in my own health care and knowing I was doing everything in my power to help myself brought me a level of confidence and peace of mind that motivated me to fight perhaps just a little bit harder.

Chapter One

Cancer:

A Thief in the Night

Cancer is a disease that takes years to develop, yet it can plunge you and your family into upheaval the instant it takes the doctor to deliver the news no one wants to hear: "What we've found is a malignancy."

At the time my cancer was discovered in 1991, I'd never been seriously ill in my life. By then I was six years removed from daily politics, busy running my own consulting firm in Washington. I'd entered government life back in 1970 as press secretary to the assistant U.S. Senate minority leader, Robert Griffin of Michigan, my home state. I went on to serve in the same capacity for Jacob Javits, helping to reelect him to his fourth and final term as senior U.S. senator from New York.

In 1976, I took a leave of absence from Senator Javits's office to handle press duties for President Gerald Ford's campaign committee. Coming on the heels of the Watergate scandal, the election was a debacle for the Republicans. Jimmy Carter edged out Ford for the White House, and the Democrats gained seats in both the House and the Senate. Not long afterward, I became communications director and chief spokesman for the Republican National Committee as the party set about rebuilding itself.

I'd been hooked by the excitement of a presidential race, though, and had the urge to do it again. To help shape a winning campaign and be part of moving the country in a direction you believe will benefit the American people is a dream that too few ever experience, especially someone like me—an immigrant who as a boy came to the United States from England on a battered troop-carrier ship following World War II.

George Bush, the former congressman from Texas, United Nations ambassador, and director of the Central Intelligence Agency, was gearing up for a presidential run in 1980. He was widely respected, but certainly considered a dark-horse candidate. Although I didn't know him well on a personal level, I'd admired him as a public official. So I was delighted to become his press secretary in 1979. The association was to last into his second term as vice president under Ronald Reagan.

In 1985, I decided to leave politics and launch my own business. As happens to many public servants, I was worn out from the eighteen-hour days and constant travel. It wasn't unusual for a foreign trip with the vice president to log twenty-five or thirty thousand miles over the course of three weeks as we leapfrogged from Alaska to Japan to Korea to Singapore to Australia to New Zealand to China to Hawaii before finally returning home. And the fall political campaigns frequently resembled a cross-country derby. We used to wring a few extra hours out of the day by opening with an early-morning campaign stop on the East Coast. Then we'd work our way west through the time zones, with stops in, say, Chicago, Kansas City, and Denver, before winding up in Los Angeles by nightfall.

Another reason for my departing the White House: I was newly married. While I was press secretary, I had hired Valerie Hodgson, a twenty-seven-year-old photographer for United Press International, to be the vice president's official photographer. The year was 1983.

The two of us nearly ended up being the proverbial ships that pass in the night. Valerie's first day on the job coincided with my leaving for a fellowship at the Institute of Politics at Harvard University's John F. Kennedy School of Government. Then she left the White House to pursue a freelance career shortly before I came back to Washington. But during my sabbatical, I had accompanied the vice president on a trip to California. Valerie and I struck up a conversation aboard *Air*

Force Two, went out for a late dinner that night in San Diego, and started dating. We were married on November 18, 1984, two weeks after the Reagan-Bush ticket's landslide victory for a second term.

Our daughter Randall was born in 1987, and Adrienne arrived three years later, on my fiftieth birthday. My two daughters from my first marriage were already in their twenties: Susan, a speech pathologist in Livonia, Michigan, and Laura, a communications major at Western Michigan University in Kalamazoo.

In all, it was a happy time. I had a wonderful family, and a thriving business that allowed me to enjoy them. Then everything was abruptly put on hold.

The ordeal began innocently enough: I had a dull pain in my right side. Valerie and the kids had been suffering from the stomach flu since Labor Day, so I figured I'd picked up what they had and didn't pay much attention to it. But after it persisted for a few days, I went to our family doctor for an examination. She poked around a bit, told me not to worry, and sent me home. When the pain didn't subside, I saw her partner, with the same result.

Several days passed, and still I kept complaining—with little sympathy from Valerie, I might add. "Look," she said one night, "if you think there's something wrong, why don't you go down to the emergency room and have an X ray taken?" Which I did. My doctor read the films the next day and assured me she saw nothing unusual.

"But there's obviously something bothering you," she continued. "So I'm going to schedule you for an MRI scan tomorrow afternoon." No sooner did I return home from the imaging procedure than the phone rang. It was my doctor. "I want you to get over to the hospital," she said urgently, naming a nearby community hospital. "You've got an inflamed appendix, and you need to have it taken out now.

"I've checked you in. A surgeon will meet you there and remove it right away. I'll see you in the recovery room."

I tossed some clothes into an overnight bag, called a taxi, and went off to have an appendectomy, or so I thought.

The next thing I remembered was waking up in a darkened hospital room. Though still drowsy from the anesthesia, I knew it was late at night, perhaps 2:00 or 3:00 A.M. Three hospital attendants were hoisting me into a bed. I hurt badly all over and sensed something was seriously wrong. But I was too exhausted to pursue the thought. I just wanted to sleep.

At about 7:30 in the morning, the bedside phone rang, jarring me partially awake.

"Teeley! How ya feeling?"

It was George Bush calling.

"I really feel bad, I'm sorry, I can't talk now," I mumbled, and dropped the receiver back into the cradle.

Christ, I thought to myself, *I just hung up on the president of the United States.*

Later that morning the surgeon would explain how he'd been surprised to discover a tumor and had to remove a one-foot section of large intestine, along with the appendix and the lymph nodes for biopsy. The pathology report, which came back a few days later, noted that three nodes out of twenty-two tested positive for cancer.

"I'd never for an instant worried that the doctor would find anything other than an appendix that needed to be removed," Valerie recalls. "So to be told that Peter had cancer was shocking. It was unreal."

The entire situation grew stranger still. A week to the day after the first surgery, a Friday, I went under the knife again, this time to untangle the twisted colon. "It'll take twenty minutes," the surgeon informed me. "Don't worry about it." Apparently, he had failed to mention to the anesthesiologist that I'd been throwing up black bile all week. When it happened again during the operation, the fluid slipped into my lung, essentially drowning me and causing aspiration pneumonia to set in. Though it's no longer the threat it once was, pneumonia is still the fifth deadliest disease in the United States.

For the second time in a week, Valerie was sitting in the waiting room, relatively unconcerned about what had been presented to us as a simple operation, only to be approached by the surgeon with news of a major complication. This time the anesthesiologist accompanied him.

"In a very calm fashion, they were trying to explain to me what had happened," she remembers. "I was lulled by their voices, and thought, *Okay . . . okay, this will be fixed, too . . .*"

Valerie was allowed to see me briefly in the recovery room while the medical team prepared to move me up to the intensive-care unit. "It was awful," she says with a shudder. "Peter was unconscious and on a mechanical respirator. When they took him off the machine, he started convulsing because he wasn't getting any oxygen. I just kind of stood there, not knowing what to do." Then the doctors and nurses took their places on either side of the gurney. Looking much like a bobsled team, they hastily wheeled it and me out the doors and down the hall, leaving Valerie standing there alone in a daze.

The story takes an almost comical turn—at least in hindsight: A nurse came huffing and puffing up to Valerie, brandishing an inflatable air mattress we'd purchased for the hospital bed. "When are you going to get this thing and all these flowers out of your husband's room?" the woman demanded. Perhaps she figured I was destined for the morgue anyway and wouldn't be needing them.

"I don't care what you do with the flowers!" Valerie snapped. "Besides, the doctors said the pneumonia won't last long, and he may be back in his room tomorrow." Hardly. Despite massive doses of intravenous antibiotics, the pneumonia held fast. The night that the pulmonologist conceded that I might not survive, Valerie went to bed assuming she was about to become a thirty-five-year-old widow with two young children. She recalls thinking to herself, *They'll call me if Peter dies. And if I wake up in the morning, and no one's called, I'll know he's still alive.*

What upset her most of all was my being kept on continuous sedation. "My husband is totally knocked out and doesn't know what's going on!" she appealed to the pulmonologist. "Pete's a fighter. You have to allow him to wake up. You have to give him a chance." The doctor agreed to lower the dosages.

"I don't know if I did that more for Peter or for me," Valerie reflects. "But it really bothered me that he could die without ever being awake again."

Finally, after seven days, I regained consciousness, once again to find her on the edge of my bed.

"You've been through a terrible time," she said, smiling, "but you made it. You're going to be all right." Because of the breathing tube down my throat, I couldn't talk.

"It's Friday," she added.

Friday, I thought. *The day of the operation.*

"Friday *a week later.*"

The Friday after that, October 11, I left the hospital, intent on never going back there again. Valerie had brought the girls. As an attendant wheeled me out to our van, it struck me how brisk the air was compared to the balmy Indian summer day when I'd checked in three weeks before. The trees had now taken on their fall colors. Other than taking a few walks around the neighborhood to rebuild my strength, I relaxed over the weekend, grateful to be home.

In the aftermath of a cancer diagnosis, many men and women go into shock, perhaps believing that there's been some mistake: The pathologist must have misinterpreted the slides. Or the radiologist is going to call any minute with the glorious news that what had appeared on X ray to be a cancerous lesion was nothing more than scar tissue.

It doesn't take long, though, for the reality to sink in, setting off a chain reaction of emotional distress, anxiety, depression, numbness, worry, and an overwhelming sense of powerlessness. Your mind plays out the endless variables: What am I going to do next? If I need chemotherapy, is it going to make me sick? How are the kids going to handle this? *Am I going to die?* So I suppose you could say my reaction was atypical, for despite everything I'd just been through, I felt strangely confident that I was going to survive.

There is no script to follow in the wake of a cancer diagnosis. No timetable. No way you "should" feel. But in a common pattern, after a week or two most patients resolve to do what they can to fight their disease, and they begin to focus on pursuing a treatment plan. That in itself is bound to improve your outlook.

One lesson politics teaches you is not to dwell on such setbacks as an election defeat but to assess the situation and move ahead. The week following my discharge from the hospital, I got down to the task of researching where and how to have my cancer treated. I knew I'd have to make a lot of decisions, and quickly.

Chapter Two

The Basics: What Every Patient Needs to Know About Cancer

V alerie is a voracious reader. Whenever there's a problem or question at home—the kids, needlepoint, decorating—"I go to the bookstore," she says, "and buy everything written on the subject." Once I was out of immediate danger, she purchased an armload of books about cancer, and we began poring through them.

Learning about your disease and being able to envision the battle raging inside your body is the first step to regaining a semblance of control. And brushing up on this chapter's basic biology and key medical terms will give you the confidence to assert yourself with doctors and to take part in the decisions that will shape your medical care.

The Multiple Personalities of Cancer

T he first thing you learn about cancer is that it encompasses as many as two hundred related yet distinct diseases, which raises an important point: Inevitably, along the way, concerned friends and relatives will draw you aside to recount their or someone else's cancer experience. Or they'll relate fragments of some report about cancer treatment they caught on the evening news. Frankly, even most patients don't know the specifics about their medical care. We're not suggesting that you dismiss well-meaning advice out of hand: Just be selective when considering information from sources who aren't medical professionals. Ask questions and make sure that what's being said pertains to *your* medical situation.

"My father had cancer, and according to the doctor . . ."

Which type of cancer? Melanoma is cancer. Acute myeloid leukemia is cancer. The former is a solid tumor of the skin, calls for surgery, and generally carries a highly favorable prognosis if discovered early. The other is a notoriously virulent "liquid" malignancy of the blood and bone marrow for which chemotherapy and bone-marrow transplantation comprise the main arm of treatment.

"Why is your doctor saying you have to have a radical hysterectomy? My sister also had cervical cancer, and she didn't need an operation . . ."

What stage was the cancer? Meaning, how extensive was it? A tumor confined to the cervix and one that has infiltrated surrounding tissue require radically different approaches to treatment: in the first example, surgery alone—and possibly a minor procedure at that—versus radiation therapy with or without chemotherapy.

Knowing the type and stage doesn't necessarily complete the picture. Other factors add crucial elements that may determine the course of treatment: the family of cells that make up the tumor, the cancer's aggressiveness, and a patient's age and general health. An oncologist might recommend prostate surgery for an otherwise healthy fifty-five-year-old man whose cancer has not spread outside the gland. Given the identical tumor in a seventy-five-year-old diabetic also suffering from chronic heart disease, the most sensible strategy might be no therapy at all, since prostate cancer progresses slowly, and an elderly person with other medical problems might not be expected to withstand radiation, much less an operation.

Our point is this: You can't necessarily draw conclusions about treatment based on other people's experiences with the disease, not even when their medical situation seems very much like yours. With so much material to wade through, who needs to get sidetracked by information that's outdated, incomplete, or simply not applicable to your condition?

Types of Cancer

Table 2.1 lists the twenty-five most common forms of cancer, from cancer of the prostate to cancer of the small intestine. Combined, they ac-

TABLE 2.1   The 25 Most Common Types of Cancer

Type of Cancer	Estimated Number of New Cases in 1999	Estimated Number of Deaths in 1999
1. Prostate	179,300	37,000
2. Breast[1]	176,300	43,700
3. Lung	171,600	158,900
4. Colorectal	129,400	56,600
5. Lymphomas	64,000	27,000
Non-Hodgkin's lymphomas	56,800	25,700
Hodgkin's disease	7,200	1,300
6. Bladder[2]	54,200	12,100
7. Melanoma[3]	44,200	7,300
8. Uterine	37,400	6,400
9. Leukemia	30,200	22,100
10. Kidney	30,000	11,900
11. Pancreatic	28,600	28,600
12. Ovarian	25,200	14,500
13. Stomach	21,900	13,500
14. Liver, gallbladder, and bile ducts	21,700	17,200
15. Oral cavity	21,500	6,000
16. Thyroid	18,100	1,200
17. Brain	16,800	13,100
18. Multiple myeloma	13,700	11,400
19. Cervical	12,800	4,800
20. Esophageal	12,500	12,200
21. Laryngeal	10,600	4,200
22. Pharyngeal	8,300	2,100
23. Soft-tissue sarcomas	7,800	4,400
24. Testicular	7,400	300
25. Small Intestine	4,800	1,200

[1] Carcinoma in situ of the breast accounts for an additional 36,900 new cases each year.
[2] Includes carcinoma in situ of the bladder.
[3] An additional 21,000 cases of melanoma carcinoma in situ are diagnosed annually.

Source: American Cancer Society, Surveillance Research, 1999.

Medical Terms You're Likely to Hear

Adenocarcinoma: The most common type of cancer, adenocarcinomas occur in the lining of *glands*—clusters of cells that discharge chemical substances. *Endocrine* glands release hormones, while mucus, saliva, digestive juices, and other secretions come from *exocrine* glands. Among the glands that most often play unwilling host to cancer are the prostate, pancreas, ovaries, testicles, and thyroid. Glandular tissue is found in organs as well, including the stomach, liver, intestines, esophagus, and breasts. Cancers that form glandlike structures are also considered adenocarcinomas.

count for about 95 percent of the estimated 1,221,800 new cases in 1999. (Absent from the list, and not discussed in *The Complete Cancer Survival Guide,* is the most prevalent cancer of all: nonmelanoma skin cancer, a highly curable disease that affects over 900,000 men and women each year.)

Cancers are classified according to the type of tissue and the type of cell in which they originate. Nine in ten take hold in the *epithelium,* the membranous tissue that forms the inner lining and outer covering of organs, glands, and vessels, as well as the surface layer of the skin. These tumors are called *carcinomas.* The remaining 10 percent of cancers belong to one of five other categories:

Sarcomas—cancers of the body's connective tissues, including hard tissues such as bone and cartilage, and soft tissues like muscle and vessels

Leukemias—cancers of the blood and the bone marrow, where blood cells are manufactured

Lymphomas—cancers of the lymph nodes scattered along the network of vessels known as the lymphatic system

Melanomas—cancers found exclusively in the skin cells that produce the pigment responsible for skin color

Gliomas—cancers of the nerve tissue. The term is often applied to all cancers of the brain and spinal cord.

Some organs contain more than one type of tissue. For instance, virtually all cancers of the uterus are carcinomas, because they grow in the *endometrium,* the mucous membrane that lines the womb. But a small number of uterine sarcomas are seen in the uterus's outer layer, which is made of muscle. Although both fall under the heading of "uterine cancer," they are different diseases with different treatment plans.

Classifying the cell type reveals additional important information about cancer. This is done by *biopsying* a small piece of malignant tissue through one of several methods (described in Chapter Three, "How Cancer Is Diagnosed and Staged"). A medical specialist known as a *pathologist* then studies the sample under a microscope to make the identification. Cancers of the same organ, and even the same tissue line, may spring from different cells. Once again, using the uterus as an example, three in four endometrial tumors are adenocarcinomas, and another one in five are *adenosquamous* carcinomas—a mixture of adenocarcinoma cells and *squamous* cells. These scalelike cells also make up the epithelium, but not the glandular (adeno-) epithelium.

Think of cell type as your cancer's "psychological profile." Some cells grow faster and behave more aggressively than others. Knowing which type of cell a tumor stems from helps your oncologist select the best course of treatment.

How Cancer Begins

All cancers, regardless of where they arise, share the same humble origin: a defect in a single *gene,* a linear thread of chemical substances known as *DNA* (deoxyribonucleic acid). Each of the body's trillions of microscopic cells contains approximately 140,000 genes, which are arranged along twenty-three X-shaped pairs of biologic units called *chromosomes.*

The genes program every one of our physical, biochemical, and physiologic traits, from hair color to body functions. One of their many duties is to regulate the continuous process of cell division. As the body needs replacements, genes signal their cell to replicate itself, creating twins with genetic codes that are identical—most of the time. For reasons scientists don't fully understand, about once in every 1 million divisions a copying error occurs, and one descendant departs with part of its DNA jumbled or missing.

This by itself doesn't cause cancer. In fact, it may have no medical consequences whatsoever. Since all cells—except for the human sperm and egg cells—claim duplicates of each gene, often a cell can press on with one normal copy. But if the cell needs both twins healthy in order to carry out its tasks, or if the other copy's DNA also becomes altered, the cell ceases to function properly.

Cancer develops when the genetic mechanism that controls a cell's proliferation goes awry, allowing it to multiply recklessly. For this to happen, however, a cell has to acquire a number of mutations in its DNA, usually over many years. In carcinoma of the lung, for instance, "it probably takes a minimum of ten to twenty genetic aberrations in order for the cancer to occur," says Dr. David Johnson, associate director of the Vanderbilt Cancer Center in Nashville, Tennessee. That is why cancer is often referred to as a disease of aging: The older you are, the greater the odds that one cell will have accumulated enough defects to change into a cancer cell. The median age of cancer patients at the time of diagnosis is sixty-seven.

Some men and women are born with a defective gene, which places them one step closer to cancer. But most mutations come about as a result of prolonged or repeated exposure to a *carcinogen:* any agent known to cause cancer. Tobacco smoke, certain viruses, and the radioactive gas radon are three examples of *initiators,* carcinogens capable of crippling genes on their own. *Promoters,* such as alcohol, cannot trigger cancer directly. Rather, they complete the process by converting damaged cells to malignant cells, in the way that alcohol works in tandem with tobacco to cause the majority of cancers of the oral cavity, larynx, throat, and esophagus.

Classes of Cancer-Predisposition Genes

Since the 1970s, researchers have discovered four major classes of genes that in their mutated form set the cancer process in motion: *oncogenes, tumor suppressor genes, mismatch repair genes,* and *telomerase genes.* Remarkably, microbiologists are able to pinpoint the genetic culprits behind many cancers. The ever-expanding roster includes the p53 gene, located on chromosome 17. It has been implicated in six in ten human cancers, including colon cancer, stomach cancer, melanoma, leukemia, and lymphoma.

Dr. Johnson, himself a survivor of lymphoma ("diagnosed on St. Patrick's Day 1989," he says proudly), observes that, "although not every cancer has been linked to a particular genetic abnormality, we believe that all cancers are somehow genetic aberrations."

Oncogenes and Cancer
Most cells carry what are known as *proto-oncogenes.* In their undamaged state, these genes help oversee cell growth and other vital functions. Or they exert no influence at all. But a break or mutation in a proto-oncogene's DNA may transform it into an oncogene. In its malevolent new guise, the gene instructs the cell to multiply at an accelerated rate, one of the hallmarks of cancer.

Tumor Suppressor Genes and Cancer

The p53 gene is one of many tumor suppressor genes. As the name implies, TSGs inhibit aberrant cells from dividing and becoming cancerous; or they destroy the cells outright. If contact with a carcinogen or some other molecular event disables a suppressor gene (also referred to as an antioncogene), then oncogenes seize control of the cell.

Mismatch Repair Genes and Cancer

Normally, this third class of genes enables a cell to repair errors in its DNA before it replicates and passes on the error to the next generation of cells. Once again, a mutation causes mismatch repair genes to malfunction, thus freeing the defective cell to copy itself. The aberrant mismatch repair genes MSH2 and MLH1 are responsible for the majority of hereditary nonpolyposis colon cancers, while most cases of noninherited colon cancer stem from a faulty GTBP gene.

Telomerase Genes and Cancer

The ends of chromosomes are tipped with DNA segments called *telomeres,* which see to it that cells divide only so many times. With each replication, the caps become shorter and shorter, until eventually the cell can no longer proliferate. In 1999, scientists discovered that cancer occurs when errant telomerase genes get switched on and begin to produce an enzyme that the cells use to rebuild their telomeres. The ongoing repairs enable the cells to divide indefinitely.

The Result: A Cancer Cell

Whichever class of altered gene is to blame, the result is a cancer cell with jagged borders and a sinister crablike shape, unlike a normal round cell. Its appearance under the microscope conveys a great deal about its probable behavior. Cancer cells that essentially resemble their noncancerous counterparts and can still perform some of their normal functions are described as *well differentiated.* In general, *poorly differentiated* cells—identifiable by their disorganized structure—divide more rapidly and chaotically.

Medical Terms You're Likely to Hear

Lesion

Malignancy

Mass

Neoplasm

. . . words the doctor may use instead of "tumor"

The haywire cell and its descendants proceed to grind out copies of themselves faster than old cells die off, until eventually they form a mass of excess tissue called a *tumor.* A *benign* growth, made up of cells that are abnormal but not cancerous, cannot invade normal tissue. It generally poses no serious health threat—unless it manifests in the brain, which sits hemmed in against the skull. In most cases, the benign lesion is removed surgically, and the patient receives a clean bill of health.

A malignant tumor, however, enlarges and begins to encroach upon surrounding tissue. It is this *invasive* feature, along with uncontrolled growth, that distinguishes a cell as a cancer cell. If not arrested, the expanding mass will crowd out normal cells, deprive them of nutrients, and in time destroy them. Ultimately, the cancer may disrupt the functions of the organ or system it touches—and, should it spread, multiple organs or systems.

When Cancer Spreads

A *localized* tumor remains confined to the original, or *primary,* location. Cancer that spreads does so in two ways. It can grow straight through the primary organ and directly into adjacent tissue, as my tumor did. You may hear this referred to as *local extension,* or *regional* disease. In *metastatic* cancer, a colony of malignant cells breaks away and rides the circulatory system to nearby lymph nodes or a distant organ, where it forms a *secondary* cancer. The brain, bones, lung, liver, and lymph nodes are the most common sites of *metastasis.*

A lot of patients and families find this confusing at first. "The doctor said I have a tumor in my liver; I thought I had cervical cancer." Right. A person in this situation is said to have cervical cancer (primary tumor) metastatic to the liver (secondary tumor). Not liver cancer. And an important distinction is that the malignancy in the liver consists of cervical-cancer cells. Most cervical tumors are squamous-cell carcinomas, characterized by thin, flat cells, whereas the majority of liver cancers are adenocarcinomas, with cells that grow in columnlike patterns. If a sample of diseased liver tissue were examined under a microscope, the cells would bear squamous-cell carcinoma's unmistakable shape.

Medical Terms You're Likely to Hear

Refractory cancer: disease that resists conventional methods of treatment.

The Lymphatic System: Cancer Courier

The *lymphatic system* belongs to both the circulatory system and the immune system. Lymphatic vessels branch throughout the body like blood vessels and are responsible for returning tissue fluid to the bloodstream. Along this route lie tiny bean-shaped organs called lymph nodes, which form in clusters in the neck, armpits, chest, abdomen, and groin.

The nodes filter out waste products, germs, and, ironically, cancer cells. Along with the spleen, another component of the lymphatic system, they also produce infection-fighting white blood cells called *lymphocytes.* Most cancers can potentially spread to nearby nodes—never a welcome development, since there's always the danger that the lymphatic vessels may smuggle malignant cells elsewhere in the body.

Sometimes, despite batteries of tests, a metastatic tumor is diagnosed but no primary cancer can be found. When this happens, the cancer is declared a *cancer of unknown primary* origin, or CUP. In determining how to treat it, oncologists piece together other clues—cell type and appearance, tumor location, the presence of certain telltale biochemical substances—to narrow down the possibilities of the original location.

A cancer that *recurs* after a period of *remission,* when no trace of disease can be detected, is also classified as local, regional, or metastatic. In either situation, an initial diagnosis or a *recurrence,* it's preferable for cancer to be caught when it is localized. The cure rates for ten major forms of cancer at that stage range from 90 to 100 percent. We hasten to add that cancers that have spread are often highly treatable. I am proof of that.

What Does "In Situ" Mean?

Of the major cancers, several go through a precancerous stage before becoming malignant. In cervical cancer, that stage is called *dysplasia,* meaning "abnormal growth," a reference to the early changes in the size, shape, and number of cells that make up the organ's surface layer. Cancer of the uterus is preceded by a step known as *hyperplasia,* in which unruly cells overmultiply ("hyper" is Greek for "over") but remain normal in appearance. And a type of lung cancer called squamous-cell carcinoma progresses through both hyperplasia and dysplasia.

Carcinoma *in situ,* Latin for "in its normal place," isn't precancerous, nor does it meet the true definition of cancer. "The cancer is there," explains Dr. Mitchell Morris of M. D. Anderson Cancer Center in Houston, "but it hasn't invaded any normal tissue yet." Dr. David Johnson compares it to "a moment in time: like taking a picture of a waterfall, with the water splashing out in midair before it hits the pond.

Medical Terms You're Likely to Hear

Microinvasive: a carcinoma in situ containing malignant cells that have superficially invaded surrounding tissue.

"The good news," he adds, "is that carcinoma in situ is cancer at its absolute earliest. Once treated, in all probability it will be gone forever." Not all cancers have an in situ stage. In some cases, it's because they don't pause long enough in this stage to be caught in situ. Or in other cases, they don't give rise to symptoms, so that a diagnosis comes about only when an unrelated medical condition brings a patient to the doctor and the nonmalignant tumor is detected by chance.

Warning Signs and Symptoms of Cancer

The warning signs and symptoms of cancer are as varied as the organs or systems affected by the disease, but one or more of these classic symptoms frequently is the first to arouse suspicion:

- A change in bowel or bladder habits

- A sore that won't heal

- Unusual bleeding or discharge

- A thickening or lump in the breast or other part of the body

- Indigestion or difficulty in swallowing

- An obvious change in a wart or mole

- Persistent coughing or hoarseness

Any one of these symptoms could signify a far less serious ailment. For example, blood in the stool, a common indicator of colon cancer, might prove to be nothing more than bleeding hemorrhoids. Because cancer symptoms are often vague, people don't necessarily rush off to the doctor the moment they notice something unusual. Two other fea-

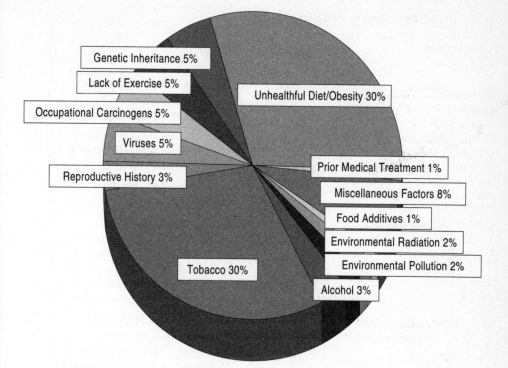

tures of colon cancer are fatigue and abdominal pain. In my case, I blamed both symptoms on the flu.

Cancers of the lung, pancreas, ovary, liver, stomach, and esophagus can be especially insidious because these so-called silent diseases tend not to bring on symptoms right away. As a result, they frequently evade detection until they have already spread.

The Causes (Etiology) of Cancer

In many respects, cancer is the ultimate quirk of fate, an unfortunate convergence of a genetic error and an environmental insult. Environment, in this context, refers to any external cause, not just the air, water, and soil. In fact, contrary to what many people believe, cancer is not "all around us." Only 2 percent of deaths from the disease can be tied to environmental pollution. The predominant factor, by far, is human behavior—smoking, unhealthy eating habits, lack of exercise—which accounts for four in five cancers.

TABLE 2.2   Causes of Cancer

Cause	Percentage of Cancer Deaths	Associated with These Cancers
Tobacco	30%	Lung · Esophageal · Laryngeal · Throat · Oral cavity · Bladder · Kidney · Pancreatic
Unhealthy diet and obesity	30%	Breast · Colorectal · Prostate · Endometrial (uterus) · Ovarian · Small intestine
Lack of exercise	5%	Colon · Prostate · Breast · Endometrial (uterus) · Ovarian
Genetic inheritance	5%	Breast · Ovarian · Colon · Prostate · Lung · Pancreatic · Kidney · Stomach · Thyroid · Melanoma · Basal-cell carcinoma · Brain · Soft-tissue sarcomas · Liver · Leukemia · Lymphomas
Viruses and other infectious agents	5%	Liver · Cervical · Hodgkin's disease and Non-Hodgkin's lymphomas · Nasopharyngeal · Soft-tissue sarcomas · Stomach · Leukemia
Occupational carcinogens	5%	Lung and pleura (the membrane that encases each lung and lines the chest cavity) · Bladder · Skin · Laryngeal · Nasal cavity · Leukemia · Throat · Lymphomas · Soft-tissue sarcomas · Liver
Excessive alcohol consumption	3%	Liver · Oral cavity · Laryngeal · Throat · Esophageal · Breast
Reproductive history	3%	Breast · Endometrial (uterus) · Cervical · Ovarian
Environmental pollution	2%	Lung
Environmental radiation: Solar radiation	2%	Melanoma · Basal-cell carcinoma · Squamous-cell carcinoma
Radon		Lung
Salt, other food additives, and contaminants	1%	Stomach · Liver · Small intestine

Prior Medical Treatments: 1%	
Radiation therapy	Leukemia ▪ Thyroid ▪ Breast ▪ Brain
Cancer chemotherapy	Leukemia ▪ Bladder
Immunosuppressants	Lymphomas ▪ Soft-tissue sarcomas
Hormone therapy	Endometrial (uterus) ▪ Breast
Miscellaneous other factors 8%	

How Do They Cause Cancer?

Tobacco (30%)—Of the more than four thousand chemical compounds in tobacco, forty-three are confirmed carcinogens. Although the bloodstream brings cigarette smoke's tars and gases in contact with many organs, 90 percent of the toxic chemicals become entrapped in the lungs. Tobacco is responsible for about 135,000 lung-cancer deaths each year, as well as mortalities from cancers of the larynx, oral cavity, esophagus, kidney, bladder, and pancreas.

Unhealthful diet and obesity (30%)—Obviously, a high-fat diet and obesity are interrelated, along with lack of exercise (see below). A high-fat diet is one that derives more than 30 percent of its total daily calories from fat, while obesity is generally defined as having a *body mass index* (BMI) of 30 or above. (Examples: The BMI for a person who stands five feet four and weighs 150 pounds is 25.7; 175 pounds, 30.1; 200 pounds, 34.2.) Severely overweight women exhibit higher rates of cancers of the breast, ovary, and the lining of the uterus.

What's the connection? Fatty tissue metabolizes the female sex hormone *estrogen*, which stimulates cell growth in all three organs. As for a direct association between a fat-heavy diet and these cancers, fatty foods are believed to cause the large intestine to allow estrogen to be reabsorbed into the bloodstream.

A similar mechanism may explain the connection between fat and prostate cancer. Fat, it is hypothesized, overstimulates production of *testosterone*. An imbalance of this male sex hormone spurs the growth of cancer cells in the prostate. Obese men have a 40 percent greater chance than leaner men of developing prostate cancer. Both genders see their risk of colon cancer rise in proportion to their body mass index, although the exact reason is not well understood.

Lack of exercise (5%)—Inactivity has been linked to cancers of the breast, ovary, endometrium, prostate, and colon, and not just because a sedentary lifestyle contributes to weight gain. The evidence is strongest with regard to colon cancer. The theory is that exercise speeds the transit time of waste products through the bowel, thereby reducing the opportunity for any carcinogens to come into contact with the intestine's inner lining. Inactivity's influence on the risk of the other cancers isn't as compelling. But it is believed that physical activity lowers production of estrogen in women and testosterone in men. By not exercising regularly, a person may therefore be losing this protection and consequently increasing his risk.

Genetic inheritance (5%)—Roughly one in twenty people who die of cancer inherited flawed DNA from their parents. We receive our genes in pairs: half from our mother, half from our father. As has already been explained, a single wayward cell can set the stage for the disease. But when a genetic mutation occurs in a male sperm cell or a female egg cell—the two cells that create human life—the child they produce will have that defect repeated in every cell in her body.

The first hereditary cancer-susceptibility gene identified was *RB1*, located on chromosome 13. A tumor suppressor gene, its defective form is responsible for four in ten cases of retinoblastoma, a children's cancer of the eye. A decade later, more than two dozen other familial cancer genes had been fingered. In addition, there are about two hundred documented hereditary cancer syndromes—ominous patterns of cancers that shadow certain families—still waiting for their genes to be discovered.

Not everyone who acquires a cancer-predisposition gene at birth will go on to develop a malignant tumor—remember, the faulty genes have to be activated in order to start down the path to cancer—but the odds are heightened considerably. The odds that a woman with the mutated version of *BRCA2* gene will develop breast cancer by age fifty are 60 percent, more than seven times higher than normal; by age seventy, the likelihood of the disease catching up to her rises to 77 percent. She also faces a 16 percent chance of incurring ovarian cancer by age seventy, when the occurrence rate among the general population is less than 2 percent. According to a 1999 report published in the *Journal of the National Cancer Institute,* the gene's presence also elevates the risk of five other cancers anywhere from two and a half times to five times.

TABLE 2.3   Inherited Cancer Predisposition Genes Discovered to Date[1]

Defective Gene	Implicated Mainly in These Cancers	Year Discovered
RB1	Retinoblastoma[2], sarcomas, others	1986
WT1	Wilms' tumor[2]	1990
p53	Breast, sarcomas, brain	1990
NF-1	Brain, sarcomas	1990
APC	Colon	1991
NF-2	Brain, others	1993
VHL	Kidney, brain, others	1993
RET	Thyroid, others	1993
TSC2	Kidney, brain	1993
MSH2	Colon, ovarian, endometrial, stomach, others	1993
MLH1	Colon, ovarian, endometrial, stomach, others	1994
PMS1	Colon, ovarian, endometrial, stomach, others	1994
PMS2	Colon, ovarian, endometrial, stomach, others	1994
CDKN2 (also known as p16, INK4a, or MTS1)	Melanoma	1994
BRCA1	Breast, ovarian	1994
ATM	Breast, non-Hodgkin's lymphomas, leukemia, liver, others	1994
BRCA2	Breast, ovarian, pancreatic, stomach, gallbladder, melanoma, prostate	1995
CDK4 (also known as p15, INK4b, or MTS2)	Melanoma	1996

Defective Gene	Implicated Mainly in These Cancers	Year Discovered
EXT2	Chondrosarcoma, a soft-tissue sarcoma	1996
PTCH	Skin, brain (in children)	1996
TSC1	Kidney, brain	1996
MET	Kidney	1997
MSH6 (also known as *GTBP)*	Colon, endometrial, stomach	1997
MEN1	Endocrine tumors, carcinoid tumors	1997
PTEN	Breast, thyroid	1997
CDH1	Stomach	1998
TGFBR2	Colon	1998
LKB1 (also known as *STK11)*	Colon, breast, pancreatic, testicular, ovarian	1998
SMAD4 (also known as *DPC4)*	Colon	1998
KIT	Gastrointestinal stromal tumors	1998

[1] As of January 1, 1999.
[2] Retinoblastoma and Wilms' tumor are children's cancers.

The biological roll of the dice depends largely on whether the gene is *dominant* or *recessive. Adenomatous polyposis coli* (APC), which causes about one in one hundred cases of colorectal cancer, is an example of a dominant gene, meaning that it prevails over its healthy counterpart in the unaffected parent's genetic composition. Therefore, a father who harbors the abnormal APC gene has a fifty-fifty chance of passing along the defect to each of his children. Most of the inherited adult-cancer genes that have been pegged to date, including BRCA1 and BRCA2, are dominant.

A recessive gene expresses itself only if both parents transmit an abnormal copy. Thus, a mother and father may each carry a recessive cancer-predisposition gene yet never get the disease themselves. As for each of their children, the odds fall this way:

- A one in four chance of not acquiring either parent's recessive gene

- A one in two chance of acquiring one parent's recessive gene

- A one in four chance of acquiring both parents' recessive genes—and with them the genetic disorder

Most recessive disease genes aren't "cancer genes" per se; they typically cause disorders that may have cancer as one feature. For example, the *ATM* gene, on chromosome 11, touches off a rare, crippling neurological disease of childhood called ataxia telangiectasia. One in ten people with ataxia also develop lymphoma, leukemia, or cancer of the breast, brain, or other organ.

In some family trees, cancer worms its way from one branch to another. Science has yet to determine exactly why the disease may spare one generation (though at least one family member unknowingly carries the genetic mutation), only to stalk the next. A doctor's ears should perk up if a family history reveals one or more key traits of hereditary cancers:

1. Cancer that strikes fifteen to twenty years earlier than average
2. Several close relatives who have had cancer
3. One or more close relatives who have had more than one form of cancer
4. Multiple generations in the family who have had cancer

Viruses and other infectious agents (5%)—Viruses and bacteria were virtually disregarded as a cause of cancer until 1967, when scientists linked the hepatitis B virus to liver cancer. Since then, seven other infectious agents have been documented as instigators. *Helicobacter pylori,* the first bacterium associated with cancer, may be a factor in as many as 80 percent of all carcinomas of the stomach.

Cervical cancer is caused almost exclusively by one of three sexually transmitted infections. Several subtypes of the more than seventy human papillomaviruses are at the root of nine in ten cases, while genital herpes (herpes simplex virus) and the human immunodeficiency virus, too, promote the disease. HIV, the precursor to AIDS (acquired immunodeficiency syndrome), can give rise to non-Hodgkin's lymphomas as well as Kaposi's sarcoma—a soft-tissue cancer of the blood-vessel walls that riddles the skin with blue, brown, or purple lesions.

Occupational and environmental carcinogens (5%/2%)—Fears that pollutants of the air and water cause cancer are all but unfounded in the United States. The Environmental Protection Agency estimates that air pollution is responsible for about one percent of the 175,000 or so

TABLE 2.4   Viruses and Bacteria Known to Cause Cancer

Infectious Agent	Type of Cancer	Estimated Proportion
Human papillomaviruses (HPV)	Cervical	90%
Epstein-Barr virus (EBV)	Nasopharyngeal (upper throat)	40%–70%
	Hodgkin's disease	35%–50%
	Non-Hodgkin's lymphomas	10%–15%
Chronic hepatitis B virus (HBV)	Liver	40%–60%
Chronic hepatitis C virus (HCV)	Liver	20%–30%
Human lymphotropic virus type I (HTLV-I)	Adult T-cell leukemia/ lymphomas[1]	5%
Helicobacter pylori bacterium	Stomach	50%–80%
Herpes simplex virus (HSV)	Cervical	No estimate available
Human immunodeficiency virus (HIV)	Cervical	No estimate available
	Non-Hodgkin's lymphomas	
	Kaposi's (soft-tissue) sarcoma	

[1] Adult T-cell leukemia/lymphomas are a group of rare lymphomas unrelated to the types typically seen in the United States.

Source: *Cancer Causes & Control,* November 1996, vol. 7, supplement 1, *Harvard Report on Cancer Prevention,* vol. 1, *Causes of Human Cancer.*

cases of lung cancer per year. This figure doesn't include probably the most pernicious source of air pollution both at home and in the workplace: smoke from other people's cigarettes. The EPA places secondhand smoke right alongside asbestos and radon as a class A carcinogen that is confirmed to trigger cancer.

Occupational carcinogens present a greater danger, though safety measures imposed since 1950 or so have probably halved the number of job-related fatal cancers. Today occupational exposures account for less than 5 percent of cancers in men and no more than 1 percent of cancers in women, with malignancies of the lung, bladder, and skin topping the list.

Excessive alcohol consumption (3%)—According to a study by the American Cancer Society, drinking two or more alcoholic beverages per day is enough to increase a person's risk of cancer. While not a direct carcinogen, alcohol is a highly synergistic *co*carcinogen, meaning that it enhances the damaging effects of other cancer-inducing substances. The combined effects of alcohol and tobacco, for instance, cause three in four oral and throat cancers, as well as tumors of the larynx and esophagus.

Alcohol contributes to liver cancer by impairing the organ's ability to deactivate other carcinogens. Even moderate consumption appears responsible for a small percentage of breast cancers: Alcohol elevates the levels of the hormone estrogen in the circulation, which in turn stimulates breast-cell division, which in turn can lead to cancer.

Reproductive history (3%)—We've seen how external factors such as obesity, a fat-heavy diet, and overindulgence of alcohol can subject women to excess estrogen, predisposing them to several cancers. A woman's menstrual history also influences her risk of developing breast and endometrial cancers.

During the first two weeks of the monthly menstrual cycle, the ovaries secrete estrogen, which goes to work on the endometrium to prepare a hospitable environment for the arrival of a fertilized egg should conception occur. Midway through the cycle, the estrogen level peaks, and another hormone, progesterone, takes over the task. The estrogen level rises, then falls; rises, then falls. This takes place every month for years and years.

The longer a woman menstruates, the greater her exposure to estrogen. Therefore, women who begin to menstruate early, before the age of twelve, and/or cease menstruating later than average, after age fifty, exhibit higher rates of these two cancers.

Neither early *menarche* (the time of life when menstruation begins) nor late *menopause* (the cessation of menstruation, which closes the curtain on the ability to bear children) has much of an effect on ovarian cancer. In fact, delayed menopause seems to confer something of a protective benefit. With the onset of menopause, a gland at the base of the brain releases high levels of yet another hormone, gonadotropin, which is believed to increase the risk of ovarian cancer.

Pregnancy diminishes gonadotropin secretion; therefore, never having given birth predisposes a woman to cancer of the ovary. Pregnancy also safeguards against cancers of the uterus and breast, though for a different reason. Estrogen levels actually rise throughout gestation. But it is believed that during this time the tissue in the breast and the uterus somehow grows resistant to carcinogens, and to estrogen. This does not mean, however, that a pregnant woman cannot develop cancer.

Hormones exert little impact on the other gynecologic malignancy, cervical cancer. The focus here is on sexual history. Since sexually transmitted diseases (STDs) produce the vast majority of cervical-cancer cases, it stands to reason that having unprotected sex with multiple partners boosts the odds of contracting the human papillomavirus or another STD. Becoming sexually active and/or pregnant during puberty heightens a woman's risk because the cervical tissue is undergoing many changes that may leave the area more vulnerable to cancer.

Environmental radiation (2%)—Solar radiation from the sun damages skin cells sufficiently to cause well over 90 percent of the nearly 1 million cases of skin cancer diagnosed annually. Basal-cell carcinoma and squamous-cell carcinoma are rarely fatal, but malignant melanoma can be a virulent foe if not detected and treated promptly.

Radon, a colorless radioactive gas produced by the natural disintegration of uranium in the ground and water, is the second leading cause of lung cancer. Most people are unwittingly exposed to it in their own homes; the unwelcome intruder frequently slips inside through cracks in walls, solid floors, and the foundation, or any number of other entranceways, including the water supply. The Environmental Protection Agency estimates that as many as one in fifteen U.S. homes are plagued by hazardous levels of radon.

Food additives and contaminants (1%)—Eating the occasional hot dog or bologna sandwich isn't going to give anyone cancer. But a diet high in these and other foods that are salt-cured, salt-pickled, or smoked can promote cancers of the esophagus, stomach, and small intestine. The reason: They contain a preservative called nitrates, which the body converts to nitrites, then nitrosamines, a known carcinogen. Aflatoxins, a group of chemicals produced by a mold that sometimes contaminates peanuts, grains, seeds, and other foods, have been shown to cause liver cancer.

Prior medical treatments (1%)—Ironically, certain medications and medical procedures, including those used to treat cancer, predispose patients to a slight—we emphasize, slight—risk of cancer. These include radiation therapy; chemotherapy; tamoxifen, a hormonal agent proven to be effective against breast cancer; and the immunosuppressant drugs given to patients following bone-marrow transplantation.

An area of great concern for many women once they reach menopause is whether or not to go on *hormone replacement therapy* (HRT). With the cessation of menstruation, estrogen production trails off dramatically. Restoring the lost estrogen with oral supplements not only relieves the hot flashes, itching, and vaginal dryness that menopausal women often experience for several years, it also protects against the progressive bone-thinning disease osteoporosis, as well as cardiovascular disease.

In the late 1960s, long-term estrogen replacement therapy (ERT) sparked a rash of endometrial cancers. Use tumbled by nearly half. After years of study, manufacturers began in the 1980s to supplement the estrogen with a dose of progesterone. When both hormones are taken, a woman's risk of endometrial cancer is all but normal. The U.S. Food and Drug Administration recommends hormone replacement therapy over plain estrogen for menopausal women who have not undergone a hysterectomy to remove the uterus. For women who opt to take estrogen alone, the odds of developing this cancer multiply up to tenfold.

A number of contradictory patient studies have stirred confusion as to whether or not adding progesterone to the regimen offsets the danger of incurring breast cancer—or, for that matter, if "unopposed" ERT is associated with breast cancer in the first place. Should a risk exist, it certainly is modest, and, one could argue, more than offset by the protective benefits. After all, a woman is ten times more likely to have a heart attack than to develop breast cancer. Ultimately, it's up to each woman to discuss the pros and cons of hormone replacement therapy with her doctor and weigh all the factors before coming to a decision.

The oral contraceptive's relationship to cancer follows a similar story line. Birth control pills, introduced in 1960, originally delivered nothing but estrogen for the first half of a woman's menstrual cycle, then added one week of progesterone to the sequence. As with estrogen replacement therapy, higher-than-average rates of gynecologic cancers were the result. The FDA yanked the "sequential" pills off the market in 1976. The subsequent "combination" oral contraceptives, which administer estrogen and progesterone simultaneously throughout the cycle, actually lower a woman's chances of developing cancer of the uterus and cancer of the ovary. Accordingly, never having taken birth control pills is considered a risk factor for both of those diseases.

The 25 Most Common Types of Cancer

Cancer of the Prostate

Predominant cell type: adenocarcinoma

RISK FACTORS

Lifestyle-Related
- Fatty diet • Obesity • Lack of exercise

Family Medical History
- Family history of prostate cancer

Personal Medical/Health History
- No association positively identified

Environmental/Occupational Carcinogens
- No association positively identified

WARNING SIGNS/SYMPTOMS
- Weak or interrupted urine flow • Unusually frequent urination • Difficulty in holding back urine or starting urination • Pain or a burning sensation upon urinating • Blood in the urine or semen • Inability to urinate • Painful ejaculation

IF NOT CONTROLLED, PROSTATE CANCER MAY SPREAD TO:
- Lymph nodes • Bone • Liver • Lung • Bladder • Rectum

Prostate cancer, considered rare in the early 1900s, is now the most commonly seen form of cancer in the United States. Two reasons for this are improved screening techniques, which pick up the cancer before symptoms emerge, and heightened awareness. Hearing public figures like former U.S. Senator Bob Dole and comedian Jerry Lewis speak candidly about their brushes with the disease sent thousands of men to their doctors for a blood test called PSA (prostate specific antigen). Much in the same way, when Betty Ford and Happy Rockefeller talked about their mastectomies in the mid-1970s, they persuaded countless women to have mammograms.

Prostate cancer is what's called an *indolent* cancer. That's good news, because it means that the tumor grows extremely slowly, sometimes taking as long as two to four years to double in size. Because the median age at diagnosis is seventy-two, a doctor and patient may elect to forgo aggressive treatment in favor of surveillance, or "watchful waiting." Even with no therapy at all, says Dr. Donald Urban, a urologic oncologist at the University of Alabama at Birmingham Comprehensive Cancer Center, "patients can live for many years."

About the Prostate

The chestnut-sized prostate occupies a strategic position in the male anatomy, not to mention the male psyche. Located just below the bladder, it wraps snugly around the upper part of the *urethra,* the thin tube that carries urine from the bladder to the tip of the penis. The sex gland's primary job is to produce seminal fluid.

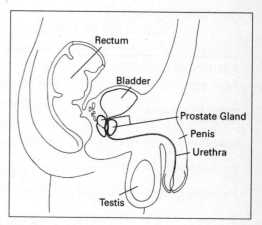

Testosterone: Fueling the Fire

At around the time that men enter into their fifties, the testicles suddenly begin to secrete *testosterone,* the key male sex hormone. The rising tide stimulates the prostate to grow, just like the last eruption of testosterone, during puberty.

The gland may increase in size by nearly half every ten years. More than 50 percent of men between the ages of sixty and seventy suffer from a noncancerous condition called *benign prostatic hyperplasia* (BPH). "As the prostate enlarges, or hypertrophies," explains Dr. Urban, "it compresses the urethra and the channel for urine to pass through." The symptoms of benign prostatic hyperplasia mirror those of prostate cancer. Men typically find themselves making repeated trips to the bathroom, but without being able to empty their bladder. Not only is this exhausting and frustrating, the obstruction can make urination painful.

The testosterone, meanwhile, doesn't differentiate between normal cells and malignant ones. Should a cell in the prostate turn into cancer, and a tumor eventually form, the hormone spurs its growth like gasoline feeding a fire. As long as the testicles keep producing testosterone, the cancer will continue to grow and spread. Accordingly, one treatment strategy is to cut off the supply, either by surgically removing the testicles or by administering other hormones that either halt testosterone production or block its effect.

How Prostate Cancer Is Typically Detected

Early-stage prostate cancer produces no symptoms. By the time a tumor is large enough to cause urinary problems, it may have spread beyond the gland.

Thanks to the PSA blood test, about two-thirds of all cases are now diagnosed while the disease is still local. "The majority of patients are asymptomatic," notes Dr. Urban. "They have this test as part of their annual physical exam." Before the widespread use of PSA, only one in three prostate cancers were caught early.

See Chapter Three, "How Cancer Is Diagnosed and Staged."

PROSTATE CANCER/ At Diagnosis	
EXTENT OF DISEASE AT THE TIME OF DIAGNOSIS	
Local disease	57% of cases
Regional disease	17% of cases
Metastatic disease	14% of cases
Unstaged	12% of cases

Cancer of the Breast

Predominant cell types: duct-cell carcinoma and lobular carcinoma

RISK FACTORS

Lifestyle-Related
- Obesity ▪ Lack of exercise ▪ Excessive alcohol consumption

Family Medical History
- Breast cancer ▪ Breast-ovarian cancer syndrome, in which patients develop ovarian cancer and breast cancer at an

unusually early age, and with a high incidence of tumors in
both breasts

Personal Medical/Health History

• Previous cancer in the other breast • Lobular carcinoma in situ •
Moderate or atypical hyperplasia, a benign condition in which
normal breast-tissue cells proliferate at an abnormally high rate •
Papilloma, a nonmalignant tumor of the milk ducts or skin of
the breast • Any medical condition that required large doses of
radiation to the chest • Early menarche/late menopause • Never
having given birth, or first giving birth after age thirty

Environmental/Occupational Carcinogens

• No association positively identified

WARNING SIGNS/SYMPTOMS

• Persistent lump or thickening in the breast or armpit •
Change in the breast's size or contour • Change in the color of
the breast or areola • Dimpling, puckering, scaling, or similar
change in the skin's texture • Discharge from the nipple that
appears milky, bloody, green, or clear and sticky • Retraction of
the nipples

IF NOT CONTROLLED, BREAST CANCER MAY SPREAD TO:

• Lymph nodes • Bone • Lung • Liver • Skin • Central
nervous system • Thyroid

Probably no disease is more dreaded by most women than breast
cancer, the leading form of cancer among females. The fear of mortality is compounded by anxiety over the prospect of possibly losing a
breast to surgical masectomy.

The percentage of women who die from breast cancer has actually
been on the decline since 1989, a fact that Dr. Larry Norton, chief of
breast-cancer medicine at Memorial Sloan-Kettering Cancer Center in
New York, wishes more patients were aware of. "The modern means of
detection and therapy now cures most people with breast cancer," he
points out. You should also know that if a tumor is diagnosed while still

localized to the breast—as are the majority of breast cancers—under most circumstances you would be considered a candidate for breast-conservation therapy. Instead of removing the entire breast, only the tumor and usually some nearby lymph nodes are taken out. Patients then receive six weeks of radiation therapy on an outpatient basis. "The cure rate," says Dr. Norton, "is exactly the same as it is for mastectomy."

About the Breast

Each breast has approximately fifteen to twenty fan-shaped sections called *lobes,* which are surrounded by fatty tissue and a patchwork of blood and lymph vessels. The lobes, in turn, contain many smaller *lobules* that culminate in tiny bulbous milk glands. A system of thin

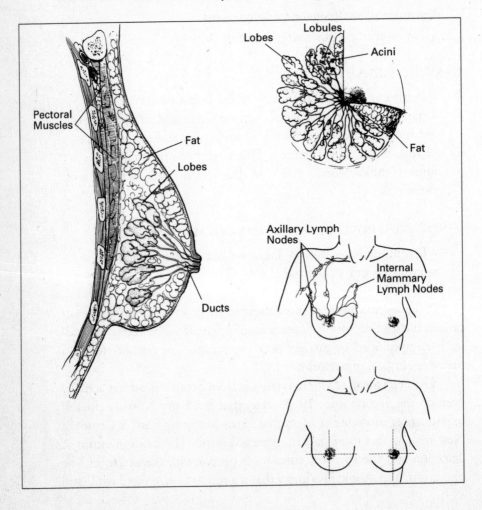

duct tubes carries the milk to the nipple located in the center of the darker-pigmented *areola*. The breast itself has no muscles, although breast cancer sometimes spreads to the chest muscle separating the breast from the rib cage.

Types of Breast Cancer

About three in four breast cancers are *ductal carcinomas*. They originate in milk ducts, whereas *lobular carcinomas* arise in either the lobes or the lobules. A third type, the rare *inflammatory breast cancer,* materializes in the lymph vessels in the skin of the breast. Its symptoms are markedly different from the other two.

"Inflammatory breast cancer resembles an infection," explains Dr. Norton. "The skin becomes thick, raised, and red. And instead of a discrete lump, it usually involves the whole breast." A fast-growing disease, inflammatory breast cancer is prone to metastasis. Of the three types, lobular carcinoma is the one most likely to occur in both breasts, or *bilaterally.*

Ductal Carcinoma In Situ (DCIS) and Lobular Carcinoma In Situ (LCIS)

One in seven breast cancers are discovered when they haven't yet infiltrated normal breast tissue. "Ductal carcinoma in situ is cancer in its earliest possible stages," says Dr. Norton. It is 97 percent curable. "Lobular carcinoma in situ, on the other hand, isn't generally considered cancer. It is a sign that the breast forms tumors and has a high probability of forming a cancer." A woman diagnosed with LCIS often faces a one-in-four chance of developing cancer in either breast sometime in the next twenty-five years.

Dr. Norton, an oncologist since 1974, adds, "In the 'old days,' when masectomies were routinely performed for breast cancer, it was not uncommon for women with a diagnosis of lobular carcinoma in situ to go for elective bilateral prophylactic masectomies"— having both breasts surgically removed as a precaution. The current standard, however, is stepped-up surveillance. At Sloan-Kettering, for instance, women with LCIS are advised to have their breasts examined by a doctor three times a year, as compared to the normal yearly screening.

How Breast Cancer Is Typically Detected

In the past, most breast cancers were diagnosed after a woman noticed a lump or swelling and brought it to her doctor's attention. Four in five breast lumps, incidentally, turn out to be benign. According to Dr. Norton, "Nowadays more cases are being picked up by mammography than by self-examination."

See Chapter Three, "How Cancer Is Diagnosed and Staged."

BREAST CANCER/ At Diagnosis	
EXTENT OF DISEASE AT THE TIME OF DIAGNOSIS	
Local disease	58% of cases
Regional disease	32% of cases
Metastatic disease	6% of cases
Unstaged	3% of cases

Cancer of the Lung

Predominant cell types: squamous-cell carcinoma, adenocarcinoma, small-cell carcinoma, and large-cell carcinoma

RISK FACTORS

Lifestyle-Related

- Smoking

Family Medical History

- Lung cancer

Personal Medical/Health History

- Chronic emphysema or bronchitis • Lung scarring from tuberculosis or other conditions • Any medical condition that required large doses of radiation to the chest

Environmental/Occupational Carcinogens

- Exposure to a number of industrial/environmental pollutants

WARNING SIGNS/SYMPTOMS

- A new cough that won't subside, or a worsening chronic cough, such as smoker's cough • Difficulty in breathing • Wheezing • Coughing up blood • Increased mucus production • Chest pain • Recurrent pneumonia or bronchitis

Less Common

- Persistent hoarseness • Difficulty in swallowing • Back pain

IF NOT CONTROLLED, LUNG CANCER MAY SPREAD TO:

- Lymph nodes • The opposite lung • Bone • Central nervous system • Liver • Trachea (windpipe) • Heart • Esophagus • Thyroid

Lung cancer, far and away the leading cause of death from cancer, scarcely attracted notice at the turn of the twentieth century, when it was almost always misdiagnosed as tuberculous, then the scourge that lung cancer is today. Tobacco use is to blame for 85 percent of all lung cancers. The other 15 percent stem mainly from occupational and environmental exposures to radon, asbestos, and secondhand cigarette smoke. Although the death rate for men has declined since the 1980s, in 1987 the disease overtook breast cancer as the foremost killer of women as well, a trend directly related to the rising number of female smokers.

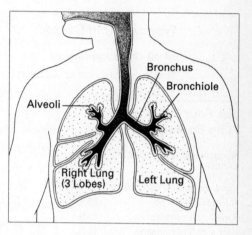

About the Lungs

The lungs, two saclike breathing organs made up of spongy, pinkish-gray tissue and an intricate network of blood vessels, lie on either side of the heart. The right lung, the larger of the pair, has three sections, or *lobes* (the left lung has two), and handles 60 percent of our respiratory function.

With every breath we take, air enters each lung by way of a large tube called the *mainstem bronchus*. The two bronchi feed smaller *bronchioles,*

Medical Terms You're Likely to Hear

Mediastinum: the compartment between the lungs that contains the heart, esophagus, trachea (windpipe), bronchi, lymph nodes, and blood vessels.

Pulmonary: pertaining to the lungs, as in *pulmonary oncologist.*

Thoracic: pertaining to the chest, as in *thoracic surgeon.*

which branch out and end in millions of tiny air sacs known as *alveoli.* The lungs expand to accommodate the inrushing air. Next they draw off waste products from the recirculated blood routed to them by the heart, reoxygenate the blood, and return it to the heart so that it can be pumped out to all the body's tissues via the arterial system. Then both lungs contract like a bellows to expel carbon dioxide and other waste gases back up the windpipe, past the larynx, and out the nose and mouth. Elapsed time: four seconds.

Types of Lung Cancer

Small-Cell Lung Cancer

Small-cell carcinoma is also referred to as *oat-cell cancer* because the diminutive cells, when viewed under a microscope, do in fact resemble oats. The tumor, which typically occurs in the central portion of the lung, is extraordinarily virulent.

The Four Types of Lung Cancer	
PERCENTAGE OF ALL CASES OF LUNG CANCER	
Squamous-cell carcinoma	33%
Adenocarcinoma	25%
Small-cell carcinoma	25%
Large-cell carcinoma	16%

"It tends to grow rapidly and spread to the lymph nodes and to other organs extremely quickly," explains Dr. Kasi Sridhar, a lung-cancer specialist at the Sylvester Comprehensive Cancer Center in Miami. "Without treatment, small-cell carcinoma is usually fatal within a month or two at most." However, the tumor is far more responsive to chemotherapy and radiation therapy than non-small-cell lung cancers.

Non-Small-Cell Lung Cancer

Three cell types belong to the more common form of lung cancer:

- *Squamous-cell carcinoma* frequently takes root in the bronchi. It spreads more slowly than any other type of lung cancer.

- *Adenocarcinoma,* the most common form of lung cancer in people who never smoked, typically begins along the outer perimeter of the lungs and under the bronchial lining.

- *Large-cell carcinomas,* so named for their large, abnormal-looking cells, are a group of cancers that, like adenocarcinomas, are usually found along the lung's outer border.

How Lung Cancer Is Typically Detected

"Early-stage tumors usually produce few symptoms or none at all," observes Dr. Sridhar. Because it is not standard practice to order chest X rays for patients who are asymptomatic, it is a fortuitous accident for a cancer to be discovered while still limited to the lung: perhaps when a patient comes in for an annual physical or needs a chest X ray for an unrelated reason.

LUNG CANCER/ At Diagnosis	
EXTENT OF DISEASE AT THE TIME OF DIAGNOSIS	
Local disease	15% of cases
Regional disease	26% of cases
Metastatic disease	44% of cases
Unstaged	15% of cases

In seven of ten diagnoses, the disease has already spread to neighboring lymph nodes or to other organs outside the chest. Consequently, "symptoms can vary so widely, almost any complaint can result in a diagnosis of lung cancer," says Dr. Sridhar. "The physician has to accurately distinguish which of the symptoms and abnormalities are from cancer and which are not." Besides the coughing, labored breathing, and other respiratory complications that can be brought on by a tumor in the lung, patients may exhibit symptoms that don't seem related to lung cancer at all, such as fatigue, appetite loss, or weight loss.

"A patient could present with seizures or a stroke, due to a metastatic lung tumor in the brain," explains Dr. Sridhar. "Or he could have pain due to cancer that has spread to the bone." Some lung tumors will impinge on adjacent nerves, sending pain shooting down the shoulder, arm, or hand; pressing on nearby large blood vessels can cause the face and neck to swell. Then there is an array of neurological and neuromuscular symptoms referred to collectively as *paraneoplastic syndrome*. Certain lung-cancer cells emit substances that deplete the blood of the mineral sodium. The resulting imbalance can give rise to muscle weakness, twitching, abdominal cramping, confusion, convulsions, and coma.

See Chapter Three, "How Cancer Is Diagnosed and Staged."

Cancer of the Colon or Rectum

Predominant cell type: adenocarcinoma

RISK FACTORS

Lifestyle-Related
- High-fat, low-fiber diet • Obesity • Lack of exercise

Family Medical History
- Colorectal cancer or polyps • Breast cancer, ovarian cancer, or endometrial cancer • Any of the following hereditary syndromes: (1) hereditary nonpolyposis colorectal cancer (HNPCC), (2) familial adenomatous polyposis (FAP), (3) Gardner's syndrome, an inherited disorder similar to FAP

Personal Medical/Health History
- Colorectal polyps • Inflammatory bowel diseases such as ulcerative colitis or Crohn's disease • Previous cancer of the breast, ovary, endometrium, or small bowel

Environmental/Occupational Carcinogens
- No association positively identified

WARNING SIGNS/SYMPTOMS
- Bloody stool • Cramping, bloating, gas pains • Abdominal pain • Persistent change in bowel habits, such as diarrhea, constipation, or narrow stools • Chronic fatigue and other symptoms of anemia, due to intestinal bleeding

IF NOT CONTROLLED, COLORECTAL CANCER MAY SPREAD TO:
- Lymph nodes • Liver • Lung • Brain • Bone • Kidney • Bladder

Colorectal cancer refers to cancer of the *large intestine,* a tubular digestive organ that curves around the abdominal cavity. The first five feet of the intestine, or *bowel,* is called the colon, and the last six to eight inches, the rectum. Because it can sometimes be difficult to pinpoint the location of a tumor in the large bowel, the colon and rectum are frequently grouped together as the *colorectum.*

Colorectal cancer is one of the few types that can be screened effectively. Since the mid-1980s, the death rate from this disease has fallen steadily, a trend attributed to improved methods for early detection, such as colonoscopy, sigmoidoscopy, and the fecal occult-blood test.

About the Colon and Rectum

After the small intestine has completed the process of digestion, it sends its contents on to the colon, which is divided into four segments. The organ's muscular walls contract and expand in a wavelike motion to nudge the indigestible fluid and nutrients up the *ascending colon,* across the *transverse colon,* and down the *descending colon.* Along the way, any remaining water gets absorbed. What is left, semisolid waste matter, or stool, collects in the *sigmoid colon* and rectum before being excreted out the *anus.*

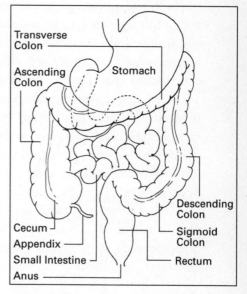

Polyps and Colorectal Cancer

Ninety-nine percent of all colorectal cancers stem from *adenomatous polyps,* small round or mushroom-shaped masses of tissue that form on the colon's inner lining, or *mucosa.* "They can be found in the rectum, too," says Dr. Peter Rosen, director of solid oncology at the Jonsson Comprehensive Cancer Center in Los Angeles. One in twenty polyps will evolve into carcinoma in situ, then invasive cancer over five to ten years.

Polyps are present among two in three men and women over age sixty-five. Most of the time they are benign and completely harmless. The problem is that the only way to ascertain if a growth is potentially malig-

> **Medical Terms You're Likely to Hear**
>
> **Gastroenterologist:** a doctor specializing in diseases of the digestive tract. *GI* (gastrointestinal) *oncologist* refers to a physician who diagnoses and treats cancers of the GI tract.

nant is to remove it and examine it microscopically. Normally, this can be done nonsurgically, says Dr. Rosen. "For small polyps, the most common technique by far is *polypectomy*," in which a flexible fiber-optic scope is inserted into the rectum and carefully advanced up the colon's twists and turns. Then a wire loop is passed through the instrument and over the polyp's head or stalk. Generating a painless electric current eliminates the mass. "Sometimes surgery is still required," says Dr. Rosen, "for example, if the polyp is too large to be removed safely."

Polypectomy drastically reduces the odds of getting colorectal cancer. Still, one in three patients go on to develop new growths. Anyone with a history of polyps should see a gastroenterologist at least annually, with periodic colonoscopies. The screening guidelines for men and women who have no known elevated risk of colorectal cancer is a colonoscopy every three to five years, beginning at age fifty.

More than 15 percent of cancers of the large intestine can be traced to inherited disorders. In families beset by *hereditary nonpolyposis colorectal cancer* (HNPCC), the most common of all congenital cancer-predisposition syndromes, several relatives are diagnosed with polyps, and often colon cancer, at an unusually early age. They are also in danger of developing cancers of the ovary, uterus, stomach, and still other organs. In another disorder, *familial adenomatous polyposis* (FAP), patients express literally thousands of polyps beginning around puberty. Their odds of cancer are so astronomically high, it is usually recommended that they have their large intestine removed as a preventive measure.

How Colorectal Cancer Is Typically Detected

Although screening tests are designed to diagnose disease in the absence of clinical features, "most patients," says Dr. Rosen, "are picked up by symptoms. The most frequent warning sign, blood in the stool,

COLORECTAL CANCER/At Diagnosis		
EXTENT OF DISEASE AT THE TIME OF DIAGNOSIS		
	Colon	Rectal
Local disease	36% of cases	37% of cases
Regional disease	38% of cases	37% of cases
Metastatic disease	21% of cases	19% of cases
Unstaged	5% of cases	6% of cases

is not always heeded, by patients or by doctors. "Many patients," he notes, "have been misdiagnosed as having bleeding hemorrhoids, because they are so common, and a cancer gets overlooked."

See Chapter Three, "How Cancer Is Diagnosed and Staged."

Lymphomas

Predominant cell type: lymphocytes

RISK FACTORS

Lifestyle-Related
- No association positively identified

Family Medical History
- No association positively identified

Personal Medical/Health History
- Epstein-Barr virus (EBV) - Human lymphotropic virus type I (HTLV-I) - Human immunodeficiency virus (HIV) - Immunosuppressant drug therapy following organ transplantation surgery - End-stage renal disease

Environmental/Occupational Carcinogens
- Occupational exposure to chemicals such as those used in the rubber industry and petroleum refining, among others

WARNING SIGNS/SYMPTOMS
- Painless swelling of the lymph nodes in the neck, underarm, or groin - Enlarged spleen - Fatigue - Fevers - Night sweats - Weight loss - Itchy, reddened skin

Less Common
- Nausea and vomiting - Abdominal pain

IF NOT CONTROLLED, LYMPHOMAS MAY SPREAD TO:
- Other lymph nodes - Bone marrow - Spleen - Liver - Central nervous system - Nose - Lung - Bone - Skin

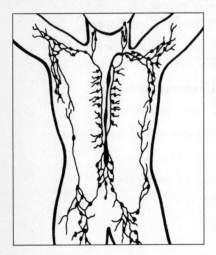

Therapy for Hodgkin's disease stands as one of the triumphs in the war on cancer. "When I first started in medicine," says Dr. Paul Carbone, an oncologist since 1960, "there was less than a 15 percent cure rate. Now it's 80 percent." High-dose radiation therapy and combination chemotherapy are two of the treatment advances he credits for this transformation.

"In non-Hodgkin's lymphomas, we've had the most success with the 'large-cell' lymphomas. Again, in the past, these were very rarely curable; now at least 30 to 40 percent can be cured. That's a good start. We just need to keep pushing and raise that envelope."

Hodgkin's disease and the group of cancers known collectively as non-Hodgkin's lymphomas are malignancies of the *lymphatic system,* a network of vessels and organs charged with defending the body against infection. Hodgkin's originates in the *lymph nodes,* as do some of the non-Hodgkin's lymphomas. The nodes, which are interspersed along the branches of lymphatic vessels, act as tiny sieves, skimming toxins from the straw-colored *lymph fluid* as it flows through. In addition, they and the *spleen,* another component of the lymphatic system, circulate crucial disease-fighting white blood cells called lymphocytes.

In lymphoma, the lymphocytes cease to function effectively. Like all cancer cells, they overproliferate—crowding out and damaging healthy lymphocytes—so that as the disease disseminates, patients become increasingly vulnerable to infection. Lymphomas, along with leukemia, are classified as *hematopoietic* malignancies: cancers of tissues that form blood cells.

Completing the lymphatic system are the bone marrow, the tonsils, and an organ called the *thymus,* where undeveloped lymphocytes mature and reproduce. Lymphoid tissue can be found in many other parts of the body too, including the intestines, stomach, liver, and skin. In contrast to Hodgkin's, non-Hodgkin's lymphomas often form in these and other *extranodal* sites—that is, lymphoid tissues other than

TABLE 2.5	Types of Non-Hodgkin's Lymphomas
Low-Grade (Indolent) Lymphomas: Types Include	**High-Grade (Aggressive) Lymphomas: Types Include**
Follicular small cleaved-cell lymphoma	Diffuse mixed-cell lymphoma
Follicular mixed-cell lymphoma	Diffuse large-cell lymphoma
Follicular large-cell lymphoma	Immunoblastic large-cell lymphoma
Diffuse small cleaved-cell lymphoma	Lymphoblastic lymphoma
Small lymphocytic lymphoma	Diffuse small noncleaved-cell lymphoma and Burkitt's lymphoma
Cutaneous T-cell Lymphoma	

the nodes. (An unusual type of low-grade lymphoma accounts for about 15 percent of small-intestine cancers.) With the lymphatic vessels serving as an expressway for tumor cells, lymphomas can metastasize all too readily.

See "Cancer of the Small Intestine," page 113, and "Primary Central Nervous System Lymphoma," page 93.

Types of Lymphomas

Hodgkin's Disease

Hodgkin's disease, named for Thomas Hodgkin, the nineteenth-century English physician who first described it, typically afflicts two age groups: young people between the ages of fifteen and thirty-four, and men and women over fifty-five. Under the microscope, the cancer is easily distinguishable from the non-Hodgkin's variety by the presence of unique large cells called *Reed-Sternberg* cells. In general, the fewer the number of these cells, the better the prognosis. One reason Hodgkin's is so treatable is that the disease usually travels slowly and predictably down the body: from nodes in the neck to those in the chest, then farther down to nodes in the abdomen and pelvis.

Non-Hodgkin's Lymphomas

The eleven main types of non-Hodgkin's lymphomas are grouped according to how aggressively they spread—low grade (indolent) or high grade (aggressive)—and also according to the tumor cells' shape and size: small, large, follicular, diffuse, and so on. *Cleaved* cells are referred to as such because the membrane surrounding the nucleus of each cell bears a distinctive cleft.

Compared to Hodgkin's, these malignancies tend to advance rapidly and follow a less predictable course. Yet it is possible for low-grade lymphoma to proceed all the way to stage IV—at which point the disease has spread to organs outside the lymphatic system—without producing any symptoms. Dr. Carbone, director of the University of Wisconsin Comprehensive Cancer Center in Madison, Wisconsin, tells of a patient who came to him for a consultation after having been to two other hospitals.

"She was diagnosed with stage II non-Hodgkin's lymphoma," he recalls. "When I looked at her throat, I couldn't see anything or feel anything. Yet we looked at the slides and concluded she had cancer. Rather than treat her, I said, 'Let's just watch you for a little while.' It's been twelve years now, and she's never had a recurrence and never been treated."

Lymphomas and Immunosuppression

Just as lymphomas compromise a person's immunity, an immuno-compromised state appears to lead to lymphoma. People with AIDS, the retrovirus that progressively destroys the immune system, are sixty times more likely than the general population to develop non-Hodgkin's lymphoma. Likewise, kidney recipients, who receive drugs intended to suppress the immune system so that it doesn't reject the transplanted organ, run a 40-fold to 100-fold risk of non-Hodgkin's lymphoma. These cancers often attack the brain and central nervous system.

How Lymphomas Are Typically Detected

"The first thing patients usually feel," according to Dr. Carbone, "is a painless lump in the neck, armpit, or groin area from one or more enlarged lymph nodes." Swollen nodes in the chest will produce vague respiratory symptoms, like shortness of breath or coughing.

Fever, night sweats, and weight loss can accompany lymphomas, Dr. Carbone observes, adding that physicians used to regularly mistake Hodgkin's disease for an infection. Such features usually signal that the cancer has already spread. "In general,

**LYMPHOMAS/
At Diagnosis**

EXTENT OF DISEASE AT THE TIME OF
DIAGNOSIS

Percentages of lymphoma patients diagnosed with local, regional, or metastatic disease are not available. Non-Hodgkin's lymphomas are classified according to the cells' appearance and behavior.

most patients present with what's called limited disease. But 30 percent or more will have extensive disease."

See Chapter Three, "How Cancer Is Diagnosed and Staged."

Cancer of the Bladder

Predominant cell type: transitional-cell carcinoma

RISK FACTORS

Lifestyle-Related
- Smoking

Family Medical History
- No association positively identified

Personal Medical/Health History
- Previous cancer treatment incorporating the drug cyclophosphamide (brand name: Cytoxan) • End-stage renal disease

Environmental/Occupational Carcinogens
- Occupational exposure to chemicals used in the rubber industry and the manufacturing of magenta and auramine, among others

WARNING SIGNS/SYMPTOMS
- Bloody urine ranging in color from bright red to rusty • Frequent urination • Painful urination • Inability to urinate • Fever

IF NOT CONTROLLED, BLADDER CANCER MAY SPREAD TO:
- Lymph nodes • Liver • Lung • Prostate • Uterus • Vagina • Abdominal wall • Pelvic wall

Men are more than twice as likely as women to develop bladder cancer, the most common malignancy of the urinary tract. In three out of four cases that are diagnosed early—a number of those as carcinoma in situ—bladder cancer is eminently treatable. But the chances of superficial disease recurring anywhere on the organ's inner lining can range as high as 60 percent.

"Once you've had a diagnosis of bladder cancer, you're always at risk for a new tumor in the bladder," explains Dr. Michael Cooper, a specialist in *genitourinary oncology* at Duke University Medical Center in Durham, North Carolina, "unless you've had your bladder taken out surgically. If the tumors do recur, hopefully they will continue to be superficial. But occasionally, the cancer does come back as an invasive tumor. In fact, there are some who think that if we followed patients long enough—in other words, if they didn't die of other causes—all of them would eventually develop invasive disease."

About the Bladder

Every few seconds a pair of tubes called the *ureters* deliver urine from the *kidneys* to the bladder, a hollow receptacle barely the size of a baby's fist. When it is time to urinate, the sphincter muscles around the opening to the narrow *urethra* relax and the bladder walls contract. This expels the urine down through the urethral opening.

Most cancers occur in the bladder wall's *mucosa,* the innermost of its three layers. The tumor, sometimes referred to as a *papillary tumor,* often resembles a tiny mushroom, its stalk attached to the inner lining. "The key issue in bladder cancer," says Dr. Cooper, "is whether the disease remains confined to the lining [stage I] or invades the muscular wall and perhaps extends into the surrounding fatty tissue [stages II and III]. Once it has infiltrated the bladder wall, consideration must be given to removing the bladder or to initiating combination radiation and chemotherapy."

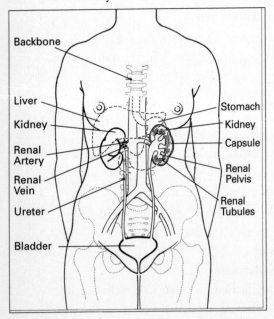

Backbone
Liver
Kidney
Renal Artery
Renal Vein
Ureter
Bladder
Stomach
Kidney
Capsule
Renal Pelvis
Renal Tubules

How Bladder Cancer Is Typically Detected

A tumor can grow in the bladder for some time without raising suspicion. Even so, "it is very rare for a patient to be diagnosed with widespread metastatic disease," says Dr. Cooper. "Most of these tumors are picked up due to urinary-related symptoms caused by the local presence of disease in the bladder."

See Chapter Three, "How Cancer Is Diagnosed and Staged."

BLADDER CANCER/ At Diagnosis	
EXTENT OF DISEASE AT THE TIME OF DIAGNOSIS	
Local disease	74% of cases
Regional disease	18% of cases
Metastatic disease	3% of cases
Unstaged	5% of cases

Melanoma

Predominant cell type: melanoma

RISK FACTORS

Lifestyle-Related

- Overexposure to the sun's ultraviolet rays, particularly during the first ten to fifteen years of life • A blistering sunburn

Family Medical History

- Melanoma • Any of the following genetic skin disorders: (1) xeroderma pigmentosum, (2) albinism, (3) multiple basal-cell carcinoma syndrome, (4) dysplastic nevus syndrome, (5) familial atypical multiple mole melanoma (FAMMM) syndrome

Personal Medical/Health History

- Fair complexion • Blond or red hair • Blue eyes • Freckles • An inability to tan • Sensitivity to the sun • A large mole present since birth • A compromised immune system, perhaps due to taking immunosuppressive drugs following a bone-marrow transplant or organ transplant • Prior history of melanoma

Environmental/Occupational Carcinogens

- No association positively identified

WARNING SIGNS/SYMPTOMS

- A mole that meets any of the "ABCD" criteria for melanoma:

  A = **a**symmetrical shape
  B = ragged, notched, or blurred **b**order
  C = uneven **c**olor that may change over time
  D = wider than ¼ inch in **d**iameter or a change in size

- A mole that itches, oozes, or bleeds
- Change in a mole's texture; it may become hard, lumpy, or scaly

IF NOT CONTROLLED, MELANOMA MAY SPREAD TO:

> • Lymph nodes • Liver • Lung • Central nervous system •
> Bone • Other locations in the skin

From the early 1970s to the mid-1990s, the incidence rate of melanoma among white men and women more than doubled. (African Americans, while not invulnerable to the potential hazards of solar radiation, are twenty times less likely to incur the disease.) Yet over the same period, the five-year survival rate rose from 68 to 88 percent, a testament to early detection and to heightened public awareness of the sun's harmful effects.

Dr. Allan Oseroff, chairman of the department of dermatology at the Roswell Park Cancer Institute in Buffalo, New York, observes, "It's an enormous pleasure to go to the beach nowadays and see people wearing hats and sunscreen and swimming in sun-protective clothing. Five years ago, I didn't see that at all."

About the Skin

Melanoma arises in the *melanocytes,* one of three types of cells that make up the skin's outer layer, or *epidermis*. Melanocytes produce *melanin,* the *pigment* that lends skin its color. Moles, the tan or brown spots also known as *nevi,* are nothing more than benign clusters of melanocytes.

Roughly 10 percent of all men and women have one or more moles that appear abnormal in size, shape, or color. Dermatologists call these *dysplastic nevi*. Most are harmless and never change into melanoma; in fact, the disease rarely takes hold in preexisting moles of any kind. But they are more likely than ordinary cells to become cancerous.

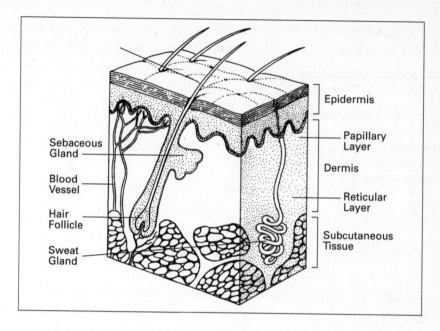

Sebaceous Gland

Blood Vessel

Hair Follicle

Sweat Gland

Epidermis

Papillary Layer

Dermis

Reticular Layer

Subcutaneous Tissue

More often, melanoma materializes as a new growth with any of the characteristics described in "Warning Signs/Symptoms." (Generally, you acquire all the moles you're going to have before age forty.) Men tend to develop the disease on the trunk, head, and neck; women, on the trunk and lower legs. When melanoma does afflict people with dark skin, it often forms on the palms of the hands, the soles of the feet, or under the fingernails or toenails.

In addition to the more than forty-four thousand cases of invasive melanoma detected in 1999, another twenty-three thousand people were diagnosed with melanoma in situ. The cure rate for this nonmalignant stage exceeds 99 percent. However, if the disease is not controlled early on, it may burrow deep into the inner layer of the skin, home to hair follicles and glands. Also running through the *dermis* are blood vessels and lymphatic vessels, which can whisk the cancerous cells throughout the body.

How Melanoma Is Typically Detected

Occasionally, a doctor comes across a melanoma during a routine physical exam. But more often than not, it's the patient who points out the suspicious-looking lesion to the doctor—frequently after a spouse or other loved one has noticed it and brought it to the patient's attention.

In other cancers, tumor size is often a crucial prognostic indicator. "But in melanoma," says Dr. Oseroff, "the most important factor is the depth, or thickness. The number of lymphatic vessels and capillaries increases the deeper you go into the skin. So the more a tumor penetrates, the greater the chance of encountering one of these pathways to other locations."

See Chapter Three, "How Cancer Is Diagnosed and Staged."

MELANOMA/At Diagnosis

EXTENT OF DISEASE AT THE TIME OF DIAGNOSIS

Local disease	82% of cases
Regional disease	8% of cases
Metastatic disease	4% of cases
Unstaged	6% of cases

Cancer of the Uterus (Endometrial Cancer)

Predominant cell types: adenocarcinoma and adenosquamous-cell carcinoma

RISK FACTORS

Lifestyle-Related

- Obesity - Lack of exercise

Family Medical History

- Hereditary nonpolyposis colorectal cancer (HNPCC), which increases a person's risk of developing cancers of the large intestine, endometrium, ovary, stomach, and other organs

Personal Medical/Health History

- Uterine polyps - Fibroid tumors that have not been surgically removed - A precancerous condition known as atypical uterine hyperplasia - Diabetes - Hypertension - Previous cancer of the large intestine, ovary, or breast - Prolonged estrogen replacement therapy - Hormone therapy using tamoxifen as a treatment for breast cancer - Never having taken oral contraceptives - Early menarche/late menopause - Never having given birth

Environmental/Occupational Carcinogens

- No association positively identified

WARNING SIGNS/SYMPTOMS

▪ Vaginal bleeding between periods or after menopause ▪ Lower abdominal and back pain

IF NOT CONTROLLED, ENDOMETRIAL CANCER MAY SPREAD TO:

▪ Cervix ▪ Ovary ▪ Vagina ▪ Bladder ▪ Colon ▪ Lymph nodes

Endometrial carcinoma, the third most common malignancy among women, boasts one of the highest cure rates of any cancer. Since more than nine in ten uterine tumors form in the organ's inner layer, or *endometrium,* doctors routinely refer to all cancers of the uterus as endometrial cancer. *Uterine sarcoma,* which accounts for less than 5 percent of cases, occurs in the uterus's muscular outer layer—the *myometrium*—or its supporting tissues.

About the Uterus

The hollow uterus, also called the *womb,* consists of two main sections. Its bottom half tapers into a narrow opening called the *cervix,* which leads to the vagina. Though the main body, or *corpus,* is no larger than a pear, during pregnancy the myometrium expands up to one thousand times its normal size in order to accommodate the growing fetus.

Throughout a woman's reproductive years, each month the spongy endometrium grows and thickens in preparation for a fertilized egg to emerge from either of the two *fallopian tubes* that branch out from the uterus's dome-shaped crown (the *fundus).* If the male sperm has indeed fertilized the female egg, the embryo embeds itself

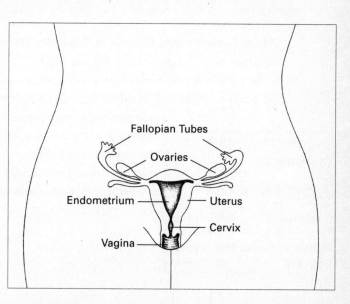

Fallopian Tubes

Ovaries

Endometrium — — Uterus

— Cervix

Vagina —

in the womb to begin its approximately forty weeks of gestation. But when fertilization fails to take place, the uterus sheds the excess endometrial tissue through the vagina, along with blood and fluid. This process, *menstruation,* is repeated until a woman reaches *menopause,* when her cycles end permanently.

Atypical Uterine Hyperplasia

Unlike cervical cancer, endometrial carcinoma has no noninvasive stage. One reason is that carcinoma in situ of the uterus is rarely seen. But a second reason is that the only way for a gynecologic oncologist to tell if a cancer meets the definition of malignant disease is to surgically remove the uterus—the treatment that would be carried out for early cancer.

"What we do see," says Dr. Michael Hogan, chief of gynecologic oncology at Philadelphia's Fox Chase Cancer Center, "are precancers of the endometrium." In *atypical uterine hyperplasia,* normal endometrial cells multiply out of control until they build up, causing the uterine lining to thicken. Depending on the degree of hyperplasia, says Dr. Hogan, "a woman will have anywhere from a 5 to 30 percent chance of progressing to endometrial cancer over the next five to ten years." Though atypical uterine hyperplasia is not cancer, it is treated as such, with either surgery or hormone therapy, depending on whether or not the patient is *postmenopausal,* or no longer biologically capable of bearing children. Most patients fall into that category, for endometrial cancer occurs mainly in women between the ages of fifty and sixty-four, and eighty and older.

How Endometrial Cancer Is Typically Detected

Endometrial cancer usually reveals itself with abnormal bleeding from the vagina. Since postmenopausal women no longer menstruate, *any* bleeding is abnormal. It often begins as a watery blood-tinged discharge, then later contains more blood. According to Dr. Hogan, for women just beginning menopause, "a change in their bleeding pattern usually alerts them that something is wrong and causes them to contact a physician."

See Chapter Three, "How Cancer Is Diagnosed and Staged."

ENDOMETRIAL CANCER/ At Diagnosis	
EXTENT OF DISEASE AT THE TIME OF DIAGNOSIS	
Local disease	73% of cases
Regional disease	13% of cases
Metastatic disease	10% of cases
Unstaged	4% of cases

Leukemia

Predominant cell types: myeloid cells and lymphoid cells

RISK FACTORS

Lifestyle-Related

- No association identified

Family Medical History

- No association identified

Personal Medical/Health History

- Human lymphotropic virus type I (HTLV-I) - Previous cancer treatment using a class of chemotherapy drugs known as alkylating agents - Any medical condition requiring high doses of radiation therapy

Environmental/Occupational Carcinogens

Symptoms of Blood Disorders Associated with Leukemia

Leukopenia (low white-cell count)
- Recurrent infections
- High-grade fever and chills

Anemia (low red-cell count)
- Chronic fatigue, weakness
- Profuse perspiration and/or night sweats
- Headache, dizziness
- Pale complexion

Thrombocytopenia (low platelet count)
- Excessive bleeding and unexplained bruising
- Tiny red spots under the skin

- Significant exposure to radiation - Occupational exposure to chemicals used in the rubber industry and petroleum refining, among others

WARNING SIGNS/SYMPTOMS

Acute Leukemias

- Leukopenia, anemia, thrombocytopenia (see box) - Enlarged lymph nodes, spleen, liver - Joint and bone pain - Swelling of the testicles - Skin sores - Sores on the eye - Complications from disease of the central nervous system: headaches, vomiting, confusion, loss of muscle control, seizures

Chronic Leukemias

- Enlarged lymph nodes, spleen, liver - General feeling of ill health - Fatigue, lack of energy - Appetite loss - Weight loss -

Night sweats • Leukopenia, anemia, thrombocytopenia (see box on page 65) • Headaches • Bone pain or tenderness

IF NOT CONTROLLED, LEUKEMIA MAY SPREAD TO:

• Lymph nodes • Spleen • Kidney • Liver • Central nervous system • Testicle • Bone

Leukemia, derived from the Greek, means "white blood," a literal description of its effect. This cancer of the tissues that form blood cells causes the *bone marrow, lymph nodes,* and *spleen* to inundate the circulation with ineffective white blood cells *(leukocytes),* which are unable to defend the body against infection and other harmful agents.

The spongy red bone marrow found in the cavities of the large bones serves as the factory for all three components of the blood—white cells, *red cells,* and *platelets*—although a type of leukocyte called *lymphocytes* matures in the marrow or in lymphatic tissues such as the nodes and spleen. In addition to decimating the immune system, leukemia disrupts the marrow's production of the other two types of blood cells. The red blood cells (RBCs), or *erythrocytes,* ferry life-sustaining oxygen throughout the body and carry off carbon dioxide to be excreted out the lungs. A deficiency of RBCs brings on anemia. The platelets *(thrombocytes),* disc-shaped clotting cells, converge on wounds to control bleeding. People with leukemia often suffer excessive bleeding and bruising, because their platelet level falls dangerously low.

> **Medical Terms You're Likely to Hear**
>
> **Hematologist:** a physician who specializes in diseases of the blood.
>
> **Hematopoiesis:** the process of blood-cell formation and development. Leukemia and lymphomas are sometimes referred to as *hematopoietic* cancers.

Chemotherapy, the initial treatment for leukemia, further suppresses immunity. A subsequent bone-marrow transplantation ultimately holds many patients' best hope for a cure. In preparation for this costly, risky procedure, high doses of chemotherapy and often full-body irradiation are used to eradicate the diseased marrow, which leaves the person without an immune system.

Thus, medical care for leukemia patients must focus not only on conquering the disease but on safeguarding them from potentially fatal complications such as infections and internal hemorrhaging. In the opinion of Dr. Fred Appelbaum, head of clinical research at Seattle's Fred Hutchinson Cancer Research Center, "good supportive care is probably more essential in leukemia than in any other type of tumor." This is a crucial point to bear in mind when you're deciding on where to undergo therapy.

Types of Leukemia

The four main types of leukemia are divided into two broad categories—acute and chronic—then further classified according to the type of white cell affected: *granulocyte* or *lymphocyte.*

Myeloid leukemias begin in immature myeloid cells—*myeloblasts*—which develop in the bone marrow; normally, they grow into mature granulocytes. *Lymphocytic* leukemias take root in *lymphoblasts,* the immature white cells that "come of age" primarily in the lymphatic tissues. *(Monocytic* leukemia involves the third type of white blood cell, *monocytes,* but it is as rare as the monocytes are few in number.)

As for the difference between chronic and acute disease, Dr. Appelbaum explains: "Even though the leukemic cells are abnormal, some may still have the capacity to develop all the way up to mature granulocytes or mature lymphocytes, in which case we call them *chronic myeloid leukemia* [CML] or *chronic lymphocytic leukemia* [CLL]." The mature white cells manage to function somewhat normally early in the disease, but over time they become more abnormal and dysfunctional.

"Other leukemic cells may remain in a very primitive form," Dr. Appelbaum continues, "able to divide but not mature or function. Those are the acute leukemias." The undeveloped blast cells characteristic of *acute myeloid leukemia* (AML) or *acute lymphocytic leukemia* (ALL) do not behave at all like normal white cells.

"In functional terms, acute and chronic leukemias are very different, because the average life expectancy of a patient with untreated acute leukemia is less than two months, whereas the average life expectancy of a patient with chronic leukemia, even if untreated, is measured in years."

Prevalence of Leukemia by Type

ESTIMATED NUMBER OF CASES DIAGNOSED IN 1999

Acute myeloid leukemia (AML)	10,100
Chronic lymphocytic leukemia (CLL)	7,800
Chronic myeloid leukemia (CML)	4,500
Acute lymphocytic leukemia (ALL)	3,100
Miscellaneous rare types	4,600
Monocytic leukemia	
Hairy-cell leukemia	
Promyelocytic leukemia	
Erythroleukemia	
Others	

Medical Terms You're Likely to Hear

Granulocytic

Myelocytic

Myelogenous

. . . words the doctor may use instead of "myeloid"

How Leukemia Is Typically Detected

Chronic Leukemias

Unlike solid tumors, leukemia is a systemic disease, so that even at diagnosis, the cancer has scattered throughout the body. Nonetheless, as many as one in four people with CLL or CML display "absolutely no symptoms whatsoever," says Dr. Appelbaum, "in part because the chronic leukemias develop so slowly. They often get picked up accidentally, when blood is drawn for a routine physical, and *voilà!*, the person's white count is found to be slightly elevated."

LEUKEMIA/At Diagnosis
EXTENT OF DISEASE AT THE TIME OF DIAGNOSIS
Percentages of leukemia patients diagnosed with local, regional, or metastatic disease are not available. As a cancer of the blood and blood-forming tissues, leukemia is by nature metastatic.

The symptoms that do emerge are rarely dramatic. Many times patients assume they're merely run-down or gripped by a lingering flu. Their malaise may stem from anemia, as red blood cells get crowded out by aberrant leukocytes. But also, explains Dr. Appelbaum, "because white cells are extremely rapidly dividing cells, the body expends a lot of energy to produce them. Patients feel fatigued and have night sweats, as if they're constantly exercising, though they're not." Appetite loss, a common early feature, is often due to an accumulation of white cells in the spleen, causing it to enlarge. Nine in ten people with CML are found to have a swollen spleen, or *splenomegaly*, at the time of diagnosis.

Acute Leukemias

In contrast to chronic leukemias, ALL and AML produce severe symptoms that come on suddenly, although here, too, the early effects may be mistaken for the flu. The organ enlargement from the buildup of rapidly dividing white cells—in the spleen and nodes, as well as the liver and men's testicles—can be painful. Joint and bone pain are also frequently seen. Forty percent of ALL patients develop leukemia of the central nervous system, which can interfere with their motor skills and cognition, and trigger headaches and seizures.

See Chapter Three, "How Cancer Is Diagnosed and Staged."

Cancer of the Kidney (Renal-Cell Carcinoma)

Predominant cell type: adenocarcinoma

RISK FACTORS

Lifestyle-Related

- Smoking

Family Medical History

- Kidney cancer

Personal Medical/Health History

- End-stage renal disease

Environmental/Occupational Carcinogens

- No association positively identified

WARNING SIGNS/SYMPTOMS

- Bloody urine • Pain in the abdomen or side • Fatigue • Appetite loss • Unexplained weight loss • Recurrent fever

IF NOT CONTROLLED, KIDNEY CANCER MAY SPREAD TO:

- Lung • Liver • Colon • Pancreas • The other kidney • Lymph nodes • Thyroid

Eighty-five percent of all adult kidney cancers originate in the lining of the *tubules,* hairpin-shaped collecting channels that run throughout each organ. These cancers are called *renal-cell carcinoma.* A second, rare form, *transitional-cell carcinoma,* arises in the funnel-shaped *renal pelvis,* located in each kidney's midsection. Transitional-cell cancer more closely resembles bladder cancer than renal-cell cancer and is treated in much the same way. The term "kidney cancer" almost always applies to renal-cell carcinoma, the type we focus on here.

About the Kidneys

The two bean-shaped kidneys lie on either side of the spine, just above the waist. Though only four inches long and two inches wide, each organ contains over 1 million *nephrons,* microscopic units that

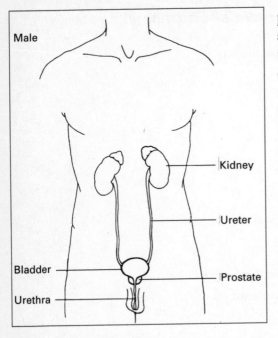

Male

Kidney

Ureter

Bladder

Prostate

Urethra

purify the blood. Then their slender tubules carry the filtered waste products and excess water, or urine, to the renal pelvis. The urine pools there before draining into the long *ureter* tubes and beginning its winding journey out of the body.

In addition to refining the blood, the kidneys help to control blood pressure and regulate the formation of oxygen-bearing red blood cells. Their versatility is equaled by their efficiency: A single kidney is capable of providing far more renal function than the body needs. Should you require surgery to remove your cancerous kidney, the primary treatment for renal-cell carcinoma, its healthy twin easily takes over cleansing all the blood. As Dr. Jim Mohler, director of urologic oncology at the UNC Lineberger Comprehensive Cancer Center in Chapel Hill, North Carolina, tells patients scheduled to undergo this operation, "God gave you two kidneys so that you could have an entire kidney removed, plus *half* the other kidney, and still have a normal life expectancy."

How Kidney Cancer Is Typically Detected

"The medical textbooks," says Dr. Mohler, "describe a classic triad of symptoms: blood in the urine, abdominal pain, and a palpable mass in the flank. But only 5 to 10 percent of kidney cancers actually present that way." Seven in ten patients will go to their doctors with nondescript, subtle symptoms that mimic many other diseases: indigestion, malaise, blood in the urine.

Among oncologists, notes Dr. Mohler, renal-cell cancer has earned the sobriquet "the internist's tumor" because pinning down the

KIDNEY CANCER/
At Diagnosis

EXTENT OF DISEASE AT THE TIME OF DIAGNOSIS

Local disease	45% of cases
Regional disease	23% of cases
Metastatic disease	25% of cases
Unstaged	7% of cases

diagnosis can be exasperating. "Often," he says, "out of frustration, a physician will order a CT scan, and lo and behold, there's a mass in the kidney."

See Chapter Three, "How Cancer Is Diagnosed and Staged."

Cancer of the Pancreas

Predominant cell type: duct-cell carcinoma

RISK FACTORS

Lifestyle-Related
- Smoking

Family Medical History
- Any of the following hereditary syndromes: (1) hereditary nonpolyposis colorectal cancer (HNPCC), (2) Peutz-Jeghers syndrome, marked by the development of potentially malignant polyps in the gastrointestinal tract, (3) hereditary pancreatitis, an inflammation of the pancreas, (4) hereditary breast cancer associated with the BRCA2 gene, (5) ataxia-telangiectasia, a rare neurological disease, (6) familial atypical multiple mole melanoma (FAMMM) syndrome

Personal Medical/Health History
- Diabetes

Environmental/Occupational Carcinogens
- No association positively identified

WARNING SIGNS/SYMPTOMS
- Jaundice · Nausea · Appetite loss · Unexplained weight loss · Weakness · Upper abdominal pain · Back pain

IF NOT CONTROLLED, PANCREATIC CANCER MAY SPREAD TO:
- Lymph nodes · Bile duct · Liver · Stomach · Small intestine · Spleen · Colon · Lung

Pancreatic cancer presents a formidable challenge, both to patients and their doctors. The pancreas will silently abide the presence of a growing cancer for some time. When symptoms finally do manifest, they frequently mirror those of other disorders, such as hepatitis, gallstones, and diabetes, so that by the time the tumor is identified, in three out of four cases it has spread beyond the pancreas.

Still, the last few decades have brought several promising advances in therapy, such as safer surgical techniques and the use of chemotherapy and radiotherapy both preoperatively and postoperatively. "Pancreatic cancer is not necessarily a death sentence," emphasizes Dr. Charles J. Yeo, director of the pancreas-cancer center at Johns Hopkins University School of Medicine in Baltimore. "There are patients who are cured."

About the Pancreas

The wing-shaped pancreas, measuring six inches by two inches, is said to have four parts: head, neck, body, tail. Its rounded head wedges into the crook formed on the right side of the upper abdomen by the C-shaped *duodenum,* the portion of the small intestine that receives partly digested food from the stomach. To the left of the head is the neck, then the body. The pancreas tapers into a narrow tail, ending at the *spleen.*

This organ is composed of two types of tissue, each with its own function. The *exocrine* portion, which makes up 99 percent of the pancreas, releases a mixture of water, enzymes, and salts that aids digestion. These *pancreatic juices* flow down the long *pancreatic duct* to the duodenum, where they help break down nutrients and neutralize acids. Pancreatic cancer occurs in the lining of that duct.

The *endocrine* cells, found within the substance of the pancreas in clusters known as the *islets of Langerhans,* belong to the hormonal system. They secrete *insulin* and *glucagon,* chemical transmitters responsible for regulating the level of sugar *(glucose)* in the blood. Insulin instructs the body's cells to burn glucose for fuel. It also signals the liver to deposit excess glucose as *glycogen,* to be withdrawn as needed. Glucagon exerts the opposite effect: When the blood sugar is low, it converts the glycogen back to glucose.

More than 95 percent of pancreatic cancers arise in the exocrine tissue. Cancer of the endocrine pancreas, also referred to as *islet-cell carcinoma,* strikes fewer than a thousand patients per year. The tumor is not as aggressive as exocrine pancreatic cancer and tends to have a more favorable prognosis. This book looks at cancer of the exocrine pancreas only.

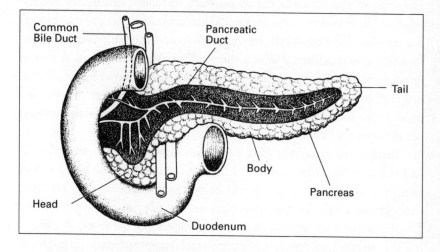

How Pancreatic Cancer Is Typically Detected

"When discussing symptoms," says Dr. Yeo, "it's important to distinguish between cancers on the right side of the pancreas and cancers on the left side, because their clinical presentations are a bit different."

About three-fourths of all exocrine malignancies originate on the right, in the head or neck of the pancreas. "Patients with those tumors," says Dr. Yeo, "typically present with jaundice." A complication of gallstones and several other diseases besides cancer, *jaundice* turns the skin and eyes yellow, due to an accumulation of *bile* in the bloodstream. Bile, produced in the liver and stored in the gallbladder, is a yellow or orange digestive fluid not unlike the pancreatic juices. When needed, it is conveyed to the small intestine by way of the *common bile duct,* which passes through the right side of the pancreas and joins the pancreatic duct. A tumor can obstruct the flow of bile, causing it to enter the circulation.

"Tumors in the body or tail of the pancreas are far away from the common bile duct, so they typically don't trigger jaundice early," Dr. Yeo explains. "Those cancers can become quite large, and they are associated more with abdominal pain and pressure."

PANCREATIC CANCER/ At Diagnosis

EXTENT OF DISEASE AT THE TIME OF DIAGNOSIS

Local disease	8% of cases
Regional disease	23% of cases
Metastatic disease	48% of cases
Unstaged	21% of cases

The Link Between Pancreatic Cancer and Diabetes

About one in fifteen newly diagnosed patients will be found to have developed *diabetes* in addition to cancer. In diabetes, either the islet cells of the pancreas fail to produce sufficient insulin, or the insulin it does make is ineffective. Glucose builds up in the bloodstream—a condition called *hyperglycemia*—and the body is deprived of its chief energy source. "When the pancreas has a tumor in it that is growing or causing the gland to become inflamed," says Dr. Yeo, "some of the islet cells won't be able to function normally. Therefore, insulin production is not up to snuff, and patients may present with elevated blood sugar and diabetes."

Surgery to excise the entire pancreas leaves patients permanently diabetic and dependent on daily injections of insulin. The operation to remove part of the organ can also bring about diabetes, says Dr. Yeo, though this is rare. People with diabetes must learn a new way to eat. The emphasis is on maintaining normal blood-glucose levels by parceling out sugars and starches (carbohydrates) appropriately throughout the day. If you should become diabetic, ask your primary doctor to refer you to a registered dietitian or *endocrinologist* who can tailor a diet plan for you based on how efficiently your body metabolizes carbs, protein, and fats.

See Chapter Three, "How Cancer Is Diagnosed and Staged."

Cancer of the Ovary

Predominant cell type: epithelial carcinoma

RISK FACTORS

Lifestyle-Related
- Obesity • Lack of exercise

Family Medical History
- One of the following cancer patterns: (1) ovarian cancer, (2) hereditary nonpolyposis colorectal cancer (HNPCC), which predisposes women to ovarian cancer, as well as to cancers of the large intestine, endometrium (uterus), stomach, and other organs, (3) breast-ovarian cancer syndrome

Personal Medical/Health History

- Diabetes - Hypertension - Previous cancer of the large intestine, endometrium (uterus), and/or breast - Benign breast disease - Ovarian cysts - Never having given birth - Never having taken oral contraceptives

Environmental/Occupational Carcinogens

- No association positively identified

WARNING SIGNS/SYMPTOMS

- Indigestion - Flatulence - Nausea or vomiting - Abdominal discomfort or pain, swelling, or bloating - Diarrhea - Constipation - Appetite loss - Unexplained weight loss - Frequent urination - Abnormal bleeding from the vagina - Shortness of breath

IF NOT CONTROLLED, OVARIAN CANCER MAY SPREAD TO:

- Lymph nodes - Liver - Uterus - Fallopian tube - Colon - Bladder - Lung - Peritoneal membrane - Diaphragm

Because the two ovaries are located in the spacious pelvic cavity, a tumor in either or both can become sizable before producing discernible pressure or pain. Cancer typically arises in the ovary's outer lining, or *epithelium*. A rare form, *ovarian germ-cell tumor*, takes hold in the female germ cells (better known as human reproductive cells, egg cells, or the *ova*), which are produced, stored, and ripened in the ovaries. This cancer, not discussed here, tends to strike young women and adolescent girls, whereas ovarian epithelial cancer generally isn't seen until after age sixty.

About the Ovaries

The saclike ovaries, each about the size and shape of an almond, lie on either side of the uterus. Approximately every twenty-eight days one ovary discharges a mature egg (on occasion, two or more) into the opening of the adjoining *fallopian tube,* where conception takes place. Should a male sperm cell unite successfully with the female ovum sometime in the next forty-eight hours or so, the now fertilized egg makes its way down the tube and implants itself in the lining of the uterus, marking the start of pregnancy.

The ovaries also serve as the main source of female hormones. *Estrogen* and *progesterone* govern the development of a woman's secondary sexual physical traits: breasts, body shape, body hair, and so on. In addition, they control the menstrual cycle and act upon the reproductive system to create an environment conducive to fertilization and gestation.

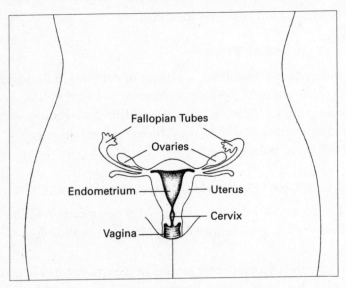

How Ovarian Cancer Is Typically Detected

Dr. Larry Copeland, chair of the department of obstetrics and gynecology at Ohio State University in Columbus, has been treating gynecologic malignancies since 1979. "The main problem with ovarian cancer," he says, "is that three in four patients aren't diagnosed until the tumor is advanced. Even once ovarian cancer has spread, it can be very subtle in its presentation.

"Women will go to their doctor and say, 'I have indigestion.' 'I've been having a lot of gas.' 'My clothes don't fit right.'" Few general practitioners or gynecologists, he observes, are likely to suspect cancer immediately based on these and other mild, nondescript symptoms. However, what may seem like run-of-the-mill constipation or frequent

**OVARIAN CANCER/
At Diagnosis**

EXTENT OF DISEASE AT THE TIME OF DIAGNOSIS

Local disease	23% of cases
Regional disease	15% of cases
Metastatic disease	56% of cases
Unstaged	6% of cases

urination could be the work of a large ovarian tumor constricting the bowel or bladder. Abdominal swelling? Many patients with this cancer develop *ascites:* an abnormal buildup of fluid in the abdomen. If the cancer has metastasized to the *diaphragm,* the dome-shaped muscle wedged up against the bottom of the lungs, fluid can collect there as well, leaving a person short of breath.

Low-Malignant-Potential Ovarian Tumor (LMP)

About one in fifteen ovarian-cancer patients will be diagnosed with a borderline epithelial malignancy identified as *low-malignant-potential ovarian tumor,* or LMP for short. Dr. Copeland describes it as "somewhere between a benign growth and cancer." What distinguishes LMP from non-LMP ovarian cancer is its *grade:* When tissue from the tumor is assessed under the microscope, it looks more like a normal cell than a cancer cell. Consequently, these malignancies behave far less aggressively than higher-grade ovarian tumors.

Seventy-five percent of LMP tumors are discovered while still localized to one ovary or both. "They tend to have a very good prognosis," says Dr. Copeland, who serves as the chief of staff at OSU's Arthur G. James Cancer Hospital and Research Institute. Even if the cancer has metastasized to the lymph nodes or to the surface of the liver or the intestines—stage III on a scale of I to IV—"those tumors also respond very well to treatment."

See Chapter Three, "How Cancer Is Diagnosed and Staged."

Cancer of the Stomach

Predominant cell type: adenocarcinoma

RISK FACTORS

Lifestyle-Related

- A diet high in salt-cured, smoked, and salt-pickled foods

Family Medical History

- Stomach cancer - Hereditary nonpolyposis colorectal cancer (HNPCC), which predisposes women to stomach cancer, as well as to cancers of the large intestine, endometrium (uterus), ovary, and other organs - Type A blood

Personal Medical/Health History

▪ Any of the following gastric disorders, which can damage the stomach's inner layer and/or the glands that secrete acid and mucus: (1) pernicious anemia, (2) chronic atrophic gastritis, (3) achlorhydria or hypochlorhydria, (4) Ménétrier's disease ▪ Having undergone an operation to remove a portion of the stomach ▪ Chronic *Helicobacter pylori* infection

Environmental/Occupational Carcinogens

▪ No association positively identified

WARNING SIGNS/SYMPTOMS

▪ Abdominal pain ▪ Chronic indigestion, including heartburn ▪ Appetite loss ▪ Unexplained weight loss ▪ Bloated feeling after meals ▪ Fatigue ▪ Nausea and vomiting ▪ Diarrhea ▪ Constipation ▪ Bloody vomit or stool

IF NOT CONTROLLED, STOMACH CANCER MAY SPREAD TO:

▪ Lymph nodes ▪ Esophagus ▪ Small intestine ▪ Colon ▪ Liver ▪ Pancreas ▪ Diaphragm ▪ Lung ▪ Ovary ▪ Spleen ▪ Kidney

The incidence of stomach cancer in the United States is just one-fourth what it was in the 1930s, when the disease reigned as the leading cause of death among men. Credit for the decline goes not so much to strides in medicine as to improved home refrigeration. With more and more families able to afford an icebox, foods no longer had to be preserved through salt-curing, smoking, or pickling, processes all linked to *gastric* cancer. In addition, fruits and vegetables, believed to lower the risk of stomach cancer, could be eaten fresh year-round.

About the Stomach

When empty, the saclike stomach is no bigger than a large sausage. But upon receiving food or liquid from the esophagus, its four-layer walls stretch to hold as much as one and a half quarts. Muscles in the wall contract in rhythm, generating a rippling, wavelike motion that propels food from the upper end to the lower end. This action, *peristalsis,* also churns the food into smaller particles and mixes it with digestive juices secreted by glands in the inner lining, until the partially digested contents are reduced to a thick liquid. Over the next one to four hours, depending on the amount and type of food, the ever-intensifying contractions empty the soupy mixture into the *small intestine,* where digestion continues.

The stomach, which is shaped like a **J**, is divided into four regions. While cancer of the lower half has decreased, the 1980s and 1990s witnessed a rise in tumors of the *gastroesophageal junction*—the gateway between the stomach and the gullet—and the surrounding area known as the *cardia.*

How Stomach Cancer Is Typically Detected

Because stomach cancer is now relatively uncommon in America, doctors don't routinely screen asymptomatic patients, and so most diagnoses tend to be advanced. Nor are most primary-care physicians well versed in the warning signs of gastric tumors, which can be as nonspecific as heartburn.

In Japan, where the rate of stomach cancer ranks among the world's highest, preventive screening is so commonplace, notes Dr. Harinder Garewal, a gastrointestinal oncologist at the University of Arizona Cancer Center in Tucson, "they even have mobile units that perform endoscopic exams in parking lots." *(Gastroscopy* enables physicians to view the stomach through a flexible, lighted scope that is inserted down the throat and esophagus.) Gastric cancer in Japan is frequently diagnosed as carcinoma in situ, which is more than 90 percent curable. "But in this country," says Dr. Garewal, "we don't usually see in situ cancer of the stomach unless it's picked up accidentally."

Gastric tumors can grow along the stomach wall into the adjoining esophagus or small intestine. More often, though, the cancer protrudes through the wall to infiltrate other organs. Metastatic stomach cancer of the ovaries has a special name: *Krukenberg's tumor.*

See Chapter Three, "How Cancer Is Diagnosed and Staged."

STOMACH CANCER/ At Diagnosis	
EXTENT OF DISEASE AT THE TIME OF DIAGNOSIS	
Local disease	18% of cases
Regional disease	32% of cases
Metastatic disease	36% of cases
Unstaged	14% of cases

Cancer of the Liver

Predominant cell types: hepatocellular adenocarcinoma and cholangio-cellular adenocarcinoma

RISK FACTORS

Lifestyle-Related
- Excessive alcohol consumption

Family Medical History
- No association positively identified

Personal Medical/Health History
- Cirrhosis of the liver • Hepatitis B (HBV) or hepatitis C (HCV) • End-stage renal disease

Environmental/Occupational Carcinogens
- Occupational exposure to the industrial toxic chemicals vinyl chloride or polychlorinated biphenyls

WARNING SIGNS/SYMPTOMS

- Jaundice • Enlarged liver • Fatigue and weakness • Appetite loss • Unexplained weight loss • Vague pain that begins in the upper abdomen on the right side and extends to the back and shoulder

IF NOT CONTROLLED, LIVER CANCER MAY SPREAD TO:

- Lymph nodes • Bone • Lung

As a refinery and repository for the body's blood, the liver is fertile ground for secondary tumors from other organs, surpassed only by the lungs. Primary liver cancer, though, is relatively uncommon.

Complicating treatment for this cancer is the fact that often the diagnosis has been preceded by years of chronic liver disease; primarily *cirrhosis, viral hepatitis,* or both, since hepatitis B and C can lead to cirrhosis. In the United States, chronic alcoholism is to blame for more than half of all cases of cirrhosis.

"The main prognostic factor in liver cancer

Medical Term You're Likely to Hear

Hepatoma: any tumor of the liver.

is whether or not the tumor is surgically removable," explains Dr. Ted Lawrence, a radiation oncologist at the University of Michigan Comprehensive Cancer Center in Ann Arbor. "And that is determined by the tumor's location and how healthy the organ is." Normally, the dark red liver is rich with blood. Cirrhosis, a degenerative disease, damages liver cells, leaving behind extensive scar tissue. As the blood flow to the organ encounters more and more obstructions, the number of dying cells mounts.

"Whereas a healthy person might tolerate a large resection, a highly cirrhotic patient would not be a candidate for surgery. From a functional point of view," Dr. Lawrence adds, "the liver damage produced by hepatitis is the same as from cirrhosis." Aside from surgery, "there is no standard therapy for primary liver cancer."

About the Liver

The liver, the body's largest internal organ, filters and stores blood. It also figures prominently in metabolism by converting the nutrients, vitamins, and minerals from food into usable forms, and stockpiling fats and *glycogen*. Glycogen is the stored form of sugar, or *glucose,* our principal source of fuel. Whenever the body's cells demand quick energy, the liver converts glycogen back to glucose and discharges it into the bloodstream.

Large Intestine — Bile Duct
Duodenum — Esophagus
Gallbladder — Pancreas
Liver — Stomach

Types of Liver Cancer

Most hepatomas are *hepatocellular adenocarcinomas*. A subtype known as the *fibrolamellar variant,* which is seen particularly in young women, generally carries a better prognosis. Not only are the odds of a cure higher for surgically resectable fibrolamellar tumors, but should the cancer prove inoper-

**LIVER CANCER/
At Diagnosis**

EXTENT OF DISEASE AT THE TIME OF DIAGNOSIS

Local disease	20% of cases
Regional disease	22% of cases
Metastatic disease	24% of cases
Unstaged	34% of cases

able, these patients are more likely to be considered for liver transplantation surgery.

Among the chemicals and substances produced by the liver is the digestive fluid *bile,* which it transmits to the small intestine via a passageway called the *hepatic bile duct.* Cancer that develops in the portion of the duct within the liver is called *cholangiocellular adenocarcinoma* or *intrahepatic bile-duct carcinoma.* It is the second most common form of liver cancer.

Tumors can also materialize in the *extrahepatic duct,* as well as the *gallbladder,* a small pear-shaped sac that lies on the undersurface of the liver, hidden behind other abdominal organs. The gallbladder serves as a reservoir for bile. Like the liver, it releases the fluid to the small intestine as needed. Cancer of the gallbladder is usually discovered after the organ has been removed for other medical reasons. If the tumor hasn't spread, patients are generally pronounced cured, with no further therapy needed.

How Liver Cancer Is Typically Detected

According to Dr. Lawrence, "Liver cancer can present in a couple of different ways. Often the only symptoms are fatigue and a mild pain in the right side, just below the ribs." Sharp pain, a rare feature, is thought to occur as a result of bleeding in the tumor. "Other times," he says, "patients will notice a mass"—actually feel a lump or hardness—"in their side."

See Chapter Three, "How Cancer Is Diagnosed and Staged."

Cancers of the Lip and Oral Cavity

Predominant cell type: squamous-cell carcinoma

RISK FACTORS

Lifestyle-Related
- Smoking or chewing tobacco • Excessive alcohol consumption

Family Medical History
- No association positively identified

Personal Medical/Health History
- End-stage renal disease

Environmental/Occupational Carcinogens
- No association positively identified

WARNING SIGNS/SYMPTOMS

- Lump in the cheek or on the floor of the mouth that may eventually become painful and/or bleed • Painful or painless mouth sore that won't heal • White or red patch on the gums, tongue, or lining of the mouth • Difficulty in opening the mouth • Difficulty in chewing, swallowing, speaking • Numbness of the lower lip, due to a tumor involving a nerve in the jaw • Dentures may no longer fit properly • Pain in the roof of the mouth or the ear, from a tumor pressing on a nerve • Toothache or loose teeth • Foul breath

IF NOT CONTROLLED, ORAL CANCER MAY SPREAD TO:

- Neck • Lung • Lymph nodes • Liver • Bone

Compared to some other cancers, a diagnosis of oral cancer doesn't always elicit the same response as forms perceived to be more life-threatening. Perhaps it's because the lesion is often clearly visible inside the mouth, or the fact that the mouth isn't generally thought of as a "vital" organ.

"Many patients will feel, 'It's just a small bump in my mouth, I'll get it taken care of,'" observes Dr. Rocco Addante, an *oral and maxillofacial surgeon* at Norris Cotton Cancer Center in Lebanon,

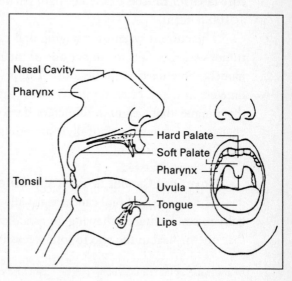

New Hampshire. Treating early-stage cancers of the lip and oral cavity with surgery or radiation therapy generally does have a high success rate; and with advances in reconstructive surgery, the operations are far less disfiguring than they were in years past.

But under certain circumstances, even relatively minor oral surgery could interfere with eating, speaking, or swallowing, as in the case of someone no longer able to wear dentures. The mouth may not seem like a vital organ, notes Dr. Addante, "until you realize all the things you use it for."

About the Oral Cavity

The oral cavity consists of various structures, including:

1. The lining inside the lips and cheeks (the *buccal mucosa*)
2. The front two-thirds of the tongue *(anterior tongue)**
3. The floor of the mouth, under the tongue
4. The roof of the mouth *(hard palate)*
5. The upper and lower gums *(gingiva)*
6. The small space behind the wisdom teeth *(retromolar trigone)*

Two pivotal factors in the outcome of this disease are tumor location and depth. Malignancies of the tongue and the floor of the mouth are most likely to spread to the neck, and possibly beyond, whereas the cure rates for cancers of the lip, hard palate, and upper gum go as high as 100 percent.

The current system for staging oral cancer takes into account the tumor's size but fails to answer one of the most important questions—namely, how deep is the lesion? "Tumors that are two to three millimeters in depth often do pretty well," says Dr. Addante. "A lesion of the tongue that's eight millimeters deep is going to have a greater chance of problems, even if there are no lumps in the neck and no obvious chest metastases."

How Oral Cancer Is Typically Detected

The first sign of oral cancer is usually a bump in the mouth, difficulty in swallowing or chewing, or a canker sore or burn on the tongue that doesn't heal in the two to four weeks it normally takes.

*A malignancy of the rear third of the tongue is considered cancer of the *oropharynx*, the middle portion of the throat.

But not everyone experiences symptoms. "There are lesions that don't hurt," says Dr. Addante. "Plus, the mouth accommodates everything from lumps to new dentures very nicely. So people can get slow-developing growths and not be aware of them.

"Many patients get picked up during a routine examination by the dentist, who will observe a swollen area or a flat red or white lesion inside the mouth, and send the person for a biopsy." White patches that won't rub off, referred to collectively as *leukoplakia,* could be nothing more serious than an inflammation or fungal infection, but some are premalignant; roughly one in twenty of these will progress to cancer. "*Erythroplakia,* a red spot with a velvety surface, is far more ominous than a white one," notes Dr. Addante. "And lesions that are a blend of both red and white have a higher incidence of being precancerous."

ORAL CANCER/ At Diagnosis	
EXTENT OF DISEASE AT THE TIME OF DIAGNOSIS	
Local disease	36% of cases
Regional disease	43% of cases
Metastatic disease	9% of cases
Unstaged	12% of cases

See Chapter Three, "How Cancer Is Diagnosed and Staged."

Cancer of the Thyroid

Predominant cell types: papillary carcinoma, follicular carcinoma, medullary carcinoma, and anaplastic carcinoma

RISK FACTORS

Lifestyle-Related
- No association positively identified

Family Medical History
- Medullary thyroid cancer

Personal Medical/Health History
- Radiation exposure or radiotherapy to the head and neck during childhood

Environmental/Occupational Carcinogens
- No association positively identified

WARNING SIGNS/SYMPTOMS

. Swelling or hard lump in the neck . Difficulty in breathing or swallowing . Hoarseness

IF NOT CONTROLLED, THYROID CANCER MAY SPREAD TO:

. Lymph nodes . Lung . Bone . Neck

Thyroid cancer, the most common *endocrine* tumor, is one of the most curable forms of cancer. If detected while still localized, which describes three in five patients with the disease, it has a 100 percent five-year survival rate.

It's not known why thyroid cancer affects nearly three times as many women as men. One risk factor that can be explained, however, is a history of radiation therapy to the head and neck during childhood. Before the hazards of radiation exposure were known, doctors used radiotherapy to treat benign conditions such as enlarged tonsils and lymph nodes, and even acne. In this group of patients, thyroid malignancies have appeared anywhere from five to more than twenty years after treatment.

About the Thyroid

The butterfly-shaped thyroid wraps around the front of the windpipe, just below the Adam's apple in men. Dr. Colin Paul Spears, a senior clinical research physician at Eli Lilly and Company, the pharmaceutical manufacturer, likens the thyroid to a thermostat, for the two main hormones it secretes into the circulation, *triiodothyronine* (T3) and *thyroxine* (T4), help to regulate heart rate, blood pressure, body temperature, and the pace at which food is converted into energy. You may hear T3 and T4 referred to collectively as *thyroid hormone*. In order to produce these hormones, the thyroid needs a small but con-

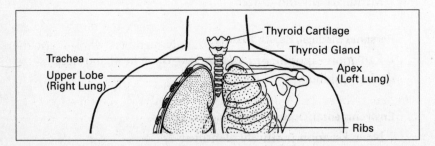

stant supply of *iodine,* a mineral most of us get in sufficient amounts from iodized table salt, shellfish, and other foods.

"The thyroid," Dr. Spears explains, "is part of a feedback loop to maintain internal stability, or *homeostasis."* Whenever the *pituitary* gland at the base of the brain senses a shortage of thyroid hormone in the blood, it releases *thyrotropin,* also called *thyroid-stimulating hormone* (TSH). As its name implies, TSH stimulates the thyroid to discharge more thyroid hormone. If the blood contains too much thyroid hormone, the pituitary responds by halting TSH production entirely, bringing the level down. Normally, thyroid-stimulating hormone contributes to good health. But when cancer invades the thyroid, says Dr. Spears, formerly of Los Angeles's Kenneth Norris Jr. Comprehensive Cancer Center, "TSH can stimulate growth of the tumor."

Types of Thyroid Cancer

Papillary Thyroid Cancer

Papillary thyroid cancer's name alludes to one of its distinguishing features: *papillae,* small nipple-shaped protuberances that give the tumor a fernlike appearance when viewed under the microscope. This type of thyroid cancer is slow to grow and highly treatable, even if it has invaded neighboring lymph nodes.

Follicular Thyroid Cancer

Like papillary cancer, the malignant cells in *follicular* thyroid carcinoma tend to resemble normal cells—a factor that bodes well for the success of treatment. Follicular tumors, seen more in older men and women, are covered by a thin capsule of tissue. While more aggressive than the papillary form, they are considered treatable in most circumstances.

The Four Main Types of Thyroid Cancer	
PERCENTAGE OF ALL CASES OF THYROID CANCER	
Papillary	60%
Follicular	17%
Medullary	5%
Anaplastic	18%

Medullary Thyroid Cancer

One in ten cases of *medullary* thyroid cancer, the rarest type, are hereditary. According to Dr. Spears, family members who inherit the faulty *RET* oncogene "have a 90 percent chance of developing medullary carcinoma over the course of their lifetime." (A blood test can determine whether or not a person possesses the errant gene.) The familial form of the disease almost always arises in both the left and the right *lobes,* the two winged portions of the thyroid.

Anaplastic Thyroid Cancer

Metastasis to other organs, common in medullary thyroid cancer, is all but a foregone conclusion in *anaplastic* thyroid carcinoma, which usually strikes people over sixty. Characterized by extremely aberrant cells, the disease is described by Dr. Spears as "explosive in its growth and aggressive in its pattern of spread."

How Thyroid Cancer Is Typically Detected

"Occasionally," Dr. Spears explains, "the thyroid malignancy produces enough thyroid hormone that patients will present with all the symptoms of an overactive thyroid *[hyperthyroidism]:* a fast heartbeat, anxiety, heat intolerance, irregular menstruation, and excessive perspiration." Much of the time, though, the attentive pituitary gland lowers its production of TSH to keep the thyroid hormone level within a normal range. Most patients first sense a problem when they feel a hard lump in the throat (although 90 percent of the time, thyroid nodules are benign). The thyroid frequently attracts metastases from the lungs, breast, and kidneys, but rarely do these secondary cancers give rise to symptoms.

THYROID CANCER/ At Diagnosis

EXTENT OF DISEASE AT THE TIME OF DIAGNOSIS

Local disease	59% of cases
Regional disease	32% of cases
Metastatic disease	5% of cases
Unstaged	5% of cases

See Chapter Three, "How Cancer Is Diagnosed and Staged."

(Adult) Cancers of the Brain

Predominant cell types: glial and meningeal

RISK FACTORS

Lifestyle-Related

- No association positively identified

Family Medical History

- Any of the following hereditary syndromes, all of them extremely rare: (1) Li-Fraumeni syndrome (LFS), (2) familial adenomatous polyposis (FAP), (3) tuberous sclerosis, (4) neurofibromatosis, (5) von Hippel-Lindau disease

Personal Medical/Health History

- High-dose radiation therapy during childhood • End-stage renal disease

Environmental/Occupational Carcinogens

- No association positively identified

WARNING SIGNS/SYMPTOMS

- Persistent headaches • Dizziness • Seizures • Changes in behavior and personality • Memory loss • Nausea and vomiting • Confusion • Gradual weakness or paralysis • Impaired vision, hearing, speech, smell, balance, motor skills

IF NOT CONTROLLED, BRAIN CANCER MAY SPREAD TO:

- The leptomeninges, the two thin membranes that surround the brain and spinal cord. • Spinal cord

Nearly half of all primary brain tumors are benign. In most parts of the body, nonmalignant lesions rarely prove harmful. But because the brain is confined by the rigid skull, there's no room to accommodate any mass. Thus, benign growths as well as cancers can wreak serious or life-threatening neurological damage, depending on their location. A tumor displacing vital nerve tissue could interfere with whatever functions that area of the brain controls: speech, movement, cognitive ability, and so on. Or, if it should exert pressure on one of the intracranial vessels, blood flow to the brain could be blocked, triggering the equivalent of a stroke. The site of the tumor also dictates whether or not it can be removed surgically, the primary therapy for most brain tumors.

Although theories abound as to the origins of brain cancer, the disease remains very much a mystery. Only two causes have been established, with less than 10 percent of cases laid to genetic inheritance, and a fraction more to high dosages of radiation therapy during childhood.

Thankfully, advances in treatment have come more readily. "Surgery is so much better today," remarks Dr. Michael Gruber, director of neuro-oncology at New York University Medical Center. "It used to be where a priest would give last rites before a patient underwent a brain operation, and that's no longer the case." He estimates that 95 percent of the patients he sees emerge from brain surgery without any significant neurological damage.

Most people diagnosed with brain cancer—or any cancer, for that matter—realize they have a serious disease. Meningiomas, one type of brain tumor, "are for the most part curable," says Dr. Gruber. With other types, depending on location and other factors, the promise of a permanent remission may not be realistic. But as Dr. Gruber emphasizes, "the majority of patients can function and be independent for most of the time they have left." For some, he adds, that can be a long time.

About the Brain and Central Nervous System

The *central nervous system* (CNS), consisting of the brain and the *spinal cord,* orchestrates everything we do, from conscious actions like walking and talking to involuntary functions such as breathing and digestion. Our five senses, emotions, thoughts, memory—all are generated within the brain as electrical impulses.

The brain is a spongy, wrinkled mass of nerve cells, supportive tissue, and blood vessels protected by a three-layer membrane called the *meninges.* Four interconnected hollow cavities within the brain, the *ventricles,* produce a continuous stream of *cerebrospinal fluid* (CSF). This fluid flows from the ventricles into the *subarachnoid space* between the innermost and middle layers of the meninges, so that the brain literally floats inside the skull. Besides serving as a shock absorber, the CSF delivers nutrients from the blood and withdraws waste products.

Yet another way in which a tumor can be destructive is if it impedes the normal flow of cerebrospinal fluid within the ventricular system, causing it to build up and the brain to swell. This condition, *hydrocephalus,* increases the intracranial pressure, which in turn damages the fragile brain tissue.

The brain has three major structures: the *cerebrum, cerebellum,*

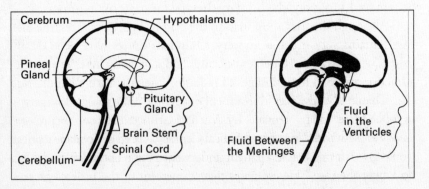

and *brain stem.* While they are interrelated, each oversees specific activities. The largest, the cerebrum, occupies most of the upper skull. A deep indentation down its middle splits the cerebrum into halves, or *hemispheres.* The left cerebral hemisphere controls voluntary muscle movements on the right side of the body; the right cerebral hemisphere governs the left side. Additional fissures divide each hemisphere into four sections—*frontal lobe, parietal lobe, temporal lobe,* and *occipital lobe*—each of which is assigned a group of functions. Memory, speech, reading, writing, hearing, behavior, sensation, emotions, and the abilities to think and reason also take place in the cerebrum.

Just below the occipital lobe, nestled at the base of the skull, lies the shell-shaped cerebellum, where the complex muscular coordination necessary for walking and talking is handled. The cerebellum connects to the stalklike brain stem, the regulatory center for such basic life-sustaining functions as heartbeat, respiration, and blood pressure.

The brain stem joins the spinal cord, a thick cable of nerve fibers that runs through a canal in the bony spinal column. It, too, is encased by the meninges and cushioned by cerebrospinal fluid. Twelve pairs of *cranial nerves* transmit orders directly from the brain to the eyes, ears, facial muscles, and other parts of the head. Messages to the rest of the body are relayed by the thirty-one pairs of *spinal nerves* that emanate from the spinal cord. Only about one in ten primary CNS tumors occur in the spinal cord.

While the brain and spinal cord act as magnets for secondary cancers from other organs, primary tumors of the brain rarely venture beyond the central nervous system.

Types of Brain Tumors

Neuro-oncologists classify primary brain tumors according to their cell type and location. Some are broken down further into subtypes based on how normal or abnormal their cells appear. As in other forms of cancer, well-differentiated brain tumors grow less rapidly and tend to carry a better prognosis than *anaplastic* tumors, which are distinguished by poorly defined, irregularly shaped cells.

Gliomas

About half of all brain tumors are gliomas, a group of cancers originating in the *glial* cells that form the supportive tissue of the central nervous system.

Astrocytomas—The most prevalent adult brain tumor, astrocytomas take hold in star-shaped glial cells called *astrocytes*. How this cancer is treated depends on the grade.

Grade	May Also Be Called	Characteristics
Well-differentiated astrocytomas	Low grade Grade I	Slow growing; rarely metastasize
Anaplastic astrocytomas	Intermediate grade Grade II	Grow more rapidly; cells exhibit malignant traits
Glioblastoma multiforme	High grade Grade III	Very rapidly growing malignant tumors that invade surrounding tissue

Brain-stem gliomas—Representing about 5 percent of adult brain tumors, these gliomas are usually comprised of astrocytomas, though sometimes the tumors contain other types of cells as well.

Ependymomas—These tumors occur in the ependymal cells found in the lining of the brain's hollow cavities and the central canal of the spinal cord. Although about 85 percent of ependymomas are benign, "the malignant forms of these tumors have a great likelihood of spreading up and down the spine via the spinal fluid," says Dr. Gruber.

Oligodendrogliomas—These form in another type of glial cell: oligodendrocytes, which nourish the cells that transmit nerve impulses. These tumors generally grow so slowly that it is not unusual for an oligodendroglioma to lurk undetected for a number of years.

Mixed gliomas—These contain two or more types of glial cells—usually astrocytes and either oligodendrocytes or ependymal cells. "The oligo cell is a marker for a better outcome," says Dr. Gruber, "because it is highly sensitive to chemotherapy. A mixed tumor where most of it is astrocytic and only a small component is oligo tends to do much better than a pure astrocytic tumor, even if the astrocytic portion is high grade." The most malignant element of the mix determines the course of therapy, so that a brain tumor comprised of well-differentiated astrocytic cells and anaplastic ependymal cells would be treated as if it were anaplastic ependymoma.

Meningiomas

About one in five brain tumors are meningiomas, materializing in the meningeal membrane that covers the brain and spinal cord. According to Dr. Gruber, "Ninety-five percent of meningiomas are benign." Once eradicated, they rarely recur.

Craniopharyngioma

This benign tumor, seen more in children and adolescents than in adults, develops in the vicinity of the *optic nerve* and the *pituitary gland.* Accordingly, a craniopharyngioma may bring on visual impairment and hormonal imbalances. It can also encroach upon the nearby *hypothalamus,* the part of the brain that regulates body temperature, hunger, and thirst.

Adult Pineal Parenchymal Tumors

The *pineal gland* is a tiny, cone-shaped structure located deep within the brain. As a result, tumors in this region are not always accessible surgically. *Pineocytomas* and *pineoblastomas,* two of the more common pineal tumors, belong to a group known as *primitive neuroectodermal tumors* (PNET for short), which stem from primitive cells that remain from early development of the central nervous system. Of the pair, "pineoblastoma is much more aggressive," says Dr. Gruber.

Another group of tumors seen near the pineal gland are the *germ-cell tumors—germinoma, teratoma, embryonal carcinoma,* and *choriocarcinoma*—comprised of maturing sex cells. "They can be very aggressive," Dr. Gruber notes, "or very sensitive to treatment." Nine in ten patients with germinoma, the most common cancerous pineal tumor, are curable.

Primary Central Nervous System Lymphoma

With the advent of the AIDS epidemic in the early 1980s, neurologists began to see a rise in the incidence of this lymphoma, which tends to occur most frequently in the cerebrum. Dr. Gruber, who estimates that the Kaplan Cancer Center at NYU diagnoses two or three new cases every month, calls primary CNS lymphoma "the most common tumor in immunocompromised patients." In addition to people with AIDS, that includes transplant recipients taking immunosuppressive drugs to reduce the risk of graft rejection. "Interestingly," says the doctor, "there's also been a marked increase of this disease in patients who are not immunocompromised."

TABLE 2.7A   **Effects of Brain Tumors, by Location**

In the Cerebrum

Frontal-Lobe Tumors
- Paralysis on one side of the body
- Impaired short-term memory • Impaired judgment
- Lack of concentration • Visual impairment
- Impaired sense of smell • Seizures • Altered behavior and personality • Awkward, unsteady gait

Parietal-Lobe Tumors
- Seizures • Speech disturbances
- Confusion between left and right, and up and down • Difficulty with expressing thoughts in writing • Difficulty with calculating numbers

Occipital-Lobe Tumors
- Visual impairment, such as double vision, blindness in one direction, or partial visual loss in one or both eyes • Seizures

Temporal-Lobe Tumors
- Impaired ability to understand speech • Seizures
- Memory impairment • Personality changes • Temporal tumors typically do not produce symptoms unless the cancer attains a significant size.

In the Cerebellum

- Tremors
- Awkward, unsteady gait
- Headaches, nausea, and swelling of the optic nerve, due to increased pressure within the skull
- Nerve irritation, generating pain in the back of the head

In the Brain Stem

- Vomiting
- Awkward, unsteady gait
- Difficulty in swallowing and speaking
- Hearing loss on one side
- Visual disturbances

How Brain Cancers Are Typically Detected

A brain tumor can mimic other neurological disorders, such as a stroke. The symptoms may occur due to the mass effect a tumor's presence brings to bear on the brain, or they may be traced to a specific damaged nerve center.

See Chapter Three, "How Cancer Is Diagnosed and Staged."

Multiple Myeloma

Predominant cell type: plasma cell

BRAIN CANCERS/ At Diagnosis	
EXTENT OF DISEASE AT THE TIME OF DIAGNOSIS	
Local disease	24% of cases
Regional disease	8% of cases
Metastatic disease	1% of cases
Unstaged	67% of cases

RISK FACTORS

- Causes unknown

WARNING SIGNS/SYMPTOMS

- Bone pain, often in the back or ribs • Broken bones • Constipation • Difficulty in urinating • Weakness or numbness in the legs • Symptoms of hypercalcemia: appetite loss, nausea, thirst, fatigue, muscle weakness, restlessness, confusion • Symptoms of anemia: chronic fatigue, weakness, profuse perspiration and/or night sweats, headaches, dizziness, pale complexion • Symptoms of thrombocytopenia: excessive bleeding and unexplained bruising, tiny red spots under the skin • Symptoms of leukopenia: recurrent infections

IF NOT CONTROLLED, MULTIPLE MYELOMA MAY SPREAD TO:

- Other bones

Multiple myeloma is a cancer of *plasma cells,* a type of *white blood cell* that manufactures *antibodies.* These proteins travel through the bloodstream and bind with foreign substances such as bacteria for the purpose of destroying them.

Like all other blood cells, the plasma cells begin their development in the red bone marrow, the spongy tissue that fills the cavities of the large bones. In multiple myeloma, aberrant plasma cells reproduce uncontrollably and inundate the marrow. If you have the disease, your marrow contains not only too many plasma cells but also an overabundance of the unique antibody they produce. It is through detecting this *monoclonal protein* (M protein) in the blood or urine that multiple myeloma is diagnosed.

Typically, multiple-myeloma cells collect in the marrow and the hard outermost layer of several bones, creating multiple tumors. In the rare related cancer *plasmacytoma,* the malignant cells accumulate in one bone to form a single mass. We're going to restrict our discussion to multiple myeloma, which accounts for 94 percent of all plasma-cell neoplasms.

The glut of plasma cells and antibodies can trigger an array of serious medical problems. But its main effect is on the bones, especially the spine and rib cage. As the cancer cells proliferate, they stimulate the activities of other cells that eat away at bone. Skeletal X rays of myeloma patients often reveal gaping black holes, called *lytic lesions.* These eroded spots leave the bone weak and prone to fracture. Bone pain and broken bones are often the first indicators of the disease.

An important distinction: Although multiple myeloma attacks bone, it is not bone cancer, because it originates in plasma cells. Numerous theories exist regarding the disease's causes, but its etiology has thus far eluded scientists. The same is true of a cure. However, multiple myeloma can be treated, with some patients living for decades.

About Plasma Cells

Plasma cells come from *B lymphocytes,* a type of white blood cell. They also come in many different forms, each programmed to respond to a specific foreign invader, or *antigen.* When a B cell is alerted to the presence of its designated foe—let's use a bacterial cell as an example— it mobilizes. Most of the activated B cells become plasma cells, which proceed to churn out antibodies. Jettisoned into the circulation, each protein affixes itself to the trespasser, then selects any of a number of ways to eradicate the bacterium.

Normally, plasma cells make up less than 5 percent of the bone marrow's cells. A person with multiple myeloma will have at least double that. Sometimes the disease's incursion is so extensive that less than 10 percent of the normal cells remain.

How Multiple Myeloma Is Typically Detected

Although multiple myeloma is occasionally stumbled upon through a routine blood test, seven in ten patients are diagnosed after complaining of bone pain, usually in the back. The deluge of plasma

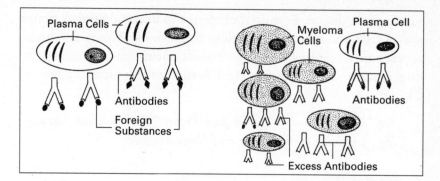

cells can also unleash a tidal wave of severe systemic effects that must be managed along with the cancer.

Hypercalcemia

Calcium, the most abundant mineral in the body, makes up the hard, dense material of the bone. "Because multiple myeloma erodes the bone," explains Dr. Jill Lacy of the Yale Cancer Center in New Haven, Connecticut, "calcium is released into the blood and can build up in large amounts." Three in ten patients present with nausea, thirst, fatigue, or other symptoms of hypercalcemia, a common complication of many cancers.

See "Hypercalcemia" in Chapter Eight, "Take Control: Managing Symptoms, Side Effects, and Complications."

Blood Disorders

As malignant plasma cells pervade the marrow, explains Dr. Lacy, "the normal marrow elements are crowded out and aren't able to produce their usual cells." These include not only white cells but the other two solid components of the blood: *red cells* and *platelets*. Red cells deliver oxygen to all the body's tissues and cart off waste products; platelets adhere to small breaks in vessels to prevent hemorrhaging.

A deficiency of red cells brings about the fatigue, shortness of breath, and lethargy of *anemia. Thrombocytopenia,* too few platelets in the bloodstream, leads to excessive bleeding and bruising. The white blood cells safe-

> **MULTIPLE MYELOMA/ At Diagnosis**
>
> EXTENT OF DISEASE AT THE TIME OF DIAGNOSIS
>
> **Percentages of multiple myeloma patients diagnosed with local, regional, or metastatic disease are not available. Multiple myeloma is staged according to the number of cancer cells that have spread throughout the body; the amount of M proteins in the blood or urine; and the disease's impact on red blood cells, calcium, and bones.**

guard against disease. Because your marrow is manufacturing defective plasma cells, you may find yourself getting sick more often. Infections associated with multiple myeloma include pneumococcal pneumonia, streptococcus, staphylococcus, and herpes zoster, better known as shingles.

See "Blood Disorders" in Chapter Eight, "Take Control: Managing Symptoms, Side Effects, and Complications."

Kidney Impairment

In three in four patients, the plasma cells also manufacture a substance that gets excreted in the urine. These so-called *Bence-Jones proteins,* named for the nineteenth-century British scientist who discovered them, can clog the narrow tubules of the kidneys and damage the organs.

"Patients sometimes present with extremely impaired renal function and have to go on kidney dialysis while they're being treated for the cancer," says Dr. Lacy, adding that the kidney failure may be permanent, "but it is usually reversible with treatment." Most of the time, however, the kidneys sustain minimal damage or none at all.

See Chapter Three, "How Cancer Is Diagnosed and Staged."

Cancer of the Cervix

Predominant cell type: squamous-cell carcinoma

RISK FACTORS

Lifestyle-Related
▪ Multiple sex partners ▪ Intercourse before age sixteen ▪ First pregnancy before age eighteen ▪ Multiple pregnancies

Family Medical History
▪ No association positively identified

Personal Medical/Health History
▪ The sexually transmitted disease human papillomavirus (HPV), or, to a lesser extent, herpes simplex virus II (HSVII) or

the human immunodeficiency virus (HIV) • Exposure to the drug diethylstilbestrol (DES) while in the womb • Dysplasia, a precancerous condition, of the cervix, vagina, or vulva

Environmental/Occupational Carcinogens
- No association positively identified

WARNING SIGNS/SYMPTOMS
- Abnormal vaginal discharge • Unusual vaginal bleeding or spotting • Pain in the pelvic region • Pain during intercourse

IF NOT CONTROLLED, CERVICAL CANCER MAY SPREAD TO:
- Vagina • Lymph nodes • Pelvic connective tissue • Bladder • Large intestine • Bone • Lung • Liver • Ureter

From the mid-1970s through the mid-1990s, the incidence of cervical cancer plummeted by about half, due largely to the widespread use of a simple screening procedure called a Pap smear. "Because of the Pap smear," says Dr. Mitchell Morris, a gynecologic oncologist at Houston's M. D. Anderson Cancer Center, "we are usually able to detect cervical lesions before they even become cancerous."

Cervical cancer is unique in that it is caused primarily by sexually transmitted viruses; in particular, the *human papillomavirus* (HPV). Millions of women are infected with HPV, which usually causes benign genital warts. Two other sexually transmitted diseases, *genital herpes* and the *human immunodeficiency virus* (HIV), are also associated with cervical cancer.

About the Cervix
The narrow, necklike cervix forms the canal that leads from the lower end of the uterus to the vagina. In reading about this cancer, you may sometimes see it referred to as the uterine cervix or cervix uteri. During ovulation, mucus secreted by glands in the cervical lining expedites the male sperm's journey through the cervix to one of the *fallopian tubes,* where fertilization takes place. Remarkably resilient, during birth the rubbery cervix can expand fifty times its normal width to allow the baby to pass from the womb and into the birth canal.

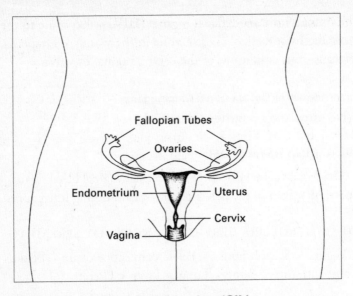

Squamous Intraepithelial Lesion (SIL)

Nine in ten cervical cancers form in squamous cells. The disease evolves extremely slowly, beginning with abnormal changes in some of the cells in the surface epithelium. This is classified as *low-grade squamous intraepithelial lesion* (SIL) or *mild dysplasia.*

"In the mild form, only the lowermost cells are growing abnormally," explains Dr. Morris. "Once the entire thickness of the cervical epithelium becomes involved, we call that *high-grade SIL* or *carcinoma in situ* [CIS], meaning that cancer is there, but it hasn't broken through the epithelium to the underlying stromal tissue, or the 'meat' of the cervix." The cure rate at this stage is 95 percent.

"It's a steady progression that we arbitrarily apply neat names to—mild dysplasia, severe dysplasia, carcinoma in situ—but it's all part of the same continuum."

Some low-grade lesions vanish on their own. But up to half will progress into cancer eventually. It's not unusual for ten to twelve years to pass before untreated cervical carcinoma in situ becomes invasive, although one in ten cases of CIS make the transition in under a year.

Medical Terms You're Likely to Hear

Cervical intraepithelial neoplasia (CIN 1)

Mild dysplasia
. . . words the doctor may use instead of "low-grade SIL"

Carcinoma in situ

CIN 2 or 3

Moderate or severe dysplasia
. . . words the doctor may use instead of "high-grade SIL"

How Cervical Cancer Is Typically Detected

Neither carcinoma in situ nor its precursor signals the presence of cervical cancer. Even early-stage cervical tumors can be asymptomatic.

"Once cervical cancer has established itself," says Dr. Morris, "women will experience symptoms like irregular bleeding from the vagina, bleeding after intercourse, and sometimes a vaginal discharge." Pain in the pelvic region, a rare feature, "is usually a sign of advanced disease."

See Chapter Three, "How Cancer Is Diagnosed and Staged."

CERVICAL CANCER/ At Diagnosis	
EXTENT OF DISEASE AT THE TIME OF DIAGNOSIS	
Local disease	51% of cases
Regional disease	33% of cases
Metastatic disease	8% of cases
Unstaged	7% of cases

Cancer of the Esophagus

Predominant cell types: squamous-cell carcinoma and adenocarcinoma

RISK FACTORS

Lifestyle-Related

- Smoking • Excessive alcohol consumption

Family Medical History

- No association positively identified

Personal Medical/Health History

- Chronic or severe heartburn(gastroesophageal reflux disease) • Barrett's esophagus • Untreated achalasia, a disorder that brings about progressive indigestion and frequent vomiting • Caustic injury to the esophagus, such as swallowing a corrosive substance

Environmental/Occupational Carcinogens

- No association positively identified

WARNING SIGNS/SYMPTOMS

- Difficult or painful swallowing • Chronic indigestion • Persistent heartburn • Coughing • Hoarseness

IF NOT CONTROLLED, ESOPHAGEAL CANCER MAY SPREAD TO:

▪ Lymph nodes ▪ Lung ▪ Liver ▪ Bone ▪ Trachea (windpipe) ▪ Stomach ▪ Neck

Half the cases of esophageal cancers are squamous-cell carcinomas; the other half are adenocarcinomas. Squamous-cell tumors, initiated largely by the combined effects of tobacco and alcohol, begin in the upper and middle portions of the gullet. The incidence of esophageal adenocarcinoma, which grows in the lower third, "is increasing at a faster rate than any other cancer in the United States," observes Dr. Charles Fuchs, a specialist in gastrointestinal cancers at Dana-Farber Cancer Institute in Boston.

Since the entire esophagus is lined with squamous-cell tissue, and adenocarcinomas stem from glandular tissue, how can that be? The reason is a related disorder called gastroesophageal reflux disease (GERD), in which stomach acid backs up into the gullet. Men and women with this condition experience chronic, severe heartburn and frequent regurgitation.

> **Medical Terms You're Likely to Hear**
>
> **Barrett's metaplasia:** another name for Barrett's esophagus. *Metaplasia* is when a tissue's cells metamorphose to a form abnormal for that tissue.

Occasional heartburn is no cause for alarm. But in GERD, the backup of stomach acid into the esophagus persists over a long period of time. The lining of the gullet is made up of flat, scalelike squamous cells. Chronic irritation from the acid can cause them to assume the columnlike cell architecture of the stomach's glandular lining. This transformation is considered normal, unless it advances more than three centimeters up the esophagus, or about one and a quarter inches. At that point it takes on a new identity as *Barrett's esophagus,* a precursor of cancer.

Of the 15 million Americans who suffer from gastroesophageal reflux disease, about one in ten will go on to develop Barrett's esophagus. One in twenty cases of Barrett's will progress to dysplasia, then carcinoma in situ, then esophageal adenocarcinoma.

The controversy among gastroenterologists is whether or not to regularly biopsy these patients, "with the expectation that if we saw dysplasia or carcinoma in situ," says Dr. Fuchs, "we would resect a portion of their esophagus. The surgery is extraordinarily successful when the cancer is found early. The problem is, we don't find it early often enough." Unlike in countries such as Japan, screening asymptomatic patients for upper gastrointestinal-tract cancers is not routine in the

United States. Consequently, this cancer rarely gets picked up in its premalignant or noninvasive stages.

About the Esophagus

The esophagus leads from the back of the throat to the stomach. When we eat, the tube's muscular walls contract to move food down its ten-to-twelve-inch length, while glands in the lining secrete mucus to facilitate swallowing and to moisten the passageway. As food approaches the esophagogastric junction, a muscular ring called the *cardiac sphincter* opens, permitting it to proceed into the stomach.

How Esophageal Cancer Is Typically Detected

"The most common manifestations that bring people to the doctor," says Dr. Fuchs, "are difficulty swallowing and heartburn." Swallowing problems may take the form of fullness, pressure, or a burning sensation in the upper chest. At times, it may seem as if the food gets lodged behind the breastbone. Initially, patients may experience this with bread, meat, and other coarse foods. As the tumor grows, narrowing the space for food to pass, softer foods—and even liquids—may be difficult or painful to get down.

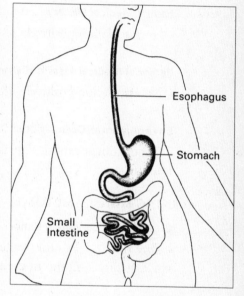

A mass in the gullet usually doesn't bring about symptoms until it has reached sizable proportions. "For somebody to have difficulty swallowing from esophageal cancer," says Dr. Fuchs, "more than 60 percent of the circumference of the esophagus has to be affected by the tumor. And when a person has that degree of involvement, you're usually talking about extension into the adjacent lymph nodes or other structures, and possibly metastases."

See Chapter Three, "How Cancer Is Diagnosed and Staged."

ESOPHAGEAL CANCER/ At Diagnosis

EXTENT OF DISEASE AT THE TIME OF DIAGNOSIS

Local disease	24% of cases
Regional disease	23% of cases
Metastatic disease	27% of cases
Unstaged	26% of cases

Cancer of the Larynx

Predominant cell type: squamous-cell carcinoma

RISK FACTORS

Lifestyle-Related
- Smoking • Excessive alcohol consumption

Family Medical History
- No association positively identified

Personal Medical/Health History
- No association positively identified

Environmental/Occupational Carcinogens
- Occupational exposure to asbestos, sulfuric-acid mist, nickel, mustard gas

WARNING SIGNS/SYMPTOMS

Supraglottic Laryngeal Cancer
- Sore throat • Painful swallowing • Ear pain • Change in voice quality • Lump in the throat or neck

Glottic Laryngeal Cancer
- Hoarseness and other voice changes

Subglottic Laryngeal Cancer
- Hoarseness • Shortness of breath • Noisy breathing

IF NOT CONTROLLED, LARYNGEAL CANCER MAY SPREAD TO:
- Lymph nodes • Lung • Liver • Bone • Throat *(pharynx)* • Neck • Back of the tongue

Since the early 1960s, the pattern of mortalities from laryngeal cancer has mirrored that from lung cancer. While fewer men die of this disease today, the mortality rate for women has risen sharply—a testament to the unfortunate increase in women smokers.

About the Larynx

The triangular larynx, perched atop the windpipe *(trachea)*, is a two-inch-long passageway made of muscle and flexible cartilage. Two bands of muscle, the vocal cords, stretch across the voice box, forming a **V**. When we speak, the bands tighten and vibrate as the lungs force air through the gap between them. This produces a sound—our voice—which the tongue, lips, and teeth then shape into words. During breathing, however, the vocal cords relax, allowing air to pass in either direction without generating any sound.

The larynx is also instrumental in swallowing. At its entrance hangs a flap of cartilage called the *epiglottis*. So that we don't inhale food or liquid into our lungs, with every swallow the epiglottis closes off the windpipe, routing food or drink into the proper tube, the esophagus.

Cancer can arise in any one of the larynx's three regions: the *glottis* (the middle section, site of the vocal cords), the *supraglottis* (the upper section, where the epiglottis is located), and the *subglottis* (the lower section, connecting to the trachea). The most common site is the glottis, followed by the supraglottis and the subglottis.

An ear, nose, and throat specialist would be most concerned to find a tumor below the vocal cords, "for several reasons," says Dr. William Richtsmeier, chief of otolaryngology head and neck surgery at Duke Comprehensive Cancer Center in Durham, North Carolina. "One, the pattern of spread from that area may well be down and to the lower part of the neck, which is a more difficult area to operate on. Two, because the vocal cords form a sort of shelf when viewed from above, they can hide a cancer that's growing in the subglottis. And three, subglottic lesions tend not to cause symptoms early, so they usually present in a more advanced stage than tumors in the glottis or supraglottis."

How Laryngeal Cancer Is Typically Detected

The success rate of treatment is highest for glottic laryngeal cancer, says Dr. Richtsmeier, primarily because "even a tiny tumor there can cause hoarseness and get the patient to the doctor for early diagnosis."

In subglottic cancer, "a few patients present with shortness of breath, from an obstruction of the airway," while tumors above the vocal cords most often inflict pain. "The pain can manifest in several different ways," he explains: "chronic sore throat, pain when swallowing, or pain in the ear."

See Chapter Three, "How Cancer Is Diagnosed and Staged."

LARYNGEAL CANCER/ At Diagnosis

EXTENT OF DISEASE AT THE TIME OF DIAGNOSIS

Local disease	49% of cases
Regional disease	32% of cases
Metastatic disease	12% of cases
Unstaged	6% of cases

Cancer of the Throat (Pharyngeal Cancer)

Predominant cell type: squamous-cell carcinoma

RISK FACTORS

Lifestyle-Related
- Smoking • Excessive alcohol consumption

Family Medical History
- No association positively identified

Personal Medical/Health History
- Epstein-Barr virus (EBV) (nasopharyngeal cancer only)

Environmental/Occupational Carcinogens
- Occupational exposure to mustard gas, formaldehyde

WARNING SIGNS/SYMPTOMS

- Chronic sore throat • Lump in the neck, throat, back of the tongue, or nose • Difficulty in breathing, speaking, and/or hearing • Difficulty in swallowing • Frequent headaches • Change in voice • Pain or ringing in the ears • Headache

IF NOT CONTROLLED, THROAT CANCER MAY SPREAD TO:

- Lymph nodes • Larynx • Lung • Liver • Bone • Neck • Nerves in the head • Nose

Cancer of the throat, or *pharynx*, is divided into three types according to location: *nasopharyngeal, oropharyngeal,* and *hypopharyngeal.* Nasopharyngeal carcinoma is unique in that it is the only head and neck malignancy not associated with tobacco and alcohol use. The Epstein-Barr virus (EBV) is suspected of causing up to 70 percent of all nasopharyngeal cancers.

"Tumors of the throat tend to be far more serious than cancer of the larynx or the oral cavity," says Dr. Randal Weber, director of the head and neck cancer center at the University of Pennsylvania in Philadelphia, "mainly because they have a higher risk of metastasis." Hypopharyngeal carcinoma, the most common of the three types, is also the most likely to spread to distant sites.

About the Pharynx

The throat is a five-inch tube that starts behind the nose and extends down the neck, where it joins the esophagus. Both food and air pass through the pharynx on the way to the stomach and lungs, respectively. While food and liquid travel straight through, air flows into the adjoining larynx and then down the windpipe *(trachea).* From top to bottom, the three areas of the throat are called the *nasopharynx,* the *oropharynx,* and the *hypopharynx.*

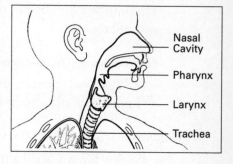

How Throat Cancer Is Typically Detected

"One of the most common early symptoms of this cancer is a chronic sore throat that isn't relieved by gargles or any of the usual medical remedies," explains Dr. Weber. Another frequent feature, he says, "is a mass in the neck due to spread to lymph nodes in the neck."

See Chapter Three, "How Cancer Is Diagnosed and Staged."

THROAT CANCER/
At Diagnosis

EXTENT OF DISEASE AT THE TIME OF DIAGNOSIS

Local disease	36% of cases
Regional disease	43% of cases
Metastatic disease	9% of cases
Unstaged	12% of cases

Soft-Tissue Sarcomas

Predominant cell type: many different cell types

RISK FACTORS

Lifestyle-Related

- No association positively identified

Family Medical History

- No association positively identified

Personal Medical/Health History

- Immunosuppressant drug therapy following transplantation •
Human immunodeficiency virus (HIV) • Neurofibromatosis, an
inherited condition that produces flat, brown patches on the
skin and benign tumors called neurofibromas; approximately
fifteen in one hundred of these patients develop
neurofibrosarcoma

Environmental/Occupational Carcinogens

- Occupational exposure to chlorophenols in wood preservatives
and phenoxyacetic acid in herbicides

WARNING SIGNS/SYMPTOMS

- Painless lump • As the tumor grows, pain or soreness

IF NOT CONTROLLED, SOFT-TISSUE SARCOMAS MAY SPREAD TO:

- Lung • Lymph nodes

Soft-tissue sarcoma is a tumor of any body tissue that connects,
supports, or envelops other structures and organs. This includes muscles, tendons, fibrous tissues, fat, joints, and circulatory vessels. Because surgery is the primary treatment for these cancers, the type of
tissue affected is less important than the cancer's size and site—two
factors that greatly determine the surgeon's ability to completely excise
the tumor.

Dr. Kenneth Yaw is chief of the division of musculoskeletal oncology at the University of Pittsburgh Cancer Institute. Compared to

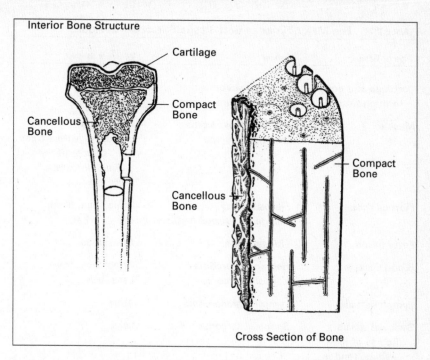

Interior Bone Structure

Cartilage

Compact Bone

Cancellous Bone

Compact Bone

Cancellous Bone

Cross Section of Bone

malignancies in the head, neck, or torso, "tumors in the extremities are more readily removed without sacrificing otherwise vital anatomic parts," he explains. Fifty-five percent of soft-tissue sarcomas develop in the limbs, particularly the legs. Thirty percent occur in the trunk (shoulders, chest, abdomen, hips), and another 15 percent in the head and neck. As Dr. Yaw notes, tumor site influences the prognosis in another way: "The cancer can grow to a larger size in the torso and abdomen before it becomes detectable than a tumor, say, on the wrist."

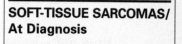

SOFT-TISSUE SARCOMAS/ At Diagnosis

EXTENT OF DISEASE AT THE TIME OF DIAGNOSIS

Percentages of soft-tissue sarcoma patients diagnosed with local, regional, or metastatic disease are not available.

TYPES OF SOFT-TISSUE SARCOMAS

There are more than a dozen different forms of soft-tissue sarcomas, each named for the type of cell from which it derives (see table 2.7).

One interesting trait of soft-tissue sarcomas is that should they spread, rarely do they metastasize to sites other than the lung. Of the major types, the only exception is synovial sarcoma, which may seed the lymph nodes as well as the lungs.

TABLE 2.7	The Major Types of Soft-Tissue Sarcomas in Adults	
Type of Tissue	**Cancer**	**Where It Strikes**
Cartilage and bone-forming tissues	*Chondrosarcoma*	**Legs**
	Osteosarcoma	**Bones**
Muscle	*Rhabdomyosarcoma*	**Arms, legs**
	Leiomyosarcoma	**Uterus, digestive tract**
		See "Cancer of the Small Intestine," page 113.
Fibrous tissue	*Fibrosarcoma*	**Arms, legs, trunk**
	Malignant fibrous histiocytoma	**Legs**
Fatty tissue	*Liposarcoma*	**Arms, legs**
Blood vessels	*Hemangiosarcoma*	**Arms, legs, trunk**
	Kaposi's sarcoma	**Legs, trunk**
Lymph vessels	*Lymphangiosarcoma*	**Arms**
Synovial tissue (linings of joint cavities, tendon sheaths)	*Synovial sarcoma*	**Legs**
Peripheral nerves	*Neurofibrosarcoma*	**Arms, legs, trunk**

Source: National Cancer Institute.

How Soft-Tissue Sarcomas Are Typically Detected

"Most patients," says Dr. Yaw, "will present with a lump. Some will have pain, some won't." Often, he notes, men and women with a soft-tissue sarcoma will have been aware of the lump or the pain "at least for a matter of months, and occasionally for a year or two."

See Chapter Three, "How Cancer Is Diagnosed and Staged."

Cancer of the Testicle

Predominant cell type: germ cell

RISK FACTORS

Lifestyle-Related
- No association positively identified

Family Medical History
- No association positively identified

Personal Medical/Health History
- An undescended or partially descended testicle, even if it has since been corrected surgically

Environmental/Occupational Carcinogens
- No association positively identified

WARNING SIGNS/SYMPTOMS
- Lump in either testicle • Enlarged testicle • Heavy sensation in the scrotum • Dull ache in the groin or lower abdomen • Sudden collection of fluid in the scrotum • Pain or discomfort in a testicle or in the scrotum • Breast enlargement or tenderness

IF NOT CONTROLLED, TESTICULAR CANCER MAY SPREAD TO:
- Lung • Liver

Testicular cancer is the leading malignancy among men aged fifteen to thirty-four, though it is by no means restricted to that age group. Medicine's increased success in treating this disease constitutes an impressive victory in the war against cancer. From the mid-1970s to the mid-1990s, the death rate from testicular cancer dropped by 71 percent, making this one of the most curable of all cancers. It's a point cancer specialist Dr. Bruce Redman regularly emphasizes to his patients at the University of Michigan Comprehensive Cancer Center in Ann Arbor.

"If treated appropriately, testicular cancer is highly curable, no matter what the stage," says Dr. Redman. "Every day I see patients while they're undergoing therapy. I'll sit next to them and say, 'John, why are we doing this?' 'Because this is curable.' " Even when the tumor has metastasized to other organs, such as the lungs, three in four patients can be cured.

About the Testicles
The testicles, also referred to as the *testes* or *gonads,* occupy the pouchlike *scrotum* behind and below the penis. These two glands man-

ufacture and store sperm. In addition, the testicles serve as the body's chief source of *testosterone* and other male hormones, which control the development of the reproductive organs and male physical characteristics such as facial hair and deep-pitched voice.

Types of Testicular Cancer

Doctors divide the several kinds of testicular tumors into two categories: *seminomas* and *nonseminomas*. Seminomas, which make up about 40 percent of all cases, usually occur in men thirty-five and older; those between fifteen and twenty-four tend to develop nonseminomas. "In order for a tumor to be a seminoma," Dr. Redman explains, "it has to be a pure seminoma." If a tissue sample is found to contain any other element, it is classified as a nonseminomanous germ-cell tumor. These distinctions are important, because the two malignancies call for different treatment strategies. About 90 percent of nonseminomanous cancers contain two or more of the following cell types: *embryonal carcinoma, teratoma, choriocarcinoma, yolk-sac tumor*—and seminoma.

How Testicular Cancer Is Typically Detected

Testicular cancer is rarely diagnosed before it induces symptoms, though not because seminomas and nonseminomas are particularly aggressive.

"The reason," explains Dr. Redman, "is that the disease is most common in young men, and that group as a whole doesn't go for checkups.

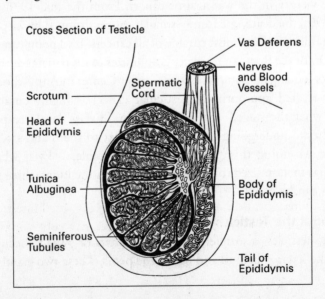

Cross Section of Testicle

Vas Deferens

Nerves and Blood Vessels

Spermatic Cord

Scrotum

Head of Epididymis

Tunica Albuginea

Body of Epididymis

Seminiferous Tubules

Tail of Epididymis

The majority of patients come in with some symptoms, usually a lump in the testicles. It may be painful or painless." It's recommended that men visit a physician if any of the warning signs of testicular cancer persists for two weeks. But Dr. Redman says that "when we ask our patients, 'When did you first notice this symptom?,' on average they'll say, 'Oh, about six months ago.' "

TESTICULAR CANCER/ At Diagnosis	
EXTENT OF DISEASE AT THE TIME OF DIAGNOSIS	
Local disease	66% of cases
Regional disease	20% of cases
Metastatic disease	13% of cases
Unstaged	3% of cases

Other complaints, such as back pain or (infrequently) difficulty in breathing, indicate metastatic disease to abdominal lymph nodes and the lungs, respectively. Oddly enough, a person can be diagnosed with carcinoma in situ—a superficial tumor in a testicle—and yet have multiple pulmonary nodules. "It's rare," says Dr. Redman, "but it does happen. We almost never have a palpable testicular mass that is pure carcinoma in situ."

See Chapter Three, "How Cancer Is Diagnosed and Staged."

Cancer of the Small Intestine

Predominant cell types: adenocarcinoma, carcinoid, leiomyosarcoma, and lymphoma

RISK FACTORS

Lifestyle-Related

. Fatty diet . A diet high in red meat and salt-cured, smoked, and salt-pickled foods

Family Medical History

. No association positively identified

Personal Medical/Health History

. Colorectal cancer or polyps . Polyps in the small intestine . Inflammatory bowel diseases such as ulcerative colitis or Crohn's disease . Adult celiac disease, a disorder of the small bowel also known as celiac sprue or nontropical sprue . Human immunodeficiency virus (HIV)

Environmental/Occupational Carcinogens
- No association positively identified

WARNING SIGNS/SYMPTOMS
- Abdominal pain • Nausea and vomiting • Diarrhea • Appetite loss • Weight loss • Fever • Intestinal bleeding

IF NOT CONTROLLED, SMALL-INTESTINE CANCER MAY SPREAD TO:
- Liver • Lung • Other abdominal organs

Cancer of the small intestine, a rare tumor, afflicts equal numbers of men and women. Four types—*adenocarcinoma, lymphoma, leiomyosarcoma,* and *carcinoid*—account for the majority of small-intestine cancers, though according to Dr. Frederick Richards of the Comprehensive Cancer Center of Wake Forest University in Winston-Salem, North Carolina, "as many as thirty or forty different malignancies may affect the small bowel."

About the Small Intestine

Digestion of food takes place mainly in the coiled small intestine, which breaks down carbohydrates, proteins, and fats into products the body can use. At twenty feet in length, the bowel is the longest part of the gastrointestinal tract—and in a sense, it is even longer than that. The organ's inner lining, or *mucosa,* contains deep circular folds, so that the thick liquid mixture received from the stomach travels a total of one hundred square feet. All along the way, tiny tubular projections called *villi* absorb the digested nutrients as quickly as they are produced and pass them along to the liver for distribution to the rest of the body, while what is left—bulky waste—proceeds to the colon or large intestine.

The bowel is divided into three sections: the C-shaped *duodenum,* which connects to the bottom of the stomach; the *jejunum,* the longest portion; and the narrow *ileum.* About twice as many cancers form in the ileum as in either the duodenum or the jejunum.

Types of Small-Intestine Cancer

Leiomyosarcoma and lymphoma are the least common small-bowel cancers. Adenocarcinomas make up a shade under 50 percent of all cases, while another 20 percent or so are carcinoid tumors, the most curable type.

"Carcinoid is somewhat different from the others," says Dr. Richards, a medical oncologist, "in several respects." This *neuroendocrine* tumor originates in hormone-secreting cells found mainly in the small intestine, but also—in descending order—in the appendix, rectum, lung, colon, stomach, pancreas, and liver. Its name was coined to reflect the fact that a carcinoid is one of the few tumors to fall midway between being malignant (in this instance, a carcinoma) and benign (an *adenoma,* a noncancerous glandular growth). Two in five carcinoid tumors grow in the small bowel, the most frequent site. Roughly one in five of these will spread, usually to the liver.

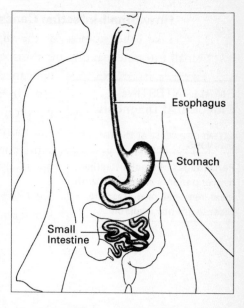

Cancer cells can produce hormones. Metastatic carcinoids that release large quantities of hormones and other substances may be accompanied by an assortment of symptoms referred to as *carcinoid syndrome:* flushing of the face, diarrhea, abrupt drops in blood pressure, swelling *(edema),* an excess accumulation of fluid in the abdomen *(ascites),* and bronchospasms not unlike an asthma attack. "Carcinoid syndrome can be very debilitating," says the doctor.

"By and large, most people with carcinoid syndrome also have liver metastasis. They may well have *extensive* liver metastasis. The other unusual thing about carcinoids is that even when patients have widely metastatic disease in the liver, the cancer may follow a very indolent course, especially in the elderly." The tumor often grows so slowly that in lieu of treatment, an oncologist may recommend what's called watchful waiting.

Tumors of the Small Intestine	
Type	**Occurs Mostly in the . . .**
Adenocarcinoma	**Duodenum**
Carcinoid	**Ileum**
Lymphoma	**Ileum**
Sarcomas	**Jejunum**

"I've got one woman patient I've been following for eight years, and a gentleman I've been following for six years," says Dr. Richards. "Neither one has shown evidence of any progression over that time. In other patients, though, the carcinoid tumor behaves very aggressively."

How Small-Intestine Cancer Is Typically Detected

Like other tumors of the digestive tract, the warning signs of small-intestine cancer are nonspecific and frequently mistaken for noncancerous conditions such as peptic ulcers. In addition to gastrointestinal-related symptoms such as diarrhea, abdominal pain, and nausea and vomiting, a patient may become anemic due to internal bleeding from the small bowel.

See Chapter Three, "How Cancer Is Diagnosed and Staged."

SMALL-INTESTINE CANCER/At Diagnosis

EXTENT OF DISEASE AT THE TIME OF DIAGNOSIS

Percentages of small-intestine cancer patients diagnosed with local, regional, or metastatic disease are not available.

How Cancer Is Diagnosed and Staged

First-rate cancer care begins with an accurate diagnosis. We're not implying that misdiagnoses are rampant, but Maureen Sawchuk, nursing coordinator at the Lombardi Cancer Center, says that "mistakes can be made," particularly if a medical institution sees relatively few cases of a certain type of cancer. "You not only want the best doctor, you want the best pathologist and the best radiologist," she emphasizes. A pathologist is a physician trained to diagnose cancer by studying tumor cells under a microscope; a *radiologist* is a doctor who specializes in interpreting X-ray films.

Even if you've already been definitively diagnosed with cancer, this chapter's information on testing is valuable. You may be awaiting further tests to *stage* the size and extent of the tumor. Or perhaps you plan to seek a second opinion, in which event the referral facility will undoubtedly order its own tests—possibly including repeats of procedures you've been through already. And, looking ahead, you'll undergo some of these tests as part of your follow-up visits to the oncologist for years to come.

Wherever you stand in terms of diagnosis and staging, compare the series of tests you've completed with the recommendations here, which reflect the diagnostic workup a patient would likely receive at a major cancer center. Were you evaluated properly and thoroughly, using state-of-the-art techniques? In detecting stomach cancer, for instance, the gold standard today is upper-GI endoscopy rather than an imaging study, "because endoscopy allows us to biopsy the lesion at the same time," explains Dr. Harinder Garewal of the Arizona Cancer Center. "If we sent someone for a radiology workup and a mass was found, we'd have to perform the endoscopy and biopsy anyway."

Before you submit to any medical test, we suggest asking the doctor or nurse questions such as those listed below. Having some idea of what to expect enables patients not only to prepare themselves mentally—which many find helps to ease pretest jitters—but to make other, practical preparations. Let's say you're scheduled for a magnetic resonance imaging scan, which, your doctor explains, entails lying inside a narrow chamber while the machine takes three-dimensional pictures. If you're prone to claustrophobia, you might ask him to prescribe a mild short-acting sedative in advance. By being an informed patient, you've just spared yourself needless anxiety.

Questions to Ask . . . About Upcoming Tests

- What is the purpose of this test?
- Are there any alternatives to this test?
- Is this an outpatient procedure? If so, will I need to have someone drive me to and from the appointment?
- Is this an inpatient procedure? If so, how long can I expect to be hospitalized?
- Are any preparations necessary beforehand, such as fasting, bowel cleansing, or discontinuing medications?
- Can a family member or friend stay with me during the procedure?
- How long does the test usually take?
- Can I anticipate any pain, discomfort, or claustrophobia? If so, what can be done to make me more comfortable?
- Will I require sedation and/or local or general anesthesia? Can I request either one if I wish?

- Are there any common side effects or complications? If so, how are they managed?

- Are there any serious health risks involved? What can go wrong?

- Are there any complications that I should be aware of once I'm home? Under what circumstances should I call you [the doctor] or go to a hospital emergency room?

- How much does the procedure cost? Based on your experience with my medical insurer, will it be covered? (Not that you wouldn't proceed with a diagnostic test because it's expensive, but isn't it better to know this ahead of time than to stare in shock at the medical bill months later?)

- When will I receive the test results?

- If the test indicates that I have cancer, who will talk to me about my treatment options? (Explain that should the results come back positive for cancer, you will probably pursue a second opinion.)

- How definitive and accurate is the test? Will further testing be necessary?

- Will a follow-up appointment be necessary? With whom? The doctor who performed the procedure? My primary oncologist? My general practitioner?

Types of Diagnostic and Staging Tests

The tests used to detect cancer can be grouped into five basic categories: physical exams; laboratory tests; imaging studies; endoscopic procedures; and biopsies, the definitive diagnostic tool. There's more than one route to a diagnosis. If signs and symptoms strongly suggest a tumor, a doctor may order the most conclusive test straightaway. Otherwise, a diagnostic workup is likely to begin with less invasive (and less expensive) procedures, to rule out other, less serious conditions. Which tests a patient undergoes also depends on her physician's preferences and ex-

Medical Terms You're Likely to Hear

Screening: Tests and exams that can pick up cancer early in the course of the disease, before it produces symptoms. Men and women considered to be at a heightened risk of cancer are advised to undergo various screening procedures at regular intervals. For instance, the screening guidelines for prostate cancer recommend that asymptomatic men aged fifty and older have a digital rectal exam and a PSA blood test every year.

perience. When imaging the pancreas, for instance, one doctor might rely on ultrasound first, while a colleague might favor the CT scan. Either approach is sound.

Once a diagnosis has been confirmed, additional tests are carried out to determine the tumor's size and whether or not it has spread. These staging procedures, too, vary from patient to patient, although typically a doctor will want to image the lungs, liver, bones, and/or brain, the most common sites of metastasis. Not all cancers can be staged *clinically*—that is, on the basis of physical exams, lab tests, and radiologic and endoscopic studies. Often it isn't until the operation to take out the cancer that the medical picture comes fully into focus. *Surgical staging* may reveal that the tumor is actually larger than was shown on X ray or that it has invaded adjacent structures. The surgeon frequently samples area lymph nodes and perhaps tissue from other organs, which the pathologist then examines for cancer, in what is called *pathologic staging.*

Physical Exams

For all the advances in medical technology, physicians still acquire much of the information needed to form a diagnosis the old-fashioned way: by sitting down with patients and discussing their symptoms, taking a thorough medical history and family medical history, and conducting a physical examination.

Except for cancers of the skin or readily accessible body cavities such as the mouth, throat, and vagina, most tumors cannot be seen. Depending on the site, the doctor will often *palpate,* or probe, the suspicious area with his fingers, as well as feel for swollen lymph nodes. Experienced physicians can sometimes discern masses in the breast, liver, and other parts of the body this way.

The physical exam may include an internal examination. By inserting a lubricated, gloved finger into the rectum, a doctor can feel for tumors of the large intestine, bladder, and prostate. Similarly, in a pelvic exam, the gynecologist explores the female reproductive organs with her fingers for abnormalities in shape and size. An ovary large enough to be felt digitally could indicate cancer or merely a cyst.

Laboratory/Specimen Tests

The blood, as well as bodily fluids and excretions, sometimes holds valuable clues. A lab test may analyze a specimen for the presence of actual cancer cells—as in a lumbar puncture, which involves withdrawing a sample of cerebrospinal fluid from the lower spine—or for other substances that indicate cancer directly or indirectly. For example, liver-function blood tests don't pick up cancer in the liver per se. But they do shed light on whether the problem is one of liver damage, brought on by progressive diseases such as hepatitis or cirrhosis, or one of liver obstruction. Should the tests point to a blockage, the probable culprit would be either a tumor or gallstones.

What Are Tumor Markers?

With certain cancers, some patients will exhibit elevated levels of proteins and other substances in the blood, urine, or tissues. These *tumor markers* may be produced by the mass itself or by the body in response to the tumor's presence. With the exception of the prostate specific antigen (PSA) test for prostate cancer, the monoclonal (M) protein test for multiple myeloma, and the alpha-fetoprotein (AFP) test for malignancies of the testicle and the liver, oncologists generally rely on tumor markers more to track the course of cancer after it has been treated than as a diagnostic tool. Not only can other diseases trigger a rise in one of these substances, but a person with, say, ovarian cancer can still test normal for the CA-125 tumor marker. Other tumor markers are currently being studied.

Imaging Studies

Radiologists can choose from an ever-expanding array of imaging techniques to take still films or moving pictures of internal structures, which are scrutinized for evidence of a tumor.

The venerable X ray, still a highly useful diagnostic tool, has been joined by newer radiographic studies such as CT scans, mammograms, and radionuclide scans. Magnetic resonance imaging, or MRI, differs from these in that it uses radio waves and a magnetic field as its energy source. Ultrasound, another imaging technique that doesn't expose patients to ionizing radiation, produces pictures on a monitor screen through sound waves.

TABLE 3.1   Laboratory Tests Used in Diagnosing and Staging Cancer

Blood Tests

Test	Description	Commonly Used to Help Detect/Stage These Cancers
Blood chemistry tests	A battery of laboratory tests that measures the levels of twenty different substances in the blood, such as electrolytes, proteins, enzymes, and glucose. May include many if not all of the chemical tests used to determine liver function and/or kidney function.	Kidney
Calcitonin test	Measures the blood level of the hormone *calcitonin.*	Thyroid
Calcium test	Measures the amount of calcium in the blood. *Hypercalcemia,* an over-abundance of calcium, is a frequent complication of many cancers.	Multiple myeloma Metastatic bone cancer
Complete blood count (CBC) *Includes white blood count (WBC), red blood count (RBC), hematocrit (HCT), and hemoglobin (HGB)*	Measures the numbers of red blood cells, white blood cells, and platelet cells in a cubic milliliter of blood; a *differential white-cell count* specifies the various types of white cells. A CBC also evaluates the total amount of *hemoglobin,* the substance in red cells that carries oxygen, and the percentage of whole blood that is made up of red blood cells, or *the hematocrit.*	Leukemia Multiple myeloma Stomach
Comprehensive metabolic panel	Measures the blood levels of more than a dozen substances, including calcium, proteins, and enzymes. May include many if not all of the chemical tests used to determine liver function and/or kidney function.	Thyroid

Blood Tests

Test	Description	Commonly Used to Help Detect/Stage These Cancers
Erythrocyte sedimentation rate (ESR)	Measures the rate at which red cells settle to the bottom of a test tube of blood. Helps to detect inflammation, infection, and many other conditions.	Hodgkin's disease
Glucose test	Measures the blood concentration of *glucose,* the simple sugar that the body converts to fuel. An abnormally high level *(hyperglycemia)* may be due to a tumor in the pancreas.	Pancreatic
Kidney-function tests	Measures the blood levels of *creatinine* and *urea nitrogen* (BUN). Abnormally elevated concentrations of both substances indicate that the kidneys are not working properly. A *creatinine-urine test* and *creatinine clearance test* complete the picture. *See "Other Laboratory Tests,"* page 126.	Multiple myeloma
Liver-function tests	Measures the blood levels of the liver enzymes alkaline phosphatase (ALP), aspartate aminotransferase (AST), and alanine transaminase (ALT). An elevated concentration of ALP signifies that the flow of bile fluid is being blocked within or outside the liver, perhaps by a tumor; AST and ALT are abnormally high in people with hepatitis or another form of liver disease. Similarly, the *bilirubin test* determines whether a buildup of bilirubin in the liver is due to an obstruction of the bile ducts or due to liver disease. There are two types of bilirubin: *conjugated* and *unconjugated.* If the blood	Liver

Blood Tests

Test	Description	Commonly Used to Help Detect/Stage These Cancers
	contains an excessive amount of conjugated bilirubin, the physician can rule out liver disease and continue testing to identify the cause of the blockage.	
Thyroid-function tests	Measures the amount of thyroid hormone (T3 and T4) in the circulation. Abnormally high blood levels of T4 and, less commonly, T3, may point to thyroid cancer.	Thyroid
Uric acid test	Measures the concentration of uric acid in the blood. People with leukemia often have higher-than-normal levels *(hyperuricemia)*.	Leukemia

Tumor-Marker Blood Tests

Tumor Marker	Description	Commonly Used to Help Detect These Cancers
Alpha-fetoprotein (AFP)	A protein produced by the developing fetus; production drops after birth, and remains low in healthy children and adults.	Liver Testicular
Beta-2 microglobulin	The level of beta-2 microglobulin, a protein discharged by the cells involved in multiple myeloma	Multiple myeloma
Carbohydrate antigen 19-9 (CA-19-9)	A substance that has been identified in patients with cancers of the large intestine, liver, stomach, and, especially, pancreas	Pancreatic
Cancer antigen 125 (CA-125)	A protein produced primarily by ovarian cancer cells	Ovarian

Tumor-Marker Blood Tests

Tumor Marker	Description	Commonly Used to Help Detect These Cancers
Carcinoembryonic antigen (CEA)	A protein normally found in low levels in the blood of healthy men and women	Colorectal Pancreatic
Human chorionic gonadotropin (HCG)	A hormone	Testicular
Monoclonal (M) protein	A type of antibody produced by plasma cells; people with multiple myeloma have an overabundance of plasma cells.	Multiple myeloma
Neuron-specific enolase (NSE)	An enzyme that has been associated with several tumors but is used as a marker primarily for small-cell carcinoma of the lung and the children's cancer neuroblastoma. The NSE level indicates the extent of the disease and also provides information about the patient's prognosis and probable response to therapy.	Small-cell lung cancer
Prostatic acid phosphatase (PAP)	A protein present in the prostate and many other tissues	Prostate
Prostate specific antigen (PSA)	A protein produced by both normal and abnormal prostate cells	Prostate
Thyroglobulin tumor-marker blood test	The level of *thyroglobulin,* a protein manufactured by papillary and follicular thyroid tumors. Some patients develop antibodies to thyroglobulin, producing negative test results even when cancer is present. To avoid a "false negative," a *thyroglobulin-antibody blood test* should also be performed. (A "false positive" refers to a test result that incorrectly diagnoses a disease.)	Thyroid

Other Laboratory Tests

Test	What Does It Evaluate?	Commonly Used to Help Detect These Cancers
Dilation and curettage (D&C)	Cells scraped from the lining of the uterus	Endometrial
Endocervical curettage (ECC)	Cells scraped from inside the opening of the cervix	Cervical
Fecal occult-blood test	A stool sample for microscopic traces of blood	Colorectal Stomach
Lumbar puncture (spinal tap)	Cerebrospinal fluid withdrawn through a syringe from the spinal canal	Leukemia Brain
Pap smear	Cells scraped or brushed from the cervix and upper vagina	Cervical
Sputum cytology	Cells found in mucus expelled from the lungs	Lung
Thoracentesis	Pleural fluid withdrawn through a syringe from the space between the two-layered pleural membrane that surrounds the lungs	Lung
Urine tests Creatinine clearance test	Measures the amount of fluid filtered by the kidneys per minute, based on two urine samples given twenty-four hours apart. Lower-than-normal results may indicate kidney impairment.	Multiple myeloma
Creatinine urine test	Measures the level of creatinine in urine, based on two urine samples given twenty-four hours apart. Abnormally high or low results may indicate kidney impairment.	Multiple myeloma
Hematuria urine test	Measures the number of red cells in a given volume of urine. An abnormally high result may indicate cancer.	Bladder Kidney Prostate

Other Laboratory Tests		
Test	What Does It Evaluate?	Commonly Used to Help Detect These Cancers
Urinalysis	Analyzes the urine for evidence of infections, kidney disease, and other conditions	Multiple myeloma Prostate Testicular
Urine cytology	Urine test to detect abnormal-looking cells.	Bladder Kidney Other cancers of the urinary tract

Why and When: CT Scan Versus MRI Scan Versus Ultrasound

"A CT scan and an MRI scan provide different tissue information," explains radiologist Rebecca Zuurbier, director of breast imaging at the Lombardi Cancer Center. Of the two imaging studies, she says, "a CT scan is usually the way to start out. The pictures tend to be crisper than an MRI and less subject to motion artifact." An artifact is a spot or distortion on the film. For that reason alone, the CT scan is generally considered superior for visualizing moving organs, such as the heart, the lungs, and the stomach, intestines, and other digestive organs that propel food through the GI tract with an undulating motion.

Magnetic resonance imaging is often the preferred method for viewing the central nervous system, head, spine, liver, soft tissue, and blood vessels. A radiologist might also order an MRI scan if a patient is pregnant and wants to avoid radiation. As for ultrasound, although it has been supplanted in many situations by the more accurate CT scan, it is frequently used to study the prostate, ovaries, and other soft tissues that tend not to X-ray clearly.

The Informed Patient:
How to Make Sure You Receive a High-Quality X Ray

"Two elements are critical to getting a good X ray," says Dr. Zuurbier. "One is good equipment. But secondly, an X ray is only as good as the person that's reading it." So if you're slated for a chest X ray, for example, "you can help yourself by going to a facility that has modern technology and a radiologist who specializes in chest radiology."

As a general rule, "newer equipment is better," says Dr. Zuurbier, but that is not to say older models kept in good repair and monitored regularly for film quality don't take high-caliber pictures. Likewise, while X-ray and mammography machines manufactured by Toshiba, Philips, General Electric, Fisher, Fuji, Du Pont, and Low Rad are considered top-of-the-line, lesser known brands aren't necessarily lacking in quality. Realistically, most of us probably aren't going to call a radiology department prior to an X ray and grill the person at the other end about the make, model, and year of the equipment anyway. (Though it is certainly your right to know. "If anyone gives you grief, you shouldn't be having your X ray there," Dr. Zuurbier states flatly.)

> **Medical Terms You're Likely to Hear**
>
> **Fluoroscope:** an X-ray machine that projects a moving image onto a TV-type monitor. *Fluoroscopy* enables physicians to observe an organ or physiological process in motion. Surgeons often use fluoroscopy to guide them while performing needle biopsies, among other procedures.

A simpler solution is to go to a busy medical center. As she explains, "Places that perform a lot of procedures will usually have better equipment than a small hospital, which perhaps can't justify investing in a new piece of equipment." Incidentally, this applies across the board, not just to radiology, and should be one more consideration when deciding on where to receive treatment.

Next: How do you exercise some control over who interprets the study? "You might not be able to do that on the first go-round," says Dr. Zuurbier. Her recommendation is to call back another day and request that a specialist within the department examine the film. If you underwent a mammogram, an X ray of the breast, ask that the lead mammographer read it. Radiology departments have their own internal hierarchies. At Lombardi, for instance, Dr. Zuurbier evaluates the majority of mammograms. "I frequently have patients who will say to another mammographer, 'After you're done reading it, would you please have Dr. Z. look at this?'

"The person who reads the most films is the best," she says. "It's not because we're smarter, it's just that over time we develop an eye for spotting problems." Should the department not have a radiology specialist on staff, seek a second opinion at a facility that does.

See "Obtaining Medical Records," page 322.

Endoscopic Exams

Another way to view the inner lining of hollow organs and body cavities is through a flexible lighted instrument known as an *endoscope*. A *cystoscope* is for inspecting the bladder; a *laryngoscope*, the larynx; a *bronchoscope*, the air passages of the lungs; and so on.

The scopes vary in length. A *sigmoidoscope* is twenty-five inches long and can reach midway up the colon; a *colonoscope* is approximately twice as long and allows for examination of the entire bowel. Endoscopes can be equipped with a tiny video camera, suction pump, electrode tips for cauterizing, and other accessories.

The physician feeds the scope through one of the body's orifices— nose, mouth, anus, urethra, or vagina—or through a small incision in the chest or abdomen. Then it's lights, camera, action: Both doctor and patient (if you wish) watch on a video monitor as the physician maneuvers the scope through the body's corridors. A tiny brush or a cutting tool connected to a long cable can be passed through the hollow instrument to biopsy tissue samples.

Biopsies

Although there are times when a cancer diagnosis is made based solely on clinical evidence, the only decisive method for identifying the disease is to remove either a partial tissue specimen or the entire lesion, and then have a pathologist evaluate the cells under a microscope.

The long-standing old wives' tale that to pierce or cut into a tumor can scatter malignant cells throughout the body is categorically untrue—with a few exceptions. When tests suggest cancer in an ovary or testicle, the organ must be cut out whole. In fact, most of the time the affected organ itself is excised. A needle biopsy of the pancreas carries the slight risk of dragging cells through the abdomen as the doctor withdraws the instrument. Therefore, when the pancreas is sampled at all, which is rare, it's with a tiny brush passed through an endoscope. Perforating or cutting into the spleen, a reservoir for blood, is ill-advised, because to do so could induce serious bleeding. The preferred method is to surgically remove the organ intact.

Types of Biopsies

Needle Biopsy (also called *percutaneous biopsy)*—In a *fine-needle aspiration biopsy,* the doctor numbs the area with an injection of local anesthetic, then inserts a thin-gauge hollow needle into the mass and withdraws anywhere from dozens to thousands of cells into an attached syringe. Should the physician suspect cancer, but the aspiration biopsy turns out to be negative, she might progress to a more accurate *core-needle biopsy,* which uses a larger needle with a special cutting edge. For difficult-to-reach organs like the liver, physicians frequently rely on fluoroscopy, ultrasound, or a CT scan to help guide them in positioning the needle.

◆ Most often used to diagnose cancers of the bone, bone marrow, breast, liver, lung, pancreas, prostate, soft tissue, thyroid, and uterus.

See "Stereotactic Core-Needle Biopsy of the Breast," page 139, and "Stereotactic Biopsy of the Brain," page 166.

Endoscopic Biopsy—the most common form of biopsy. By running a double-bladed cutting instrument called a *forceps* through an endoscope, the doctor can snip off a tiny piece of tissue from the inner lining of hollow structures.

◆ Most often used to diagnose cancers of the large intestine, small intestine, stomach, esophagus, larynx, bladder, abdominal cavity, chest, windpipe, and lung.

Incisional Surgical Biopsy—A small surgical knife *(scalpel)* or cookie-cutter-like tool called a punch is used to cut out a portion of a lump.

◆ Most often used to diagnose cancers of the cervix, oral cavity, skin, soft tissue, throat, and, rarely, breast.

See "Loop Electrosurgical Excision Procedure (LEEP) · Cone Biopsy," two biopsy techniques for diagnosing cervical cancer, page 171

Excisional Surgical Biopsy—Before resorting to an excisional biopsy, in which the entire mass is removed, physicians will usually try to obtain a specimen through one of the less invasive methods. Why subject a patient to an operation when the growth may turn out to be nonmalignant? However, swollen lymph nodes must be examined intact in order to achieve an accurate diagnosis. For a similar reason, some surgeons favor excisional biopsies for small breast masses measuring one inch or less in diameter. As we've already noted, the ovaries and testicles are virtually always biopsied whole, in part to eliminate the slight risk of disseminating tumor cells. In addition, surgical biopsy may be necessary when other methods fail to produce conclusive results.

Since an excisional biopsy removes the entire tumor, it can qualify as both a diagnostic procedure and a form of treatment. For early-stage testicular cancer and some types of in situ carcinoma, no further therapy may be necessary. In taking out a mass, the surgeon looks to also excise a border, or *margin,* of surrounding tissue. Depending on the type and extent of the cancer, this may be done during the biopsy. The more common practice is for the doctor to schedule a second, definitive operation.

♦ Most often used to diagnose cancers of the breast, larynx, lung, lymph nodes, oral cavity, ovary, skin, spleen, and testicle.

Surgical biopsies vary considerably in terms of the operation itself. A woman set to undergo an excisional breast biopsy can expect to be on her way home an hour later. The same cannot be said about a surgical chest biopsy to detect lung cancer, which entails a two-to-five-day hospital stay, plus four to six weeks of recuperation at home.

It is common during a surgical biopsy for the surgeon to send a tissue sample off to the pathology lab for what's called a *frozen section,* in which the specimen is fast-frozen, cut, stained, and studied under the microscope. Frozen sections aren't as accurate as *permanent sections,* a more involved method of processing that takes several days. Nor do they provide a complete profile of the cells. But within thirty minutes or so, they answer the question foremost in everyone's mind: Is the tumor benign or malignant?

With the patient already anesthetized, the surgical team may then proceed to harvest lymph nodes and tissue from other organs as part of staging, to see if they, too, contain cancer. Or they may commence with treatment right then and there, as in the case of a woman who has signed a consent form authorizing a mastectomy should the surgical breast biopsy come back positive. This is called a *one-step procedure.* Most women opt for a *two-step procedure,* with the operation scheduled a week or two later. The same set of circumstances could arise for people with other cancers, such as tumors of the lung or the head and neck.

Other Questions Answered by the Biopsy

A permanent section reveals additional vital details about cancer, including:

Tumor Histology—*Histology* refers to a tumor's cellular composition, which is variable even within each form of cancer. To give you an example, while roughly 85 percent of kidney cancers begin in a type of cell known as a renal cell, 7 percent stem from a different kind: transitional cells. Treatment for the less common of the two mirrors treatment for bladder cancer, the histology of which is predominately transitional-cell carcinoma.

Histology may also provide clues regarding a tumor's aggressiveness. Carcinomas of the lung are divided among four main cell types: squamous cell, adenocarcinoma, small cell, and large cell. Not only are they not all treated the same way, but their aggressiveness varies. Squamous-cell lung cancer spreads less rapidly than the other three; small-cell lung cancer is the most virulent.

Tumor Grade—Grade, expressed in numbers from 1 to 4, denotes the degree to which the malignant cells resemble their healthy counterparts.

How Cancer Is Graded	
G1	Well differentiated
G2	Moderately well differentiated
G3	Poorly differentiated
G4	Undifferentiated
GX	Grade cannot be assessed

Source: American Joint Commission on Cancer.

"Grade I tumors have tissue patterns similar to the normal cell pattern," explains Dr. Larry Copeland of Ohio State University Comprehensive Cancer Center, "whereas at stage III the tissue architecture is disorganized and bizarre looking." When a tumor contains two or more grades of cells, as is often the case, the most malignant cell discovered on biopsy determines the grade of the whole tumor. Grade, along with stage (more about staging shortly), is a key piece of prognostic information. As a rule, low-grade, or well-differentiated, malignancies behave less aggressively than high-grade, or undifferentiated, ones.

Hormone-Receptor Status—For a tumor of the breast or endometrium to test positive for *hormone receptors* indicates that hormones such as estrogen and progesterone stimulate its growth and that the patient is likely to respond to hormone therapy.

See "Cancer of the Breast," page 138, and "Cancer of the Uterus," page 149.

Other Tumor Characteristics—Additional sophisticated lab analysis can reveal valuable details about the tumor. Example: Nearly one in three breast-cancer patients have an altered version of an oncogene known as *Human Epithelial Growth Factor Receptor-2* or *HER-2* for short. Instead of the normal two HER-2 genes per cell, each of their tumor cells contains multiple copies. The aberrant genes instruct the malignant cells to multiply wildly and spread to other organs; in fact, the greater the number of altered HER-2 genes, the more rapidly the tumor grows and metastasizes. HER-2, which has several aliases—*C-ERBb2, B2,* and *C2*—is also associated with ovarian, endometrial, small-cell lung, and oral carcinomas, though it is considered most significant in breast cancer.

Testing biopsy specimens for other biological markers "has not yet proven so beneficial that it has entered standard practice," observes Dr. Jeffrey Abrams, a clinical research scientist at the National Cancer Institute. In hospitals and independent labs where cancer research is not a high priority, this level of tumor analysis "isn't likely done at all." And at research-oriented cancer centers, there's no established protocol as to which tests should be performed. "It depends on the research going on there," Dr. Abrams explains.

Personally, I'd want to be treated at a cancer facility that armed my oncologist with as much information as possible; anything to perhaps give me an advantage. So add "research" to your list of treatment centers' desirable features.

See "Cancer of the Breast," page 138.

The Importance of an Expert Pathologist

For many people with cancer, just choosing a doctor is a major step in taking charge of their own medical care. How many of us, though, give much thought to the qualifications of the pathologist performing the biopsy—upon which other physicians will largely base their recommendations for therapy?

According to the College of American Pathologists, a medical society that accredits more than five thousand medical laboratories, although all labs are certified or licensed by the government, many meet only the minimal standards of laboratory management. A number of facets enters into establishing an accurate cancer diagnosis, more so with some forms of the disease than with others. As we mentioned at the beginning of this chapter, patients are sometimes misdiagnosed and, consequently, treated improperly.

"Let me tell you a story about a patient of mine," says Dr. Paul Carbone, director of the University of Wisconsin Comprehensive Cancer Center, and a specialist in lymphomas. "She presented with an enlarged lymph node in the neck, was diagnosed as having stage II Hodgkin's disease, and was about to receive chemotherapy and radiation therapy.

"She happened to be a hairdresser. One of her customers told her she ought to get a second opinion, so she came to see me. We looked at the original biopsy slides, and it turned out they had been misread. She didn't have Hodgkin's disease, she had a mild inflammation. She's never been treated, and five years later she's doing fine.

"The moral here? Interpretation of pathology slides is extremely critical in terms of reaching the right diagnosis." Dr. Carbone goes on to cite a study of lymphoma patients carried out by the Eastern Cooperative Oncology Group (ECOG), a consortium of hundreds of hospitals and medical centers that engage in cancer research, when he was its chairman. "About 5 to 10 percent of the time the original pathologists were wrong," he notes. In addition to being staged and graded, non-Hodgkin's lymphomas are classified according to their cells' shape and size. "Perhaps 30 to 40 percent of the time," he adds, "they misclassified the disease."

Questions to Ask . . . Before a Biopsy

The College of American Pathologists suggests asking your primary physician these questions to help ensure that your biopsy is evaluated by qualified professionals:

- What is the name of the laboratory, and where is it located?
- Is the pathologist performing the biopsy board-certified?
- Is the laboratory accredited by an agency that performs on-site inspections? The College of American Pathologists is one of several.
- When was the last inspection?
- Do you [the doctor] communicate well with the pathologist at the laboratory analyzing my biopsy?
- Can I see a copy of my pathology report, and will you explain the findings to me?

We would additionally recommend asking if the pathologist subspecializes in diagnosing diseases of the organ that was biopsied (lung, breast, liver, and so forth). Though these are not formal subspecialties, a pathologist may come to concentrate in a particular area. Therefore, if you were being tested for rectal cancer, ideally you would want your biopsy to be examined by a *dedicated* gastrointestinal pathologist: one who studies GI biopsies exclusively. What you're looking for is reasonable assurance that cases similar to yours have crossed his desk before.

Should your slides be read by a nonspecialist, consider seeking a second opinion, particularly if questions arise about the diagnosis, or if the cancer under suspicion is relatively uncommon, or simply if doing so would ease your mind. According to Dr. William H. Hartmann of the American Board of Pathology, "Any patient or physician should feel comfortable suggesting to the pathologist that they get another opinion." Chances are, your doctor or the referring pathologist will know of a dedicated pathologist, probably at a major cancer center or university hospital.

The Informed Patient:
Is the Laboratory Accredited?

To find out if the laboratory processing your biopsy is accredited by an agency that conducts on-site inspections, call:

> The College of American Pathologists (CAP): 800-522-5678
> The Joint Commission on Accreditation of Healthcare Organizations (JCAHO): 630-792-5000

Laparotomy

Sometimes the only way to definitively stage, or even diagnose, cancers of the ovary, pancreas, small intestine, and lymph nodes is through exploratory surgery, which enables the surgeon to physically examine the organ in question as well as others. The broad term *laparotomy* refers to an incision in the abdomen. A laparotomy to stage Hodgkin's disease, for example, typically consists of removing the spleen and any suspicious lymph nodes, and biopsying the liver. In a staging laparotomy for ovarian cancer, the surgeon's mission is to both stage and treat the disease: Nodes and other tissues in the pelvis and abdomen are evaluated and biopsied, and the malignant ovary(ies) taken out, along with any other reproductive organs the tumor may have invaded.

Diagnostic and Staging Tests for Each of the 25 Most Common Types of Cancer

What You Should Know About the Biopsy Procedure and Blood Tests That Pertain Specifically to Diagnosing or Staging Your Cancer

Cancer of the Prostate

You may undergo any number of these diagnostic procedures:
- Physical exam • Digital rectal exam

Laboratory Tests
- Prostate specific antigen (PSA) tumor-marker blood test • Prostatic acid phosphatase (PAP) tumor-marker blood test • Urine tests, to detect blood, pus, or abnormal cells

Imaging Studies
- Transrectal ultrasound • Intravenous pyelogram (IVP) of the kidneys and ureters

Endoscopic Exams
- Cystoscopy

Biopsy
- Transrectal needle biopsy

Any number of these staging procedures may be performed next:
Laboratory Tests
- Repeated PSA tumor-marker blood test

Imaging Studies (TYPICALLY OF THE BONES, LIVER, LUNGS, RECTUM)
- Radionuclide bone scan • Transrectal ultrasound, if not performed previously • CT scan • MRI scan • Chest X ray

---

Diagnosing and Staging Prostate Cancer: What You Should Know

PROSTATE SPECIFIC ANTIGEN (PSA) TUMOR-MARKER BLOOD
TEST

The *PSA* tumor-marker blood test, recommended annually for men
aged fifty and older (forty and older if anything in their medical history places them at high risk for prostate cancer), measures the level of
a specific protein shed into the blood by the prostate. If cancer is present, more PSA enters the circulation. "The standard normal range is
zero to four nanograms per milliliter," explains Dr. Donald Urban of
the University of Alabama at Birmingham Comprehensive Cancer
Center, "with adjustments sometimes made for age or for race." A
nanogram (ng) is one-billionth of a gram.

While a finding of 4ng/ml or higher warrants a full diagnostic
workup, a single elevated value below that level might prompt the doctor to merely follow a patient and keep an eye out for trends on subsequent PSA tests. In Dr. Urban's view, further testing should be
considered "if a person's level begins in the normal range but progressively increases over time."

Because common conditions such as benign prostatic hyperplasia
can also raise PSA levels, the test is a stepping-stone to other procedures, typically a transrectal needle biopsy. (Ejaculation, too, can
nudge up the PSA temporarily; therefore men are asked to refrain from
sexual activity two days prior to testing. For the sake of accuracy, the
procedure should be postponed if you are suffering from an inflamed
prostate [*prostatitis*] or an acute urinary tract infection.)

Another tumor-marker lab test, for *prostatic acid phosphatase*
(PAP), is rarely performed nowadays, since it usually doesn't sound an
alarm until prostate cancer is advanced. What's more, its specificity
leaves much to be desired; malignancies involving the bone can also elevate blood levels of PAP.

TRANSRECTAL NEEDLE BIOPSY OF THE PROSTATE

The thought of having a needle inserted in his prostate is enough to
turn almost any man's knees to jelly. Relax.

With the advent of a spring-loaded needle
"gun," the procedure has become—if not
completely free of discomfort—painless
enough that the majority of patients don't re-

Typical setting:	**outpatient**
Anesthesia:	**local**
Sedation:	**not required**

quire anesthesia or sedation. The only medications typically given be-forehand are an *antibiotic,* to prevent the remote chance of an infection, and an injection of local anesthetic. "Most patients feel pressure for an instant," says Dr. Urban, "but not a sharp sensation."

To guide him, the physician inserts a tiny ultrasound transducer in the rectum. This generates images on a monitor. Then he carefully passes a spring-loaded core needle into a sheath attached to the ultra-sound probe, up against the prostate. A squeeze of the trigger, and the needle darts in and out through the rectum wall, taking with it a tiny piece of prostate tissue. Most urologists, says Dr. Urban, collect about six samples from various sites, "to get a sense of how involved the prostate is," though some, he notes, "advocate taking as many as twenty biopsies at a time."

If your urologist feels that the transrectal route may lead to com-plications, the older, *transperineal* approach can be used. Under ultra-sound guidance, the needle is inserted through the *perineum* and into the prostate. The perineum is the smooth patch of skin that extends from the anus to the scrotum.

Cancer of the Breast

You may undergo any number of these diagnostic procedures:
- Physical exam • Clinical breast exam

Imaging Studies
- Ultrasound (often shows whether a lump is a solid mass or a benign cyst filled with fluid) • Mammogram

Biopsy
- Needle biopsy • Stereotactic core-needle biopsy • Mammographic localization with biopsy • Incisional surgical biopsy • Excisional surgical biopsy

Any number of these staging procedures may be performed next:
Laboratory Tests
- Blood tests

Imaging Studies (TYPICALLY OF THE LIVER, LUNGS, BONES)
- Chest X ray • CT scan • MRI scan

Biopsy

- Excisional surgical biopsy of lymph nodes under the arm, performed as part of the operation to treat the cancer

---

Diagnosing and Staging Breast Cancer: What You Should Know

STEREOTACTIC CORE-NEEDLE BIOPSY OF THE BREAST

Four in five abnormalities picked up by a mammogram turn out to be benign. *Stereotactic core-needle breast biopsy,* a virtually painless procedure, spares women from having to undergo a surgical biopsy, and at one-third the cost. It is also more accurate and quicker than incisional or excisional biopsies, with the results often available the next day.

Typical setting:	outpatient
Anesthesia:	local
Sedation:	not required

For a stereotactic biopsy, you lie facedown on a padded table designed with an opening to accommodate the breast. To help pinpoint the lesion, a special grid is applied to the breast, and then a new mammogram taken. Unlike a standard mammogram, the image appears on a computer screen instead of X-ray film.

Once the doctor has confirmed the position, the site is numbed with an injection of local anesthetic. Then she aims and "fires" an automated hollow needle, which extracts a tissue sample in a split second. At least four more specimens are taken from the same area.

Cosmetically, two advantages of this technique over surgical biopsy are that it leaves no scarring—as opposed to a two-inch incision—and withdraws no surrounding tissue. "Because no margins are taken, stereotactic core biopsy is not definitive," points out Dr. Larry Norton of Memorial Sloan-Kettering Cancer Center. "It doesn't tell us whether or not we've excised the whole mass." Should the lump prove to be malignant, either of two operations, lumpectomy or mastectomy, will follow.

MAMMOGRAPHIC LOCALIZATION WITH BIOPSY

Not all health-care facilities offer stereotactic core-needle biopsy, which is relatively new. Its predecessor, *mammographic localization with needle biopsy,* or needle localization, is still used when a mammogram reveals a breast abnormality that the doctor can't feel with her fingers.

Typical setting:	outpatient
Anesthesia:	local
Sedation:	not required

This procedure calls for you to sit upright in a chair. Following an injection of local anesthetic, a wire with a tiny barbed end is temporarily implanted in your breast to mark the biopsy site. Here, too, the physician relies on mammography to guide her. Next you are taken to the operating room, where a surgeon excises the tissue surrounding the wire. This is done under local anesthesia, either alone or in combination with a mild sedative. Then the wound is sutured closed and a dressing applied.

EXCISIONAL SURGICAL BIOPSY OF THE BREAST

Incisional surgical breast biopsy, to remove part of a lump, is performed only for extremely large abnormal breast masses that cannot be cut out completely. Far more common is excisional breast biopsy, also known as a *lumpectomy*, which can be either diagnostic or therapeutic, or both.

Typical setting:	**outpatient**
Anesthesia:	**local**
Sedation:	**usually**

Most women undergo surgical biopsies as outpatients. In the event your tissue sample reveals cancer, the oncologist will arrange for you to enter the hospital within a week or two for an operation to remove and biopsy lymph nodes under the arm, a frequent site of metastasis. This is done under general anesthesia and entails a stay of several days. There are instances when the initial outpatient procedure achieves a sufficiently clear margin that no additional breast tissue must be taken out. "But most of the time," says Dr. Norton, "patients need to have a wider excision."

> *See "Lumpectomy" under "Cancer of the Breast" in Chapter Six, "State of the Art: Your Treatment Options."*

HORMONE-RECEPTOR STATUS AND BREAST CANCER

"The most important factors in diagnosing and staging breast cancer are tumor size, tumor type, and lymph-node status," says Dr. Norton. "Then we color those with various other determinations such as grade, and whether the tumor contains estrogen receptor, progesterone receptor, or neither or both."

Hormone-receptor tests are conducted as part of the biopsy. A positive result indicates that the cancer needs estrogen and progesterone, the female hormones, in order to grow. At the same time, "the more hormone receptor a tumor contains," Dr. Norton says, "the more sensitive it is to hormone therapy," which may be given in place of or in addition to chemotherapy. "Also, tumors that contain a lot of estrogen and/or progesterone receptor tend to be more benign and have a slightly better prognosis."

HER-2 ONCOGENE STATUS AND BREAST CANCER

Breast-cancer cells that overexpress the HER-2 are extremely virulent. Initially, knowing a woman's HER-2 status was useful strictly as a predictor of the tumor's behavior. However, in 1998 came the arrival of Herceptin, a genetically engineered monoclonal-antibody therapy designed specifically to disrupt the gene's commands to reproduce. While not a cure, it can add months, and sometimes years, to the lives of patients who tested positive for the "bad" HER-2 gene.

PROLIFERATIVE FRACTION AND BREAST CANCER

In addition to testing the tumor tissue for hormone-receptor content and HER-2 status, the pathologist may assess the cells' *proliferative fraction.* It's not as complicated as it sounds. "Every cell goes through different cycles of growth," explains Dr. Jeffrey Abrams of the National Cancer Institute. "First there's a resting phase of growth, called *G0.* Next the cells move into phase *G1,* where they divide. Then they enter their most rapidly growing stage, the *S phase,* before they rest again.

"In breast cancer," he continues, "we've been able to measure how many tumor cells are in S phase. Studies show that the higher the percentage, the more aggressive the tumor."

Cancer of the Lung

You may undergo any number of these diagnostic procedures:
- Physical exam

Laboratory Tests
- Sputum cytology · Thoracentesis

Imaging Studies
- Chest X ray · CT scan

Biopsy
- Needle biopsy, guided by fluoroscopy or CT scan ·

Endoscopic biopsy performed as part of bronchoscopy or thoracoscopy ▪ Surgical chest biopsy (thoracotomy)

Any number of these staging procedures may be performed next:

Imaging Studies (TYPICALLY OF THE BONES, BRAIN AND SPINAL CORD, LIVER)

▪ Radionuclide scans of the bones, brain, and/or liver ▪ MRI scan ▪ CT scan

Endoscopic Exams

▪ Mediastinoscopy or mediastinotomy, to detect any spread to the lymph nodes in the chest compartment

---

Diagnosing and Staging Lung Cancer: What You Should Know

NEEDLE ASPIRATION BIOPSY OF THE LUNG

Aspiration biopsy of the lung is the initial choice for small lesions that are accessible by needle or are outside the range of bronchoscopy.

Typical setting:	outpatient
Anesthesia:	local
Sedation:	not required

Depending on the location of the abnormal growth, you are asked to lie prone or supine on an X-ray table or a CT scanner. The slender biopsy needle measures three to six inches long. After anesthetizing the skin and the muscle lining the chest wall, the doctor carefully inserts the needle until it has entered the mass. You are asked to hold your breath for several seconds each time she repositions the needle, checking her placement on a TV-type monitor or with still films.

Because the lung has no pain fibers, you won't feel the needle once it is all the way in. In fact, the most uncomfortable part of the procedure is the burning sensation from the injection of the anesthetic, which patients typically compare to a bee sting. You can anticipate a second sharp twinge of pain when the needle pierces the *pleura,* the double-layered membrane that envelops the lung. Next the doctor attaches a syringe, then aspirates cells and fluid, and withdraws the needle. In all, it remains in the lung no more than ninety seconds, and usually less.

One potential hazard of an aspiration biopsy is that the needle can collapse the lung like a balloon, causing air to accumulate in the space between the lung and the chest wall. This condition, called a *pneu-*

mothorax, usually subsides on its own, without the need for a chest tube to be inserted. To help avert a pneumothorax, afterward patients are asked to lie on the side that took the needle. If it was inserted through the back, you would lie faceup; through the chest, facedown. The less distance the needle has to travel through the lung to reach the suspected tumor, the less chance there is of the lung deflating.

As a precaution, many facilities will take an X ray immediately after the last tissue sample is taken, and again an hour or so later before letting patients go home. So although the biopsy itself usually takes no more than an hour, plan to spend about half a day there.

ENDOSCOPIC BIOPSIES OF THE LUNG

Bronchoscopy ▪ Thoracoscopy

There are two routes to sampling lung tissue endoscopically. *Bronchoscopy,* an outpatient procedure that requires local anesthesia, is optimal for biopsying tumors within the tracheobronchial tree or in the substance of the lung itself. For peripheral lesions near the lung's surface, which the bronchoscope cannot reach, a *thoracoscopic biopsy* may be the answer. After you've been put to sleep, two or three small incisions are made in the chest; the medical team then passes a camera and various tools through these ports. To enhance the view of the mass, the lung is deflated. Therefore, in order to be considered for thoracoscopy, you must be healthy enough to breathe on one lung.

See "Endoscopies of the Respiratory Tract," (page 199.)

SURGICAL CHEST BIOPSY (THORACOTOMY)

An open-lung biopsy is reserved for patients who would normally undergo a thoracoscopy but don't have adequate respiratory function. *Thoracotomy* affords such a clear view of the lung that nine in ten patients can be diagnosed by way of this operation alone.

As with thoracoscopy, a surgical chest biopsy is performed under general anesthesia and entails a hospital stay of two to five days.

Typical setting:	inpatient
Anesthesia:	general
Sedation:	not required
Hospital stay:	2–5 days

The major difference between the two is that thoracotomy leaves a two-inch scar, whereas the chest incisions for thoracoscopy are about half an inch each.

With the patient unconscious, a breathing tube is fed down the throat. The surgeon cuts through the chest wall and muscles, exposing the lung for tissue sampling. When all the specimens have been taken, a small incision is made for the placement of a temporary chest tube, which attaches to a machine that drains the pleural cavity. Then the wound is irrigated with *antibiotics* and sutured closed. The chest tube will remain in until just before discharge from the hospital.

The Informed Patient:
Diagnosed with Small-Cell Lung Cancer but You Never Smoked?
Time for a Second Opinion

An accurate cancer diagnosis is always crucial, but particularly so for lung cancer, where the approaches to therapy diverge like a fork in the road. Surgery, the primary treatment for non-small-cell carcinoma, has virtually no place in small-cell carcinoma, which is attacked with chemotherapy and radiation.

"Small-cell lung cancer occurs predominately in smokers," notes Dr. Kasi Sridhar of the Sylvester Comprehensive Cancer Center in Miami, Florida. "So if you've never smoked and receive a diagnosis of small-cell carcinoma, I would look further to make sure the diagnosis is correct." Small-cell lung cancer has such unique characteristics that "a qualified pathologist should have little difficulty in distinguishing it from non-small-cell lung cancer," Sridhar adds. Nevertheless, some tumors of the bronchi—the large tubes that convey air to and throughout the lungs—elude classification when viewed under a conventional light microscope. According to the National Cancer Institute, the greater magnification and resolution of an *electron-beam microscope* may make it easier for pathologists to differentiate between small-cell and non-small-cell cancers.

Now, what do you do with this information? If there appears to be some question regarding the diagnosis, find out from your attending physician whether or not the pathology lab examined the tissue sample using electron microscopy. The next step would be to arrange for a second opinion at a hospital or independent laboratory that does utilize this technology. Our recommendation: Get thee to a major medical center specializing in cancer.

See "Obtaining Medical Records" in Chapter Five, "The Next Step: Getting a Second Opinion and Deciding Where to Seek Treatment."

Cancer of the Colon or Rectum

You may undergo any number of these diagnostic procedures:
- Physical exam • Digital rectal exam

Laboratory Tests
- Fecal occult-blood test

Imaging Studies
- Lower GI series (barium enema)

Endoscopic Exams
- Sigmoidoscopy • Colonoscopy

Biopsy
- Endoscopic biopsy performed as part of sigmoidoscopy or colonoscopy

Any number of these staging procedures may be performed next:
Laboratory Tests
- Liver-function blood tests • CEA tumor-marker blood test

Imaging Studies (TYPICALLY OF THE LIVER AND LUNGS)
- Chest X ray • Ultrasound • CT scan

Diagnosing and Staging Cancer of the Colon or Rectum: What You Should Know

---

ENDOSCOPIC BIOPSIES OF THE COLORECTUM

Sigmoidoscopy • Colonoscopy

"Today a diagnosis of colorectal cancer is usually made based on a *sigmoidoscopy* or *colonoscopy,*" says Dr. Peter Rosen of the Jonsson Comprehensive Cancer Center at UCLA, "with biopsies obtained at the time of either procedure." Still, your gastroenterologist may schedule a *lower GI series* first, on the grounds that it is less invasive and less costly. The imaging study is not nearly as accurate, however, nor can it obtain biopsies. Should the barium enema prompt any questions, the next step is an endoscopy.

See "Endoscopies of the Lower GI Tract," (page 200.)

Lymphomas

You may undergo any number of these diagnostic procedures:
- Physical exam

Laboratory Tests
- Complete blood count (CBC), to detect abnormally high levels of neutrophils and eosinophils, two types of white blood cells

Biopsy
- Surgical biopsy of an enlarged lymph node

Any number of these staging procedures may be performed next:

<table>
<tr><td>

What's an Elevated Sedimentation Rate?

The normal *erythrocyte sedimentation rate* (ESR) ranges from 10mm/hr to 20mm/hr (translation: in a test tube of blood, ten to twenty millimeters of red cells settled to the bottom after one hour), denoting no discernible active inflammatory disease in the body. Each stage of Hodgkin's disease is further divided by symptoms into A and B. An ESR of 50mm/hr or higher tells the doctor you have an inflammatory disease, which may indicate the B group of symptoms: weight loss, fever, and night sweats.

</td><td>

Laboratory Tests
- Erythrocyte sedimentation rate (ESR) blood test • Lumbar puncture (spinal tap), to detect spread to the central nervous system

Imaging Studies (TYPICALLY OF THE CHEST, BONES, LIVER, SPLEEN, LYMPHATIC SYSTEM)
- Chest X ray • CT scan • Radionuclide scan • Lymphangiogram of the lymphatic system • Ultrasound • MRI scan

Biopsy
- Core-needle biopsy of the liver • Bone-marrow aspiration biopsy • Bone-marrow core-needle biopsy • Surgical biopsies of the liver and lymph nodes as part of exploratory laparotomy

</td></tr>
</table>

Diagnosing and Staging Lymphomas: What You Should Know

SURGICAL BIOPSY OF THE LYMPH NODES

In order to positively identify lymphoma, the pathologist needs to examine the architecture of an entire node, not just cells, thus ruling out a needle biopsy. As Dr. Anil Tulpule of the Kenneth Norris Jr. Comprehensive Cancer Center in Los Angeles explains, the surgeon usually takes out a single enlarged peripheral lymph node, "whichever one is the most accessible." The only time the operation would be done on an inpatient basis, he adds, "is if the node was located deep within the abdomen."

Needle biopsies do come into play once the disease is diagnosed, to see if the liver or bone marrow is affected.

Typical setting:	outpatient
Anesthesia:	local
Sedation:	not required

See "Needle Biopsy of the Liver," (page 162,) and "Bone-Marrow Aspiration and Bone-Marrow Core-Needle Biopsy," (page 203.)

EXPLORATORY LAPAROTOMY

Exploratory abdominal surgery is used to stage Hodgkin's disease (not non-Hodgkin's lymphomas) but only if clinical evaluations have put your stage at I or II. The reason, explains Dr. Tulpule, is that "patients with stage III or stage IV Hodgkin's disease are treated with systemic chemotherapy, whereas we usually use radiation alone for stages I and II." Radiation is local therapy, meaning it kills only

Typical setting:	inpatient
Anesthesia:	general
Sedation:	not required
Hospital stay:	2–3 days

those cancer cells within range of its beam. At stage III or IV, the cancer has spread far enough that the only way to get a crack at vanquishing every malignant cell is to deliver anticancer drugs directly into the bloodstream.

"Therefore, if we've staged a patient at I or II," says Dr. Tulpule, a hematologic oncologist, "we want to be absolutely sure. Because studies have shown that quite a few patients who undergo an exploratory laparotomy see their stage upgraded to III or IV."

During the operation, the surgeon removes all suspicious lymph nodes, as well as the entire spleen, and takes larger biopsies from the left and right lobes of the liver than could be obtained through a core-needle biopsy. In addition, "if a woman is of child-bearing age, the ovaries are shifted out of the expected field of radiation," to preserve her fertility.

Cancer of the Bladder

You may undergo any number of these diagnostic procedures:
- Physical exam
- Digital rectal exam and/or vaginal exam

Laboratory Tests

- Urine tests, to detect blood or abnormal cells

Imaging Studies

- Intravenous pyelogram (IVP) of the kidneys and ureters

Endoscopic Exams

- Cystoscopy

Biopsy

- Endoscopic biopsy performed as part of cystoscopy

Any number of these staging procedures may be performed next:

Imaging Studies (TYPICALLY OF THE ABDOMEN AND PELVIC REGION)

- CT scan ▪ Ultrasound ▪ MRI scan

Diagnosing and Staging Bladder Cancer: What You Should Know

IN GENERAL

Compared to many forms of cancer, diagnosing carcinoma of the bladder involves relatively few tests. *Urine cytology,* to detect malignant cells in the urine, is done as a matter of course, but it is accurate only about half the time. From there your urologist may want to order an X ray called an *intravenous pyelogram* or proceed to a *cystoscopy,* in order to view the bladder directly. "If he sees an area that looks like a tumor or an area of the bladder wall that appears abnormal," explains Dr. Michael Cooper, "he can biopsy tissue right then and there through the scope."

See "Cystoscopy," page 201.

Melanoma

You may undergo any number of these diagnostic procedures:

- A head-to-toe dermatologic exam by a dermatologist or a dermatologic oncologist

Biopsy

- Excisional surgical biopsy

Any number of these staging procedures may be performed next:
- Physical exam

Laboratory Tests
- Blood tests

Imaging Studies (TYPICALLY OF THE LUNGS, LIVER, BONES, BRAIN, LYMPH NODES)

- Chest X ray • Radionuclide scans of the liver, bones, brain, lymph nodes

---

Diagnosing and Staging Melanoma: What You Should Know

EXCISIONAL BIOPSY OF THE SKIN

Typical setting:	outpatient
Anesthesia:	local
Sedation:	not required

Because melanoma is staged based on thickness as well as whether or not it has spread, it's essential that the entire lesion be excised. "We can make the diagnosis based on biopsying just a portion of it," explains Dr. Allan Oseroff of the Roswell Park Cancer Institute, "but we really want to have the whole melanoma, to know where it is deepest."

When the disease is discovered early, this procedure rarely leaves a scar. In the definitive surgery to treat melanoma, the surgeon removes the lesion plus a rim of normal tissue measuring 1 centimeter to 3 centimeters, "depending on the size of the lesion," says Dr. Oseroff. (That's ½ inch to 1¼ inches.) For an excisional skin biopsy, "most of the time we'll take a *conservative margin,* sometimes even less than 1 centimeter. Then if pathology confirms the diagnosis, we'll reexcise the area, rather than doing it in one step and leaving a scar that may not be necessary." Thin melanomas, he notes, may not require the second surgery.

Cancer of the Uterus (Endometrial Cancer)

You may undergo any number of these diagnostic procedures:
- Physical exam • Pelvic exam

Laboratory Tests
- Pap smear
  - *Performed as part of a pelvic exam but not considered reliable for detecting endometrial cancer*

Biopsy

- Aspiration biopsy ▪ Dilation and curettage (D&C)

Any number of these staging procedures may be performed next:
Laboratory Tests

- Blood tests

Imaging Studies (TYPICALLY OF THE ABDOMEN AND LUNGS)

- Chest X ray ▪ CT scan ▪ Ultrasound

Diagnosing and Staging Endometrial Cancer: What You Should Know

ASPIRATION BIOPSY OF THE ENDOMETRIUM

In this procedure, also referred to as *suction curettage,* the gynecologist inserts a thin tube through the vagina and into the uterus, then suctions out a small amount of tissue. Dr. Michael Hogan, chief of gynecologic oncology at Philadelphia's Fox Chase Cancer Center, calls the procedure "relatively pain free." At most, you may experience cramping during and afterward.

Typical setting:	outpatient
Anesthesia:	local; not required
Sedation:	not required

DILATION AND CURETTAGE (D&C)

Most women tolerate an aspiration biopsy well. However, a condition called *cervical stenosis* may make this method of endometrial sampling physically impossible. Cervical stenosis, a narrowing of the cervix, "is a problem related to age and estrogen deficiency," Dr. Hogan explains. Though the suctioning instrument is only two millimeters in diameter, "we may still have difficulty getting it inside the canal. Those women would require a D&C."

Typical setting:	outpatient
Anesthesia:	local or general
Sedation:	not required

Dilation and curettage uses tiny graduated rods to expand the cervical opening, after which the gynecologist gently scrapes tissue from the uterine lining with a spoon-shaped *curette.* Increasingly, D&C is performed through a flexible fiber-optic *hysteroscope.* Some cases, says Dr. Hogan, call for local anesthesia, and "there are times when we even have to go to the operating room to do it."

SCREENING PROCEDURES FOR OTHER CANCERS
Mammogram ▪ Lower GI Series ▪ Sigmoidoscopy

"Most women with this cancer are fifty or older," Dr. Hogan points out. "Once we've got a diagnosis, we generally try to make sure the patient has been screened for the other cancers common in that age group. She'll have a mammogram, if she hasn't had one in the prior year, to rule out any concomitant breast cancer. Many of the women we see haven't had a colorectal-cancer screening, so we'll do a contrast barium enema, then a sigmoidoscopy at the time of the operative procedure. Assuming those tests are negative, the patient will undergo her surgery." Endometrial cancer is typically treated by removing the uterus and the cervix, and often the ovaries, fallopian tubes, and possibly the upper portion of the vagina.

See "Mammogram," page 189; "Lower GI Series," page 195; and "Endoscopies of the Lower GI Tract," page 200.

HORMONE-RECEPTOR STATUS AND ENDOMETRIAL CANCER
Analyzing the biopsy specimen for hormone receptors yields important information about the cancer. "Studies show that endometrial tumors with high levels of progesterone tend to be well differentiated and less invasive, and have a better prognosis," says Dr. Hogan. One study, conducted at the University of North Carolina, cited progesterone-receptor content as "the single most important prognostic indicator" for women with early-stage disease. In the study, more than nine in ten of the participants with progesterone-receptor levels of 100 or higher were still alive after three years, as compared to fewer than four in ten of the women with receptor levels below 100.

Hormone-receptivity status doesn't influence the strategy for treating endometrial cancer to the degree that it does for breast cancer, another tumor frequently spurred by hormones. It is, however, a factor in metastatic or recurrent disease, when surgery is no longer an option in most cases. "If a patient had a high progesterone-receptor level," says Dr. Hogan, "it would then make sense to put her on a progestational drug."

Leukemia

You may undergo any number of these diagnostic procedures:
- Physical exam
  - ◆ *The doctor feels for swelling in the liver, the spleen, and the lymph nodes under the arms, in the neck, and in the groin.*

Laboratory Tests
- Complete blood count (CBC), to detect abnormally high levels of white cells and abnormally low levels of red cells and platelets ▪ Uric acid blood test, to detect an abnormally high level of uric acid

Biopsy
- Bone-marrow aspiration biopsy

Any number of these staging procedures may be performed next:
Laboratory Tests
- Lumbar puncture (spinal tap), to test for spread to the central nervous system

Imaging Studies
- Chest X ray

Diagnosing and Staging Leukemia: What You Should Know

BLOOD TESTS AND BONE-MARROW ASPIRATION BIOPSY

Leukemia frequently signals its presence by inducing some abnormality of the blood. Blood tests can pick up the disease, but in order to pinpoint the type of leukemia, "bone-marrow aspiration biopsy is routinely needed," says Dr. Fred Appelbaum of the Fred Hutchinson Cancer Research Center. In this outpatient procedure, a needle is inserted into the rear of either hip, or sometimes the breastbone, and a small sample of marrow withdrawn.

Additional laboratory analysis called *immunophenotyping* is performed on leukemic cells from either the bloodstream or the marrow. Each type of leukemia cell wears distinctive proteins *(antigens)* on its surface. Staining the antigens with colored dyes further helps the pathologist identify the form of leukemia.

Chronic Leukemias

One cubic millimeter of a healthy person's blood contains about four thousand granulocytes, the white blood cells that mature in the marrow. In someone with chronic myeloid leukemia (CML), it's not unusual for the white-cell count to soar to 1 million per cubic millimeter, a condition you may hear referred to as *leukocytosis.* CML also tends to depress the number of red blood cells.

The telltale indicator of this disease is a chromosomal defect called the *Philadelphia (Ph) chromosome,* seen in 90 percent of CML patients. About one in three adults with acute lymphocytic leukemia (ALL) also possess the aberrant chromosome, which is usually more detectable in a bone-marrow biopsy than in a blood sample.

Chronic lymphocytic leukemia (CLL) also inundates the bloodstream with white cells, but in this case with lymphocytes, the type of white cell that matures in lymphoid tissue, not in marrow. Whereas normally a cubic millimeter of blood holds roughly 2,500 lymphocytes, a person with CLL will have more than 15,000. The medical term for this is *lymphocytosis.*

CLL primarily afflicts men and women fifty or older. In people of that age group, the sighting of three antigens unique to chronic lymphocytic leukemia is often sufficient evidence for diagnosing the disease.

Acute Leukemias

Acute leukemias typically drive down the blood's numbers of normal white cells, platelets, and *hemoglobin,* the protein in red cells that transports oxygen; a blood test may also reveal the intrusion of immature blast cells. Yet as many as one in ten patients diagnosed with acute myeloid leukemia (AML) or acute lymphocytic leukemia (ALL) have normal levels of all three blood components. Biopsying the bone marrow, therefore, is the definitive method of identifying the disease.

The blast-cell content of normal marrow is less than 5 percent. In a person with either AML or ALL, anywhere from 30 to 100 percent of the marrow may be taken up by these undeveloped cells. Because the number of abnormal cells isn't always uniform within the marrow, several specimens may have to be sampled in order to accurately evaluate the extent of the disease.

As noted above, the flawed Philadelphia chromosome turns up in the marrow of about one-third of adult ALL patients. Another characteristic of acute lymphocytic leukemia, revealed during immunophenotyping, is the presence of an antigen known as the *"common ALL antigen"* (CALLA, for short) on roughly half the lymphocytes. When the marrow cells house rod-shaped granules called *Auer rods,* the pathologist knows he's looking at acute myeloid leukemia.

> *See "Bone-Marrow Aspiration and Bone-Marrow Core-Needle Biopsy," page 203, and "Blood Disorders" in Chapter Eight, "Take Control: Managing Symptoms, Side Effects, and Complications."*

Cancer of the Kidney (Renal-Cell Carcinoma)

You may undergo any number of these diagnostic procedures:
- Physical exam

Laboratory Tests
- Complete blood count (CBC), to detect an abnormally high level of red blood cells ▪ Blood chemistry, to detect abnormally high levels of calcium and the enzymes alanine transaminase (ALT) and alkaline phosphatase (ALP) ▪ Urine tests, to detect blood or abnormal cells

Imaging Studies
- Intravenous pyelogram (IVP) of the kidneys and ureters ▪ CT scan ▪ Ultrasound ▪ Arteriogram ▪ MRI scan ▪ Nephrotomogram

Any number of these staging procedures may be performed next:
Imaging Studies (TYPICALLY OF THE LUNGS, LIVER, LYMPH NODES, MAJOR BLOOD VESSELS)
- Chest X ray ▪ CT scan ▪ MRI scan

Diagnosing and Staging Kidney Cancer: What You Should Know

IS A NEEDLE BIOPSY OF THE KIDNEY NECESSARY?

No, according to Dr. Jim Mohler of the UNC Lineberger Comprehensive Cancer Center. "The reason," he explains, "is that if a person has a solid mass in the kidney, 90 percent of the time it's kidney cancer. If we performed a biopsy and it came back negative for cancer, we usually wouldn't believe it, and so biopsies are very rarely done." This is a point to raise with your physician should he schedule a renal biopsy to verify a suspected malignancy.

THE ROLE OF MRI SCANNING IN STAGING RENAL-CELL CARCINOMA

A chest X ray and a CT scan generally reveal whether or not kidney cancer has disseminated to the lungs or the liver, the two most common sites of metastasis. "If there's no evidence of distant spread," says Dr. Mohler, "next we want to know if the tumor is resectable. This involves evaluating the regional lymph nodes and more importantly, the major vascular structures.

"About 10 percent of these cancers," he explains, "will grow 'tongues' of tumor through the renal vein and into the *inferior vena cava,* and sometimes as far as the heart." The inferior vena cava is the trunklike vein that returns blood from the lower half of the body to the heart. "This can be addressed with a high-quality CT scan, an MRI, or duplex ultrasonography. All are quite reliable in ruling out any vascular involvement."

Cancer of the Pancreas

You may undergo any number of these diagnostic procedures:
- Physical exam

Laboratory Tests
- Glucose blood test, to detect an abnormally high level of sugar in the blood
- Liver-function blood tests
  - *Depending on the levels of certain chemical markers, these tests point the doctor in one of two directions. Either the problem is due to liver damage from a disease such as hepatitis, or it is the result of obstruction caused by gallstones or a tumor.*

- CEA and CA-19-9 tumor-marker blood tests

Imaging Studies
- CT scan ▪ Ultrasound ▪ MRI scan ▪ Percutaneous transhepatic cholangiogram

Endoscopic Exams

- Endoscopic retrograde cholangiopancreatogram (ERCP), with or without a brush biopsy ▪ Laparoscopy

Any number of these staging procedures may be performed next:

Imaging Studies (TYPICALLY OF THE LUNGS, LIVER, INTESTINES, LYMPH NODES, BLOOD VESSELS)

- Chest X ray ▪ CT scan ▪ Angiogram of the blood vessels ▪ MRI scan

Endoscopic Exams

- Laparoscopy ▪ Endoscopic ultrasound

Biopsy

- Needle biopsy of the liver

Surgical Procedures

- Exploratory laparotomy at the time of definitive surgery to remove part or all of the pancreas

---

Diagnosing and Staging Pancreatic Cancer: What You Should Know

---

IS A NEEDLE BIOPSY OF THE PANCREAS NECESSARY?

"Most medical centers would not percutaneously biopsy the pancreas," says Dr. Charles Yeo of the Johns Hopkins University School of Medicine. "There definitely are places that do, and I think they're foolish to do so unless they are contemplating chemoradiation prior to the operation." One reason for not doing so, he explains, is that "in most cases, the knowledge gained from a preoperative percutaneous biopsy does not alter our ultimate surgical decision-making."

Besides, says Dr. Yeo, if a mass in the pancreas is visible by way of imaging or endoscopy and it appears solid, "it ought to come out, whatever it is, so long as the patient is fit and a reasonable risk for the surgery.

"Not only is a biopsy unnecessary," he continues, "it can be risky." It is believed that the needle can break the tumor capsule, spreading malignant cells throughout the abdomen. "There are also cases of patients having fatal episodes of bleeding as a result of the biopsy." One risk-free technique is to harvest cells with a tiny brush during an endoscopic exam called an *endoscopic retrograde cholangiopancreatogram* (ERCP) in which a flexible fiber-optic tube is passed down the throat, through the digestive tract, and into the pancreas. But this is rarely done.

Nearly half of all men and women with pancreatic cancer will be diagnosed with metastatic disease, usually to the liver, at which point strategy shifts from attempting to treat the cancer to keeping the patient comfortable. You could say that stage IV pancreatic cancer is diagnosed "backward." The liver, in contrast to the pancreas, is easily accessible by needle. Therefore, if tests indicate a lesion in both the pancreas and the liver, a needle liver biopsy is performed and the cells analyzed to see if they are pancreatic-cancer cells.

See "Needle Biopsy of the Liver," page 162.

EXPLORATORY LAPAROTOMY

With no biopsy of the pancreas to rely on, exploratory *laparotomy* is the only way to definitively diagnose, stage, and resect pancreatic cancer that hasn't metastasized to distant sites. This is done during the surgical treatment to resect part or all of the organ, never as a separate operation.

Typical setting:	inpatient
Anesthesia:	general
Sedation:	yes
Hospital stay:	6–12 days

*See "Surgery" under "Cancer of the Pancreas" in Chapter Six,
"State of the Art: Your Treatment Options."*

EXPLORATORY LAPAROSCOPY

The less invasive *laparoscopy* is performed infrequently; mainly to examine tumors of the left side of the pancreas (the body or tail), which make up one in four pancreatic cancers. The purpose is to avoid unnecessary major surgery. While all stage IV pancreatic cancers are considered inoperable, patients with tumors of the right side (the head of the organ)

Typical setting:	inpatient
Anesthesia:	general
Sedation:	yes
Hospital stay:	0–2 days

sometimes require bypass surgery because the lesion is blocking the bile duct—inducing jaundice—or the stomach.

Left-side tumors do not obstruct either route, though according to Dr. Yeo, many spread to the liver. "Therefore, we'll usually do a laparoscopy," he says, "simply because if a patient is found to have metastatic disease, no further surgery is necessary. By diagnosing stage IV pancreatic cancer with laparoscopy, we've spared them a large laparotomy incision, and they spend only one or two nights in the hospital."

Cancer of the Ovary

You may undergo any number of these diagnostic procedures:
- Physical exam ▪ Pelvic exam

Laboratory Tests
- Pap smear
  ◆ *Performed as part of a pelvic exam but not considered reliable for detecting ovarian cancer.*

- CA-125 tumor-marker blood test

Imaging Studies (TYPICALLY OF THE OVARIES, LIVER, COLON, RECTUM, KIDNEYS, URETERS)
- Transvaginal ultrasound ▪ CT scan ▪ Lower GI series (barium enema) of the colon and rectum ▪ Intravenous pyelogram (IVP) of the kidneys and ureters

Any number of these staging procedures may be performed next:
Surgical Procedures
- Exploratory laparotomy at the time of definitive surgery to remove the cancerous ovary(ies)

Diagnosing and Staging Ovarian Cancer: What You Should Know

EXPLORATORY LAPAROTOMY

Unless ovarian cancer has spread beyond the abdomen, exploratory *laparotomy* is the sole method for assessing the extent of the disease. The operation has a dual purpose: to definitively diagnose and stage as well as to treat.

Ovarian tumors are never biopsied with a needle or cut into, because doing so may allow malignant cells to escape. After the surgeon makes an incision in the abdomen, the ovary

Typical setting:	inpatient
Anesthesia:	general
Sedation:	not required
Hospital stay:	5 days

(or ovaries) in question is removed intact and sent off to the pathology lab. If it tests positive, the least extensive surgery calls for taking out the adjacent fallopian tube. But usually, by the time ovarian cancer is discovered, it has spread to other organs within the pelvis. In the most common operation, the surgeon takes out both ovaries and fallopian tubes, plus the uterus and cervix. The one situation where the cancerous ovary can possibly be preserved, and only the tumor excised, is if the patient is a young woman with a borderline or low-grade cancer.

"A number of other factors enter into surgical staging," says Dr. Larry Copeland of the Arthur G. James Cancer Hospital and Research Institute. "We sample the linings of the pelvis and the abdomen, in various areas, and lymph nodes. We often remove the *omentum,* which is a pad of fat that hangs down from the stomach over the upper colon.

"We also do *cellular washings* from different parts of the abdominal and pelvic cavities. We fill a wide-barrel bulb syringe with saline [a saltwater solution], squirt it into an area, aspirate it out with a syringe, put it in a container, and send it to cytology." There it is analyzed for evidence of malignant cells.

See "Cancer of the Ovary" in Chapter Six, "State of the Art: Your Treatment Options."

Cancer of the Stomach

You may undergo any number of these diagnostic procedures:
- Physical exam

Laboratory Tests
- Fecal occult-blood test • Complete blood count (CBC), to detect an abnormally low level of red blood cells

Imaging Studies
- Upper GI series (barium swallow)

Endoscopic Exams
- Gastroscopy

Biopsy
- Endoscopic biopsy performed as part of gastroscopy

Any number of these staging procedures may be performed next:

Imaging Studies (TYPICALLY OF THE LIVER, LUNGS, PANCREAS, SPLEEN, BONES, LYMPH NODES)

- CT scan - Chest X ray - MRI scan - Ultrasound

Biopsy

- Exploratory laparotomy at the time of definitive surgery to remove part or all of the stomach

---

Diagnosing and Staging Stomach Cancer: What You Should Know

IN GENERAL

In the past, if you were suspected of having a mass in the stomach, one of your first stops would be the radiology department for an upper GI series. "These days," says Dr. Harinder Garewal of the University of Arizona Cancer Center, "it's more common to send a patient directly to endoscopy instead. If we look in the stomach and find a mass, we biopsy it right then and there through the scope." An endoscopic exam of the stomach, or *gastroscopy,* is more than 90 percent accurate in diagnosing gastric malignancies.

Sometimes stomach cancer cannot be thoroughly staged until the operation is performed to remove part or all of the stomach, at which time the surgeon takes samples of neighboring lymph nodes and possibly other organs. The normal preoperative workup would certainly include a CT scan, Dr. Garewal says, "primarily of the upper abdomen, to see whether or not there's any involvement of the nodes or the liver." Since the lungs and the esophagus are also common sites of metastasis, "almost all stomach-cancer patients will have a CT scan of the chest, or at least a conventional chest X ray. Staging beyond that would be driven by symptoms. If the patient had headaches or pain in the bones, we would want to scan those areas too."

See "Endoscopies of the Upper GI Tract," page 199.

Cancer of the Liver

You may undergo any number of these diagnostic procedures:
- Physical exam

Laboratory Tests
- Liver-function blood tests ▪ Alpha-fetoprotein tumor-marker blood test

Imaging Studies
- CT scan ▪ Radionuclide scan ▪ Angiogram of the blood vessels

Biopsy
- Needle biopsy

Surgical Procedures
- Laparoscopy

Any number of these staging procedures may be performed next:
Imaging Studies (TYPICALLY OF THE LUNGS, BONES, LYMPH NODES)
- Chest X ray ▪ CT scan ▪ MRI scan ▪ Radionuclide bone scan

Diagnosing and Staging Liver Cancer: What You Should Know

LIVER-FUNCTION BLOOD TESTS

"The term 'liver-function tests' is a misnomer," says Dr. Ted Lawrence, a liver-cancer specialist at the University of Michigan Comprehensive Cancer Center. These blood tests don't assess the liver's efficiency. Dr. Lawrence explains that what they do is "distinguish between the two main causes of liver dysfunction," those being an obstruction, as from a tumor in the liver or gallstones lodged in the bile ducts, and damage brought on by liver diseases such as hepatitis.

Liver-function tests measure the blood content of several liver enzymes and *bilirubin,* the orange pigment that combines with an acid in the liver to form the pigment excreted in bile fluid. Bilirubin is classified as being either *conjugated (direct)* or *unconjugated (indirect).* Unconjugated bilirubin has yet to enter the liver; conjugated bilirubin has already passed through and merged with the acid. Elevated amounts of conjugated bilirubin and the enzyme *alkaline phosphatase* in the circulation point to a blockage, which the physician will then attempt to X-ray. "Usually," says Dr. Lawrence, "a CT scan is the definitive test for showing the lesion."

ALPHA-FETOPROTEIN (AFP) TUMOR-MARKER BLOOD TEST

More than most of the tumor markers associated with other cancers, the *alpha-fetoprotein blood test* is a reliable indicator of liver carcinoma. As many as seven in ten men and women diagnosed with the disease have increased levels of AFP. According to Dr. Lawrence, "There are doctors who say that if the alpha-fetoprotein content is greater than 1,000* and the clinical setting is right"—meaning the physical exam, other lab tests, and imaging studies all suggest liver cancer—"nothing else other than a hepatoma can produce that constellation." Some physicians, in fact, will forgo a liver biopsy and diagnose a patient on that basis alone "if they think there's any danger in performing the procedure. But the standard," he says, "would be to do a biopsy."

NEEDLE BIOPSY OF THE LIVER

For a needle biopsy of the liver, you lie on your back. "Once the skin and muscle have been numbed," Dr. Lawrence explains, "a syringe needle is

Typical setting:	outpatient
Anesthesia:	local
Sedation:	not required

introduced into the tumor—usually under guidance from a CT scan or ultrasound—and a small specimen removed. While the liver itself has no pain sensors, the sac that surrounds it does. My patients frequently tell me they feel a 'stabbing' sensation the moment the needle enters the surface of the liver."

Cancers of the Lip and Oral Cavity

You may undergo any number of these diagnostic procedures:
- Oral exam using a mirror and lights
  - *The dentist or physician also uses his fingers to probe the inside of the mouth.*

*Alpha-fetoprotein is measured in international units per milliliter (IU/ml).

Biopsy

- Incisional or excisional surgical biopsy

Any number of these staging procedures may be performed next:
- Physical exam
  - *The doctor feels the neck for swollen lymph nodes.*

Imaging Studies (TYPICALLY OF THE HEAD AND NECK, LUNGS, LIVER, BONES)

- Dental X rays ▪ X rays of the head and chest ▪ CT scan ▪ Ultrasound ▪ MRI scan ▪ Radionuclide scans of the liver and/or bones

---

Diagnosing and Staging Lip and Oral-Cavity Cancers: What You Should Know

---

INCISIONAL SURGICAL BIOPSY OF THE ORAL CAVITY

It is typically a dentist who notices a lump or abnormal area in the mouth during a dental exam, then sends the patient to an *oral surgeon* or an *ear, nose, and throat surgeon* for a biopsy.

Typical setting:	outpatient
Anesthesia:	local
Sedation:	not required

Sometimes the surgeon can simply scrape enough cells from the surface of the oral cavity for the cancer to be diagnosed on the basis of cell cytology. "The problem with that," notes Dr. Rocco Addante, an oral and maxillofacial surgeon at the Norris Cotton Cancer Center, "is that it's not always definitive. The gold standard is a tissue sample."

Unless your doctor is reasonably certain the lesion is malignant, he will perform an incisional biopsy, cutting out a small piece as opposed to the entire growth. An ulcer inside the mouth may be cancer and thus require a *wide excision:* the removal of the tumor as well as a section of normal tissue around it. "But the ulcer could also be caused by a chronic irritation or many other things that merit only a minimal excision," Dr. Addante explains. The prevailing wisdom is that it is preferable for a patient to perhaps return for wide-excision oral surgery in the event the specimen does contain cancer than to lose tissue from the tongue, lip, or gums unnecessarily.

EXCISIONAL SURGICAL BIOPSY OF THE ORAL CAVITY

"On the other hand," Dr. Addante continues, "if someone has a smooth, round, firm mass the size of a chickpea protruding from the inside of the cheek, we might very well be tempted to excise it, because to do an incisional biopsy would only disrupt this well-contained lump." In the case of salivary-gland cancer, he adds, no further surgery may be warranted. Other times the surgeon has to schedule a second operation, to widen the margin. Barring complications, excisional biopsy is often a same-day procedure.

Typical setting:	outpatient or inpatient
Anesthesia:	general
Sedation:	not required

Cancer of the Thyroid

You may undergo any number of these diagnostic procedures:
- Physical exam

Laboratory Tests
- Thyroid-function blood tests • Comprehensive metabolic panel • Thyroglobulin-antibody blood test and thyroglobulin tumor-marker blood test (papillary and follicular thyroid cancers only) • Calcitonin blood test, to detect an abnormally high level of the hormone calcitonin (medullary thyroid cancer only)

Imaging Studies
- Radionuclide scan/iodine uptake test • Ultrasound

Biopsy
- Needle biopsy

Any number of these staging procedures may be performed next:
Imaging Studies (TYPICALLY OF THE LUNGS, BONES, NECK, THE CHEST COMPARTMENT KNOWN AS THE MEDIASTINUM)
- CT scan • MRI scan • Chest X ray • PET scan • Radionuclide bone scan

Diagnosing and Staging Thyroid Cancer: What You Should Know

NEEDLE BIOPSY OF THE THYROID

Because the thyroid gland sits just beneath the surface of the skin, local anesthesia usually isn't administered for a needle biopsy, unless you request it. The procedure is simple: With the patient lying on her back, the skin at the base of the throat is cleansed and disinfected, a needle is inserted into the mass in the thy-

Typical setting:	outpatient
Anesthesia:	not required
Sedation:	not required

roid, and cells are withdrawn. Dr. T. S. Greaves, the pathologist who evaluates most of the thyroid biopsies performed at the Los Angeles County/University of Southern California Medical Center, compares the fleeting discomfort you may feel to that of "having blood drawn; nothing more."

(Adult) Cancers of the Brain

You may undergo any number of these diagnostic procedures:

- Physical exam
- Neurological exam
  - ◆ *The neurologist typically tests: (1) eye movements, eye reflexes, and pupil reaction; (2) reflexes; (3) hearing; (4) sense of touch; (5) movement; (6) balance and coordination; (7) mental capacity and memory; (8) strength; (9) symmetry of the face.*

Laboratory Tests

- Lumbar puncture (spinal tap)
  - ◆ *A lumbar puncture, in which a needle is used to withdraw a small amount of cerebrospinal fluid from the spinal cavity in the lower back, is never performed initially if the doctor suspects a brain tumor may be causing pressure to build up within the skull.*

Imaging Studies

- MRI scan ▪ CT scan ▪ PET scan ▪ Radionuclide scan ▪ Angiogram of the brain's blood vessels

Other Studies

- Electroencephalogram (EEG)

Biopsy

- Stereotactic biopsy

Any number of these staging procedures may be performed next:

Laboratory Tests

- Lumbar puncture (spinal tap), if not done previously

Imaging Studies

- MRI scan of the spine

Diagnosing and Staging Brain Cancers: What You Should Know

STEREOTACTIC BIOPSY OF THE BRAIN

Because of their location, some brain tumors cannot be sampled safely. For instance, when faced with an apparent brain-stem glioma, many times a physician will identify the cancer solely from symptoms and a CT scan or an MRI scan. Of the two imaging studies, "MRI is clearly the better modality," asserts Dr. Michael Gruber of the Kaplan Cancer Center at New York University Medical Center.

Typical setting:	inpatient
Anesthesia:	not required
Sedation:	yes
Hospital stay:	2 days

Most brain tumors, however, can be biopsied, due in part to the expanding use of stereotactic instrumentation, which affords access to almost anywhere in the brain. In a *stereotactic biopsy,* Dr. Gruber explains, "the patient has a halo-shaped metal frame attached to his skull bone. He is then sedated and taken to an operating room with a CT scanner. By putting patients in the scanner, we can get a three-dimensional co-ordinate for the surgeon, who drills a tiny hole in the skull, inserts a needle precisely, and takes the biopsy from the exact area we're interested in." In contrast, surgical biopsy, also referred to as an "open" biopsy, calls for removing part of the skull and cutting out a small piece of brain tissue.

In addition to accuracy, Dr. Gruber says that another major advantage of stereotactic, or "closed," biopsy is safety. The rate of complications, primarily hemorrhaging from the needle site, is around 1 percent.

Plan to spend one night in the hospital, although some medical centers now perform stereotactic brain biopsy on an outpatient basis.

Multiple Myeloma

You may undergo any number of these diagnostic procedures:
- Physical exam

Laboratory Tests

- M protein tumor-marker blood test • Urinalysis to measure the level of M protein

Imaging Studies

- Whole-body X rays of the entire skeleton

Biopsy

- Bone-marrow aspiration biopsy or bone-marrow core-needle biopsy

Any number of these staging procedures may be performed next:
Laboratory Tests

- Tumor-marker blood test to measure *beta-2 microglobulin,* a protein shed by B lymphocytes, the cells that become plasma cells
  - *Beta-2 microglobulin, a normal product of cells, will be abnormally elevated in a person with multiple myeloma. The higher the level, the more severe the disease.*
- Complete blood count (CBC), to detect abnormally low levels of red cells, hematocrit, white cells, and platelets
- Calcium blood test, to detect an abnormally high level of calcium
- Kidney-function blood tests
  - *Heightened concentrations of the substances creatinine and blood urea nitrogen (BUN) in the blood denote impaired renal function.*

Imaging Studies (OF THE BONES)

- Whole-body X rays of the entire skeleton • Whole-body CT scan of the entire skeleton • MRI scan of a particular bone or area

Diagnosing and Staging Multiple Myeloma: What You Should Know

M PROTEIN BLOOD TEST

Since most people with multiple myeloma first complain of back pain, they are usually sent to radiology straightaway. Seventy percent of the time, X rays will show holes in the bones (lytic lesions), prompting a blood test to detect the monoclonal protein secreted by both benign and malignant plasma cells. There are several different M proteins, but each patient has one specific type. By far the most common is *immunoglobulin G,* abbreviated as *IgG;* the next most common is *IgA.*

The sample undergoes a process called *electrophoresis,* in which an electric current tugs at the assorted proteins floating in the blood serum. Then the results are charted. If you have multiple myeloma, the M protein will appear as a sharp spike, indicating an abnormally high level. A positive blood test, in combination with one of the other factors spelled out below, is enough to diagnose the disease.

M PROTEIN URINE TEST

Bence-Jones proteins frequently turn up in the urine, which is also subjected to electrophoresis.

BONE-MARROW ASPIRATION BIOPSY/BONE-MARROW CORE-NEEDLE BIOPSY

The procedure for withdrawing marrow from the hip, also used to diagnose leukemia and to stage lymphomas, is described in this chapter's glossary of tests. Should plasma cells make up more than 10 percent of a marrow specimen—more than twice the normal proportion—multiple myeloma is presumed to be the culprit.

See "Bone-Marrow Aspiration and Bone-Marrow Core-Needle Biopsy," page 203.

HOW MULTIPLE MYELOMA IS DIAGNOSED

For the diagnosis to be confirmed, a patient must meet at least two of four criteria:

1. A positive M protein blood test
2. A positive Bence-Jones protein urine test
3. A positive bone-marrow biopsy
4. Lytic lesions in at least three bones

HOW MULTIPLE MYELOMA IS STAGED

The classification system for multiple myeloma differs from that for other solid tumors, which are generally staged according to their size and extent of spread. Dr. Jill Lacy, a medical oncologist at the Yale Cancer Center, describes it as "a crude measurement of the overall tumor burden. The three stages are based on a number of different elements: the levels of M protein in the blood and urine, and whether or not the patient has lytic lesions in his bones, anemia, and/or hypercalcemia. For example, a person who had a low M protein component, no bony lesions, and wasn't anemic or hypercalcemic would be classified as stage I."

Cancer of the Cervix

You may undergo any number of these diagnostic procedures:
- Physical exam • Pelvic exam

Laboratory Tests
- Pap smear • Endocervical curettage

Endoscopic Exams
- Colposcopy with or without the Schiller test

Biopsy
- Cervical biopsy • Loop electrosurgical excision procedure (LEEP) • Cone biopsy

Any number of these staging procedures may be performed next:
- Physical exam • Pelvic exam

Laboratory Tests
- Blood test

Imaging Studies (TYPICALLY OF THE LYMPH NODES, LUNGS, LIVER, BLADDER, COLON, RECTUM, URETERS, BONES)

▪ CT scan ▪ Lymphangiogram of the lymphatic system ▪ Chest X ray ▪ Intravenous pyelogram (IVP) of the kidneys and ureters ▪ Lower GI series (barium enema) ▪ Ultrasound ▪ MRI scan

Endoscopic Exams

▪ Cystoscopy, to look for spread to the bladder ▪ Sigmoidoscopy, to look for spread to the colon or rectum

---

Diagnosing and Staging Cervical Cancer: What You Should Know

INCISIONAL BIOPSY OF THE CERVIX

Although the *Pap smear* is an enormously effective screening test—capable of divulging the presence of not only malignant cells but also abnormal cells before they progress to cervical cancer—a biopsy is necessary to diagnose the disease.

Typical setting:	outpatient
Anesthesia:	not required
Sedation:	not required

The procedure begins by having a *speculum* inserted in the vagina. If the tumor isn't visible to the naked eye, your gynecologist will use a magnifying instrument called a *colposcope* to examine the cervix for an area to sample. One technique for exposing abnormal tissue is to swab the cervix with an iodine solution, in what is called a *Schiller test.* Healthy tissue will show dark brown; abnormal tissue shows white or pink.

With the biopsy site pinpointed, the gynecologist introduces a long-handled *forceps* into the vagina and snips off a piece of cervical tissue. "Patients usually don't feel it," explains Dr. Mitchell Morris of the M. D. Anderson Cancer Center, "because the tumor doesn't have any nerves." As part of the procedure, the doctor also takes a small spoon-shaped *curette* and scrapes tissue from inside the opening of the cervix, an area that cannot be viewed during colposcopy. This is called *endocervical curettage* (ECC).

OTHER BIOPSIES OF THE CERVIX

Loop Electrosurgical Excision Procedure (LEEP) ▪ Cone Biopsy

A cervical biopsy is generally sufficient for establishing a diagnosis. However, sometimes the results are inconclusive. "Then we would want to take a bigger sample," says Dr. Morris, a gynecologic oncologist, "with either a surgical cone biopsy or a loop electrosurgical excision procedure, which is a form of cone biopsy." Each of these methods is more commonly employed to treat cervical carcinoma in situ.

LEEP	
Typical setting:	outpatient
Anesthesia:	local
Sedation:	not required
Cone Biopsy	
Typical setting:	outpatient
	or inpatient
Anesthesia:	general
Sedation:	not required

LEEP, an office procedure, uses an electric wire loop to slice off a thin, round piece of tissue. For a *cone biopsy,* the patient is put to sleep and the doctor cuts out a cone-shaped tissue sample. Because conization takes place in the operating room, requires the services of an anesthesiologist, and may involve hospitalization, it is the most expensive form of cervical biopsy. What's more, bleeding often occurs. To stem the flow, your physician may make several stitches in the cervix before taking the specimen and may *cauterize* the wound with an electric current afterward.

The Informed Patient:
The Controversy over Routine Surgical Staging for Cervical Cancer

---

Compared to other forms of cancer, the testing for determining the extent of cervical carcinoma is strikingly low-tech. The most important element? "A pelvic exam," says Dr. Morris. "Because the primary way that cervical cancers spread is by direct extension, meaning they grow larger. So we want to carefully feel the tumor. How big is it? Has it invaded any of the tissues adjacent to the cervix, those being the bladder above and the rectum below? We also feel the connective tissues and ligaments that hold the cervix in place, along with the rest of the uterus."

The second most common route of metastasis is the lymphatic system. A CT scan or the lesser-used lymphangiogram vividly depicts the pelvic and abdominal lymph nodes, the ones most frequently affected. Often, no further staging needs to be done beyond the pelvic exam and CT scan, although a woman diagnosed with a large tumor may have her bladder and rectum examined endoscopically as a precaution.

According to Dr. Morris, some gynecologic oncologists believe in staging all their patients surgically, by removing and biopsying the pelvic and abdominal nodes. The logic behind performing this operation is to help define the ideal area to receive radiation therapy, the primary treatment for cervical cancer once it has grown beyond the cervix.

"A lot of us in the field don't think it's right to routinely surgically stage patients," says Dr. Morris. "There has never been a study to show that it saves lives or provides any meaningful information." At the M. D. Anderson Cancer Center, "we surgically stage only a very small group of patients: those whose CT scan shows cancerous lymph glands down in the pelvic area." The concern would be that microscopic tumors might be hiding in the abdomen. "In that case," he explains, "we'd want to take out the lymph nodes and see, because that would change the way we give radiation." If your oncologic gynecologist recommends this surgery without having any radiologic evidence of nodal involvement, a second opinion is certainly in order.

Cancer of the Esophagus

You may undergo any number of these diagnostic procedures:
- Physical exam

Imaging Studies
- Upper GI series (barium swallow)

Endoscopic Exams
- Esophagoscopy

Biopsy
- Endoscopic biopsy performed as part of esophagoscopy

Any number of these staging procedures may be performed next:
Imaging Studies (TYPICALLY OF THE LUNGS, LIVER, LYMPH NODES)
- CT scan ▪ MRI scan

Endoscopic Exams
- Endoscopic ultrasound ▪ Mediastinoscopy ▪ Thoracoscopy ▪ Bronchoscopy ▪ Laryngoscopy

Biopsies

- Taken during any of the above endoscopic exams

Diagnosing and Staging Esophageal Cancer: What You Should Know

IN GENERAL

Diagnosing esophageal cancer is usually a two-step process. "The first test typically ordered is a barium swallow," says Dr. Charles Fuchs of the Dana-Farber Cancer Institute. From there you'd proceed directly to an *esophagoscopy,* which Dr. Fuchs calls "the gold standard, because we can not only look at the esophagus but take brushings and biopsies of the lesion."

Your staging may now include a relatively new approach, *endoscopic ultrasound,* in which an ultrasound probe is attached to a flexible endoscope and lowered down the gullet. "This allows us to actually look at the tumor's depth of penetration," explains Dr. Fuchs, "as well as the possibility of spread to the adjacent lymph nodes. It's really quite good for assessing local involvement." In order to look for distant metastasis, most often to the lungs or the liver, a CT scan is commonly ordered.

As reliable as the CT scan and endoscopic ultrasound are overall, either test may fail to show lymph-node involvement, says Dr. Fuchs. Therefore, during the surgery to remove part or all of the esophagus, a patient originally classified as having stage II cancer may be found to actually have stage III disease. Accordingly, Dana-Farber and other major referral centers frequently add *mediastinoscopy* or *thoracoscopy* to the battery of staging exams. Here, two or three small incisions are made in the chest and an endoscope is put in to assess the lymph nodes and, if necessary, take biopsies. As part of the same procedure, says Dr. Fuchs, "sometimes we'll also do a laparoscopy, to see if the liver and any other structures in the abdomen are involved."

See "Endoscopies of the Upper GI Tract," page 199.

Cancer of the Larynx

You may undergo any number of these diagnostic procedures:
- Physical exam

Imaging Exams
- CT scan ▪ MRI scan

Endoscopic Exams
- Indirect laryngoscopy ▪ Direct laryngoscopy

Biopsy
- Endoscopic biopsy performed as part of direct laryngoscopy

Any number of these staging procedures may be performed next:
Imaging Studies (TYPICALLY OF THE LUNGS, LYMPH NODES, LIVER)
- Chest X ray ▪ CT scan ▪ MRI scan

Diagnosing and Staging Laryngeal Cancer: What You Should Know

---

IN GENERAL

"The evaluation typically begins with an office examination of the larynx," says Dr. William Richtsmeier of Duke Comprehensive Cancer Center. In what is called an *indirect laryngoscopy,* your doctor inspects the larynx using a long-handled mirror. Does it look abnormal? Do the vocal cords move properly? "The vast majority of laryngeal cancers arise from the surface epithelium and have a pretty typical appearance," explains Dr. Richtsmeier.

The physician then passes a flexible laryngoscope through the nose or mouth and down the throat. At Duke, patients are usually put to sleep for *direct laryngoscopy,* but other centers may give you a local anesthesic to prevent gagging and a mild sedative to help you relax. During the outpatient procedure, the doctor obtains a biopsy specimen through the scope and may or may not evaluate the larynx with an imaging study. Some early-stage malignancies are small enough that they can be excised completely, in which case the biopsy doubles as therapy. But according to Dr. Richtsmeier, that is fairly unusual.

See "Endoscopies of the Respiratory Tract," page 199.

Cancer of the Throat (Pharyngeal Cancer)

You may undergo any number of these diagnostic procedures:
- Physical exam ▪ Visual exam using a mirror and lights

Imaging Studies
- X rays of the skull ▪ CT scan ▪ MRI scan

Endoscopic Exams
- Nasopharyngoscopy

Biopsy
- Incisional surgical biopsy

Any number of these staging procedures may be performed next:
- Physical exam ▪ Oral exam using a mirror and lights

Imaging Studies (TYPICALLY OF THE LYMPH NODES, LUNGS, LIVER, BONES)
- Chest X ray ▪ CT scan ▪ MRI scan ▪ Angiogram ▪ Upper GI series (barium swallow)

Endoscopic Exams
- Nasopharyngoscopy ▪ Laryngoscopy ▪ Esophagoscopy

Diagnosing and Staging Throat Cancer: What You Should Know

INCISIONAL SURGICAL BIOPSY OF THE PHARYNX

The throat can be viewed indirectly by reflecting a bright light off a small mirror, illuminating the throat. Or your *otolaryngologist* may elect to inspect the pharyngeal walls directly through a flexible *nasopharyngoscope,* which she inserts into a nostril and advances down the throat. In contrast to many other cancers that can be examined endoscopically, biop-

Typical setting:	outpatient
Anesthesia:	general
Sedation:	not required

sies are rarely harvested this way, says Dr. Randal Weber, a surgeon at the University of Pennsylvania Cancer Center.

"The tumor has to be in the direct line of sight in order for us to get a biopsy," he explains. "Most of the time, the patient is put to sleep, and a forceps is used to take a small sample from the tumor."

IF YOU'VE BEEN DIAGNOSED WITH THROAT CANCER

It is essential that your oral cavity, esophagus, and larynx be examined thoroughly. With cancers of the lower two-thirds of the throat (the oropharynx and the hypopharynx), about 10 to 15 percent of patients will be found upon further testing to have a second primary tumor of the head and neck—not a secondary metastatic tumor spawned from the first, but another, separate malignancy.

Soft-Tissue Sarcomas

You may undergo any number of these diagnostic procedures:
- Physical exam

Imaging Studies
- X ray ▪ MRI scan ▪ CT scan

Biopsy
- Needle biopsy ▪ Incisional surgical biopsy ▪ Excisional surgical biopsy

Any number of these staging procedures may be performed next:
- Physical exam

Imaging Studies (TYPICALLY OF THE LUNGS)
- Chest X ray ▪ CT scan of the chest

Diagnosing and Staging Soft-Tissue Sarcomas: What You Should Know

---

NEEDLE BIOPSY OF THE SOFT TISSUE

When deciding between a needle biopsy and a surgical biopsy of soft tissue, an orthopedic surgeon's top two considerations are "the anatomic site" and "the level of confidence he has in his pathologist," according to Dr. Kenneth Yaw. A needle biopsy, performed under local anesthesia in the doctor's office, yields little tissue; some pathologists aren't comfortable interpreting such a small specimen.

Typical setting:	outpatient
Anesthesia:	local
Sedation:	not required

SURGICAL BIOPSY OF THE SOFT TISSUE

A soft-tissue lesion is excised whole only if it is small and if X rays and an MRI scan have convinced the surgeon beyond a doubt that it is benign. Most of the time, you will be put to sleep, and a small piece will be cut out and sent for cell analysis. Either way, in this era of managed-care insurance coverage, you can

Typical setting:	outpatient
Anesthesia:	general
Sedation:	not required

anticipate going home the same day, although you may be admitted to the hospital for several hours of observation.

The Informed Patient:
Why the Biopsy Should Be Performed Only by a Cancer Surgeon

Biopsying soft tissue is fraught with potential hazards, the most serious being an improperly placed needle or incision. "In the extremities, a poorly planned or poorly performed biopsy can make an otherwise resectable tumor unresectable and cost the patient a limb," Dr. Yaw says bluntly. The Musculoskeletal Tumor Society goes so far as to recommend that at nonacademic medical centers the procedure be performed exclusively by a cancer surgeon experienced in resecting soft-tissue sarcomas.

"In order to plan a biopsy correctly," says Dr. Yaw, "a doctor needs to know where the incisions for surgery would have to be made," in the event that the pathologist discovers cancer. "When we do a biopsy, all the tissue we expose—whether by passing a needle through it or by cutting it open and looking at it—has to be resected during the operation in order for us to achieve a wide margin." Consider that a surgeon operating to remove a sarcoma measuring about two inches in diameter ideally plans to also take out at least another three-fourths inch of tissue in all directions. Look at your arm or your leg and you can see how the loss of any additional tissue—perhaps a major nerve or a tendon severed because of a bungled biopsy—could result in a potentially devastating physical impairment.

The axiom among orthopedic surgeons is to avoid cutting across a limb *(transversely,* in medical jargon) or at an angle *(obliquely).* "If a doctor orients an incision transversely to the long axis of a leg or arm," explains Dr. Yaw, "that entire biopsy tract has to be removed. At the very least, that usually creates a soft-tissue defect that requires elaborate reconstructive surgery. And more often than not, if it's a large transverse incision, we have to do an amputation."

This disturbing scenario affects a minority of patients, he emphasizes. "But it's a common enough problem that everybody has seen it, and we dread it." Other problems can arise from biopsies of soft-tissue tumors, including infection and obstinate surgical wounds that take a long time to heal. A study conducted by the Musculoskeletal Tumor Society reported that biopsy-related complications forced doctors to change the preferred treatment plan for nearly one in five patients. According to the authors, such developments were three to more than five times less likely to occur when the procedure was carried out at a treatment center rather than at a referring medical facility.

To dramatically reduce your risk, ask your doctor for a referral to an orthopedic cancer surgeon in private practice or (our preference) on staff at an academic medical center. Or, in the event your orthopedic surgeon does not subspecialize in musculoskeletal malignancies, insist that he confer with a seasoned professional regarding how the biopsy should be placed.

Soft-tissue sarcomas are uncommon enough, says Dr. Yaw, that if your biopsy is being read at a medical facility that hasn't treated many cases, "after you get the pathology report, always seek a consultation with a physician who sees lots of them."

Cancer of the Testicle

You may undergo any number of these diagnostic procedures:
- Physical exam

Laboratory Tests

- Tumor-marker blood tests for alpha-fetoprotein (AFP) and beta human chorionic gonadotropin (HCG) • Urine tests, to detect the presence of blood

Imaging Studies

- Ultrasound • Chest X ray

Biopsy

- Excisional surgical biopsy

Any number of these staging procedures may be performed next:
- Physical exam

Laboratory Tests

- Blood tests

Imaging Studies (TYPICALLY OF THE LYMPH NODES, LIVER, KIDNEYS, URETERS)

- CT scan ▪ Intravenous pyelogram (IVP) of the kidneys and ureters ▪ Lymphangiogram of the lymphatic system ▪ MRI scan

---

Diagnosing and Staging Testicular Cancer: What You Should Know

ALPHA-FETOPROTEIN (AFP) AND BETA HUMAN CHORIONIC GONADOTROPIN (HCG) TUMOR-MARKER BLOOD TESTS

Simply put, if an imaging exam such as ultrasound shows a mass in one of the testicles, and your blood contains elevated levels of the tumor markers *alpha-fetoprotein* and *beta human chorionic gonadotropin,* it's testicular cancer, says Dr. Bruce Redman of the University of Michigan Comprehensive Cancer Center.

What's more, an abnormally high concentration of AFP establishes that the tumor is a nonseminoma as opposed to a seminoma. This is a crucial distinction, because the two histologic types of testicular cancer are treated differently. While the hormone HCG is associated with both types, "seminoma tumors *never* produce alpha-fetoprotein," says Dr. Redman. "I always tell our resident doctors that if a pathologist claims a tumor is a seminoma, but the blood test shows AFP elevation—and it's not due to another condition, such as liver inflammation or hepatitis—it should be treated as nonseminoma cancer."

The two tumor markers continue to prove their worth after the cancerous testicle is removed. Normally, the levels of AFP and HCG in the blood serum gradually diminish, beginning about a week or so following surgery. "Under normal circumstances, men never secrete alpha-fetoprotein or beta human chorionic gonadotropin," explains Dr. Redman. "So if the markers remain elevated—even though the CT scan of the abdomen is negative and the chest X ray is negative—we know there's still persistent, active cancer."

EXCISIONAL SURGICAL BIOPSY OF THE TESTICLE

Until about 1980, the testicles were biopsied by inserting a needle through the scrotum. This approach has since been abandoned in

Typical setting:	outpatient
	or inpatient
Anesthesia:	general
Sedation:	not required

favor of *inguinal orchiectomy,* in which the testicle is taken out whole via an incision in the groin. The older method, *transscrotal needle biopsy,* has two major drawbacks: the potential for scattering malignant cells locally and—the more serious flaw—sampling error. "Without the doctor being able to hold the testicle in his hand and palpate it," Dr. Redman explains, "he's not sure if he's putting the needle into the right area. Those of us who treat testicular cancer cringe whenever we hear a patient had a transscrotal biopsy, though fortunately it's very rare nowadays."

One instance in which an incisional biopsy may be taken is if the tumor markers test negative and the ultrasound exam is inconclusive. In order to spare the testicle should the mass prove to be benign, the surgeon cuts into the groin, pulls up the testicle from within, and biopsies it outside the body. It is still connected to the *spermatic cord* and vein and is able to be returned to the scrotum. However, according to Dr. Redman, such situations are rare.

For patients with seminoma tumors, inguinal orchiectomy constitutes their only surgery. If you are diagnosed with nonseminoma testicular cancer, you may have to return for another operation to dissect the *retroperitoneal lymph nodes* in the abdomen, although a new, equally effective strategy is to simply monitor patients and treat any recurrences with chemotherapy.

> *See "Surgery" under "Cancer of the Testicle" in Chapter Six, "State of the Art: Your Treatment Options."*

Cancer of the Small Intestine

You may undergo any number of these diagnostic procedures:
- Physical exam

Imaging Studies

- Upper GI series (barium swallow) ▪ CT scan ▪ MRI scan ▪ Ultrasound

Endoscopic Exams

- Esophagogastroduodenoscopy ▪ Laparoscopy

Biopsy

- Endoscopic biopsy performed as part of esophagogastroduodenoscopy or laparoscopy

Surgical Procedures

- Exploratory laparotomy at the time of definitive surgery to remove a portion of the small intestine

Any number of these staging procedures may be performed next:
Imaging Studies (TYPICALLY OF THE LUNGS, ABDOMEN)

- Chest X ray ▪ CT scan

Diagnosing and Staging Small-Intestine Cancer: What You Should Know

---

EXPLORATORY LAPAROTOMY

Esophagogastroduodenoscopy is of limited use in diagnosing cancer of the small bowel, because the endoscope reaches only as far down as the duodenum, the first of the small intestine's three portions. "Occasionally," says Dr. Michael Sterchi of Baptist Hospital in Winston-Salem, North Carolina, "the jejunum and the ileum can be endoscoped through the mouth too." Patients receive a spray of local anesthetic at the back of the throat, plus intravenous sedation.

Typical setting:	inpatient
Anesthesia:	general
Sedation:	not required
Hospital stay:	5–7 days

"But generally," says the doctor, a specialist in gastrointestinal surgery, "small-bowel cancer is diagnosed through exploratory laparotomy, usually as part of the same operation to resect the small bowel." Your physician may contemplate ordering an exploratory *laparoscopy.* Though also a surgical procedure, it typically doesn't require hospitalization, as compared to the nearly weeklong stay for patients who undergo exploratory *laparotomy.* But since laparoscopy is strictly diagnostic, it is usually passed over in favor of the more extensive surgery, at which time the tumor is not only biopsied but removed.

> See *"Endoscopies of the Upper GI Tract," page 199, and "Surgery" under "Cancer of the Small Intestine" in Chapter Six, "State of the Art: Your Treatment Options."*

Other Tests Commonly Used to Diagnose and Stage Cancer

What to Expect ▪ What the Test Can Tell Your Doctor

Physical Exams

CLINICAL BREAST EXAM

Used in detecting cancer of the breast.

You are positioned lying on your back.

The doctor, who should be skilled at palpating women's breasts for lumps, feels each breast, as well as the neck and under the arms, while you are asked to raise your arms over your head, then let them hang at your sides, and then press them against your hips. Should a lump be discovered, she will note its size, texture, and firmness.

Typical setting:	**outpatient**
Anesthesia:	**not required**
Sedation:	**not required**

The best time to schedule a breast exam is seven to ten days after your menstrual flow begins, when the breasts tend to be less lumpy and tender.

DIGITAL RECTAL EXAM

Used in detecting cancers of the colon, rectum, bladder, prostate, and ovary.

You are positioned lying on your side.

Typical setting:	outpatient
Anesthesia:	not required
Sedation:	not required

Inserting a gloved, lubricated finger in the rectum enables the doctor to feel several organs for irregularities in shape and size.

PELVIC EXAM

Used in detecting cancers of the cervix, ovary, uterus, fallopian tube, vagina, vulva, bladder, and rectum.

You are positioned lying on your back, with your knees apart and your feet in stirrups.

Typical setting:	outpatient
Anesthesia:	not required
Sedation:	not required

The doctor, wearing rubber gloves, inspects the vulva before inserting a plastic instrument called a *speculum* into the vagina to afford a clear view of the upper vagina and cervix. Next she digitally examines the uterus, ovaries, and fallopian tubes for any abnormalities that could indicate a tumor. When feeling the ovary or bladder, two fingers may be used, one in the rectum and one in the vagina. A Pap smear, described in this section under "Laboratory/Specimen Tests," is taken as part of the exam.

NEUROLOGICAL EXAM

Used in detecting cancers of the central nervous system.

A basic neurological exam assesses:

- Eye movement and reflexes, and pupil reaction
- Changes in hearing
- Neuromuscular reflexes
- Gag reflex

Typical setting:	outpatient
Anesthesia:	not required
Sedation:	not required

- Movement of the head, tongue, and facial muscles
- Sense of touch

- Balance and coordination
- Mental ability, memory, abstract thinking
- Strength
- Facial symmetry

Laboratory/Specimen Tests

VENIPUNCTURE

Anyone undergoing chemotherapy can count on having regular blood drawings, or *phlebotomies,* usually from a vein near the crook of the elbow. A phlebotomy nurse cleanses your skin with antiseptic, wraps a rubber tourniquet around your upper arm, then puts in the needle. He may ask you to repeatedly clench and unclench your fist, to speed matters along, while the attached vial fills with blood.

Typical setting:	outpatient
Anesthesia:	not required
Sedation:	not required

See *"Methods of Delivery: Venipunctures" in Chapter Seven, "What You Can Expect During Treatment."*

PAP SMEAR

Used in detecting cancer of the cervix.

You are positioned lying on your back, with your knees apart and your feet in stirrups.

The simple, painless Pap smear, performed as part of a woman's pelvic exam, is a highly effective screening test for cervical cancer, but not for carcinomas of the uterus or ovary. Using a plastic or wooden *spatula,* the doctor obtains a thin layer of cells from the outer surface of the cervix; next she twirls a miniature brush inside the cervical opening, for the same purpose. The specimens are placed on a slide and sent to the pathology lab, where they are classified as normal, low-grade lesion, or high-grade lesion, the latter term a synonym for cervical carcinoma in situ.

Typical setting:	outpatient
Anesthesia:	not required
Sedation:	not required

The best time to schedule a Pap smear is about two weeks after the first day of your menstrual period. Beginning two days before the test, you should refrain from sexual intercourse, and avoid using douches, spermicidal foams, creams, or jellies, and vaginal medicines, unless your physician instructs otherwise.

FECAL OCCULT-BLOOD TEST

Used in detecting cancers of the colon, rectum, and stomach.

This home test, conducted over a three-day period, is for detecting hidden *(occult)* traces of blood in the stool. At your initial doctor's visit, you're given a set of slides impregnated with a substance that undergoes a chemical reaction when it comes into contact with blood.

Typical setting:	home test
Anesthesia:	not required
Sedation:	not required

Each day, you smear a small sample of fecal matter on a slide and close the cover. The slides, returnable by mail, are then tested in a laboratory. A developing liquid is added to each. Should the stool contain blood, the substance, called *guaiac*, will turn blue.

To ensure accuracy, it is recommended that you eat plenty of raw vegetables, fruits, and cereals and avoid red meat, aspirin, vitamin C, and iron supplements the day before testing begins and continuing through day three.

SPUTUM CYTOLOGY

Used in detecting cancer of the lung.

Analyzing the mucus for cancer cells can draw attention to centrally located lung tumors before they give rise to symptoms. For three to five consecutive mornings, upon waking up you brush your teeth and rinse your mouth, then cough deeply and expectorate into a wide-mouthed jar with a snap-on lid, which you either return to the doctor's office or mail directly to a processing lab.

Typical setting:	home test
Anesthesia:	not required
Sedation:	not required

LUMBAR PUNCTURE (SPINAL TAP)

Used in detecting cancers of the central nervous system.

You are positioned lying on your side, with your knees drawn up to your chest and your arms wrapped around them.

Cancer cells—lymphomas and leukemia in particular—can infiltrate the *cerebrospinal fluid* that bathes the brain and spinal cord. The purpose of a lumbar puncture is to with-

Typical setting:	outpatient
Anesthesia:	local
Sedation:	not required

draw a small amount of the fluid though a hollow needle that the doctor inserts between two vertebrae in the lower spine. Your position—curled up as if performing a cannonball dive—eases his task by widening the space between the bones. (In a *cisternal puncture*, which is rarely done, the sample is aspirated from the base of the brain, with the syringe introduced into the back of the neck.)

The notion of having a four-inch needle stuck in your backbone isn't a pleasant one, especially if you've never gone through a spinal tap before. However, the skin on the back is less sensitive than the skin on, say, the arm, so most of the time the procedure is surprisingly pain free. Should you feel the bendable needle graze the bone or a nerve as it enters the spinal canal, tell the doctor, who can reposition the instrument.

The needle remains in for several minutes, because unlike blood, cerebrospinal fluid trickles out slowly. After it is removed, you may experience a headache from the temporary decrease in fluid to cushion the brain. Most medical facilities will have you lie flat on your back for fifteen minutes or so, by which time your body has already made back a quarter of the fluid taken out.

Except in a medical emergency, a lumbar puncture should not be performed if you are suspected of having increased pressure within the skull, as from a brain tumor or abscess. As a precaution, a physician will often want to image the brain beforehand.

THORACENTESIS

Used in detecting cancer of the lung.

You are seated facing the back of a chair.

In thoracentesis, the doctor uses a thin needle to tap fluid from the shallow cavity between the two layers of the *pleural membrane* that encases the lungs. Prior to the procedure, an X ray is usually taken to determine where to place the needle. Then you straddle the chair and lean forward, resting your arms and head

Typical setting:	outpatient
Anesthesia:	local
Sedation:	not required

on the back. This "stretches" the rib cage, giving the physician a wider target for inserting the needle between the bones.

An injection of local anesthetic numbs the skin and muscle, but you may experience momentary pain as the needle penetrates the pleura to draw out a small quantity of fluid. Afterward, plan on remaining at the hospital for at least an hour of observation. If a follow-up X ray shows no sign of a collapsed lung *(pneumothorax)*—an occasional but readily correctable complication—you may go home.

Imaging Studies

The Informed Patient:
What You Should Know Before Undergoing
a Contrast-Medium Imaging Study

To enhance the picture from a conventional X ray, CT scan, or MRI scan, you may be administered a solution that fills the organ(s) or vessel(s) being studied and produces highlighted images. The *contrast* agent collects more in diseased tissue than in healthy tissue, to outline abnormalities such as tumors.

Usually, contrast is injected into a vein in the arm or an artery in the groin, though it may also be given orally or rectally, as in an upper or lower GI series. "Right after the dye is injected, patients will typically feel a sensation of warmth or an odd taste in the mouth," says Dr. Rebecca Zuurbier, a radiologist at the Lombardi Cancer Center. "Some become nauseous from the contrast moving through them." These effects, she adds, usually pass within a matter of minutes.

Severe itching, difficulty in breathing, and a drastic drop in blood pressure, on the other hand, signal a life-threatening allergic reaction. Rest assured that the chances of such an occurrence are slim: one in forty thousand. If you've ever reacted adversely to an injection of contrast medium in the past, be sure to alert the doctor, although one *anaphylactic* reaction doesn't necessarily mean it will happen again. Nevertheless, instead of the standard *ionic* contrast, you'll be given *nonionic* contrast, which carries a significantly lower risk of triggering a reaction. The same would hold true for men and women who have histories of severe allergies or medical conditions such as diabetes, kidney impairment, or heart failure.

Patients with no extenuating health concerns can request the safer solution if they wish—not that one-in-forty-thousand odds should cause anyone undue alarm. Just know in advance that nonionic contrast costs ten times more; your insurance company may not cover the difference in price. "Personally, that's what I would do," admits Dr. Zuurbier. "I wouldn't want to take a chance." As an added precaution, she recommends having the procedure done at a hospital, as opposed to a freestanding radiology center. This way, in the unlikely event of a crisis, you're next door to an emergency room.

CHEST X RAY

Used in detecting cancers of the lung and mediastinum.

You are positioned standing in front of a cassette containing X-ray film.

The granddaddy of radiographic studies, and still as useful as ever. An X-ray tube levels an X-ray beam at the cassette; this produces an image on the film. Two exposures are typically taken: one from the front and one from the side.

Typical setting:	outpatient
Anesthesia:	not required
Sedation:	not required

MAMMOGRAM

Used in detecting cancer of the breast.

You are positioned standing in front of the mammography machine.

Mammography screening for breast cancer has long been the subject of heated controversy. Is it beneficial for women in their forties, or only for women fifty and older? That seems to depend on which study you read. Even the National Cancer Institute has seesawed back and forth on this issue: In 1993, the agency

Typical setting:	outpatient
Anesthesia:	not required
Sedation:	not required

rescinded its recommendation that forty-to-fifty-year-old women have regular mammograms, only to reinstate it four years later. What can't be disputed is the X ray's ability to detect early breast cancer: up to two years before a woman or her physician can feel a lump.

Normally, two pictures are taken of each breast: one from the top and one from the side. But if the X ray reveals an abnormality, and you're called back for a second series, "you may get as many films as it takes to resolve the question," says Dr. Zuurbier, director of breast imaging at Lombardi. "Typically, we take two or three extra exposures, though sometimes I may have to take as many as twelve." If you've had mammograms in the past, bring the last several *original* films with you, she says. A seemingly insignificant white spot on your X ray "could increase in importance if it's different from years before."

The day of your mammogram, do not use deodorant or powder, which can produce shadows on the film.

Tips for Reducing Discomfort

In positioning you for the mammogram, a technologist sandwiches one breast between a pair of plastic plates that can be adjusted by height and angle. One consists of an X-ray tube; the other, X-ray film. The flatter the breast, the sharper the picture. Many women find the compression uncomfortable, if not downright painful, especially those with extremely large breasts.

"Mammography doesn't have to hurt," maintains Dr. Zuurbier, who advises trying your best to relax during the procedure, as well as taking an over-the-counter pain reliever such as aspirin or Tylenol prior to the visit. "But the best thing a patient can do," she says, "is to know her menstrual cycle and to avoid having a mammogram when her breasts are most tender." The optimum time to schedule your appointment is ten days after the start of menstruation.

Questions to Ask . . . Before a Mammogram

To improve the quality of mammograms around the country, in 1994 Congress passed a law requiring that all facilities be accredited and certified by the U.S. Department of Health and Human Services.

> **Is the mammography facility ACR-accredited? Find out by contacting:**
>
> American College of Radiology:
> 800-227-5463
> National Cancer Institute's
> Cancer Information Service:
> 800-422-6237
> American Cancer Society:
> 800-227-2345

As the lead mammographer at a major referral center, Dr. Zuurbier often reads films that were taken elsewhere. According to her, "I still see a variation in the quality of mammograms that is of some concern."

One way to ensure that you receive a high-quality mammogram is to find out if the radiology facility is certified by the American College of Radiology (ACR), which evaluates the caliber of equipment, personnel, and procedures. The ACR's program is voluntary, however, and not all facilities—including some very good ones—choose to seek accreditation. The National Cancer Institute recommends that before you arrange to have a mammogram at a non-

ACR-approved center, call and ask the following five questions. A single "no" answer, and you should be looking elsewhere.

1. Do you use only *dedicated* mammography machines, equipment designed specifically for taking mammograms and for no other purpose?
2. Is the technologist who performs the mammograms state-licensed and/or certified by the American Registry of Radiological Technologists?
3. Is the radiologist who interprets the mammograms certified by either the American Board of Radiologists or the American Osteopathic Board of Radiology? And how many mammograms does she review per year? (For a point of comparison, the American College of Radiology's minimum requirement is 480 films annually.)
4. Does the facility conduct mammograms as part of its regular practice? The ACR recommends that you consider only a facility that performs at least ten per week.
5. Is the mammography equipment calibrated at least once a year, so that measurements and doses are accurate?

As reliable as mammograms are, they are not foolproof. Ten to 15 percent of breast cancers will not show up on the film. The procedure is most likely to miss small tumors in women under age fifty who have dense breast tissue. If you're considered to be at higher-than-average risk for breast cancer, or the doctor feels something suspicious upon a manual exam, it's wise to request that the mammogram be supplemented with a sonogram.

COMPUTED TOMOGRAM (CT SCAN)
Used in detecting many forms of cancer.

You are positioned lying down on the CT scanner's padded mechanical table.

The portable platform draws you inside a roomy oval cylinder while the scanner rotates 360 degrees around you. A regular CT-scan machine X-rays at set intervals: You're

Typical setting:	outpatient
Anesthesia:	not required
Sedation:	not required

asked to hold your breath; *bzzzzzzzzzzz*, it takes a picture; now breathe, as the table moves you to the next position. The one shortcoming of this type of equipment is that if the patient breathes differently from one exposure to the next, a crucial "slice" of the full image may be lost.

With the newer *helical* CT scanners, available since the early 1990s, all the information is gathered at once. "You move through at a constant rate," Dr. Rebecca Zuurbier of the Lombardi Cancer Center explains, "while the machine acquires information in a corkscrew fashion. Then the computer puts all that information into regular slices, giving us clear, crisp pictures."

NEPHROTOMOGRAM

Used in detecting cancer of the kidney.

Nephrotomography is similar to computed tomography, except that the single-plane images of the kidneys are formed without the aid of a computer. You will be given contrast intravenously.

MAGNETIC RESONANCE IMAGING (MRI)

Used in detecting many forms of cancer.

You are positioned lying down on the MRI scanner's padded mechanical table.

Magnetic resonance imaging employs a powerful magnetic field and computer-generated radio waves to visualize body structures without X rays. The table pulls you headfirst into a narrow open-ended chamber—actually the center of a large circular magnet housed inside a square unit that measures approximately seven feet by seven feet.

Typical setting:	outpatient
Anesthesia:	not required
Sedation:	not required but can be requested

The tunnel is four feet long. If it's your abdomen that's being scanned, you should be able to peek out the other end, whereas someone undergoing an MRI of the brain spends the entire procedure inside the tube. According to Lombardi's Dr. Rebecca Zuurbier, patient complaints typically concern the grating noises generated by the device. She compares it to the sound of "being inside a garbage can while somebody bangs on it." Patient-friendly centers usually supply earplugs or headphones.

If you are prone to claustrophobia, alert the radiology department in advance, so you can be given a short-acting sedative. Dr. Zuurbier estimates that perhaps one in twenty of her patients require medication to combat anxiety or restlessness. (She herself claims to have *fallen asleep* during her one MRI scan, but then concedes, "I was a resident doctor at the time; you fall asleep anywhere.")

Who Cannot Have an MRI Scan?

Having an implanted prosthesis containing metal precludes you from taking an MRI scan, because the machine's potent magnetic field could disrupt the device's function or cause it to shift inside your body. Examples include cardiac monitors, artificial heart valves, pacemakers, cerebral aneurysm clips, insulin pumps, neurostimulators, and intrauterine contraceptive devices (IUDs). Today most implants are made of a nonferromagnetic material and generally don't present a problem. In determining whether or not you are suitable for MRI, a nurse takes an in-depth history, medical and otherwise. Even the fact that you once worked in an industry where metal shavings might have entered your eyes could remove you from consideration.

RADIONUCLIDE SCAN

Used in detecting cancers of the bone, brain, liver, thyroid, and lymphatic system.

You are positioned lying beneath a gamma camera.

Standard radiographic studies rely on an external source to beam X rays through the body and onto specially sensitized film. In radionuclide imaging, also referred to as *nuclear scanning* and *radioisotope scanning,* a minute amount of short-lived radioactive material is injected into the bloodstream.

Typical setting:	outpatient
Anesthesia:	not required
Sedation:	not required

Then a circular *gamma camera* about two feet in diameter moves in an arc over you, recording the gamma rays emitted by the radioisotope. In addition to producing an image, the device compiles computer data on the distribution of radioactivity within the organ being studied.

The principle behind radionuclide scanning is that various organs absorb specific minerals or hormones undetectable on regular X rays. Adding the radioisotope highlights these substances. Too little or too much could indicate the presence of a tumor, as might a high concentration in one area but not in others.

"Will I glow in the dark?" Patients ask that all the time, says radiologist Dr. Rebecca Zuurbier. Her answer: an emphatic no. In fact, a nuclear scan exposes patients to less radiation than do many X-ray studies, and allergic reactions to the intravenous radionuclide are virtually unheard-of.

POSITRON EMISSION TOMOGRAM (PET SCAN)

Used in detecting cancers of the brain and thyroid.

You are positioned lying down.

Positron emission tomography looks at organ activity rather than structure. "It is a very important research tool," says Dr. Zuurbier. A radionuclide is chemically coupled to a "tracer," such as the simple sugar *glucose,* then injected into a blood vessel.

Typical setting:	**outpatient**
Anesthesia:	**not required**
Sedation:	**not required**

"The premise of PET scanning," she explains, "is that cancer cells tend to metabolize substances at a higher rate than normal cells." Glucose, the body's fuel, is converted into energy. A malignant tumor would consume more of the radioactive glucose and consequently give off more gamma rays. The PET scanner not only detects the radioactivity but also feeds the information into a computer to produce an image. PET scanning is not widely available at present because few hospitals own the expensive equipment needed to conduct the test.

ULTRASOUND

Used in detecting many forms of cancer.

You are positioned lying down.

The doctor rubs conducting jelly onto the area to be examined, then passes a handheld probe resembling a microphone over the skin. This probe, or *transducer,* pulses high-frequency sound waves, inaudible to humans, into the body. As the waves ricochet off various internal structures, the echo pattern is

Typical setting:	**outpatient**
Anesthesia:	**not required**
Sedation:	**not required**

translated into a picture, or *sonogram,* which the physician views on a monitor screen.

Ultrasound can also be done internally. Here the doctor inserts a tiny transducer, less than an inch in diameter, into an orifice such as the vagina *(transvaginal ultrasound)* or rectum *(transrectal ultrasound)* and beams sound waves off a particular organ. Another route is through the mouth and down the esophagus, by affixing the probe to a flexible endoscope *(endoscopic ultrasound).*

Duplex/Doppler ultrasound, used to help diagnose tumors that have infiltrated blood vessels, employs Doppler technology. In addition to viewing images, the physician can listen to recordings of the blood as it courses through the vessels: The sound grows louder as the blood approaches the transducer, then fainter as it continues through the circulatory system. A tumor occluding the vein or artery would slow down the blood flow and hence the sound pattern.

UPPER GI SERIES (BARIUM SWALLOW)

Used in detecting cancers of the esophagus, stomach, and small intestine.

LOWER GI SERIES (BARIUM ENEMA)

Used in detecting cancers of the large intestine.

You are positioned lying on a tilting X-ray table.

Both of these fluoroscopic–X-ray studies utilize *barium sulfate,* a white, opaque contrast medium. For an upper GI series, you force down a cupful of the chalky solution, which will undoubtedly be described to you as tasting like a vanilla or strawberry milkshake. Don't believe it. Sometimes a water-soluble liquid may be used instead. "Patients usually find that more palatable," says radiologist Dr. Rebecca Zuurbier, "because it can be mixed in Kool-Aid or iced tea to disguise the taste a bit."

Typical setting:	outpatient
Anesthesia:	not required
Sedation:	not required

In a lower GI series, an enema bag filled with barium is instilled into the rectum while you're lying on your side. The procedure cannot be performed unless your large intestine is completely free of waste, and so most facilities will instruct you to observe a clear-liquid diet—no solid or semisolid foods—beginning the day before. Although preparations may vary somewhat from one institution to the next, expect to be supplied with laxatives and an enema.

Tilting and rotating the table helps distribute the contrast, which is tracked by a fluoroscope and captured on X ray. The barium enema requires that you suppress the urge to move your bowels. Once the radiologist has taken enough pictures, you'll be helped to a bathroom or handed a bedpan and asked to evacuate as much of the contrast as you can. More X rays will follow.

To provide a clearer view, air may be pumped into the colon or the stomach. This is called a *double-contrast* study. The distension causes a sensation of fullness and can also bring on moderate to severe cramping. If you find the spasms unbearable, tell the radiologist, who can give you an injectable medication called glucagon to calm the gastrointestinal tract.

ANGIOGRAM/ARTERIOGRAM

Used in detecting cancers of the liver, pancreas, central nervous system, and kidney.

You are positioned lying down.

An angiogram employs intravenous contrast dye and moving-picture fluoroscopic X rays to study veins *(angio*gram) or arteries *(arteri-*

Typical setting:	**outpatient**
Anesthesia:	**local**
Sedation:	**yes**

*o*gram). In cancer it is generally used after a diagnosis has been established, to visualize the vessels entering and exiting the tumor. The surgeon will refer to this "road map" when planning the operation to remove the cancer.

In most angiograms, the contrast is injected through a flexible *catheter* tube inserted in the large *femoral* artery in the groin, although veins, too, can be used, in the groin as well as in other parts of the body. No incision is necessary. After you've been given IV sedation and an injection of local anesthetic, the radiologist places a needle in the artery. The catheter is threaded through the needle, which should give you an idea of how thin it is. He carefully guides it through the blood vessel until it reaches the site under investigation, then injects contrast into the tube and begins taking still pictures.

Following the procedure, the radiologist presses on the wound for roughly fifteen minutes, so that it heals over, and covers it with an adhesive bandage. The next four to eight hours are spent in the recovery room, lying on your back. You must keep your leg straight, to prevent bleeding. Before discharging you, a doctor will check the puncture site. Although the sedative should have worn off by this time, many medical facilities insist that you have someone drive you home, so as not to apply pressure on the leg.

LYMPHANGIOGRAM

Used in detecting cancers of the lymphatic system.

You are positioned lying down.

Lymphangiography is gradually falling out of favor as a means of visualizing the lymphatic system. For one thing, says Lombardi's Dr. Rebecca Zuurbier, there's some question about the test's sensitivity. But also, from a technical standpoint, lymphangiograms are difficult to perform and require a one-inch incision in the back of the patient's foot.

Typical setting:	outpatient
Anesthesia:	local
Sedation:	not required

First, a blue dye is injected between the toes and given fifteen to thirty minutes to make its way into the lymphatic vessels of the foot. After numbing the area with an injection of local anesthetic, the physician cuts into the skin to expose a lymph vessel. Taking a needle-tipped catheter in hand, she punctures the vessel and injects contrast, which disperses throughout the lymphatic system over a period of one and a half to two hours. Once X rays have been made, the tube is withdrawn, and the incision sutured and bandaged.

It is generally recommended that for the first twenty-four hours patients rest in bed with their feet elevated, to help curtail swelling. Don't be worried if during the next two days the dye lends a bluish tinge to your skin, urine, and stool before dissipating. The contrast agent, however, remains in the body up to six months, allowing for future X rays to be taken.

INTRAVENOUS PYELOGRAM (IVP, UROGRAM)

Used in detecting cancers of the kidney, bladder, ureter, testicle, ovary, cervix, and prostate.

You are positioned lying on your back.

Through intravenous pyelography, a radiologist can spot masses in the kidneys, ureters, and bladder. The test also evaluates urinary function, something that may yield indirect clues about the activity of other forms of cancer. Because a full intestine obscures the kidneys on the X ray, you will be instructed to take a mild laxative the night before and not eat or drink anything beginning eight hours prior to the study.

Typical setting:	outpatient
Anesthesia:	not required
Sedation:	not required

The first step is an X ray of the urinary tract, followed by an injection of contrast medium into a vein in your arm. IVP tracks the dye as it travels through the kidneys, down the ureter tubes, and into the bladder, with pictures taken at regular intervals: The typical pattern is upon injection, then at five, ten, and fifteen minutes. At the five-minute mark, a cuff is wrapped tightly around your waist and two rubber bulbs slipped under it. Inflating the bulbs pushes the ureters out of the way to afford an unobstructed view of the kidneys' anatomy. Once films are made, the bulbs are deflated.

For the last part of the test, you will be asked to empty your bladder, then return to the table for a final X ray.

PERCUTANEOUS TRANSHEPATIC CHOLANGIOGRAM

Used in detecting cancer of the pancreas.

You are positioned lying down on a tilting X-ray table.

This contrast X-ray study determines whether a patient's jaundice is due to liver disease or an obstruction of a *bile duct.* Ruling out the former problem would narrow down the cause to either a tumor or gallstones and prompt further testing.

Typical setting:	outpatient
Anesthesia:	local
Sedation:	not required

Once the skin over the liver has been numbed with a local anesthetic, a long, flexible needle is inserted. You may feel momentary pain as the instrument moves deeper into the organ. The physician monitors its position on a fluoroscope. When he sees the needle has entered a bile duct, contrast dye is administered, and a series of films are made while the table rotates into different angles.

After the needle is withdrawn and a dressing is applied, you will be held for approximately six hours of observation, during which time you are asked to lie on your right side, to prevent bleeding from the puncture site.

ENDOSCOPIC RETROGRADE CHOLANGIOPANCREATOGRAM (ERCP)

Used in detecting cancers of the pancreas, bile ducts, and small intestine.

You are positioned lying on your stomach or on your side.

ERCP, a combination endoscopic-radiographic study of the ducts leading from the pancreas and gallbladder, is used to image gallstones or tumors.

After your throat has been sprayed with a topical anesthetic and an intravenous sedative has been administered, the doctor advances a flexible endoscope down your throat and esophagus, through the stomach, and into the first portion of the small intestine. If your stomach is a little overactive, you may be

Typical setting:	outpatient
Anesthesia:	local
Sedation:	yes

given a drug such as glucagon to reduce the movement, or *motility*. A long catheter is fed through the scope until it reaches the *common bile duct*. Then a contrast dye is injected through the tube as films are taken in rapid sequence by a tiny camera in the scope.

Endoscopic Exams

◆ *Biopsies or brushings may be taken during any of these procedures.*

ENDOSCOPIES OF THE RESPIRATORY TRACT

Nasopharyngoscopy ▪ Laryngoscopy ▪ Bronchoscopy

ENDOSCOPIES OF THE UPPER GI TRACT

Esophagoscopy ▪ Gastroscopy ▪ Esophagogastroduodenoscopy

You are positioned lying on your side or on your stomach with your head turned to one side.

Many patients will probably tell you that the least pleasant part of an endoscopy down the throat is the bitter taste of the topical anesthetic sprayed in the back of the mouth to numb the gag reflex. In order for the doctor to maneuver the scope past the back of the throat—ideally on the first try—you'll be instructed to tuck in your chin and swallow, though you won't be able to feel your tongue and throat muscles working.

With that hurdle cleared, you should experience no significant discomfort as the viewing instrument passes down the respiratory tract or upper digestive tract. The nurse will encourage you to breathe slowly and deeply through your nose. Should you feel a cough coming on, don't fight it. Most likely, though, you'll drift off from the intravenous sedative.

You will be observed briefly afterward—longer, obviously, if general anesthesia was used—then sent home in the company of a friend or family member who is capable of driving. If it took several attempts to insert the endoscope, you can expect to wake up the next day with a sore throat.

ENDOSCOPIES OF THE LOWER GI TRACT

Sigmoidoscopy ▪ Colonoscopy

You are positioned lying on your side, back, or stomach.

Both these endoscopic exams involve inserting a lubricated flexible scope in the rectum for the purpose of viewing the large intestine. A sig-

TABLE 3.2	Endoscopies of the Respiratory and Upper GI Tracts			
Name	Route of Endoscope	Typical Setting	Anesthesia	Sedation
Nasopharyn- goscopy	Nose ➡ throat	Outpatient	Local	Not required
Direct laryn- goscopy	Mouth ➡ throat ➡ larynx	Outpatient	General or local	Yes, if local anesthesia is used
Bronchoscopy	Nose or mouth ➡ throat ➡ larynx ➡ trachea ➡ bronchial tree of the lung	Outpatient	General or local	Yes, if local anesthesia is used
Esophagoscopy	Mouth ➡ throat ➡ larynx ➡ esophagus	Outpatient	Local	Yes
Gastroscopy	Mouth ➡ throat ➡ larynx ➡ esophagus ➡ stomach	Outpatient	Local	Yes
Esophagogastro- duodenoscopy	Mouth ➡ throat ➡ larynx ➡ esophagus ➡ stomach ➡ duodenum (the first portion of the small intestine)	Outpatient	Local	Yes

moidoscope can travel the rectum and about one-third of the way up the colon, while a colonoscope provides a tour of the entire bowel. Although the colonoscope is twice as long as the sigmoidoscope, colonoscopies are actually the less uncomfortable of the two procedures, because patients receive IV sedation.

Sigmoidoscopy	
Typical setting:	outpatient
Anesthesia:	not required
Sedation:	not required

Colonoscopy	
Typical setting:	outpatient
Anesthesia:	not required
Sedation:	yes

As with any lower GI evaluation, it is essential that the large intestine be empty. Patient preparations vary, but most medical facilities start you on a clear-liquid diet (no solid or semisolid foods) the day before, in combination with one or more enemas and/or several glasses of a bowel-cleansing solution.

The doctor briefly conducts a digital rectal exam before introducing the scope. You may feel mild cramping or pressure as it negotiates the twists and turns of the colon, more so with a colonoscopy than with a sigmoidoscopy. Breathe slowly and deeply through your mouth—this helps relax the abdominal muscles. Air instilled through the scope to expand the caterpillar-like folds of the colorectal walls frequently brings about gas pains and flatulence. Don't be embarrassed, and don't strain to control the gas. Believe me, the medical personnel won't even notice.

Should the physician find a polyp—a benign or potentially cancerous growth that forms on the large bowel's inner lining—it can be snipped with a forceps and then cauterized, or removed by generating an electric current through a wire snare. When a sigmoidoscopy reveals a polyp in the lower portion of the intestine, the doctor will usually schedule a full colorectal endoscopy, at which time the polyp seen on sigmoidoscopy is excised, along with any newly discovered ones.

Typically, patients who've undergone a sigmoidoscopy can go home after a few minutes of rest. Following a colonoscopy, you are held for observation until you are fully awake from the sedative, then discharged in the care of someone who can drive you home.

CYSTOSCOPY (CYSTOURETHROSCOPY)

Used in detecting cancers of the bladder, prostate, and ovary

You are positioned lying on your back, with your knees apart and your feet in stirrups.

Typical setting:	outpatient
Anesthesia:	local or
	general
Sedation:	not required

Before inserting the endoscope in the *urethra,* the doctor coats it with a topical anesthetic jelly. Though some urologists still use a rigid cystoscope, the trend is toward the thinner, flexible kind, which conforms more to the anatomy. Older patients tend to tolerate cystoscopy better, partly because the urethra dilates with age. Men usually experience more discomfort than women. Not only is a man's urethra longer, running from the tip of the penis to the bladder, but the prostate gland wraps snugly around the narrow tube. Advancing the scope past this point can produce pain, though only for an instant. (Memo to men: Take deep breaths and resist the urge to tighten your pelvic muscles.) Once the instrument has reached the bladder, the doctor may instill fluid through a separate channel to expand the muscular walls for a clearer view. Cystoscopy is considered conclusive for diagnosing bladder cancer.

Drinking plenty of water afterward will help to diminish the burning sensation often felt the first time you urinate.

SURGICAL ENDOSCOPIES

Laparoscopy ▪ Mediastinoscopy ▪ Mediastinotomy ▪ Thoracoscopy

Surgical endoscopies enable a doctor to examine internal organs by inserting a slender flexible tube through a small incision in the skin rather than subjecting patients to a major operation. For instance, exploratory laparoscopy of the abdomen can often be done on an outpatient basis, whereas exploratory laparotomy requires five to seven days of hospitalization.

Endoscopic technique also leaves a smaller scar and requires a briefer recuperation. Example: a half-inch incision in the chest for a thoracoscopy of the lung, as compared to the two-inch incision for open-chest exploratory surgery (thoracotomy). If lung tissue is to be sampled during a thoracoscopy, one or two other, smaller ports are made for passing instruments.

Biopsies

BONE-MARROW ASPIRATION AND BONE-MARROW CORE-NEEDLE BIOPSY

Used in detecting leukemia, lymphomas, and multiple myeloma.

You are positioned lying on your stomach.

These two needle biopsies of the bone marrow may be performed separately or in tandem. A marrow aspiration suctions out a small quantity of marrow fluid into a syringe, while in a marrow biopsy a wider instrument with a sharpened edge is used to withdraw a wedge of marrow tissue.

Typical setting:	outpatient
Anesthesia:	local
Sedation:	not required, but can be requested

The ridge in the pelvic bone usually serves as the puncture site, although the base of the spine and the breastbone are also available. First, local anesthetic is injected into the overlying skin and muscle, and down to the *periosteum,* the tough protective membrane that covers all bones. Once the area is numb, the physician introduces the biopsy needle as far as the periosteum. Penetrating it and the bone's hard outer layer requires a twist-and-push motion, as if turning a screw.

TABLE 3.3   Types of Surgical Endoscopies

Name	Site of Incision	Used in Detecting These Cancers	Anesthesia	Typical Setting and Typical Hospital Stay
Laparoscopy	In or below the navel	Small intestine Pancreatic Liver	General	Outpatient; or inpatient, 2–3 days
Mediastinoscopy	Chest, above the breastbone	Lung Mediastinal	General	Outpatient; or inpatient, 2 days
Mediastinotomy	Chest, next to the breastbone	Lung Mediastinal	General	Outpatient; or inpatient, 2 days
Thoracoscopy	Chest	Lung	General	Inpatient, 2–5 days

According to Dr. Jill Lacy of the Yale Cancer Center, patients should brace for several seconds of sharp pain "when the marrow is being aspirated out." Though inserting the larger core needle into the bone cavity is more arduous, a person having a marrow biopsy is likely to feel "a sensation of pressure but not a lot of pain."

After removing the instrument, the doctor presses on the wound to control bleeding, then applies an adhesive bandage. Dr. Lacy observes that "the level of comfort for the patient improves substantially in proportion to the experience of the person performing the procedure."

Other types of biopsies are described earlier in this chapter under the specific cancer each is used to diagnose.

Other Tests

IODINE UPTAKE TEST

Used in detecting cancer of the thyroid.

An iodine uptake test is conducted over two days. On day one, you swallow a capsule containing a small amount of radioactive iodine. When you return the next day, a technician in nuclear medicine aims a handheld probe at your neck. This device measures the radioactivity, which is proportionate to how much of the isotope was absorbed by the thyroid. The normal range is 10 to 30 percent after twenty-four hours. Increased uptake would not be consistent with thyroid cancer. To produce a picture of the gland, most patients additionally undergo a radionuclide scan before leaving.

Typical setting:	outpatient
Anesthesia:	not required
Sedation:	not required

ELECTROENCEPHALOGRAM (EEG)

Used in detecting cancer of the brain.

You are positioned lying on your back.

The *electroencephalograph,* an unimposing rectangular recorder, measures brain waves by way of disc-shaped *electrodes* that attach to the scalp with a dab of paste. So that they adhere properly, you'll be instructed to shampoo thoroughly the night before and to refrain from using hair spray or similar products the morning of your EEG. Another type of electrode attaches to the scalp with tiny needles, which can produce a prickling sensation that some patients find uncomfortable.

Typical setting:	**outpatient**
Anesthesia:	**not required**
Sedation:	**not required**

A technician places two dozen or more electrodes about the head. Don't worry about getting shocked; it's a common misconception. Wires connected to the electrodes carry minute electrical impulses *from* the body *to* the machine. Ink pens map the electrical activity from various areas of the brain on a slowly moving roll of paper. After the test is over, the electrodes are peeled off; a nurse helps you clean the paste out of your hair.

What's in a Number? How Staging Is Expressed

Staging simply provides doctors with a common language for communicating the size and extent of a patient's cancer. Thus far we've referred only to what's known as the American Joint Committee on Cancer (AJCC) classification system, which stages tumors from 0 (in situ disease) through IV (metastatic disease). While the Roman numerals give patients an idea of where they stand, the designations are so broad that two people can have the same type and stage of cancer yet be at very different places in terms of their treatment plan and prognosis.

Look at the variation within stage II breast cancer, for example:

1. The tumor is no larger than 2 centimeters but has spread to the lymph nodes located under the arm.
   Or:
2. The tumor measures between 2 and 5 centimeters and may or may not involve the nodes.
   Or:
3. The tumor is larger than 5 centimeters, but the nodes are cancer free.

**Metric/
U.S. Conversion Table**

Tumor size is expressed metrically.

Metric	Approximate U.S. Equivalent
1 centimeter	.3937 inch, or just under $\frac{1}{2}$ inch
2 centimeters	$\frac{3}{4}$ inch
3 centimeters	$1\frac{1}{4}$ inches
4 centimeters	$1\frac{1}{2}$ inches
5 centimeters	2 inches
6 centimeters	just above $2\frac{1}{4}$ inches

"So a stage II breast tumor could be 2.5 centimeters with no positive nodes, or 4.5 centimeters with twenty positive nodes," explains Dr. Larry Norton of Memorial Sloan-Kettering Cancer Center. "Or it could be anywhere in between. The smaller, node-negative tumor would most likely have a very good prognosis, whereas the larger node-positive tumor would have a poorer prognosis.

"In addition, they would be treated differently." Following surgery to remove the malignancy, the node-negative patient might be given hormone therapy; the women whose nodes tested positive for cancer, chemotherapy.

What Is TNM Staging?

Oncologists generally rely on a more precise system of staging called *TNM classification*. It's worth understanding because you may come across it in a doctor's report, or it might arise in a conversation with your physician.

TABLE 3.4 TNM Designations: What They Mean	
Tumor (T)	
TX	The primary tumor cannot be assessed
T0	No evidence of the primary tumor
TIS	Carcinoma in situ
T1, T2, T3, T4	Progressive increase in the tumor's size and the degree to which it involves other tissues
Nodes (N)	
NX	The regional lymph nodes cannot be assessed
N0	No evidence of regional lymph-node involvement
N1, N2, N3	Progressive degrees of regional lymph-node involvement
Metastasis (M)	
MX	Presence of distant metastasis cannot be assessed
M0	No evidence of metastasis
M1, M2, M3	Progressive degrees of distant metastasis

TNM really isn't all that complicated:

T stands for tumor size and involvement of adjacent tissues.
N stands for lymph nodes—is there regional nodal involvement?
M stands for metastasis—has the cancer spread to distant parts of the body, including lymph nodes?

Each letter is accompanied by a number, which denotes an ascending increase in tumor volume or degree of involvement.

Because they specify different tumor sizes and anatomic landmarks, the definitions vary considerably from cancer to cancer. Using kidney cancer and pancreatic cancer as examples, TNM staging of *T*2, *N*1, *M*0 tells the doctor the following information:

Kidney Cancer	Pancreatic Cancer
*T*2: The tumor measures more than 2.5 centimeters and is confined to the kidney.	*T*2: The tumor extends directly to the duodenum (part of the small intestine), the bile duct, or tissues around the pancreas.
*N*1: The cancer has spread to a single regional lymph node measuring 2 centimeters or less.	*N*1: The cancer has spread to regional lymph nodes.
*M*0: There is no evidence of distant metastasis.	*M*0: There is no evidence of distant metastasis.

In either case, *T*2, *N*1, *M*0 would be equivalent to stage III, though that, too, isn't the same among all forms of cancer. With carcinoma of the bladder, for instance, *N*1 lymph-node involvement puts the disease at stage IV, regardless of the tumor's size.

Now for the really confusing part: Still other staging systems exist for certain cancers. The need for a standardized classification system has been addressed but not yet rectified. For a patient's purposes, the numbers 0, I, II, III, and IV (or the letters A, B, C, D, or the terms "limited" and "extensive"—not all cancer staging is expressed the same way) tell us much of what we need to know. Bear in mind, though, that no staging system indicates the cancer's histology (cell type), grade, hormone-receptor status, and other characteristics that might influence the treatment plan and the prognosis.

See "Other Questions Answered by the Biopsy," page 132.

Staging: A Moving Target

Clinical staging, based on physical exams, lab tests, and radiologic and endoscopic studies, may change once the tumor has been surgically removed and biopsies are analyzed. For example, "even though stomach cancer may look localized on a CT scan," says Dr. Harinder Garewal, "when the surgeon operates, he'll frequently find it has spread through the stomach wall or to the lymph glands—in other words, more than what we anticipated." Yet with pancreatic cancer, the reverse is often true. According to Dr. Charles Yeo, "CT scans can overrepresent the size of the primary tumor due to pancreatic inflammation being visible around the tumor."

Staging Designations for Each of the 25 Most Common Types of Cancer

Cancer of the Prostate

STAGE I

The cancer produces no symptoms, cannot be felt during a digital rectal exam, and cannot be seen on an imaging study. It is usually discovered accidentally, as when surgery is performed to treat benign prostatic hyperplasia. Five percent or less of the tissue removed contains cancer that is well-differentiated in appearance or grade (see box).

STAGE II

(1) The cancer produces no symptoms, cannot be felt during a digital rectal exam, and cannot be seen on an imaging study. It is usually discovered accidentally, as when surgery is performed to treat benign prostatic hyperplasia. Five percent or less of the tissue removed contains cancer that is moderately differentiated or poorly differentiated in grade.

Or:

(2) The cancer produces no symptoms, cannot be felt during a digital rectal exam, and cannot be seen on an imaging study. It is usually discovered accidentally, as when surgery is performed to treat benign prostatic hyperplasia. More than 5 percent of the tissue removed contains cancer of any grade.

Or:

(3) The cancer produces no symptoms, cannot be felt during a digital rectal exam, and cannot be seen on an imaging study. It is discovered by way of a needle biopsy, after an elevated PSA blood test. Any grade.

Or:

(4) The cancer produces no symptoms, cannot be felt during a digital rectal exam, and cannot be seen on an imaging study. Any grade.

Or:

(5) The cancer, which is confined to the prostate, produces no symptoms, cannot be felt during a digital rectal exam, and cannot be seen on an imaging study. It is discovered in one or both lobes of the prostate by way of a needle biopsy, after an elevated PSA blood test. Any grade.

Or:

Grading Prostate Cancer

Tumor grade is especially significant in prostate cancer. A system of numbers from 1 to 5 is used to describe how normal or abnormal a tissue sample appears under the microscope:

1: has normal features
2–4: has intermediate features
5: has abnormal features

Because the differentiation can vary from one area of the prostate to another, the largest portion is assigned a primary grade; the next-largest portion, a secondary grade. The two grades are added together to yield a *Gleason score* from 1 to 10. The higher the number, the more aggressive the cancer.

---

(6) The cancer has extended into the capsule covering the prostate. Any grade.

STAGE III

The cancer has extended through the capsule covering the prostate. Any grade.

STAGE IV

(1) The cancer has spread to nearby organs such as the neck of the bladder, external sphincter, rectum, surrounding muscle, or the pelvic wall. Any grade.

Or:

(2) The cancer has spread to the regional lymph nodes. Any grade.

Or:

(3) The cancer has spread to one or more distant organs.

Cancer of the Breast

DUCTAL CARCINOMA IN SITU

The cancer is isolated within the breast duct and has not infiltrated other parts of the breast.

STAGE I

The cancer measures no larger than 2 centimeters (³⁄₄ inch) and has not spread outside the breast.

STAGE II

IIA: The cancer measures between 2 and 5 centimeters (³⁄₄ inch to 2 inches).

Or:

The cancer is no larger than 2 centimeters but involves the axillary lymph nodes located under the arm.

IIB: The cancer measures between 2 and 5 centimeters and has spread to the underarm lymph nodes.

Or:

The cancer is larger than 5 centimeters but has not spread to the underarm lymph nodes.

STAGE IIIA

(1) The cancer is smaller than 5 centimeters and has spread to the lymph nodes under the arm, and the lymph nodes are attached to each other or to other structures.

Or:

(2) The cancer measures larger than 5 centimeters and has spread to the underarm lymph nodes.

STAGE IIIB (INOPERABLE DISEASE)

(1) The cancer has spread to nearby tissues, such as the skin or the chest wall, including the ribs and chest muscles.

Or:

(2) The cancer has spread to lymph nodes inside the chest wall along the breastbone.

STAGE IV

The cancer has metastasized to other organs of the body or to the skin and lymph nodes inside the neck, near the collarbone.

◆ *A rare type of breast cancer called inflammatory breast cancer is staged no lower than stage III, and if it has metastasized to distant organs, stage IV.*

Cancer of the Lung

Small-Cell Lung Cancer

LIMITED STAGE

The cancer is confined to one lung and to neighboring lymph nodes.

EXTENSIVE STAGE

The cancer has spread outside the lung to other tissues in the chest or to other sites in the body.

Non-Small-Cell Lung Cancer

CARCINOMA IN SITU

The cancer is found in only a few layers of cells in a local area and has not penetrated the lung's top lining.

STAGE I

The cancer is confined to the lung.

STAGE II

The cancer has spread to nearby lymph nodes.

STAGE III

The cancer has spread to the chest wall or the diaphragm; or to the lymph nodes in the mediastinum; or to the lymph nodes on the other side of the chest or in the neck.

STAGE IV

The cancer has metastasized to other parts of the body.

Cancer of the Colon or Rectum

CARCINOMA IN SITU

Cancer cells exist in the innermost lining of the colon or rectum.

STAGE I (ALSO REFERRED TO AS DUKES STAGE A)

The cancer has spread beyond the inner lining to the second or third layer and involves the inside wall of the colon or rectum.

STAGE II (DUKES STAGE B)

The cancer has spread outside the colon or rectum to nearby tissue.

STAGE III (DUKES STAGE C)

The cancer involves nearby lymph nodes.

STAGE IV (DUKES STAGE D)

The cancer has spread to other parts of the body.

Lymphomas

Hodgkin's Disease

Each stage of Hodgkin's disease is divided into A or B, with B indicating that a patient has experienced these symptoms: (1) weight loss exceeding 10 percent of normal body weight in the previous six months, (2) fever, and (3) night sweats.

STAGE I

The cancer is found in only one region of lymph nodes or in only one area or organ outside of the lymph nodes.

STAGE II

(1) The cancer is found in two or more lymph nodes on the same side of the diaphragm.

Or:

(2) The cancer is found in only one area or organ outside of the lymph nodes and in the surrounding nodes; and other lymph nodes on the same side of the diaphragm may also have cancer.

STAGE III

The cancer is found in lymph-node regions on both sides of the diaphragm and may also have spread to an area or organ near the lymph-node areas and/or to the spleen.

STAGE IV

(1) The cancer has spread in more than one spot to an organ or organs outside the lymphatic system, and cancer cells may or may not be found in lymph nodes near these organs.

Or:

(2) The cancer has spread to only one organ outside the lymphatic system but has involved lymph nodes far away from that organ.

Non-Hodgkin's Lymphoma

STAGE I

The cancer is found in only one region of lymph nodes or in only one area or organ outside of the lymph nodes.

STAGE II

(1) The cancer is found in two or more lymph nodes on the same side of the diaphragm.

Or:

(2) The cancer is found in only one area or organ outside of the lymph nodes and in the lymph nodes around it, and other lymph nodes on the same side of the diaphragm may also have cancer.

STAGE III

The cancer is found in lymph-node regions on both sides of the diaphragm and may also have spread to an area or organ near the lymph-node areas and/or to the spleen.

STAGE IV

(1) The cancer has spread in more than one spot to an organ or

organs outside the lymphatic system, and cancer cells may or may not be found in lymph nodes near these organs.

Or:

(2) The cancer has spread to only one organ outside the lymphatic system but has involved lymph nodes far away from that organ.

Cancer of the Bladder

CARCINOMA IN SITU

The cancer is found only on the bladder's inner lining.

STAGE I

The cancer has spread a little deeper into the inner lining.

STAGE II

The cancer has spread to the inner half of the bladder's muscular wall.

STAGE III

The cancer has spread throughout the muscular wall and/or to the layer of tissue surrounding the bladder.

STAGE IV

The cancer has spread to the nearby reproductive organs or to area lymph nodes and may also have metastasized to distant sites in the body.

Melanoma

MELANOMA IN SITU

The cancer exists only in the outer layer of the skin, the epidermis.

STAGE I

The cancer, found in the epidermis and/or the upper part of the dermis, measures less than 1.5 millimeters thick (1/16 inch).

STAGE II

The cancer, measuring 1.5 millimeters to 4 millimeters (less than ⅙ inch) in thickness, has spread to the lower part of the dermis.

STAGE III

(1) The cancer measures more than 4 millimeters in thickness.
Or:
(2) The cancer has spread to the body tissue below the skin.
Or:
(3) The cancer has spawned "satellite" tumors within one inch of the original tumor.
Or:
(4) The cancer has spread to nearby lymph nodes, or satellite tumors can be found between the primary tumor and area lymph nodes.

STAGE IV

The cancer has spread to other organs or to distant lymph nodes.

Cancer of the Uterus (Endometrial Cancer)

ATYPICAL UTERINE HYPERPLASIA

A precancerous condition in which an overproliferation of normal cells causes the inner lining of the uterus to thicken.

STAGE I

The cancer is limited to the uterus.

STAGE II

IIA: The cancer has spread to the glandular tissue in the area where the uterus narrows into the cervix.

IIB: The cancer has spread deeper into the tissue of the cervix.

STAGE III

The cancer has invaded other tissues outside the uterus but remains within the pelvis.

STAGE IV

The cancer has metastasized beyond the pelvis, to other parts of the body, or to the lining of the bladder or the rectum.

Leukemia

Acute Myeloid Leukemia (AML)

There are no staging designations for AML.

UNTREATED

No treatment has been given other than to relieve symptoms. The blood and bone marrow contain excess white blood cells; additional signs and symptoms of the disease may be evident.

IN REMISSION

Following treatment, the numbers of white blood cells and other blood cells in the blood and bone marrow are normal, and there are no signs or symptoms of leukemia.

Acute Lymphocytic Leukemia (ALL)

There are no staging designations for ALL.

UNTREATED

No treatment has been given other than to relieve symptoms. The blood and bone marrow contain excess white blood cells; additional signs and symptoms of the disease may be evident.

IN REMISSION

Following treatment, the numbers of white blood cells and other blood cells in the blood and bone marrow are normal, and there are no signs or symptoms of leukemia.

Chronic Lymphocytic Leukemia (CLL)

STAGE 0

The white-cell count is elevated, but no symptoms are evident.

STAGE I

The white-cell count is elevated; lymph nodes are swollen.

STAGE II

The white-cell count is elevated; lymph nodes, the liver, and the spleen are swollen.

STAGE III

The white-cell count is elevated, the red-cell count is abnormally low; lymph nodes, the liver, or the spleen may be swollen.

STAGE IV

The white-cell count is elevated; the platelet count is abnormally low; the red-cell count may also be abnormally low; lymph nodes, the liver, or the spleen may be swollen.

Chronic Myeloid Leukemia (CML)

CHRONIC PHASE

A few blast cells are found in the blood and bone marrow.

ACCELERATED PHASE

More blast cells appear in the blood, and there are fewer normal cells.

BLASTIC PHASE

Blast cells make up more than 30 percent of the cells in the blood or bone marrow; tumors may arise in bones or lymph nodes.

MENINGEAL PHASE

Leukemia is found in the cerebrospinal fluid.

Cancer of the Kidney (Renal-Cell Carcinoma)

STAGE I

*T*1: The cancer measures less than 2.5 centimeters (1 inch) and is confined to the kidney.

*T*2: The cancer measures more than 2.5 centimeters but is still confined to the kidney.

STAGE II

The cancer has spread to the fat around the kidney but not beyond the organ's capsule.

STAGE III

The cancer involves the kidney's main blood vessel (the renal vein); or the vessel that carries the blood from the kidney to the heart (the inferior vena cava); or neighboring lymph nodes.

STAGE IV

The cancer has spread to nearby organs or to distant sites.

Cancer of the Pancreas

STAGE I

*T*1: The cancer is confined solely to the pancreas.

*T*2: The cancer has extended to the portion of the small intestine that connects to the stomach (the duodenum), the bile duct, or other neighboring tissues.

STAGE II

The cancer has spread to adjacent organs, such as the stomach, spleen, or colon but not to the lymph nodes.

STAGE III

The cancer involves the regional lymph nodes.

STAGE IV

The cancer has metastasized to distant sites, most often the liver or lung.

Cancer of the Ovary

STAGE I

IA: The cancer is confined to one ovary.

IB: The cancer is found in both ovaries.

IC: The cancer is found in one or both ovaries, but the tumor sits on the surface of the organ(s); or the tumor has ruptured the capsule(s) of the gland(s); or malignant cells are found in excess abdominal fluid known as ascites.

STAGE II

The cancer is found in one or both ovaries and has spread to other body parts within the pelvis.

IIA: The cancer has infiltrated or metastasized to the uterus and/or the fallopian tubes.

IIB: The cancer has infiltrated other tissues within the pelvis.

IIC: The cancer is either stage IIA or stage IIB, but the tumor sits on the surface of the organ(s); *or* the tumor has ruptured the capsule(s) of the organ(s); *or* malignant cells are found in excess abdominal fluid known as ascites.

STAGE III

The cancer involves one or both ovaries and has spread to other body parts inside the abdomen, such as the surface of the liver or the intestines, and possibly the lymph nodes.

IIIA: Microscopic amounts of the cancer are found on the surface of tissues in the abdomen.

IIIB: None of the cancers found on the surface of tissues in the abdomen measures more than 2 centimeters (³⁄₄ inch).

IIIC: (1) One or more of the cancers found on the surface of the tissues in the abdomen measures 2 centimeters. *Or:* (2) The cancer has spread to the lymph nodes.

STAGE IV

One or both ovaries contain cancer that has spread outside the abdomen or infiltrated the inside of the liver.

Cancer of the Stomach

CARCINOMA IN SITU

The cancer is found only in the innermost of the four layers of the stomach wall.

STAGE I

IA: The cancer has infiltrated the second or third layers of the stomach wall but not the neighboring lymph nodes.

IB: The cancer has spread to the second layer and to nearby lymph nodes.

STAGE II

(1) The cancer is in the second layer of the stomach wall and has spread to lymph nodes farther away from the tumor.

Or:

(2) The cancer is in the third layer and has spread to nearby lymph nodes.

Or:

(3) The cancer extends through all four layers but has not invaded lymph nodes or other organs.

STAGE III

(1) The cancer has reached the third layer of the stomach wall and has spread to lymph nodes farther away from the tumor.

Or:

(2) The cancer extends through all four layers and has spread to lymph nodes either very close to the tumor or farther away.

Or:

(3) The cancer is in all four layers and has spread to nearby tissues but may or may not have spread to neighboring lymph nodes.

STAGE IV

The cancer has spread to nearby tissues and to lymph nodes farther away from the tumor or has metastasized to other parts of the body.

Cancer of the Liver

LOCALIZED RESECTABLE PRIMARY LIVER CANCER

The cancer is found in one place in the liver and can be completely removed surgically.

LOCALIZED UNRESECTABLE PRIMARY LIVER CANCER

The cancer is found in one place in the liver but cannot be totally removed.

ADVANCED PRIMARY LIVER CANCER

The cancer has spread through much of the liver or to other parts of the body.

Cancers of the Lip and Oral Cavity

CARCINOMA IN SITU

Cancer cells are present, but only in the first layer of cells that make up the lining of the oral cavity.

STAGE I

The cancer measures no more than 2 centimeters (¾ inch) and has not spread to area lymph nodes.

STAGE II

The cancer measures more than 2 centimeters but less than 4 centimeters (1½ inches) and has not spread to area lymph nodes.

STAGE III

(1) The cancer measures more than 4 centimeters.
Or:
(2) The cancer is any size but has spread to only one lymph node, measuring 3 centimeters (1¼ inches) or less, on the same side of the neck.

STAGE IV

(1) The cancer has spread to tissues around the lip (bone, tongue, skin of the neck) or the oral cavity (bone, deep muscles of the tongue, skin, or the sinuses on either side of the nose), and possibly to one or more area lymph nodes.
Or:
(2) The cancer is any size and has spread to a single lymph node, measuring more than 3 centimeters but not more than 6 centimeters

(more than 2¼ inches), on the same side of the neck; *or* to multiple lymph nodes, none more than 6 centimeters in size, on the same side of the neck; *or* to lymph nodes, none more than 6 centimeters in size, on the opposite side of the neck or on both sides of the neck.

Or:

(3) The cancer has spread to other parts of the body.

Cancer of the Thyroid

Papillary Thyroid Cancer

STAGE I

The cancer is confined to one or both lobes of the thyroid.

STAGE II

If you are younger than forty-five years old: The cancer has spread beyond the thyroid.

If you are forty-five years old or older: The cancer remains confined to the thyroid and measures larger than 1 centimeter (about ½ inch).

STAGE III

The cancer, found in patients forty-five and older, is larger than 4 centimeters (1½ inches); or it has spread outside the thyroid but not outside the neck; or it has spread to the lymph nodes.

STAGE IV

The cancer, found in patients forty-five and older, has spread to other parts of the body.

Follicular Thyroid Cancer

STAGE I

The cancer is confined to one or both lobes of the thyroid.

STAGE II

If you are younger than forty-five years old: The cancer has spread beyond the thyroid.

If you are forty-five years old or older: The cancer remains confined to the thyroid and measures larger than 1 centimeter (about ½ inch).

STAGE III

The cancer, found in patients forty-five and older, is larger than 4 centimeters (1½ inches); or it has spread outside the thyroid but not outside the neck; or it has spread to the lymph nodes.

STAGE IV

The cancer, found in patients forty-five and older, has spread to other parts of the body.

Medullary Thyroid Cancer
STAGE I

The cancer measures less than 1 centimeter (about ½ inch).

STAGE II

The cancer measures between 1 and 4 centimeters (about ½ inch to 1½ inches).

STAGE III

The cancer has spread to the lymph nodes.

STAGE IV

The cancer has spread to other parts of the body.

Anaplastic Thyroid Cancer
There is no staging system for anaplastic cancer of the thyroid. All patients are considered to have stage IV disease.

(Adult) Cancers of the Brain

Brain tumors are not staged per se, but graded on the basis of how normal (well differentiated) or abnormal (anaplastic) the cells appear. In general, well-differentiated tumors grow less rapidly and tend to have a better prognosis than anaplastic tumors.

For the types and subtypes of brain tumors, see "(Adult) Cancers of the Brain" in Chapter Two, "The Basics: What Every Patient Needs to Know About Cancer."

Multiple Myeloma

STAGE I

(1) Relatively few cancer cells have spread throughout the body; (2) the blood contains normal amounts of red blood cells and calcium; (3) no tumors are found in the bone; and (4) the amount of M proteins in the blood or urine is very low.

STAGE II

A moderate number of cancer cells has spread throughout the body.

STAGE III

A relatively large number of cancer cells has spread throughout the body, and there may be one or more of the following: (1) a decrease in the number of red blood cells, causing anemia; (2) abnormally high levels of calcium in the blood; (3) more than three bone tumors; (4) high levels of M protein in the blood or urine.

Cancer of the Cervix

CARCINOMA IN SITU

The cancer is found only in the cervical lining's first layer of cells.

STAGE IA

The cancer involves the cervix but is visible only under a microscope.

STAGE IB

A larger amount of cancer is found in the cervical tissue.

STAGE IIA

The cancer has spread to the upper two-thirds of the vagina.

STAGE IIB

The cancer has spread to the tissue around the cervix.

STAGE IIIA

The cancer has spread to the lower third of the vagina.

STAGE IIIB

The cancer extends to the pelvic wall or has caused kidney distension or kidney failure.

STAGE IVA

The cancer has invaded the bladder or rectum.

STAGE IVB

The cancer has spread to distant organs.

Cancer of the Esophagus

CARCINOMA IN SITU

Cancer cells are found solely in the first layer of cells that make up the lining of the esophagus. In situ cancer of the gullet is rarely seen in the United States.

STAGE I

The cancer is confined to a small portion of the esophagus.

STAGE II

The cancer covers much of the esophagus and may have spread to nearby lymph nodes, but it has not infiltrated other tissues.

STAGE III

The cancer has spread to neighboring tissues or lymph nodes.

STAGE IV

The cancer has metastasized to other parts of the body.

Cancer of the Larynx

CARCINOMA IN SITU

The cancer is present but has not invaded laryngeal tissue.

STAGE I

Supraglottic cancer: The cancer is confined to one area of the supraglottis, and the vocal cords can move normally.

Glottic cancer: The cancer is confined to the vocal cords, which can move normally.

Subglottic cancer: The cancer is confined to the subglottis.

STAGE II

Supraglottic cancer: The cancer is in more than one area of the supraglottis, but the vocal cords can move normally.

Glottic cancer: The cancer has spread to the supraglottis, the subglottis, or both. The vocal cords may or may not be able to move normally.

Subglottic cancer: The cancer has infiltrated the vocal cords, which may or may not be able to move normally.

STAGE III

(1) The cancer has not spread outside the larynx but impairs movement of the vocal cords.

Or:

(2) The cancer has spread to neighboring tissues.

Or:

(3) The cancer has spread to one lymph node measuring no more than 3 centimeters (1¼ inches) on the same side of the neck as the cancer.

STAGE IV

(1) The cancer has spread to nearby tissues, such as the throat and possibly area lymph nodes.

Or:

(2) The cancer has spread to more than one lymph node on the same side of the neck as the cancer, or to lymph nodes on one or both sides of the neck, or to any lymph node that measures more than 6 centimeters (about 2¼ inches).

Or:

(3) The cancer has spread to other parts of the body.

Cancer of the Throat (Pharyngeal Cancer)

Nasopharyngeal Cancer

STAGE I

The cancer is found in only one part of the nasopharynx.

STAGE II

The cancer is found in more than one part of the nasopharynx.

STAGE III

(1) The cancer has spread into the nose or to the oropharynx.
Or:
(2) The cancer is in the nasopharynx or has spread to the nose or the oropharynx; and it involves only one lymph node, measuring 3 centimeters ($1\frac{1}{4}$ inches) or less, on the same side of the neck as the tumor.

STAGE IV

(1) The cancer has spread to the bones or nerves in the head, with or without any lymph-node involvement.
Or:
(2) The cancer is in the nasopharynx or has spread to the nose, another part of the nasopharynx, or the bones or nerves in the head; and it involves more than one lymph node on the same side of the neck as the tumor, or lymph nodes on one or both sides of the neck, or any lymph node that measures more than 6 centimeters ($2\frac{1}{4}$ inches).
Or:
(3) The cancer has spread to other parts of the body.

Oropharyngeal Cancer

STAGE I

The cancer measures no more than 2 centimeters ($\frac{3}{4}$ inch).

STAGE II

The cancer measures more than 2 centimeters but less than 4 centimeters (1½ inches).

STAGE III

(1) The cancer measures more than 4 centimeters.
Or:
(2) The cancer is any size but has spread to only one lymph node on the same side of the neck, *and* the cancerous lymph node measures no more than 3 centimeters (1¼ inches).

STAGE IV

(1) The cancer has spread to surrounding tissues and possibly to area lymph nodes.
Or:
(2) The cancer is any size and has spread to more than one lymph node on the same side of the neck, or to lymph nodes on one or both sides of the neck, or to any lymph node measuring more than 6 centimeters (about 2¼ inches).
Or:
(3) The cancer has spread to other parts of the body.

Hypopharyngeal Cancer

STAGE I

The cancer is in only one part of the hypopharynx.

STAGE II

The cancer is in more than one part of the hypopharynx.

STAGE III

(1) The cancer is in more than one part of the hypopharynx or has spread to adjacent tissue, *and* has invaded the larynx.
Or:
(2) The cancer is in the hypopharynx or has spread to adjacent tissue, has spread to only one lymph node on the same side of the neck, and the cancerous node measures no more than 3 centimeters (1¼ inches).

STAGE IV

(1) The cancer has spread to the connecting tissue or soft tissues of the neck and may or may not have affected area lymph nodes.

Or:

(2) The cancer is in the hypopharynx or has spread to adjacent tissue, and has spread to more than one lymph node on the same side of the neck, or to lymph nodes on one or both sides of the neck, or to any lymph node measuring more than 6 centimeters (about 2¼ inches).

Or:

(3) The cancer has spread to other parts of the body.

Soft-Tissue Sarcomas

Stages I through III of soft-tissue sarcomas are divided into A and B, with A denoting that the tumor measures 5 centimeters (2 inches) or less. B sarcomas are larger than 5 centimeters.

STAGE I

The cancer cells appear similar to normal cells.

STAGE II

The cancer cells appear somewhat different from normal cells.

STAGE III

The cancer cells appear very different from normal cells.

STAGE IVA

The cancer has spread to regional lymph nodes.

STAGE IVB

The cancer has metastasized to other parts of the body.

Cancer of the Testicle

STAGE I

The cancer is confined to the testicle.

STAGE II

The cancer has spread to the retroperitoneal lymph nodes in the back of the abdomen or the para-aortic lymph nodes in the upper abdomen. Patients who have cancerous retroperitoneal nodes larger than 5 centimeters (2 inches) are said to have *bulky* disease.

STAGE III

In nonbulky stage III, the cancer has spread to lymph nodes beyond the retroperitoneum and to the lung, but the masses are no larger than 2 centimeters (¾ inch); bulky stage III testicular cancer is characterized by extensive retroperitoneal involvement, as well as metastasis to the lung and sometimes the liver or the brain.

Cancer of the Small Intestine

Small-Intestine Adenocarcinoma

ADENOCARCINOMA IN SITU

Cancer cells exist in the innermost lining of the small bowel.

STAGE I

The cancer has invaded the layer of connective tissue beneath the mucous membrane or deeper still into the muscular layer of the bowel wall.

STAGE II

(1) The cancer has advanced through the muscular layer and into the tissue beneath the thin membrane that lines the abdominal and pelvic cavities.

Or:

(2) The cancer has advanced through the muscular layer and extended no more than 2 centimeters (¾ inch) into nearby tissue.

Or:

(3) The cancer has perforated the thin membrane that holds the abdominal organs.

Or:

(4) The cancer has extended more than 2 centimeters into nearby tissues, or has invaded the abdominal wall or the pancreas.

STAGE III

The cancer has infiltrated regional lymph nodes.

STAGE IV

The cancer has metastasized to distant organs.

Small-Intestine Lymphoma, Small-Intestine Leiomyosarcoma, Small-Intestine Carcinoid Tumor

There are no formal staging definitions for the other three types of small-bowel cancer. They are generally identified as being localized, regional, or metastatic.

What Are My Odds? Making Sense of Survival Rates

Like me, you're a reader. Undoubtedly, at some point in researching cancer, you'll come across the *survival rates* for your type of cancer. Seeing your prognosis summed up as a percentage can be upsetting. I know. Around the time that I was diagnosed with stage III colon cancer, the odds of living five years were 30 to 50 percent. I quickly computed the inverse of that: an ominous five-year mortality rate of 50 to 70 percent.

These statistics must be interpreted with caution. To start, "five-year survival" doesn't mean that five years is the longest you can expect to live. It is a yardstick for measuring the relative effectiveness of treatments. For most forms of cancer, reaching this milestone without relapsing constitutes a cure. In colon cancer, though, living beyond three years is considered a significant landmark, whereas breast cancer and melanoma can sometimes recur twenty years later. As cancer therapy improves, and more patients survive long-term, we'll begin to see more ten-year survival rates, fifteen-year survival rates, and so on.

It's also important to take into account that survival rates are *averages* based on large numbers of patients, some of whom have received less-than-optimal care. Others have had coexisting medical conditions that compromised their treatment; or didn't take care of themselves as well as they might have; or refused treatment altogether.

TABLE 3.5 Five-Year Survival Rates

Type of Cancer	Percentage of Patients Who Survive a Minimum of Five Years from the Time Their Cancer Is Diagnosed			
	Overall	Localized Disease	Regional Disease	Metastatic Disease
Prostate	93%	100%	99%	33%
Breast	85	97	77	22
Lung	14	50	20	2
Colorectal	62	91	66	9
Lymphomas	56	NA	NA	NA
Hodgkin's disease	80			
Non-Hodgkin's lymphomas	51			
Bladder	82	95	50	6
Melanoma	88	96	59	12
Uterine	84	96	66	27
Leukemia	40	NA	NA	NA
CLL	69			
ALL	56			
CML	27			
AML	11			
Kidney	61	89	62	10
Pancreatic	4	17	6	1
Ovarian	50	95	79	28
Stomach	21	60	21	2
Liver	5	15	5	2
Oral	53	82	42	20
Thyroid	95	100	94	44
Brain	29	34	32	52
Multiple myeloma	28	*Multiple myeloma is staged according to the number of cancer cells in the body:*		
		Relatively Few (Stage I) 25–40	*Moderate (Stage II)* 15–30	*Relatively Large (Stage III)* 10–25

TABLE 3.5 **Five-Year Survival Rates**				
Type of Cancer	**Percentage of Patients Who Survive a Minimum of Five Years from the Time Their Cancer Is Diagnosed**			
	Overall	**Localized Disease**	**Regional Disease**	**Metastatic Disease**
Cervical	70	91	48	11
Esophageal	12	24	12	2
Laryngeal	66	83	54	44
Throat		NA	NA	NA
Nasopharyngeal	48			
Oropharyngeal	25			
Hypopharyngeal	26			
Soft-tissue sarcomas	64	NA	NA	NA
Testicular	95	99	98	73
Small intestine	51	NA	NA	NA

NA: Figures not applicable.

Source: National Cancer Institute Surveillance, Epidemiology and End Results (SEER) Program, 1998.

Perspective

Statistics are open to interpretation. "Some people can be told they have just a 5 percent chance of survival, and they'll say, 'I'm going to be one of those 5 percent,'" observes Dr. Julia Rowland, director of psycho-oncology at the Lombardi Cancer Center. "The flip side of that are patients who are told they have a 95 percent chance of living, and they'll worry, 'I'm going to be in that 5 percent group, where it comes back.'"

As a cancer survivor, I would suggest viewing your disease in the following light: Nineteen seventy-one marked the official declaration of the "war" against cancer, in the form of the National Cancer Act. As in any war, this one is made up of individual battles. It may be a cliché—one repeated endlessly by doctors—but everybody (and every body) truly is unique.

"Statistics are statistics," says Dr. Rowland. "Maybe only 10 percent of patients with your type and stage of cancer are cured, but within that 10 percent, your odds are zero percent or 100 percent." That was how I chose to look at it: *Either I make it or I don't.*

I will tell you about the mental trick I played on myself as a way of coping. During one visit to Dr. Paul Woolley, my original attending oncologist, he was discussing my case with someone over the phone. When asked what stage of colon cancer I had, Dr. Woolley answered evasively. I assumed it was for my benefit.

"Well," he replied, "it's kind of stage II going on stage III." I remember chuckling to myself. Although Dr. Woolley had never discussed my stage with me, I'd read enough to know darn well that the cancer's having spread to the lymph nodes placed me firmly in the stage III category. But the odds of surviving stage II disease were far more encouraging: 50 to 75 percent. Since the doctor had hedged his answer, I chose to believe that I had stage II colon cancer, not stage III.

Chapter Four

How Cancer Is Treated

Only since the 1970s have the allies in the war against cancer waged a truly united effort. Until then, surgical oncologists, medical oncologists, and radiation oncologists seemed to be fighting alone on separate fronts.

"Initially, each discipline was trying to figure out what its role was," reflects Dr. Christine Berg, director of breast radiation therapy at the Lombardi Cancer Center and an oncologist since 1981. "Now that we've essentially learned how to best deliver our own modality, the strategy has evolved into combining therapies, not only to enhance the effectiveness of the overall treatment but to return patients to their normal lives as much as possible."

As an example, she points to the current use of surgery in conjunction with radiation therapy to treat certain sarcomas of the limbs. Almost without exception, a cancer of the thigh used to require amputation. Today, the surgical-radiologic approach enables doctors "to limit the extent of the operation as well as limit the extent of the radiation," says Dr. Berg. Only the tumor and the surrounding tissue must be removed, rather than the entire leg.

The question facing most cancer patients, then, isn't *which* form of treatment they'll be offered, but whether their situation calls for two—or perhaps more—therapies, and in what sequence.

The Roles and Goals of Treatment

Surgery remains the cornerstone of treatment for most cancers and virtually all solid tumors. Only 10 percent of all cancer cures can be attributed to radiation therapy alone; another 5 percent to radiation in combination with chemotherapy.

Chemo by itself rarely achieves a lasting remission, which is not to say it is ineffective. More and more, the anticancer drugs are implemented soon after the *primary* treatment—again, usually surgery, but sometimes radiation. The concept behind *adjuvant* chemotherapy, as this is called, "is to treat any remaining disease even though we can't detect it," explains Dr. Jill Lacy of the Yale Cancer Center in New Haven, Connecticut.

"For instance, in breast cancer, 'adjuvant' would imply that the patient had undergone surgery to remove the tumor. Everything else appears to be tumor free, yet we administer chemotherapy because we know the odds are very high that there is *occult* disease lurking somewhere that's ultimately going to become problematic." "Occult" means that cancer is present, but in amounts too small to be seen.

Radiation therapy, too, is used to wipe out vagrant malignant cells following surgery. But in medical vernacular, "adjuvant" typically specifies *systemic* treatments such as chemo and biological therapy, which hunt down malignant cells throughout the body's circulation. By contrast, radiation and surgery treat cancer *locally.*

One relatively new strategy in cancer care is to give select patients chemotherapy prior to surgery *(neoadjuvantly)* in order to shrink the tumor to a more operable size. Radiation may precede surgery as well. Thus the blueprint for treating, say, rectal carcinoma that has spread to neighboring lymph nodes might consist of:

1. Preoperative radiation therapy
alone or in conjunction with

2. Preoperative chemotherapy   **(Neoadjuvant therapy)**
followed by

3. Surgery to remove the tumor and   **(Primary therapy)**
area lymph nodes
followed by

4. Chemotherapy   **(Adjuvant therapy)**

Naturally, every patient and every physician hope treatment will deliver a cure. Should that outcome appear beyond reach, the object of therapy shifts to prolonging life by slowing the cancer's growth and preventing it from spreading, and/or relieving symptoms—provided, of course, that the patient wishes to pursue this course. Doctors refer to symptom management as *palliative* care, such as palliative radiation of the prostate to shrink a tumor that is interfering with urination.

Cancer Therapies

Surgery

May serve as primary therapy for most solid tumors.

Cancer surgery's benefit is twofold. Eradicating the primary tumor reduces the chances of the malignancy recurring in that part of the body. In addition, explains Dr. Marie Pennanen of the Lombardi Cancer Center, it enhances the potential performance of nonsurgical treatments against any residual cancer cells "because they're working against a lower tumor burden."

Depending, of course, on the cancer's location and size, the surgeon cuts out *(resects, excises)* as much of the tumor as possible—preferably all of it—as well as a *margin* of surrounding tissue approximately 1 centimeter wide. "Then we assess the margin under the microscope," says Dr. Pennanen, a surgeon. "Does the cancer come up to the outer edge of the tissue specimen? If not, that's a *negative margin.*" From this, the surgeon can infer that no visible cancer remains inside the patient.

"The larger the cancer, though," she says, "the more likely you are to have a *positive margin.*" Such a finding might warrant widening the border of normal tissue, unless it was felt the patient could not withstand further surgery, for any number of health reasons. "And sometimes," the doctor notes, "there's a gray zone, or what we call a *close margin,*" where the cancer treads near the rim of the specimen. "This will frequently require that additional tissue be resected in order to obtain a wider negative margin."

One exciting frontier in cancer surgery is the use of laparoscopy. As with laparoscopic biopsy, it is less invasive than conventional surgery and promises a shorter hospitalization and recuperation. The technique may not prove suitable for all cancers, but it's worth inquir-

---

Medical Terms You're Likely to Hear

Anastomosis: surgically connecting two organs, such as the small intestine and the rectum following a colectomy to remove the colon; or sewing together the severed ends of an organ as part of surgical resection.

-ectomy: a suffix meaning "surgical excision." In a mastectomy, the surgeon removes the breast; subtotal gastrectomy is an operation to resect a portion of the stomach; and so on.

Gross tumor: cancer that is visible to the naked eye during surgery.

---

ing about. Thus far, says Dr. Pennanen, "surgeons have applied laparoscopic surgery to cancers of the large intestine and the female reproductive tract."

The primary form of treatment for early-stage endometrial cancer is a total hysterectomy: the surgical removal of a woman's uterus and cervix, along with her ovaries and fallopian tubes. In the hands of an experienced laparoscopic surgeon, this can be accomplished by way of the vagina with the aid of a laparoscope that is inserted through a small incision in the belly button. The patient leaves the operating room with several small incisions instead of one large one, and goes home possibly the same day, as compared to the minimum three-day hospital stay for an abdominal hysterectomy. And the recuperation at home is about half as long.

See Chapter Seven, "What You Can Expect During Treatment."

Other Types of Cancer Surgery

Laser Surgery—The laser, a narrow beam of amplified light capable of cutting through tissue precisely, debuted in cancer surgery in 1961. It is used sparingly, mainly for vaporizing superficial lesions of the larynx, throat, and oral cavity, and as a palliative measure against tumors that obstruct the respiratory tract or digestive tract. Photodynamic therapy, described later in this chapter, destroys malignant cells by injecting them with a photosensitizing agent, then firing an arrow of laser light at the cancer.

What are the advantages of laser surgery over the quaint scalpel? There are smaller, tidier incisions. And because the heat generated by the beam seals and sterilizes the wound, there is less bleeding, swelling, and scarring, though not necessarily less pain. Now for the drawbacks. "The laser is cumbersome and extremely expensive to maintain," says Dr. Mitchell Morris, a gynecologic oncologist at Houston's M. D. Anderson Cancer Center and one of the few surgeons with experience in operating the device.

Oral and maxillofacial surgeon Rocco Addante of the Norris Cotton Cancer Center in Lebanon, New Hampshire, points out that because the beam obliterates lesions, "the doctor doesn't have tissue he can submit to a pathologist." It is conceivable, he says, that a mass believed to be noninvasive based on a previous incisional biopsy (which samples only a portion of a lump) could actually have contained cancer in other areas. But with no specimen to analyze under a microscope, "we would have no way of knowing that, and the patient would be more likely to have a recurrence." According to Dr. Morris, laser surgery has all but been put out of business as a treatment for cervical dysplasia and cervical carcinoma in situ by the comparatively simple *loop electrosurgical excision procedure* (LEEP).

◆ *May be used in treating cancers of the oral cavity, throat, esophagus, larynx, colon, lung, brain, and cervix.*

See "Photodynamic Therapy," page 276.

Electrosurgery—One example of electrosurgery is the aforementioned loop electrosurgical excision procedure (LEEP), which shears off precancerous and noninvasive lesions of the cervix with an electrically charged wire lasso. A similar technique may be used to treat early carcinomas of the bladder, colon, and rectum and inoperable prostate cancer. In these cases, the physician passes the wire snare through a flexible endoscope that has been inserted into the urethra or the anus. Another form of electrosurgery, *fulguration,* can destroy small tumors. Here an electrical probe showers sparks over the tissue, burning it away.

◆ *May be used in treating cancers of the bladder, cervix, colon, rectum, and prostate.*

Cryosurgery—Cryosurgery, killing malignant cells with extreme cold, was initially used to treat skin cancer by spraying or swabbing the area with frozen liquid nitrogen. Now it is also being employed against several noninvasive or localized internal tumors.

The liquid nitrogen circulates inside an instrument called a *cryoprobe,* which can be likened to a frozen knife. When treating unresectable liver cancer cryosurgically, the physician inserts the probe through an incision in the abdomen and directly into the tumor, freezing it. Then it is allowed to thaw. "We usually do three of these cycles," says Dr. Ted Lawrence of the University of Michigan Comprehensive

Cancer Center, adding that "each takes about twenty minutes." The tissue dies and soon sloughs off.

◆ *May be used in treating cancers of the liver, oral cavity, prostate, skin, and small intestine.*

Radiation Therapy (Radiotherapy)

May serve as primary therapy for cancers of the bladder, throat, larynx, brain, prostate, lung, rectum, oral cavity, cervix, thyroid, esophagus, and for lymphomas and inoperable localized tumors elsewhere in the body.

In *external-beam* radiation therapy, a machine levels high-energy rays directly at the tumor; or, if given after surgery has been performed, at the tumor bed, to wipe out any cells left behind. Whole-body irradiation is generally administered as a prelude to bone-marrow transplantation, though it has been tried experimentally as a treatment for advanced non-Hodgkin's lymphoma.

Depending on the type of cancer and the size and location of the tumor, the radiation oncologist planning your therapy will select one of three radiation sources: *X rays, gamma rays* from a machine containing the radioactive substance *cobalt 60,* or *electron-beam* radiation. Dr. Christine Berg offers an example: "We might use electron-beam radiation to treat a superficial skin tumor, because it penetrates little more than one inch into body tissue." X rays, on the other hand, can travel as deep as ten inches.

All three lock in on rapidly dividing cells, whether cancerous or not. To minimize the damage to surrounding tissue, you initially undergo a planning session, at which time imaging studies are taken and a *radiation therapist* defines the exact *field* to be irradiated. Sophisticated scanning techniques such as computed tomography and magnetic resonance imaging have made it possible to conform the beam precisely to the target area. What's more, says Dr. Berg, "our computers are now better able to combine the images from these scans with those from our treatment-planning computers, so that we can superimpose the images and better identify exactly how we're going to deliver the radiation."

Despite these precautions, some healthy cells get zapped. Because radiotherapy treats cancer locally, whatever side effects you may experience (and we emphasize *may*) are usually limited to the region being irradiated. For example, radiation to the abdomen can cause nausea and diarrhea, while people undergoing chest radiation may experience shortness of breath, chronic coughing, and/or difficulty in swallowing. Then there is the general fatigue that frequently sets in toward the end of treatment, lingering for weeks following the final session, as a result of the body's expending energy to heal injured cells.

How Frequently Is Radiation Therapy Given?

"Radiation is a gradual process," explains Dr. Berg. The total dose, measured in units called *grays*—and many times greater than that used for diagnostic X rays—is meted out over an extended period of time. "This allows us to give a higher total amount of radiation more safely and effectively," she says. On average, patients receive treatment Monday through Friday for six weeks. With testicular cancer, which calls for a lower dose, therapy can often be wrapped up within three weeks—roughly the same schedule as when giving radiation to alleviate symptoms rather than therapeutically.

Normal cells repair themselves faster than malignant cells, and so the weekend furloughs afford them opportunities to recover. The mortally wounded cancer cells, unable to replicate, die, and their remains are carried off by the bloodstream and excreted naturally.

See Chapter Seven, "What You Can Expect During Treatment."

> **Other Methods of Radiation Therapy**
>
> **Intraoperative radiotherapy:** a large dose of external radiation delivered to the tumor bed and neighboring tissue during surgery.
>
> **Radioprotectors:** investigational drugs sometimes given before radiation treatments, to protect normal tissue.
>
> **Radiosensitizers:** investigational drugs sometimes given before radiation treatments, to enhance their effectiveness.
>
> **Stereotactic radiosurgery:** a specialized form of radiotherapy carried out by a machine nicknamed the *gamma knife*. Used almost exclusively to treat brain tumors.
>
> See "(Adult) Cancers of the Brain" in Chapter Six, "State of the Art: Your Treatment Options."

Hyperfractionated Radiation Therapy

This experimental technique for delivering radiation rations the dose into smaller amounts that are administered every four to six hours, two or three times a day. According to Dr. Berg, "It appears to have some benefit for certain disease sites" such as head and neck cancers and other tumors that divide extremely rapidly.

Be forewarned that the accelerated timetable tends to increase side effects—not to mention infringe on one's daily schedule. Most men and women receiving hyperfractionated radiation are able to be treated as outpatients, commuting back and forth to the medical facility throughout the day. One appealing aspect to this, Dr. Berg points out, is that it shortens the total course.

Internal Radiation Therapy

Internal radiation entails surgically implanting a radioactive substance into a body cavity or directly into the tumor. The purpose, explains Dr. Berg, "is to deliver a dose of radiation continually over several days, while minimizing some of the side effects to the surrounding tissue, since we're not coming in from the outside."

Unlike external-beam radiation, the internal route does leave patients radioactive, but only for a few days. During that brief period, spent in the hospital, you can have visitors aged eighteen and older, so long as they sit at least six feet away from your bed and stay no more than forty-five minutes.

The *radionuclides* are sealed in containers such as pellets, wires, needles, and capsules, which a physician implants under general or local anesthesia. "Then we bring the patient to his room," says Dr. Berg, "and load the radiation source into the applicator, with protective shields placed around the person." You will be awake while this is being done.

◆ *May be used in treating melanoma and cancers of the prostate, lung, rectum, oral cavity, ovary, breast, uterus, thyroid, brain, cervix, and throat.*

See Chapter Seven, "What You Can Expect During Treatment."

Types of Internal Radiation

Low-Dose-Rate Implants—These are left in place for one to seven days. Afterward the doctor removes them in a bedside procedure that rarely requires the use of an anesthetic.

Permanent Implants—These remain in the body. After a few days they begin to decay, eventually losing their radioactivity.

High-Dose-Rate Remote Brachytherapy—Some physicians refer to all internal radiation as brachytherapy, which essentially means "treatment from a short distance." This method can be given on an outpatient basis. You lie alone in a room and are observed on closed-circuit TV while the brachytherapy team uses remote control to deliver a large dose of radiation through a catheter tube into the tumor. "It takes only a few minutes," says Dr. Berg, "then the catheter is removed." If necessary, high-dose-rate remote brachytherapy can be repeated several times over the next one to two weeks.

> **Medical Terms You're Likely to Hear**
>
> **Interstitial radiation:** an implant directly into the tumor.
>
> **Intracavitary radiation:** an implant into a body cavity such as the uterus.

Systemic Radiation Therapy—Injecting an unsealed radioactive substance into the bloodstream has at present several applications in cancer care. Men and women with thyroid cancer routinely receive intravenous I-131 radioiodine after surgery. Two other IV pharmaceuticals, strontium 89 (brand name: Metastron) and samarium 153 (Quadramet), have been found to relieve pain from secondary tumors of the bone. A radioactive form of phosphorus, chromic phosphate P-32 (Phosphocol P-32), is sometimes used to treat ovarian cancer. The liquid radioisotope is injected into the peritoneal sac that encloses the abdomen.

Chemotherapy

May serve as primary therapy for cancers of the bladder, leukemia, multiple myeloma, small-cell lung cancer, lymphomas, and inoperable tumors elsewhere in the body.

> **Medical Terms You're Likely to Hear**
>
> **Chemoradiation:** chemotherapy and radiotherapy administered at the same time *(concomitantly)* instead of one after the other *(sequentially)*.
>
> **Medical:** pertaining to treatment incorporating medication, as distinguished from surgery.

The word "chemotherapy" still evokes shudders, bringing to mind images of skeletally thin, balding patients racked by relentless nausea and vomiting. There's no denying that in addition to killing malignant cells throughout the body, these harsh chemicals can produce some nasty side effects. However, one of the most significant advances in cancer medicine has been the advent of effective medications for managing nausea, pain, appetite loss, and other adverse reactions. Administering symptom control prior to treatment can avert some of these complications altogether.

Nine in ten cancer patients receive chemotherapy, usually as a second act to surgery. We noted before that chemo alone rarely effects a cure, but when used adjuvantly it can bump up your chances for success. Dr. John Marshall of the Lombardi Cancer Center relies on percentages to help make the potential benefits seem more real to patients.

"Frequently, they have just come from the surgeon, who has told them, 'I've gotten it all,' " he says. "So I start by saying, 'You're probably wondering why you're here in an oncologist's office. Yes, the surgeon cut out everything he could see. But there is a chance some tumor cells were left behind. Now, what can we do to change that?'

"Then I'll tell them what the data show, using specific numbers. For example, in node-negative breast cancer and colon cancer, the benefit of chemotherapy is less than 10 percent. But it's real. So let's say your odds of surviving five years are seventy-thirty after surgery. If we can improve those odds to eighty-twenty, is that worth six months or a year of chemotherapy?"

As part of the discussion, Dr. Marshall is candid in raising the possibility that the person might not need chemotherapy at all. The problem is that there's no way of knowing for sure. If chemo was used and the cancer doesn't come back, "we'll never know if it was due to the chemotherapy or if it wasn't going to come back in the first place," he explains. "And if it does, did the chemo delay the recurrence, or was it entirely ineffective?" Dr. Marshall sets out these and other considerations to help patients make an informed decision about whether or not to proceed with this arm of treatment.

"Some will decide no," he says. "But most are willing to try anything that might help them."

Types of Chemotherapeutic Agents

Chemotherapy, defined as the treatment of illness by means of chemicals, can be said to encompass any agent used to treat cancer, including hormonal and biological therapies. Usually, though, the term applies to *antineoplastics:* medications that through one mechanism or another stop tumor cells from developing and multiplying.

Medical Terms You're Likely to Hear

Cytotoxin: in cancer treatment, chemotherapy or any other substance capable of killing malignant cells.

The largest family, *alkylating agents,* uses brute force to damage the cells' DNA. *Antimetabolites,* the next largest, disrupt the cells' metabolism. *Enzyme inhibitors,* a relatively new class of drugs, interfere with substances necessary for cancer to grow. *Protecting agents* offset the toxic effects of other chemotherapeutic agents. There are several more categories, which we've grouped under the general heading "antineo-plastics."

Like radiation therapy, the drugs hone in on rapidly dividing cells. Cancer cells bear the brunt of the assault, but normal cells that make up the hair follicles, the lining of the digestive tract, and the white blood cells are also especially vulnerable. Consequently, hair loss, assorted digestive problems, and an abnormally low white-cell count rank among chemotherapy's more common side effects.

Since chemotherapy became a mainstay of cancer treatment in the mid-1940s, more than 250,000 agents have been tested for their anti-tumor properties. Fewer than 60 have been approved as safe and effective for patients.

How Is Chemotherapy Administered?

Because the families that make up the clan of antineoplastics act on cancer cells at different stages in their life cycle, the trend has been toward combining chemotherapeutic agents. To give you an example, one standard regimen for treating acute lymphocytic leukemia consists of four drugs: vincristine (brand name: Oncovin), an *alkaloid salt* derived from the periwinkle plant; the *enzyme* asparaginase (Elspar); daunorubicin (Cerubidine), an *anthracycline;* and prednisone (Deltasone), a hormone.

Prednisone, taken by mouth, enters the blood through the lining of the stomach or intestines. But most chemotherapeutic drugs are too toxic to be ingested orally or are not readily absorbed that way. Vincristine, asparaginase, and daunorubicin must be given through a needle into a vein, usually in the hand or lower arm, or through a flexible tube surgically implanted in the upper chest or elsewhere in the body. *Intravenous* (IV) administration is the quickest and most common means of delivering chemotherapy to the circulation. The medicine is either injected (IV push) through a syringe needle, or it is diluted in a

> ### What Are Response Rates?
>
> During your research, you may come across the term *response rate* in relation to chemotherapy, particularly new agents or drug combinations being tested in patients, as in "a response rate of 75 percent."
>
> "It generally means the percentage of patients in whom the tumor shrank by at least 50 percent," explains Dr. Barnett Kramer of the National Cancer Institute. This is referred to as a *partial* response. "But for some tumors, like testicular cancer, you will see a substantial number of *complete* responses, where all evidence of the tumor is gone." Thus a 75 percent partial response rate indicates the treatment in question reduced tumor size by at least half in three-quarters of the patients studied.

TABLE 4.1   **Chemotherapy Drugs FDA-Approved for Commercial Use**

Generic Name	Brand Name	Category
altretamine	Hexalen	Alkylating agent
anastrozole	Arimidex	Antineoplastic
asparaginase	Elspar	Enzyme
bleomycin	Blenoxane	Antineoplastic
busulfan	Myleran	Alkylating agent
capecitabine	Xeloda	Antineoplastic
carboplatin	Paraplatin	Alkylating agent
carmustine (BCNU)	BiCNU	Alkylating agent
chlorambucil	Leukeran	Alkylating agent
cisplatin	Platinol	Alkylating agent
cladribine	Leustatin	Antimetabolite
cyclophosphamide	Cytoxan, Neosar	Alkylating agent
cytarabine	Cytosar-U	Antimetabolite
dacarbazine	DTIC-Dome	Alkylating agent
dactinomycin (actinomycin-D)	Cosmegen	Antineoplastic
daunorubicin	Cerubidine	Antineoplastic
docetaxel	Taxotere	Antineoplastic
doxorubicin	Doxorubicin, Adriamycin, Rubex, Doxil	Antineoplastic
epirubicin	Ellence	Antineoplastic
estramustine	Emcyt	Antineoplastic
etoposide	VePesid, VP-16	Antineoplastic
floxuridine	FUDR	Antimetabolite
fludarabine	Fludara	Antimetabolite
fluorouracil	Fluorouracil	Antimetabolite
gemcitabine	Gemzar	Antimetabolite
hydroxyurea	Hydrea	Antimetabolite
idarubicin	Idamycin	Antineoplastic
ifosfamide	IFEX	Alkylating agent
irinotecan	Camptosar	Enzyme inhibitor

TABLE 4.1   Chemotherapy Drugs FDA-Approved for Commercial Use

Generic Name	Brand Name	Category
leucovorin	Leucovorin, Wellcovorin	Protecting agent/folic acid derivative
lomustine (CCNU)	CeeNU	Alkylating agent
mechlorethamine	Mustargen	Alkylating agent
melphalan	Alkeran	Alkylating agent
mercaptopurine	Purinethol	Antimetabolite
mesna	Mesnex	Protecting agent
methotrexate	Methotrexate	Antimetabolite
mitomycin	Mutamycin	Antineoplastic
mitotane	Lysodren	Antineoplastic
mitoxantrone	Novantrone	Antineoplastic
paclitaxel	Taxol	Antineoplastic
pamidronate	Aredia	Bone resorption inhibitor
pegasparagase	Oncaspar	Enzyme
pentostatin	Nipent	Antimetabolite
plicamycin	Mithracin	Antineoplastic
procarbazine	Matulane	Alkylating agent
streptozocin	Zanosar	Alkylating agent
temozolomide	Temodar	Alkylating agent
teniposide	Vumon	Antineoplastic
testolactone	Teslac	Antineoplastic
thioguanine	Tabloid	Antimetabolite
thiotepa	Thioplex	Alkylating agent
topotecan	Hycamtin	Enzyme inhibitor
tretinoin	Vesinoid	Vitamin A derivative
uracil mustard	Uracil Mustard	Alkylating agent
valrubicin	Valstar	Antineoplastic
vinblastine	Velban	Antineoplastic
vincristine	Oncovin	Antineoplastic
vinorelbine	Navelbine	Antineoplastic

TABLE 4.2   **Special Delivery: Other Routes for Administering Chemotherapy**

Interstitial—into the tumor. One unique treatment for a highly malignant form of brain cancer is to surgically implant small dissolvable wafers infused with the chemotherapy drug carmustine (BiCNU) directly into the tumor bed.

Intra-arterial—into an artery

Intracavitary—into the abdominal cavity, pelvic cavity, or pleural cavity in the chest

Intralesional—into the cancerous area in the skin

Intramuscular—into a muscle, usually in the arms, thighs, or buttocks

Intraperitoneal—into the saclike *peritoneal membrane* that lines the abdominal and pelvic cavities. Has been used experimentally in ovarian cancer.

Intrathecal—through the sheath of the spinal cord and into the *cerebrospinal fluid* that flows within the *subarachnoid space*.

Intraventricular—another way to reach the cerebrospinal fluid is to inject the drug into a catheter that's been surgically implanted into one of the brain's four fluid-filled pockets *(ventricles)*. The tube leads to a storage receptacle called an *Ommaya reservoir,* placed just below the scalp for the purpose of receiving the shot.

Subcutaneous—under the skin

Topical—applying medication onto the skin

---

plastic bag hung from a pole and *infused* slowly (IV drip). Some patients receive *continuous infusion* by way of an external or internal pump.

Chemotherapy isn't exclusively systemic. One treatment for early bladder cancer is surgery followed by *intravesical* chemotherapy, in which a drug is instilled into the bladder through a tube inserted through the urethra. In *isolated arterial perfusion,* an experimental therapy for melanoma of the arms or legs, a tourniquet is wrapped below the armpit or groin, temporarily stopping the flow of blood to the extremity. Then chemotherapy is added directly to the artery supplying the limb, so that most of the dose reaches the tumor.

A related technique, implemented in liver cancer and soft-tissue sarcomas, is local or regional *intra-arterial* chemotherapy. Normally, anticancer drugs are introduced into a vein. But whereas a blood vessel called the portal vein feeds normal liver tissue, cancerous liver tissue latches onto the hepatic artery for the bulk of its supply. Infusing chemotherapy into that major vessel delivers a double benefit: a concentrated dose of medication to the tumor and less of a system-wide effect.

How Often Will I Get Chemotherapy and for How Long?

Oncologists dispense chemotherapy in *cycles*, with time off in between to let the body renew itself. During the six months I spent on fluorouracil and leucovorin, I received my injections five days in a row each month. Fluorouracil and levamisole, then regarded as the standard adjuvant regimen for my stage of colon cancer, called for one year of weekly cycles.

"The schedules vary tremendously," says Maureen Sawchuk, nursing coordinator at the Lombardi Cancer Center. "It could be one day a month, or it could be five days a week for three months." Chemotherapy typically spans anywhere from three months to three years. The duration and frequency of treatment are subject to adjustment, as researchers learn more about how these drugs impact on patients, not only physically but also on their daily lives. For instance, says Sawchuk, "some of our more elderly patients can't come in for chemotherapy five days in a row because of lack of transportation. So they might be put on continuous infusion at home through a home-care agency."

Your chemotherapy will be divided into three *courses.* The first, *induction,* lasts weeks or months and is designed to obliterate as many cancer cells as possible. Because the drugs' effectiveness wanes eventually, during the *consolidation* phase new agents may be substituted or added, with the intent of stalking resistant malignant cells. The goal of *maintenance,* the mildest and final stage, is to pick off any stragglers over a period of months, sometimes years.

See Chapter Seven, "What You Can Expect During Treatment."

Hormone Therapy

May serve as primary therapy for advanced cancers of the prostate, breast, and uterus.

Perhaps *"anti*hormone therapy" would be a more fitting name for this systemic treatment, since it is often administered to block a specific hormone's action. *Hormones,* the body's chemical transmitters, travel through the bloodstream to moderate or accelerate vital processes such as growth, metabolism, and sexual development. Certain hormones, though, also stimulate tumor growth in the breast, endometrium, and prostate.

For example, the female sex hormone estrogen spurs the development of breast-cancer cells, while the male sex hormone testosterone exerts an equivalent effect on prostate-cancer cells. A woman whose localized breast-tumor tissue tests positive for hormone receptors might receive tamoxifen following surgery in lieu of or in addition to chemotherapy. Tamoxifen, an *antiestrogen,* protects the cells from estrogen's influence. (It also induces a cytotoxic effect, causing some breast-cancer cells to self-destruct.) Similarly, a man with inoperable prostate cancer might be put on an *antiandrogen* such as flutamide plus a second drug that shuts down testosterone production entirely. For either cancer, the same outcome can be achieved by surgically removing the source of estrogen (the ovaries) or testosterone (the testicles).

Hormonal agents work in ways other than suppressing hormone activity. Prednisone, a widely prescribed *corticosteroid,* not only silences the body's inflammatory response to the invasion of cancer, it demonstrates a cytotoxic effect against the malignant white blood cells associated with lymphomas, multiple myeloma, and lymphocytic leukemias. A multifaceted steroid called dexamethasone reduces the swelling surrounding brain tumors, prevents diarrhea, quells nausea, and may have antitumor properties as well.

Potential side effects from hormone therapy tend to be milder than those commonly seen with chemotherapy. Men sometimes find that their sex drive has shifted into low gear; the agents can also bring about impotence, either temporarily or permanently. As for women, treatment can disrupt the menstrual cycle and lead to vaginal dryness. Patients of either gender may experience complications such as nausea and vomiting, swelling or weight gain, and infertility.

Immunotherapy

May be used in treating melanoma and cancers of the kidney, bladder, colon, and rectum; also an experimental treatment for a variety of advanced cancers.

Immunotherapy fights cancer by harnessing the body's own *immune system,* the complex network of white blood cells, proteins, and or-

TABLE 4.3   Hormonal Therapy Agents

Generic Name	Brand Name	Category
aminoglutethimide	Cytadren	Hormone inhibitor
androgens		Male hormone agents
fluoxymesterone	Halotestin	
methyltestosterone	Android	
	Oreton	
	Testred	
testosterone	Delatestryl	
betamethasone	Celestone	Corticosteroid
bicalutamide	Casodex	Antiandrogen
dexamethasone	Decadron	Corticosteroid
estrogens	Estratab	Female hormone agents
	Estrone	
	Menest	
	Premarin	
chlorotrianisene	Tace	
diethylstilbestrol	Stilphostrol	
estradiol	Estrace	
estropipate	Ogen	
	Ortho-Est	
flutamide	Eulexin	Androgen inhibitor
goserelin	Zoladex	LHRH agonist
ketoconazole	Nizoral	Antifungal[1]
letrozole	Femara	Enzyme inhibitor
leuprolide	Lupron	LHRH agonist
levothyroxine	Levothroid	Thyroid hormone
	Levoxyl	
	Synthroid	
nilutamide	Nilandron	Antiandrogen
octreotide	Sandostatin	Hormone agent

TABLE 4.3	Hormonal Therapy Agents	
Generic Name	**Brand Name**	**Category**
prednisolone (liquid	Pediapred	Corticosteroid
prednisone)	Prelone	
prednisone	Deltasone	Corticosteroid
	Prednicen	
	Sterapred	
progestins		Female hormone agents
hydroxyprogesterone	Hylutin	
	Prodrox	
medroxyprogesterone	Depo-Provera	
megestrol	Megace	
tamoxifen	Nolvadex	Antiestrogen
toremifene	Fareston	Antiestrogen

¹ Ketoconazole, an antifungal, has testosterone-lowering properties.

Medical Terms You're Likely to Hear

Biological response-modifier therapy

Biological therapy

Biotherapy

Immunological therapy

Immunomodulation

. . . words the doctor may use when referring to "immunotherapy"

gans that protects us from disease in one of two ways: the *humoral* immune response and the *cellular* immune response. In order to appreciate the concept behind this form of treatment, you'll need a basic understanding of how the body's defense system mobilizes to attack foreign invaders, or *antigens*. Hang in there—you'll get it.

The Humoral and Cellular Immune Responses

An antigen is any substance that provokes an immune response, such as bacteria, viruses, and transplanted tissue. Each antigen gives away its identity by wearing up to several hundred distinctively shaped proteins on its surface.

Think of humoral immunity and cellular immunity as two branches of the military. Either one is capable of initiating the counterattack against antigens, though they almost always join forces eventually.

Humoral Immunity

Humoral immunity, usually triggered in response to bacteria, is set in motion by *B lymphocytes.* Each B cell is programmed to mass-produce a specific *antibody,* a protein molecule that binds itself to its matching antigen.

When a B cell recognizes its prey, it consumes the antigen and displays fragments on its surface in order to attract the attention of collaborators called *helper T lymphocytes.* Chemicals secreted by the T cells cause most B cells to proliferate into *plasma cells,* tiny factories that flood the circulation with millions of identical antibodies. The antibodies apprehend the intruders until any of several types of cells reach the scene to finish off the antigens. In the most common scenario, lethal proteins called *complement* converge upon the interlocked antigen and antibody and puncture the antigen's outer membrane, destroying it.

Cellular Immunity

If B cells are analogous to the naval branch of the body's defense network, discharging antibodies into the bloodstream like torpedoes, T lymphocytes would be the infantry. They clash directly with body cells that have been hijacked by invading viruses or genetically corrupted by cancer and penetrate their outer membranes.

In the cellular immune response, a large white blood cell called a *macrophage* gobbles up an antigen, then brandishes the pieces like a trophy. A helper T cell recognizes the trespasser and rushes to embrace the macrophage. Together the two release powerful chemicals called *lymphokines.* One lymphokine, interleukin-2, instructs other helper Ts and another type of T lymphocyte, *killer T cells,* to multiply. The killer Ts shoot holes in infected or malignant body cells. Meanwhile, as in humoral immunity, the helper Ts prompt the B cells to make antibodies. These attach to free-floating antigens and mark them for death.

Mission accomplished. Finally, yet another type of T lymphocyte, *suppressor T cells,*

Immunity's Principal Players: Your White Blood Cells (Leukocytes)

Granulocytes (62%)
- **Neutrophils**
- **Eosinophils**
- **Basophils**

Lymphocytes (34%)
- **B lymphocytes**
- **T lymphocytes**
- **NK lymphocytes**

Monocytes (4%)
- **Monocytes migrate to body tissues, where they develop into antigen-devouring cells called macrophages.**

deactivates antibody production and other immune responses, while *memory B cells and T cells* stay behind like an occupying army, poised to spring into action should the same antigen strike again. The immune system has the capacity to recognize many millions of foreign molecules, then assemble the necessary components to pursue each one.

How Immunotherapy Works

The most obvious question is why don't our bodies destroy cancer the way they do other potentially harmful entities? The reason, explains Dr. Michael Hawkins, director of clinical research at the Lombardi Cancer Center, is that cancer outfoxes the immune response by commandeering a normal cell within the body "so the immune system doesn't recognize it as foreign." What immunotherapy attempts to do is to "overcome the body's tolerance and get it to reject the cancer cell just as it would a transplanted organ." Some immunologists believe that our defense mechanisms do in fact react to cancer cells—regularly exterminating them before they can evolve into a tumor—but that the disease manages to take hold during times when our immunity is down.

As of 2000, five of the nine immunological agents approved for treating cancer act on the cellular immune response. The idea, says Dr. Hawkins, "is to administer agents that activate the patient's white blood cells and get them 'angry' enough to kill cancer cells."

TABLE 4.4	Approved Immunotherapies
Generic Name	**Brand Name**
alpha-interferons	
alfa-2A	Roferon-A
alfa-2B	Intron-A
Bacillus Calmette-Guérin (BCG) live	**Theracys, Tice BCG**
denileukin diftitox	**Ontak**
interleukin-2, IL-2, aldesleukin	**Proleukin**
levamisole	**Ergamisol**
rituximab	**Rituxan**
trastuzumab	**Herceptin**
yttrium-90 radiolabeled carcinoembryonic-antigen antibody	**yttrium-90 radiolabeled CEA-Cide**

To classify levamisole and Bacillus Calmette-Guérin (BCG) as immune response modifiers may be stretching the definition somewhat. BCG, a bacterial microorganism, is considered a standard postsurgical treatment for early-stage and recurrent bladder cancer. Instilled into the bladder by way of a catheter, "it causes an intense inflammatory reaction in the bladder wall that kills off cancer cells," explains Dr. Hawkins. As for levamisole, although it appears to behave like an immunomodulator, "it is not yet clear if it is one at all," according to Dr. Peter Rosen of the Jonsson Comprehensive Cancer Center in Los Angeles. The oral agent is given along with the drug fluorouracil as an adjuvant treatment for regional colon cancer. The combination of immunotherapy and chemotherapy is referred to as *immunochemotherapy.*

Alpha-Interferon—The first biological response modifier sanctioned for cancer therapy, interferons are a family of naturally occurring proteins that stir lymphocytic activity. They may also inhibit the growth of cancer cells, in the manner of chemotherapy. Although beta-interferon and gamma-interferon have been studied for their effectiveness against cancer, alpha-interferons 2A and 2B are the only ones currently in use.

♦ *May be used in treating melanoma, multiple myeloma, leukemia, bladder cancer, kidney cancer, and AIDS-related Kaposi's sarcoma, and as an experimental therapy for non-Hodgkin's lymphomas and several other cancers.*

Interleukin-2—Originally named T-cell growth factor, interleukin-2 stimulates T cells to vanquish malignant cells. Like interferon, it, too, is produced in the body but can be made in the laboratory. Other interleukins that act on different sites of the immune system are being tested in patients.

♦ *May be used in treating melanoma, kidney cancer, and other tumors.*

Monoclonal Antibodies (MOABs)—"For the humoral side of immunity," says Dr. Hawkins, "the approach has been to clone in the laboratory antibodies that react specifically to certain antigens on the cancer cell's surface." Originally, the MOABs were engineered by injecting human cancer cells into mice, whose immune systems proceed to turn out antibodies against the cancer. Now antibodies are being genetically engineered to be half human or almost entirely human.

Next the antibody-producing cells are harvested and fused with another cell to create a hybrid capable of making great quantities of pure antibodies indefinitely. Once injected into the patient, the MOABs latch onto their assigned antigens, then signal complement and white blood cells to swarm over the cancer cell and annihilate it.

The first monoclonal antibody cleared for use against cancer was rituximab (Rituxan), in 1997, followed the next year by trastuzumab (Herceptin). Rituxan, approved for low-grade B-cell non-Hodgkin's lymphoma, binds to an antigen produced on the surface of B cells and B-cell tumors. It is known as CD20. The man-made antibody Herceptin goes after the errant HER-2 gene found in about one-third of breast cancers. Because these MOABs target specific proteins instead of attacking all rapidly growing cells like chemotherapy does, their side effects are relatively minor. Most patients compare the symptoms to a moderate case of the flu, which subsides after the intravenous drug is administered.

Scientists at the University of Pennsylvania medical center are currently in the process of developing a *double* monoclonal antibody that would affix itself to the same receptor molecules on the exterior of cancer cells. Whereas single-antibody agents slow down tumor growth—no small feat—the two-prong assault appears to destroy the malignant cells altogether.

◆ *May be used in treating non-Hodgkins lymphomas and breast cancer, and as an experimental therapy for leukemia and cancers of the large intestine and lung.*

Targeted Therapies Using MOABs or Oncotoxins—Monoclonal antibodies can be transformed into biological guided missiles by coupling them to anticancer agents, immunological response modifiers, or radioactive substances. Injected into the body, they selectively deliver the deadly payload to their corresponding antigen. Yttrium-90 radiolabeled carcinoembryonic-antigen antibody (CEA-Cide for short), the first targeted monoclonal antibody therapy, fuses the antibody against carcinoembryonic antigen (CEA) to the potent, deeply penetrating radioisotope Y-90. CEA-Cide was first given to people with pancreatic cancer; it has since been incorporated into treatment for small-cell lung cancer and ovarian cancer.

Already an improved targeted therapy has arrived. Instead of MOABs, it pairs toxic substances with long proteins that bind to specific chemical receptors on the surface of the tumor cell. Like a Trojan horse, the *oncotoxin* sneaks into the cell, then destroys it from within. Denileukin diftitox (Ontak), a novel treatment for a rare form of non-Hodgkin's lymphoma called cutaneous T-cell lymphoma (CTCL), won FDA approval in 1999. About three in five CTCL tumors bear receptors for interleukin-2. Ontak joins IL-2 and protein from the *diphtheria toxin,* which is produced by the bacteria responsible for the contagious childhood disease of the same name.

♦ *May be used in treating cancers of the lung, prostate, and ovary, and cutaneous T-cell lymphoma. Not to split hairs, but since neither method manipulates the immune system, it would be more accurate to refer to each as a biological therapy.*

Investigational Immunotherapies

Adoptive Immunotherapy—This approach, also known as *cell-transfer therapy,* calls for removing white cells from the patient's blood, bathing them in interleukin-2 in the laboratory, then infusing them back into the circulation. The process yields supercharged *lymphokine-activated killer* (LAK) T cells capable of destroying tumors while sparing healthy cells. In the mid-1980s, the same research team that developed LAK cells applied a similar technique with special cancer-killing cells taken from actual tumor tissue, on the assumption that fewer of these *tumor-infiltrating lymphocytes,* or TILs, would be needed to enhance an immune response.

♦ *May be used experimentally in treating leukemia, metastatic melanoma, and kidney cancer.*

Tumor Necrosis Factor (TNF)—Tumor necrosis factor, another chemical emitted by white cells during the body's immune response, has been tested in patients. According to Dr. Hawkins, "It has not yet proven to be a very effective anticancer drug," partly because the dose necessary for this lymphokine to rouse immunity and impair tumor cells is highly toxic.

♦ *May be used experimentally in treating several cancers.*

Therapeutic Tumor Vaccines—Vaccines have traditionally been used to prevent illnesses. Ironically, a vaccine is made up of cells from the very disease it is expected to ward off, but in a weakened, inactivated, or dead form. Though not strong enough to bring about severe illness, it leaves its imprint on the immune system for future rendezvous with the antigen.

The first vaccine, administered to a small boy by a British physician named Edward Jenner in 1796, consisted of the *vaccinia* virus—better known as cowpox, a relative of the more deadly smallpox. Once Jenner's young patient recovered from a mild case of cowpox, the doctor inoculated him with smallpox. The boy's immune system "remembered" the virus cells from the previous encounter and mounted a defense. He never contracted the disease.

Researchers are looking for ways to apply this concept of *acquired immunity* in cancer treatment. In simple terms, a vaccine is tailor-made to each patient's cancer by using molecules extracted from the tumor. Then it is injected along with an immunostimulant such as interleukin-2. The revved-up immune system destroys this "new" antigen and commits it to memory: At last the body recognizes the cancer as foreign and launches an attack. Scientists are also experimenting with vaccines containing altered genes that, once transferred to malignant cells, could cause the cells to induce an immune response to the cancer.

◆ *May be used experimentally in treating melanoma, lymphomas, and cancers of the kidney, lung, large intestine, breast, and prostate.*

See "Gene Therapy," page 259.

Immunotherapy: Is It a Realistic Option?

For two decades, many researchers have looked to immunotherapy as the next quantum leap in cancer therapy. It's easy to see why: The notion of enhancing the body's own potential to eradicate disease is an appealing one. Progress, however, has been frustratingly slow. While immunotherapy certainly has claimed a niche for itself, for the immediate future, at least, it will continue to benefit a relatively small number of patients. Except for the handful of commercially available immune response modifiers, immunological-based cancer treatment is limited to investigational studies conducted almost exclusively at major research centers.

"The agents that have been studied so far have lacked specificity in the way they stimulate the immune system," observes Dr. Hawkins, who was involved in early clinical trials evaluating alpha-interferon. Interleukin-2 and the other immune response modifiers developed to date stimulate the overall immune response rather than target a type of cancer cell.

Immunologists have faced the same problem in cloning antibodies. "It may be that an antigen is expressed only on breast-cancer cells," says Dr. Hawkins. "But more commonly, the same antigen is expressed on some normal cells in the breast, and in the colon and/or the lungs too."

This lack of specificity brings about adverse side effects that can rival those associated with chemotherapy. "In many respects, they're worse," Dr. Hawkins says candidly. "The original concept of immunotherapy was that the agents could be given without much toxicity because they would work through the body's own immune system. But the doses of interleukin-2 that were approved for use were so high that it had to be given in an intensive-care unit and had a mortality rate of 4 percent, which is hardly 'benign therapy.' The doses of interferon that were approved for use in melanoma are also fairly high. Around half the patients needed the dose reduced at some point during the course of treatment, because of side effects."

Both agents produce flulike symptoms. In fact, the fever, chills, and fatigue we associate with the flu are caused not by the virus itself, but by the activity of our immune system, which is busy secreting IL-2, interferon, and other substances to help combat the bug. "Now, many patients would say they'd gladly take the flu over the side effects from chemotherapy," Dr. Hawkins continues. "But these treatments typically need to be given over a long period of time. Would you take a year of the flu versus chemotherapy? Maybe not."

With continued progress, perhaps one day immunotherapy will fulfill its potential. "The focus now," says Dr. Hawkins, "is to make immune stimulation more specific to the patient's cancer. That's what needs to be done before we can really take immunotherapy to the next level."

Gene Therapy

May be used experimentally in treating several cancers.

Gene therapy, which is still in its infancy, attempts to stem the disease process by altering the genetic makeup of the tumor or the body itself. This is accomplished by inserting a desirable gene into the DNA of cells that have been removed from a patient. The reprogrammed cells are then injected directly into the cancer or into droplets of fat that cling to malignant cells. This revolutionary biotechnology works

TABLE 4.5	**Agents Frequently Prescribed for Each Form of Cancer**

(B) Bone-resorption inhibitor (H) Hormonal therapy (I) Immunotherapy (PS) Photosensitizer for photodynamic therapy (R) Radiopharmaceutical

Type of Cancer	Anticancer Drugs That May Be Used (Standard therapies or drugs used most commonly are in boldface.)
Prostate cancer	▪ **estrogens (H)** ▪ **leuprolide (H)** ▪ **goserelin (H)** ▪ **flutamide (H)** ▪ estramustine ▪ prednisone (H) ▪ nilutamide (H) ▪ bicalutamide (H) ▪ ketoconazole ▪ mitoxantrone ▪ cisplatin ▪ cyclophosphamide ▪ doxorubicin
Breast cancer	▪ **cyclophosphamide** ▪ **doxorubicin** ▪ **fluorouracil** ▪ **leucovorin** ▪ **methotrexate** ▪ **tamoxifen (H)** ▪ **prednisone (H)** ▪ **vincristine** ▪ epirubicin ▪ paclitaxel ▪ docetaxel ▪ thiotepa ▪ progestins (H) ▪ aminoglutethimide (H) ▪ androgens (H) ▪ testolactone ▪ estrogens (H) ▪ pamidronate (B) ▪ goserelin (H) ▪ anastrozole (H) ▪ letrozole (H) ▪ vinorelbine ▪ trastuzumab (I) ▪ capecitabine ▪ toremifene (H) ▪ cisplatin ▪ dexamethasone (H) ▪ leuprolide (H) ▪ lomustine ▪ melphalan ▪ mitomycin ▪ vinblastine
Small-cell lung cancer	▪ **doxorubicin** ▪ **etoposide** ▪ **vincristine** ▪ **cisplatin** ▪ **cyclophosphamide** ▪ **ifosfamide** ▪ **carboplatin** ▪ methotrexate ▪ lomustine ▪ paclitaxel ▪ topotecan ▪ teniposide ▪ yttrium-90 radio-labeled carcinoembryonic-antigen antibody (I)
Non-small-cell lung cancer	▪ **cisplatin** ▪ **vinblastine** ▪ **mitomycin** ▪ **doxorubicin** ▪ **cyclophosphamide** ▪ **paclitaxel** ▪ vinorelbine ▪ docetaxel ▪ topotecan ▪ irinotecan ▪ carboplatin ▪ ifosfamide ▪ gemcitabine ▪ porfimer (PS)
Colorectal cancer	▪ **fluorouracil** ▪ **leucovorin** ▪ **levamisole (I)** ▪ irinotecan ▪ methotrexate ▪ floxuridine ▪ mitomycin ▪ lomustine
Hodgkin's disease	▪ **carmustine** ▪ **chlorambucil** ▪ **cyclophosphamide** ▪ **dacarbazine** ▪ **doxorubicin** ▪ **mechlorethamine** ▪ **procarbazine** ▪ **vinblastine** ▪

TABLE 4.5   Agents Frequently Prescribed for Each Form of Cancer

(B) Bone-resorption inhibitor (H) Hormonal therapy (I) Immunotherapy (PS) Photosensitizer for
photodynamic therapy (R) Radiopharmaceutical

Type of Cancer	Anticancer Drugs That May Be Used (Standard therapies or drugs used most commonly are in boldface.)
	vincristine ▪ **bleomycin** ▪ **prednisone/prednisolone (H)** ▪ **methotrexate** ▪ lomustine ▪ etoposide ▪ dexamethasone (H)
Non-Hodgkin's lymphomas	▪ **cyclophosphamide** ▪ **vincristine** ▪ **prednisone/ prednisolone (H)** ▪ **doxorubicin** ▪ chlorambucil ▪ bleomycin ▪ etoposide ▪ mechlorethamine ▪ procarbazine ▪ methotrexate ▪ leucovorin ▪ cytarabine ▪ fludarabine ▪ cladribine ▪ dexamethasone (H) ▪ carmustine ▪ vinblastine ▪ ifosfamide ▪ teniposide ▪ thiotepa ▪ rituximab (I) ▪ alpha-interferon (I) ▪ denileukin diftitox (I) ▪ methoxsalen (PS)
Bladder cancer	▪ **Bacillus Calmette-Guérin (BCG) (I)** ▪ thiotepa ▪ doxorubicin ▪ mitomycin ▪ cisplatin ▪ carboplatin ▪ paclitaxel ▪ methotrexate ▪ alpha-interferon (I) ▪ bleomycin ▪ cyclophosphamide ▪ fluorouracil ▪ vinblastine ▪ valrubicin ▪ ifosfamide ▪ gemcitabine
Melanoma	▪ dacarbazine ▪ carmustine ▪ cisplatin ▪ vinblastine ▪ dactinomycin ▪ vincristine ▪ lomustine ▪ levamisole (I) ▪ Bacillus Calmette-Guérin (BCG) (I) ▪ interleukin-2 (I) ▪ alpha-interferon (I) ▪ tamoxifen (H) ▪ melphalan
Endometrial cancer	▪ progestins (H) ▪ doxorubicin ▪ cisplatin ▪ tamoxifen ▪ cyclophosphamide ▪ fluorouracil
Acute myeloid leukemia (AML)	▪ **cytarabine** ▪ **daunorubicin** ▪ **idarubicin** ▪ **thioguanine** ▪ etoposide ▪ **mitoxantrone** ▪ cyclophosphamide ▪ doxorubicin ▪ mercaptopurine ▪ asparaginase ▪ fludarabine ▪ methotrexate

TABLE 4.5	**Agents Frequently Prescribed for Each Form of Cancer**

(B) Bone-resorption inhibitor (H) Hormonal therapy (I) Immunotherapy (PS) Photosensitizer for photodynamic therapy (R) Radiopharmaceutical

Type of Cancer	Anticancer Drugs That May Be Used (Standard therapies or drugs used most commonly are in boldface.)
Acute lymphocytic leukemia (ALL)	▪ **asparaginase** ▪ **daunorubicin** ▪ **vincristine** ▪ **prednisone/prednisolone (H)** ▪ **methotrexate** ▪ cyclophosphamide ▪ doxorubicin ▪ cytarabine ▪ mercaptopurine ▪ thioguanine ▪ pegasparagase ▪ dexamethasone (H)
Acute promyelocytic leukemia (APL)	▪ **tretinoin**
Chronic lymphocytic leukemia (CLL)	▪ **fludarbine** ▪ **chlorambucil** ▪ **cyclophosphamide** ▪ **prednisone (H)** ▪ cladribine ▪ pentostatin ▪ mechlorethamine ▪ dexamethasone (H)
Hairy cell leukemia	▪ **pentostatin** ▪ **cladribine** ▪ alpha-interferon (I) ▪ chlorambucil
Chronic myeloid leukemia (CML)	▪ **alpha-interferon (I)** ▪ **hydroxyurea** ▪ busulfan ▪ methotrexate ▪ cytarabine ▪ vincristine ▪ prednisone (H) ▪ doxorubicin ▪ mechlorethamine ▪ cyclophosphamide ▪ daunorubicin ▪ mercaptopurine ▪ thioguanine
Kidney cancer	▪ **interleukin-2 (I)** ▪ **alpha-interferon (I)** ▪ vinblastine ▪ lomustine
Pancreatic cancer	▪ **fluorouracil** ▪ **leucovorin** ▪ **dacarbazine** ▪ **mitomycin** ▪ **gemcitabine** ▪ yttrium-90 radiolabeled carcinoembryonic-antigen antibody (I)
Ovarian cancer	▪ **paclitaxel** ▪ **carboplatin** ▪ **cisplatin** ▪ cyclophosphamide ▪ topotecan ▪ doxorubicin ▪ ifosfamide ▪ chlorambucil ▪ altretamine ▪ fluorouracil ▪ leucovorin ▪ etoposide ▪ tamoxifen (H) ▪ melphalan ▪ thiotepa ▪ chromic phosphate P-32 (R) ▪ yttrium-90 radiolabeled carcinoembryonic-antigen antibody (I)

TABLE 4.5   Agents Frequently Prescribed for Each Form of Cancer

(B) Bone-resorption inhibitor (H) Hormonal therapy (I) Immunotherapy (PS) Photosensitizer for photodynamic therapy (R) Radiopharmaceutical

Type of Cancer	Anticancer Drugs That May Be Used (Standard therapies or drugs used most commonly are in boldface.)
Stomach cancer	• **fluorouracil** • doxorubicin • mitomycin • cisplatin • methotrexate • carmustine • etoposide • leucovorin
Liver cancer	• **doxorubicin** • **cisplatin** • **floxuridine**
Oral cancer	• bleomycin • cisplatin • carboplatin • fluorouracil • vinblastine • methotrexate • leucovorin • doxorubicin • mitomycin
Thyroid cancer	• **levothyroxine (H)** • doxorubicin • cisplatin • carboplatin • paclitaxel • docetaxel • topotecan • sodium iodide I-131 (R)
Brain cancer	• **carmustine** • **lomustine** • **procarbazine** • **vincristine** • **carboplatin** • **cisplatin** • **bleomycin** • **etoposide** • **methotrexate** • **cytarabine** • cyclophosphamide • doxorubicin • prednisone/ prednisolone (H) • dexamethasone (H) • Gliadel • topotecan • temozolomide
Multiple myeloma	• **melphalan** • **prednisone (H)** • **vincristine** • **cyclophosphamide** • **doxorubicin** • **dexamethasone (H)** • carmustine • alpha-interferon (I) • pamidronate (B) • busulfan
Cervical cancer	• **cisplatin** • **carboplatin** • **fluorouracil** • paclitaxel • vinorelbine • bleomycin • ifosfamide • irinotecan
Esophageal cancer	• **fluorouracil** • **cisplatin** • mitomycin • paclitaxel • porfimer (PS)
Laryngeal cancer	• **cisplatin** • **fluorouracil** • hydroxyurea • bleomycin • doxorubicin • carboplatin • mitomycin

TABLE 4.5	**Agents Frequently Prescribed for Each Form of Cancer**

(B) Bone-resorption inhibitor (H) Hormonal therapy (I) Immunotherapy (PS) Photosensitizer for photodynamic therapy (R) Radiopharmaceutical

Type of Cancer	Anticancer Drugs That May Be Used (Standard therapies or drugs used most commonly are in boldface.)
Pharyngeal cancer	▪ **cisplatin** ▪ **fluorouracil** ▪ hydroxyurea ▪ bleomycin ▪ doxorubicin ▪ carboplatin ▪ mitomycin
Soft-tissue sarcomas	▪ **doxorubicin** ▪ **ifosfamide** ▪ dacarbazine ▪ cyclophosphamide ▪ cisplatin ▪ carboplatin ▪ vincristine ▪ alpha-interferon ▪ mesna ▪ dactinomycin ▪ mitomycin
Testicular cancer	▪ **cisplatin** ▪ **etoposide** ▪ **bleomycin** ▪ carboplatin ▪ vinblastine ▪ dactinomycin ▪ methotrexate ▪ cyclophosphamide ▪ ifosfamide ▪ plicamycin ▪ doxorubicin
Small-intestine cancer	▪ **fluorouracil** ▪ **leucovorin** ▪ **streptozocin** ▪ **cyclophosphamide** ▪ **doxorubicin** ▪ **vincristine** ▪ **prednisone (H)** ▪ **dacarbazine** ▪ octreotide (H)

Metastatic Cancers

Metastatic cancer of the bone	▪ pamidronate (B) ▪ samarium 153 (R) ▪ strontium 89 (R)
Metastatic cancer of the brain	▪ cyclophosphamide ▪ fluorouracil ▪ methotrexate ▪ tamoxifen (H)
Metastatic cancer of the leptomeninges	▪ methotrexate ▪ cytarabine ▪ thiotepa ▪ mercaptopurine
Metastatic cancer of the liver	▪ cisplatin ▪ doxorubicin ▪ floxuridine ▪ fluorouracil
Metastatic cancer of the lung	*Secondary tumors of the lung are generally treated with the same drug(s) used to treat the primary cancer.*

against tumors in one of several ways, depending on which gene is used.

For instance, biotechnologists can arm the cells with the gene that produces the cancer killer tumor necrosis factor, an approach tried experimentally to treat metastatic melanoma. In kidney cancer and prostate cancer, investigators have added the genes for inter-leukin-12 and other chemical substances known to fortify the immune system. And in clinical trials made up of patients with brain cancer, biotechnologists have implanted genes that sensitize tumors to the effects of anticancer drugs, while breast-cancer patients have had their stem cells reengineered to include a gene that offers protection against the toxic effects of chemotherapy. Theoretically, this could make it possible to administer high doses of anticancer drugs without damaging the bone marrow. Such a development would render autologous bone-marrow transplantation to restore the immune system obsolete.

Bone-Marrow Transplantation and Peripheral-Blood Stem-Cell Transplantation

May serve as primary therapy for leukemia and lymphomas; may be used experimentally in treating multiple myeloma and cancers of the breast, testicle, lung, ovary, and brain.

Bone marrow, the soft, spongy meshwork of blood vessels and fibers that fills the hollow spaces of the large bones, is the production center for blood cells. Bone-marrow transplantation (BMT) replaces diseased or damaged marrow with healthy marrow taken from the patient, or from a family member or an anonymous volunteer *donor.*

Many people think of BMT as a last resort, employed only after other measures have failed. But increasingly, the game plan for treating myeloid leukemias starts with chemotherapy—to get the cancer into remission—then proceeds to transplantation immediately, rather than waiting until the patient suffers a relapse.

In leukemia, a cancer of the marrow, BMT is often considered definitive therapy. As a prelude to transplantation, the malignant marrow is obliterated with chemotherapy and, frequently, *total-body irradiation* (TBI). Then the physician infuses the disease-free marrow into the patient's veins. In treating solid tumors affecting the breast, testicle, lung, ovary, and brain, bone-marrow transplantation has assumed a role as a companion to chemotherapy.

"What transplantation allows us to do is to try to eradicate all tumor cells by giving extremely heavy doses," explains Dr. Kenneth Meehan, acting director of the Lombardi Cancer Center's BMT program. However, doing so inevitably wipes out patients' marrow, leaving them dangerously low on oxygen-toting red blood cells, infection-fighting white blood cells, and blood platelets, the cells that prevent excessive bleeding. In what is called *high-dose chemotherapy with stem-cell rescue,* the drug regimen is followed by a transplant to replenish the marrow.

Stem cells, undeveloped blood cells, are the seeds from which all blood cells grow. They exist primarily in the marrow, but also in the peripheral blood vessels. Half of the approximately twelve thousand marrow transplants performed in the United States annually use *peripheral-blood stem cells* (PBSCs) instead of bone marrow. Unlike harvesting marrow, removing cells from the blood doesn't require anesthesia. Another advantage is that PBSC recipients' levels of red, white, and platelet cells appear to return to normal more quickly than do those of patients who receive marrow. According to the Leukemia Society of America, the origin of the stem cells—marrow or circulating blood—makes no difference in the procedure's ultimate success.

The Informed Patient:
Looking Down the Road, Planning Ahead

Collecting stem cells is the medical equivalent of panning for gold. The immature blood-forming cells are rare, comprising fewer than one in 100,000 of the cells in the bone marrow. Unfortunately, prolonged courses of *alkylating* chemotherapy to keep slowly progressing cancers in check "gradually deplete a person's stem-cell population," says Dr. Jill Lacy, a medical oncologist at the Yale Cancer Center. "This pertains particularly to low-grade lymphomas and multiple myeloma, where patients may be relatively asymptomatic for years." Alkylating agents (see box) are the harshest group of anticancer drugs.

Dr. Lacy notes, "We'll see patients with low-grade lymphoma who've been on alkylating therapy for a long period of time. When things turn sour, they're referred here for high-dose chemotherapy with stem-cell support, but by then they don't have many stem cells left."

At a facility where the different arms of treatment are integrated from the outset, chances are good that the medical team will have the foresight to ensure that patients don't find themselves in the situation described by Dr. Lacy. Still, we advise never leaving matters to chance. If you've been diagnosed with a form of cancer that could possibly benefit from high-dose chemotherapy at some point (see Chapter Six, "State of the Art: Your Treatment Options"), raise the issue with your attending physician *now.* Is there perhaps an equally effective but less toxic chemotherapy for your type and stage of disease?

Alkylating Agents Used to Treat Cancer	
busulfan	lomustine
capecitabine	mechlorethamine
carboplatin	melphalan
carmustine	procarbazine
chlorambucil	streptozocin
cisplatin	temozolomide
cyclophosphamide	thiotepa
	uracil mustard

Another question to ask: Can your oncologist offer you access to *stem-cell growth factor,* should it become necessary? Stem-cell factor, currently being tested in patients, is one of several substances that stimulate the development of blood cells, in this case peripheral-blood stem cells. But until approved for commercial use, it is available only to participants in a limited number of investigational studies.

Allogeneic Bone-Marrow Transplantations

BMTs are divided equally between *allogeneic* transplantations and *autologous* transplantations. Allogeneic transplants, in which the marrow comes from a genetically compatible donor, is the preferred method for people with leukemia. The indicator of compatibility is whether or not the donor's marrow and the patient's marrow share at least four of six

Medical Terms You're Likely to Hear
MUD: matched unrelated donor.

major *human leukocyte antigen* (HLA) proteins that reside on the surface of all cells. Three of the immunological markers are inherited from the mother and three from the father. The higher the HLA match, which is determined by a special blood test, the greater the prospects for the graft "taking."

In addition, closely matched marrow reduces the chances that the graft will reject the body, or *host,* a common and potentially fatal complication known as *graft-versus-host disease* (GVHD). According to the National Cancer Institute, 40 percent of patients infused with HLA-identical marrow develop GVHD, as opposed to 70 percent of those who receive marrow bearing two mismatched antigens.

An identical twin—endowed with the exact same set of genes, including all six antigens—might appear to make for the ideal donor. In fact, says Dr. Meehan, "allogeneic marrow from a nonidentical twin is the best." The reason? Once it settles in the bones, the marrow begins manufacturing T lymphocytes that recognize any residual leukemia cells as foreign. "In a *syngeneic* transplant," from an identical twin, "this graft-versus-leukemia effect doesn't necessarily happen." Consequently, patients infused with syngeneic marrow have a higher relapse rate than do allogeneic recipients. Given that identical twins account for a mere 0.3 percent of all births, syngeneic BMT is an option for a small minority of patients.

"In an allogeneic transplantation," continues Dr. Meehan, "the best type of marrow is from a brother or sister." Siblings are more likely than other relatives and unrelated donors to possess those crucial matching antigens. He points to the difference in survival rates between people with chronic myeloid leukemia, a disease curable only through BMT. "If the marrow comes from a sibling, the cure rate ranges from 60 to 80 percent; with a MUD transplant, it's 40 to 50 percent."

However, only about one in four patients have a sibling or parent with suitable marrow. Among the general population, the odds of finding a match plummet to one in twenty thousand, so that one-third of all patients who need bone-marrow transplantations cannot get them. On a more encouraging note, the number of volunteer donors has risen dramatically in recent years.

Who Conducts a Donor Search?

When an allogeneic BMT is chosen as the appropriate course of treatment, it falls to the patient or her loved ones to contact family members about having their marrow *typed* as soon as possible, beginning with siblings and parents. The next tier would consist of aunts, uncles, and first cousins.

If the blood tests fail to produce a match among family and relatives, the task of identifying an unrelated donor is handled by the hospital's *transplant coordinator,* who lists your name with the federally funded National Marrow Donor Program. The NMDP, established in 1987, strives to link each transplant candidate with one of the more than 3.5 million potential donors in its computerized registry. A private organization, the Caitlin Raymond International Registry, also initiates searches among its pool of more than 2.7 million volunteers.

What if no compatible unrelated donor can be found? Fifteen years after doctors at Memorial Sloan-Kettering carried out the first MUD transplant in 1973, that remained the deciding factor as to whether or not plans for a bone-marrow transplantation could proceed. One apparent solution to this dilemma was so startlingly simple, it had been overlooked all along: extract the stem cells from the blood left in the umbilical cords and placentas of newborn babies.

The procedure, performed since 1988, has given new hope to patients who might otherwise find themselves at an impasse in their cancer treatment. But umbilical-cord-blood transplants may actually be preferable to unrelated-donor-marrow transplants in several respects.

Certainly the blood-collection process is easier and safer than harvesting marrow. Once the mother delivers the placenta, usually minutes after birth, the doctor inserts a catheter into the umbilical vein of the cord and drains the blood into a soft-plastic receptacle. Neither the mother nor the baby feels any discomfort. The blood, which normally would be discarded as medical waste, is a rich source of stem cells. Just a few ounces are needed, in contrast to the quart or more of bone marrow typically withdrawn for a BMT.

Most significant of all, whereas the success of a MUD transplant usually depends on whether or not the patient and donor corre-

New Transplant Techniques, New Hope

Two innovative methods of typing and treating donor marrow, both developed overseas, could make it so that anyone who needs a bone-marrow transplant can get one, even when perfectly matching marrow can't be found.

There are six major human leukocyte antigens: HLA-*A*, HLA-*B*, HLA-*C*, HLA-*DR*, HLA-*DQ*, and HLA-*DP*. All have a number of subtypes. In a 1998 study of 440 MUD-transplant recipients, four in five of whom had leukemia, Japanese researchers found that matching the subtype of the HLA-*A* antigen nearly doubled the survival rate and significantly lowered the risk of graft-versus-host disease. The other key antigen appears to be HLA-*C*. Strangely enough, while a perfect match of this substance also decreased the chances of patients' incurring GVHD, it doubled their odds of suffering a recurrence. Disparities in the subtypes of the other four antigens had little effect on the outcome.

The second milestone in bone-marrow transplantation, reported the same week, came from Israel's Weizmann Institute of Science and Perugia University in Italy. Scientists there devised a technique for pretreating the donor marrow so that only three of the six HLA markers need correspond. Between 1995 and 1997, forty-three severely leukemic patients received mismatched marrow that had undergone this special "cleansing" process. Eighteen months after the transplant, twelve were still free of cancer. Several hospitals in the United States have implemented the Perugia-Wiezmann method.

spond on all six genetic traits, cord-blood transplants can engraft even when only five or four HLA antigens match—in some cases, as few as three. The *cord-blood stem cells* (CBSCs) are also far less likely to transmit viruses and other diseases.

The New York Blood Center in Manhattan coordinated a large study at ninety-eight hospitals across the United States and abroad. Five hundred sixty-two patients underwent cord-blood transplants after attempts at locating suitable marrow donors had been exhausted. All participants were seriously ill with cancer or another disease. The investigators published their findings in the *New England Journal of Medicine* in 1998, and the survival rates were virtually identical to those from MUD transplants in which all six HLA antigens match.

However, researchers did notice an interesting pattern that has yet to be explained: The cord-blood recipients who had chronic myelogenous leukemia, a malignancy that generally responds well to bone-marrow transplantation, fared poorly compared to the other cancer patients in the trial.

Preparation for Allogeneic BMT

In those instances where a MUD is located, it takes an average of four to six weeks between the time the request goes out and the day the donor checks into the hospital. The procedure that follows is the same for both related and unrelated donors: After a battery of routine tests, a small amount of marrow is aspirated from the hipbone under general or regional anesthesia. The donor usually goes home the next day, by which time the marrow has already been filtered and transported to the patient's treatment center. It may be frozen and stored for up to three years, although allogeneic transplants typically take place within twenty-four hours of the marrow harvest.

During the week prior to marrow-infusion day, the patient is bombarded with high-dose chemotherapy, alone or followed by total-body irradiation. Different transplant centers have their preferred *conditioning* regimens, but studies show that two agents—chemo and radiation, or combination chemotherapy—are more effective than one at reducing the odds of a recurrence. Another finding is that the addition of radiation improves the likelihood that the recipient's body will accept the graft.

With allogeneic BMT, the goal is to eliminate every last trace of the cancerous marrow "because even one malignant cell has the theoretical possibility of multiplying," explains Dr. Meehan, whose unit harvests more marrow than any other in the country. Ridding the bones of the marrow also creates room for the incoming marrow and reduces the chances of rejection. However, the interruption in blood-cell production leaves patients temporarily defenseless against infection and prone to anemia and abnormal bleeding. From the time conditioning commences until the new marrow "takes" and restores some measure of immunity, you stay in a private room equipped with special air filters. You will be instructed on how to keep yourself scrupulously clean, to ward off infection, and the medical staff and all visitors must wash their hands thoroughly before entering the transplant unit and don sterile masks, gloves, and gowns.

Allogeneic BMT: The Procedure

Compared to the events leading up to it, the actual transplant may seem somewhat anticlimactic. The stem cells are infused over the course of several hours, much like a blood transfusion. Then begins the wait for the new marrow to start forming red, white, and platelet cells. *Engraftment,* as this is called, typically occurs two to four weeks after the transplant, although regaining full immunity "may take months," says Dr. Meehan, "sometimes years." If new blood cells fail to appear after thirty days or so, a second attempt is made using stem cells stored from the time of harvest.

Graft-Versus-Host Disease (GVHD)

After an organ transplant, patients must take immunosuppressant drugs for the rest of their lives to prevent the body from attacking the newcomer. In GVHD, the reverse happens, with the donor marrow perceiving the host as foreign and attacking it.

GVHD is classified as acute or chronic. The acute form, which strikes within the first three months following transplant, "reacts against epithelial-type cells in the skin, gastrointestinal tract, and liver," explains Dr. Meehan. Common symptoms include skin rashes, jaundice, liver dysfunction, and GI complications such as nausea, vomiting, and profuse diarrhea. Chronic GVHD, seen anywhere from three months to two years posttransplant, "is more of an autoimmune type of phenomenon," in the sense that it can inflame skin and joints and cause them to thicken and harden.

Interestingly, physicians actually welcome mild graft-versus-host disease. "Patients who develop GVHD have a lower relapse rate," says Dr. Meehan, "probably because they now have a revved-up immune system better able to kill cancer cells." Mild acute or chronic reactions are highly treatable, but severe symptoms can be fatal. Consequently, the transplant team looks to stave off GVHD, starting you on immunosuppressants the day before transplantation. This can hinder recovery, as immunosuppressants and other medications used to prevent or manage the disease impair patients' already fragile immune systems. Fortunately, after about six months, the donor T cells adapt to their new environment, and the medications can be discontinued.

Another technique for averting GVHD involves eliminating the T cells in the donor marrow before infusing it. While *T cell depletion* significantly reduces the incidence of graft-versus-host disease, the absence of T cells increases the risk not only of graft failure but of the leukemia returning.

Autologous Bone-Marrow Transplantations

Solid tumors call for autologous bone-marrow or peripheral-blood stem-cell transplantation as a complement to high-dose chemotherapy. Some patients with leukemia, lymphomas, and multiple myeloma may also be candidates for this type of transplantation if, say, an allogeneic donor cannot be found. Before the green light can be given, though, the cancer must be in remission.

Since autologous BMT gives you back your own stem cells, there's no chance of rejection, and GVHD-like reactions are extraordinarily rare. What's more, with no need for immunosuppressant drugs, the immune system rebuilds more quickly. Whereas a physician would be reluctant to recommend allogeneic BMT for patients fifty-five and older, "autologous transplant can be offered to people in their seventies," says Dr. Meehan. The major drawback to autologous BMT as a treatment for leukemia is that the stem cells do not induce the graft-versus-leukemia effect, and so the relapse rates are higher than those associated with transplantation using donor marrow.

Preparation for Autologous BMT

Autologous transplant patients go through the same harvesting procedure as allogeneic donors, except that it takes place seven to ten days before transplantation so that the stem cells can be treated to eradicate any tumor cells. Not all centers believe in *purging,* however, as it has not been shown to improve the long-term prognosis.

Many prospective autologous BMT patients have had their marrow decimated by previous courses of chemotherapy. Therefore, it is routine practice to augment the harvested marrow with stem cells skimmed from the circulation. But the peripheral blood contains roughly one-tenth the amount of stem cells as is found in the marrow. To hike the numbers further, patients receive stem-cell growth factor before and during *apheresis,* the process for withdrawing blood from a vein and running it through a machine that extracts the precious PBSCs.

Conditioning in advance of autologous BMT is less intensive. The salvos of chemotherapy, at least two to ten times higher than standard chemotherapy, suppress the marrow for several days *(myelosuppression)* rather than destroy it *(myeloablation).* Total-body irradiation may also be administered.

Autologous BMT: The Procedure

Marrow infusion is the same for all three types of transplantations. You will already have had a central catheter surgically implanted in your upper chest. The stem cells drip slowly from a hanging plastic bag into the flexible tube. Barring graft failure, the transplanted marrow should begin generating new blood cells in eight to ten days, though you won't be back to full immunity for six to nine months. As with an allogeneic BMT, if engraftment doesn't occur by the fourth week, reserve cells are given.

What If the Transplantation Is Unsuccessful?

Graft failure, a relatively rare occurrence, is usually attributable to one of two causes: Either the body rejects the donor marrow or the transplanted stem cells simply never take well enough to function properly. Factors that may contribute to an abortive BMT include:

Graft Rejection

- An imperfect HLA match
- A sufficient number of the recipient's T cells survive the conditioning regimen to attack the transplanted marrow.

Graft Failure

- Previous chemotherapy has harmed or depleted the patient's stem cells

- Damage to the marrow *stroma,* the framework necessary to support new marrow
- Posttransplant infections and some of the medications used to control them
- The effects of the immunosuppressant drugs
- The use of T-cell-depleted donor marrow
- A recurrence of the leukemia

Cost and Controversy

While there is no disputing bone-marrow transplantation's value as a therapy for leukemia and other "liquid" tumors, its effectiveness against certain solid tumors has yet to be definitively established. In particular, the use of autologous BMT in breast-cancer treatment has become a battleground for disputes between patients and insurance companies that deny coverage for this prohibitively expensive procedure, which on average exceeds $60,000 and requires six to ten weeks of hospitalization.

Between 1989 and 1994, the number of women with breast cancer to undergo marrow transplants multiplied eightfold, from about five hundred to an estimated four thousand. Whether or not high-dose chemotherapy with autologous support is superior to standard chemotherapy—at $15,000 to $40,000, a far less costly option—is currently being explored in several long-term investigational trials. Until those studies are finally completed, autologous BMT is still considered an experimental treatment for breast cancer.

As a rule, private insurance companies do not pay for experimental cancer therapies. Most, however, will cover an autologous BMT under these circumstances.

A study published in the *New England Journal of Medicine* found that of some five

MONEY MATTERS

Federally Funded Insurance Programs and Coverage for Autologous BMT for Breast Cancer

- Medicaid—the state-administered program that provides medical care to people with incomes below a certain level. Coverage varies from state to state.

- Medicare—the federal program that provides health coverage primarily for the elderly. Does not cover BMT for solid tumors on the grounds that the treatment is experimental.

- CHAMPUS—the Civilian Health and Medical Program of the Department of the Uniformed Services, which insures active-duty and retired military personnel as well as their dependents and survivors. Covers BMT provided that beneficiaries enroll in one of the clinical trials being conducted by the National Cancer Institute.

hundred breast-cancer patients who sought insurance coverage for an autologous transplant, about 75 percent received approval. Still, that means one in four claims were turned down. Should you find yourself in this situation, there are steps you can take to persuade the insurer to reconsider its position—from enlisting your oncologist's help in tracking down studies and statistics supporting the benefits of the treatment, to threatening legal action. A good place to begin is the hospital's department of social work, which regularly assists patients embroiled in insurance disputes. At some major cancer centers, like Memorial Sloan-Kettering in New York, one social worker's sole responsibility is to help BMT candidates win approval and to file an appeal should the request be rejected.

See "Contesting Denied Insurance Claims" in Chapter Ten, "Getting Help When You Need It."

What to Look for in a Bone-Marrow Transplant Facility

In a word, look for experience. "The most important question a patient can ask," says Dr. Meehan, "is how many people with disease have you transplanted?" To give you a basis for comparison, "a busy unit performs about forty to forty-five bone-marrow transplants a year," says Dr. Meehan, whose own unit carries out more than one hundred annually.

Another major consideration in selecting a transplant center should be whether the nursing staff is specially trained in caring for BMT patients. Perhaps as essential as the caliber of the medical team is the quality of the supportive care to prevent and manage the many serious posttransplant complications that may arise.

> **Need help in finding a transplant center? Have questions? Call:**
>
> **National Marrow Donor Program, office of patient advocacy: 888-999-6743**
> **Caitlin Raymond International Registry: 800-726-2824**

See Chapter Five, "The Next Step: Getting a Second Opinion and Deciding Where to Seek Treatment."

Other Cancer Therapies

The following treatment methods are used sparingly in cancer care; most are still being evaluated.

Photodynamic Therapy (PDT)

May be used in treating advanced esophageal cancer, borderline non-small-cell lung cancer, and skin lesions associated with cutaneous T-cell lymphoma; may be used experimentally in treating early-stage cancers of the oral cavity, throat, larynx, ovary, brain, bladder, breast, and soft tissue.

Photodynamic therapy entails injecting a *photosensitizing agent* into the circulation, yet it treats cancer locally, not systemically. Although the drug collects in all the body's cells, it clears from nonmalignant tissue rapidly. Forty-eight hours after the shot, a red beam of argon laser light is sent coursing through a fiber-optic scope placed against the tumor, setting off a chemical reaction that destroys the cancer cells. The lone significant side effect of the approximately thirty-minute treatment is a heightened sensitivity to sunlight. For the next four to six weeks, you must wear sunscreen, protective clothing, and sunglasses whenever you venture outdoors.

PDT is used as a palliative treatment for tumors that are obstructing the esophagus and interfering with swallowing. Studies testing its effectiveness against several cancers have been promising, producing complete response rates and cure rates of up to 95 percent. The chief drawback is that the low-power argon laser penetrates only about one-third of an inch into tissue. Researchers are currently testing other drugs that are activated by light sources capable of infiltrating more deeply.

Hyperthermia

May be used experimentally in treating melanoma and cancers of the liver, brain, lip and oral cavity, and throat.

Tumor cells exhibit greater sensitivity to heat and cold than do normal cells. "The concept behind hyperthermia," explains Dr. Ted Lawrence of the University of Michigan Comprehensive Cancer Center, "is that heating cancer cells to between 40 and 43 degrees Celsius [104 and 109 degrees Fahrenheit] makes them more susceptible to both radiation therapy and chemotherapy."

A number of techniques have been developed for heating just the tumor *(local hyperthermia)*, an organ or limb *(regional hyperthermia)*, or the entire body *(whole-body hyperthermia)*:

Local Hyperthermia

- External ultrasound
- Internal probes such as heated wires, or tubes filled with warm water
- Implanted microwave antennae
- Radio-frequency electrodes

Regional Hyperthermia

- Placing magnets and other devices that produce high energy over the area
- Perfusion: removing and heating the blood, then pumping it back into the limb or organ

Whole-Body Hyperthermia

- Warm-water blankets
- Inductive coils, much like those in a heating blanket
- Hot wax
- Thermal chambers similar to an incubator

Antiangiogenesis Therapy

May be used experimentally in treating leukemia, lymphomas, and cancers of the brain, breast, stomach, lung, prostate, ovary, cervix, and pancreas.

Arterial Embolization

May be used experimentally in treating cancers of the liver and kidney.

Both *antiangiogenesis* and *arterial embolization* attempt to limit the blood supply to the tumor, effectively starving it to death. Like vampires, tumors thrive on blood and will go to extreme lengths to ensure a steady diet.

Antiangiogenesis Therapy

Virtually every cell in the body resides on the surface of one of the hair-thin blood vessels known as *capillaries*. When a healthy cell becomes abnormal and starts to divide recklessly, its descendants pile up into a mass. Eventually, the tumor reaches the in situ state, where the constant proliferation of new cells is counterbalanced by the dying off of older ones as they get nudged farther and farther away from a nearby blood vessel.

After months, sometimes years, the internal equilibrium crumbles as the in situ carcinoma releases substances that cause new capillaries to form. This is called *angiogenesis* or *neovascularization*. Its lifelines open once more, the cancer can feast on oxygen, nutrients, and growth factors, and resume expanding. The larger it grows, the more vessels it develops and the more likely it is to metastasize.

Some scientists believe that from the moment tumors form, they attempt to seize control of existing blood vessels. But anytime a vessel is abducted, the body resourcefully cuts off its blood supply. That probably kills many developing cancers. In time, though, surviving tumors sprout their own conduits for blood, and the body's defenses are overwhelmed.

Antiangiogenesis drugs are designed to interfere with this ability to forge new sources of blood, for without angiogenesis, a mass would remain the size of a pinhead and never invade neighboring tissue. The first agent tested in patients was TNP-470, in 1992. Seven years later, twenty more were in clinical trials.

"What makes antiangiogenesis therapy so attractive," says Dr. Michael Hawkins of the Lombardi Cancer Center, "is that it targets only new blood vessels." Healthy blood vessels do not replenish their cells, unlike, say, the bone marrow, hair follicles, and lining of the digestive tract, which are characterized by rapid cell turnover. "Once you're an adult," he explains, "you have all the blood vessels you need. So the therapy could potentially devastate the cancer yet have little effect on the body."

Arterial Embolization

The principle in arterial embolization is to deprive tumors of blood flow by obstructing a major existing vessel. In kidney cancer, for instance, a catheter is inserted into a tiny incision in the femoral artery in the groin and threaded through the circulation until it reaches the artery, or arteries, feeding the tumor. "Then," says Dr. Jim Mohler of the UNC Lineberger Comprehensive Cancer Center in Chapel Hill, North Carolina, "we inject a foreign substance or a preformed blood clot into the artery, which causes it to clot off."

Malignant tumors of the liver, too, are rich with blood, most of it delivered by the hepatic artery. Injecting one of several chemotherapeutic agents directly into the artery has a double-barreled effect, says Dr. John Butler, chief of surgical oncology at the Chao Family Comprehensive Cancer Center in Orange, California. Not only does chemoembolization deny entrance to the cancer, "the chemotherapy is prevented from traveling further. The result is a higher concentration of the drug where we want it most."

Thus far, arterial emobilization has proved to be minimally effective, since it is the medical equivalent of plugging a finger into a leaky dam. The main artery may be closed off, but the tumor's ability to stimulate angiogenesis endures. In time, the resourceful tumor will simply find another source of blood.

Alcohol Ablation Therapy

May be used experimentally in treating inoperable liver cancer.

In alcohol ablation, the physician injects pure alcohol directly into the tumor, relying on ultrasound or a CT scan to guide his placement of the needle. Although alcohol is effective at destroying *(ablating)* cancer cells, doctors have yet to perfect a technique for delivering the liquid so that it permeates the tumor uniformly.

What Are Clinical Trials?

Compared to most other serious diseases, cancer is atypical in that it is standard practice for oncologists to routinely rely on unapproved treatments. More than half of all patients, at some point, receive a drug *"off-label"*—that is, prescribed for a condition other than those specified on the product's lengthy package insert. Others choose to participate in experimental protocols. A number of the treatments you have just read about, in fact, are available mainly through formal research studies.

Clinical trials, as they are also known, evaluate the safety and effectiveness of new treatments in people. They're experimental, yes, but they are carefully monitored by physicians within the realm of conventional medicine. This is how new medications make their way from the research bench to the pharmacy shelf and earn acceptance (and coverage) from health insurers.

Certainly, there are clinical trials designed with the hope of achieving a cure. More commonly, however, the potential advances are less dramatic but still significant, even if they only improve a patient's chances by a slight percentage. Many research studies assess the value of modifying existing therapies: new drug combinations, new techniques for administering medications or radiation, new sequences of treatment. Others test new approaches to managing symptoms and side effects. For example, neither of the two drugs I received as a participant in a clinical trial was experimental (fluorouracil had been used to fight cancer since 1962; leucovorin since 1986), but employing them in combination as an adjuvant to surgery for stage III colon cancer was. Today the regimen is considered a standard therapy and, in the opinion of many oncologists, superior to its predecessor, fluorouracil and levamisole.

Although only five in one hundred cancer patients enroll in clinical trials, "there seems to be greater public interest in investigational therapies than ever before," says Dr. Michael A. Friedman, acting deputy commissioner of the Food and Drug Administration, the federal agency charged with regulating medicines and medical devices. "More patients, and the people who care about them, are looking into investigational options, and they want to exercise those options early." It is not unusual for oncologists at centers engaged in clinical research to propose an experimental protocol as first-line therapy, particularly in situations where no effective treatment has been developed yet.

According to Dr. Larry Norton of Memorial Sloan-Kettering Cancer Center, "A clinical trial offers the best therapy you can get," and not only because the treatment under study is thought to be at least as beneficial as approved strategies. "A number of studies have shown that participants in clinical trials do better than nonparticipants"—including the members of the group given standard cancer therapy rather than the experimental protocol. This may be explained by the fact that people in clinical trials receive first-rate follow-up care.

Research studies aren't appropriate for everyone. Nor can everyone afford to join a trial, which may not be covered by insurance. How do you know whether or not you are a suitable candidate? Ask your attending physician, preferably at the time of diagnosis. Don't assume that the doctor will raise the issue, especially if he isn't affiliated with an institution involved in clinical research. Not all oncologists have knowledge of, or access to, the latest cutting-edge therapies.

Another point to bear in mind: After reviewing your options, you and your physician might decide that your type and stage of disease warrants standard therapy. What if your condition should change? Perhaps you might benefit from an investigational protocol somewhere down the road. That's why we recommend reading on about clinical trials and finding out about studies being conducted in your area.

The Three Phases of Clinical Trials

PRECLINICAL TESTING

Average length of time: 3½ years
Goals: to assess the treatment's safety and its biological activity against cancer cells

The lengthy process of evaluating new treatments is divided into three stages. Before a drug enters phase I of human testing, its safety and anticancer action are rigorously tested in the laboratory and in animals. The institution or manufacturer sponsoring the trial then submits an investigational new drug (IND) application to the FDA. For every medication that receives the go-ahead to launch patient studies, eight hundred others are abandoned. And of those that enter human testing, only one in five will become licensed for commercial use.

PHASE I

Average length of time: 1 year
Goals: to establish the treatment's safety; define the maximum safe dose and optimal schedule of administration; and assess the value of combining the new drug with other drugs or with other forms of treatment

Phase I trials recruit from twenty to eighty patients. Some will see their condition improve as a result of the experimental protocol, but for the most part they have volunteered out of a desire to contribute to cancer research. "I've had a number of patients say, 'I don't really believe that this is going to cure me,'" remarks Maureen Sawchuk, nursing coordinator at the Lombardi Cancer Center, "'but if my doing this can help someone else one day, then I feel I've done something important.'"

PHASE II

Average length of time: 2 years
Goals: to establish the treatment's effectiveness and monitor its side effects

Phase II studies enlist one hundred to three hundred volunteers, all with the same type of cancer or related cancers. An investigational drug must elicit a significant response in at least one-fifth of the subjects in order to advance to phase III. To expedite the development and approval process, the FDA allows investigators to combine phases II and III for promising new cancer medications.

PHASE III

Average length of time: 3 years
Goals: to confirm a treatment's effectiveness by comparing it against currently accepted treatments, and to monitor adverse effects from long-term use

In a *randomized* phase III clinical trial, one thousand to three thousand patients with similar traits (such as the extent of their cancer) are randomly assigned by computer to one of two groups. The *control group* receives the best treatment currently available; the *study group* receives the standard therapy plus the experimental protocol. With the exception of a *placebo trial* or a *blinded trial* (see box), you learn beforehand which therapy you'll be getting. You have the option of leaving the study then or anytime afterward, at which point you would receive the current standard of care. This is true of all phases of clinical trials. Likewise, should an experimental treatment cause your condition to deteriorate, you would be withdrawn from the trial and switched to accepted therapy.

The Approval Process

After all three phases are completed, the sponsor submits its results to the Food and Drug Administration for approval. The agency, long criticized for moving too slowly, has slashed its approval time by more than half: from 33 months in 1987 to 15.4 months in 1996. In the interim, the therapy is made available to patients through *Group C* and *modified Group C* protocols. Though not clinical trials per se, these treatment plans serve a dual purpose, yielding additional data and getting effective medications to patients. Individual pharmaceutical manufacturers have instituted similar policies that allow continued access to a new drug while the company awaits the FDA's blessing.

> **Medical Terms You're Likely to Hear**
>
> **Placebo:** a tablet, capsule, or injection containing a harmless, inactive substance. When no treatment exists for a particular cancer, one group of patients may receive placebos; the other, the medication under investigation.
>
> **Single-blind trial:** a study in which the patient doesn't know if he's receiving experimental or standard therapy. In a *double-blind trial,* neither the patient nor the attending physician knows which combinations or doses are being given, although this information can be obtained if necessary.

"Cancer patients' access to new drugs is improving," Dr. John Marshall of the Lombardi Cancer Center notes. "In 1996 alone, five cancer drugs were introduced, when in years past it was rare to see a single new drug come out." In both 1997 and 1998, three cancer therapies were approved—including the first monoclonal-antibody therapy and the first gene therapy—plus several medications for relieving symptoms and side effects.

Once sanctioned for commercial use, the typical pattern is for new cancer therapies to move cautiously into the field of treatment. "If a standard therapy exists," explains Dr. Larry Copeland of the Arthur G. James Cancer Hospital and Research Institute, "the new drug usually gets its foot in the door by showing activity in previously treated patients whose cancer has recurred. The next step is to test the drug in first-line situations, to see whether or not it should be incorporated into standard therapy."

How to Find Out About Clinical Trials

I have to confess that I had some extra help in locating a research study. When President George Bush learned from Valerie that I was in a coma following the surgery to correct my twisted colon, he sent Dr. Larry Mohr, one of his personal physicians, to the hospital. After the crisis passed, it was Dr. Mohr who kindly called Dr. Samuel Broder, then the

TABLE 4.6 Example of Eligibility Criteria for a Clinical Trial		
Extent/Characteristics of the Disease	Extent of Prior Treatment	Physical Requirements
▪ Stage III or IV colorectal cancer, confirmed by a biopsy ▪ At least one lesion measuring 1 cm by 1 cm ▪ No metastasis to the brain	▪ No prior chemotherapy for advanced or metastatic disease ▪ No adjuvant chemotherapy therapy in the previous six months ▪ No radiotherapy in the previous twenty-one days ▪ Patients may not undergo other treatments while on the trial.	▪ The patient is aged eighteen or older. ▪ The patient is expected to live at least eight weeks. ▪ Women patients may not be pregnant or nursing. ▪ Blood tests must confirm that the patient has adequate kidney and liver function as well as acceptable levels of white blood cells and platelets.

director of the National Cancer Institute, to find out which hospitals in the Washington area were running clinical trials investigating adjuvant therapies for stage III colon cancer. One day while I was recuperating at home, Dr. Mohr stopped by, and the two of us spent several hours discussing my treatment options.

I can imagine someone reading this and thinking, "How wonderful for you, but *I* can't call the president's doctor."

You don't have to. You, me—anyone—has access to the same information about experimental therapies. The best way to learn about clinical trials is to have your attending oncologist or a trusted general practitioner make these contacts for you. A doctor can provide the mounds of medical information necessary for determining whether or not you qualify for the trial. Each participant must meet exacting *entry criteria* encompassing (1) the stage and characteristics of the cancer, (2) the type and extent of prior or concurrent treatment, and (3) the patient's age and general health.

How specific are the requirements? To give you an example, table 4.6 lists just some of the inclusion and exclusion criteria for a phase II clinical trial conducted at the Lombardi Cancer Center by my oncologist, Dr. John Marshall. The study, now completed, evaluated a new three-drug chemotherapy regimen in men and women with locally advanced or metastatic colorectal cancer.

If you'd prefer to find out about clinical trials yourself, by all means do so. Then share the information with your primary doctor. The following routes and resources are good ways to get started:

· Call the National Cancer Institute's Cancer Information Service (800-422-6237).

The NCI maintains a massive computerized database on cancer treatment, diagnosis, and prevention, called the *Physician Data Query* (PDQ), which it updates regularly. Call the toll-free number, give the information specialist your name, address, age, and type and stage of cancer, and you'll receive a thick printout detailing pertinent clinical trials within a five- or six-state radius currently accepting patients. Each summary outlines the study's objective, the medical center(s) taking part, the telephone number of the *principal investigator* (the physician in charge of directing the study) at each institution, and the protocol eligibility criteria.

For instant access, you can conduct your own search by tapping into the National Cancer Institute's "Cancer Trials" site on the World Wide Web: *http://cancernet.nci.nih.gov/trials.* The PDQ contains information on over sixteen hundred cancer clinical trials being carried out mainly at NCI-funded cancer centers and affiliated hospitals and private practitioners. Until the 1980s, the National Cancer Institute supported the vast majority of patient studies, but budget cuts have shifted the balance to pharmaceutical and biotechnology companies. Individual medical centers may also sponsor clinical trials. There is no central registry of privately funded investigational studies, which makes tracking them down a little more time-consuming.

· Contact local cancer centers or the department of oncology at local teaching hospitals.

Here's what you say: "I've just been diagnosed with stage _____ cancer, and I'm interested in learning about any open clinical trials you might be running for people with my kind of cancer. Is there someone there who could help me?" Expect to be transferred to a *clinical research nurse* or *protocol coordinator* charged with recruiting volunteers.

For the telephone numbers and Web site addresses of nearly ninety major cancer centers, see table 5.1 in Chapter Five,

"The Next Step: Getting a Second Opinion and Deciding Where to Seek Treatment."

• **Call pharmaceutical companies directly.**

The *Physicians' Desk Reference,* available in most libraries, lists addresses and telephone numbers of all prescription-drug manufacturers. For the names of companies that produce anticancer agents, look up "antineoplastics" in the "Product Category Index" at the front of this weighty reference book.

• **Local chapters of cancer-patient support organizations such as the American Cancer Society may know of open patient studies in your area.**

See Appendix A, "Cancer Organizations Offering Information and Support for Patients and Families."

• **Surf the Internet.**

A multimedia publishing company called Centerwatch hosts a Web site that posts clinical trials by disease categories, including approximately one thousand privately funded cancer research studies actively seeking patients: Its cyberspace address is *http://www.centerwatch.com.*

See "Clinical Trials Information" in Appendix B.

The Informed Patient:
If You Do Not Qualify for an Experimental Protocol

The National Cancer Institute reserves a limited number of *Treatment Referral Center* (TRC) *protocols,* which offer promising treatments to patients for whom no standard therapies exist but who do not meet the eligibility criteria for a clinical trial. TRC protocols are administered only at the 325-bed Warren Grant Magnusen Clinical Center in Bethesda, Maryland, a federally funded research facility, or at the approximately fifty NCI cancer centers around the country. Only your oncologist can enroll you in a TRC protocol; if he's unaware of the program, request that he call the Cancer Information Service for more details.

Similarly, the Food and Drug Administration has two "compassionate use" policies in place to get experimental drugs to patients who have run out of standard options and are facing immediate medical crises. Perhaps a promising medication is available through clinical trials, but no studies are being conducted for a patient's type of cancer. The *single-patient investigational new drug program* allows his or her physician to apply for what's called an "emergency IND."

Special Protocol Exceptions apply to any of the following situations: (1) A drug that could conceivably help a patient is being tested in other cancers or other diseases; (2) the patient does not qualify for a study; or (3) the patient lives too far away from the medical facility(ies) offering the trial. Under the special protocol, the medical company that applied to the FDA for an IND application "sponsors" the patient; her doctor must agree to provide the information the manufacturer needs for its investigational study.

The FDA typically responds to all applications within two days, and sometimes in a matter of hours. For more information, you or your doctor can call the agency's Rockville, Maryland, headquarters at 301-827-4460.

What Is Informed Consent?

Should you commit to joining a clinical trial, by law you must receive in writing a document of *informed consent* outlining the potential benefits and risks. The National Cancer Institute recommends that before patients sign any form, they should ask the doctor or nurse as many questions as it takes until they are satisfied that they understand exactly what is involved.

Questions to Ask . . . Before Participating in a Clinical Trial

- What is the purpose of this study?
- Who has reviewed and approved it?
- Who is sponsoring it?
- What are the credentials of the trial's investigators and medical staff?
- What information or results is this trial based on?
- How are the study's results and patient safety checked?
- Who receives the information from the study?
- How might this new treatment help me?
- Why is it believed to be superior to the current standard treatment for my cancer?

- What are my other treatment options, including standard therapies? How do they compare to the experimental protocol in terms of possible outcomes, complications, time involved, and quality of life?

- How long will I be in the study?

- What is the treatment plan?

- Please describe the tests and treatments I would undergo.

- Will I have to be hospitalized? If so, how often and for how long?

- How frequently will I have to be seen for follow-up examinations, tests, and treatments?

- What are the new treatment's potential side effects, complications, and long-term risks?

- If I were to encounter adverse side effects, to what treatment would I be entitled?

- Does the study include long-term follow-up care?

- How much will this treatment cost?

- Can I expect my health insurer to cover the expense of this treatment?

Then pose the question that no one ever asks: Can I speak to someone currently participating in the study *as well as* someone who chose to drop out? The investigators may or may not be able (or inclined) to arrange this. But if possible, you want to hear both parties' experiences as members of the trial.

After talking to Dr. Mohr, I decided to enroll in a large multicenter phase III adjuvant clinical trial for stage III colon cancer that was under way at the Lombardi Cancer Center. The Friday following my discharge from the hospital, a dismally rainy day, I received a call from Dr. Paul Woolley, the oncologist running the study.

"I've spoken to Dr. Mohr about getting you into this clinical trial," he said. "Can you come in to see me right now? I need to start you on treatment on Monday." The figurative flip of the coin had landed me in the experimental protocol.

Valerie was out with the kids, and I was still too weak to drive myself, so I called a cab and hurriedly shaved, showered, and threw on some clothes. Fifteen minutes later, a beat-up station wagon rumbled up in front of the house.

"Do you mind if I smoke?" the driver asked.

"I really don't care what you do," I said distractedly. "Just please get me to the Lombardi Cancer Center."

"You have cancer?"

I told her I'd just had an operation and needed chemotherapy.

"I used to drive this one guy to the cancer center all the time."

"Really?" I asked. "What happened to him?"

"He died."

"Thanks a lot," I grumbled, and returned my attention to the driving rain.

MONEY MATTERS

Medical Insurers and Clinical Trials

In general, insurance companies are more likely to approve coverage for an experimental cancer treatment if it is part of a clinical trial, particularly a large multicenter research study. As we explain in Chapter Ten, patients who wish to enroll in an investigational protocol should enlist the help of the medical team in compiling and submitting to their insurer the proper documentation attesting to the treatment's value. The time to do this is *before* beginning therapy, so as to avoid the risk of having your claim denied after the experimental therapy has begun.

See "Contesting Denied Insurance Claims" in Chapter Ten, "Getting Help When You Need It."

Chapter Five

The Next Step: Getting a Second Opinion and Deciding Where to Seek Treatment

Dr. Vincent DeVita, director of the Yale Cancer Center and former head of the National Cancer Institute, has counted numerous physicians among his patients. "I've never taken care of one," he notes, "who didn't get a second opinion."

Many people with cancer, however, proceed through the medical system as if on a conveyor belt, routed by their general practitioner to a local oncologist rather than to a state-of-the-art facility. "In my experience," says Dr. DeVita, "the average person goes to a doctor he trusts and accepts that doctor's view of things." All too often, referrals to centers of excellence are not made until a patient's condition takes a turn for the worse.

How much wiser it is to sort out your options at the beginning. The National Cancer Institute recommends that all cancer patients pursue a second opinion to confirm the diagnosis and review the proposed course of treatment. According to the Institute for Advanced Study in Medicine, a nonprofit organization in Atlanta, studies have shown that one in four cancer patients' treatment plans change following a second-opinion consultation. Even at a multidisciplinary institution such as Lombardi, where each case comes under the scrutiny of two, three, or more cancer specialists, "I still encourage my patients to go elsewhere for a second opinion," says Dr. John Marshall.

The window of opportunity for soliciting another physician's viewpoint prior to treatment is wider for some cancers than for others, but usually a short delay of approximately two, three, even four weeks will not compromise the outcome. "Sometimes cancers present in a way that's immediately life-threatening and has to be dealt with at once," notes Dr. DeVita. He could be talking about my case when he adds, "Even in that situation, if there's further treatment to be given once the emergency is over, there's usually time to get another opinion."

When you're a cancer survivor, people tend to seek out your advice, either for themselves or for someone they know. Inevitably, the question arises: Should I get a second opinion? And if so, where? I tell them about my experience: how doctors at the Lombardi Cancer Center were able to offer me an investigational regimen of chemotherapy that I could not have received at my community hospital, and the comfort I felt as a result. Without exception, I recommend they make an appointment at a major cancer center, such as those listed in table 5.1.

Of the nearly ninety treatment facilities, covering thirty-eight states plus the District of Columbia, forty-eight belong to the National Cancer Institute's network of clinical cancer centers and comprehensive cancer centers. (The "comprehensive" designation is awarded to facilities that excel in the areas of public outreach, education, and information services; from a standpoint of medical care, there is little or no difference between the two.) Completing the list are thirty-nine teaching institutions, all of which ranked among "America's Best Hospitals" for cancer care in one or more years from 1996 through 1999, according to *U.S. News & World Report* magazine's annual ratings.

What to Look for in a Cancer-Treatment Facility

M ost Americans live within a half-day's drive of a cancer referral center, though it's highly possible you won't have to make the trip more than once. "Fully half the patients that I see come for a single visit," says Dr. David Johnson, associate director of the Vanderbilt Cancer Center in Nashville. A medical oncologist, he and his colleagues routinely plan patients' protocols, then refer them to physicians closer to home, who will carry out the treatment.

"I know every oncologist in the state of Tennessee," says Dr. Johnson. "So I can tell someone from Soddy-Daisy, which is a small city near Chattanooga, 'This is what we think ought to be done, and Dr. X in Chattanooga is superb.'" A second opinion can also serve as a quality check. From a psychological point of view, the reassurance of knowing that a group of experts concurs with your local doctor's treatment recommendation is well worth the travel involved.

Then there are circumstances under which patients go to a state-of-the-art facility for a highly specialized inpatient procedure—perhaps stereotactic radiosurgery to eradicate a brain tumor, or mastectomy and breast-reconstruction surgery—with adjuvant therapy, if necessary, delegated to a local physician.

By no means are we implying that the hospitals in table 5.1 are the only ones in the entire United States providing first-rate cancer care. "You can find excellent care at any level," stresses Dr. Rick Ungerleider, chief of the National Cancer Institute's clinical investigations branch. "And going to the top level doesn't necessarily mean you're going to get excellent care." Choosing a cancer-treatment facility is no different from shopping for any other service. You base your decision not on reputation alone but on whether it offers the components of quality care you need, such as:

- Experience in diagnosing and treating your form of cancer, including expertise in managing symptoms and side effects
- Pain-management and palliative-care services
- Access to investigational therapies as well as advanced techniques and technology
- A multidisciplinary approach to treatment planning
- Laboratory and imaging facilities on-site
- Other patient services, such as psycho-oncology, social work, nutrition, and rehabilitation

In the box on page 299, we've arranged the various types of treatment centers according to three general categories. Overall you are more likely to find the full array of features listed above (and discussed in greater detail below) in one location at an NCI center or other large academic institution, with "large" used to describe a hospital that has roughly four hundred or more beds. Yet you can find teaching hospi-

---

TABLE 5.1   The "A" List: Top Cancer Centers in the United States

---

Σ indicates the facility was ranked as one of the top cancer hospitals in the country by
U.S. News & World Report for one or more years from 1996 through 1999.
* Indicates the facility is an NCI-designated clinical cancer center.
** Indicates the facility is an NCI-designated comprehensive cancer center.

Alabama
University of Alabama at Birmingham
Comprehensive Cancer Center **
Birmingham
205-934-5077
http://www.ccc.uab.edu

Arizona
Arizona Cancer Center ** Σ
University of Arizona Health
Sciences Center
Tucson
520-626-2900
http://www.azcc.arizona.edu

Arkansas
University Hospital of Arkansas Σ
Little Rock
501-686-6121
http://www.uams.edu/#new

California
City of Hope National
Medical Center **
Beckman Research Institute
Duarte
800-826-4673
http://www.cityofhope.org

UCSD Cancer Center * Σ
University of California at San Diego
La Jolla
858-543-3456
http://www.ucsd.edu

Loma Linda University
Medical Center Σ
Loma Linda
909-796-7311
http://www.llu.edu

Jonsson Comprehensive Cancer
Center ** Σ
UCLA
Los Angeles
800-522-6237/213-764-3000
http://www.cancer.mednet.ucla.edu

Kenneth Norris Jr. Comprehensive
Cancer Center and Hospital**
University of Southern California
Los Angeles
800-872-2273/323-865-3000
http://ccnt.hsc.usc.edu

Chao Family Comprehensive
Cancer Center **
University of California at Irvine
Orange
714-456-8000
http://www.med.uci.edu/~cancer

USC Davis Medical Center Σ
Sacramento
916-734-2011
*http://www.ucdmc.ucdavis.edu/
medical_center/index.html*

University of California
San Francisco Comprehensive
Cancer Center ** Σ
San Francisco
415-567-9980
http://cc.ucsf.edu

Stanford Hospital and Clinics Σ
Stanford
650-723-4000
http://www-med.stanford.edu

Colorado
University of Colorado
Cancer Center ** Σ
Denver
800-473-2288
*http://www.uchsc.edu/chancllr/UCCC/
UCCCwelcome.html*

Connecticut
Yale Cancer Center ** Σ
New Haven
203-785-2000
*http://www.info.med.yale.edu/ycc/
new/welcome.htm*

Delaware
Medical Center of Wilmington Σ
Wilmington
302-733-1000
http://www.christianacare.org

District of Columbia
Lombardi Cancer Center ** Σ
Georgetown University
Medical Center
202-784-4000
http://lombardi.georgetown.edu

Florida
Shands Hospital at the
University of Florida Σ
Gainesville
352-395-0552
http://www.hsc.ufl.edu/shands/sth.htm

H. Lee Moffitt Cancer Center and
Research Institute at the University
of South Florida *Σ
Tampa
813-972-4673
http://www.hlmcc.org

Georgia
Emory University Hospital Σ
Atlanta
800-753-6679/404-778-7777
*http://www2.cc.emory.edu/WHSC/
EUH/euh.html*

Hawaii
Cancer Research Center of Hawaii *
University of Hawaii at Manoa
Honolulu
808-586-3013
http://www2.hawaii.edu/crch

Illinois
Robert H. Lurie Comprehensive
Cancer Center **
Northwestern University
Chicago
312-908-5250
*http://www.nums.nwu.edu/lurie/
index.html*

Rush-Presbyterian St. Luke's
Medical Center Σ
Chicago
312-942-5000
http://www.rush.edu

University of Chicago Cancer
Research Center ** Σ
Chicago
888-824-2282/773-702-9200
http://www.-uccrc.bsd.uchicago.edu

Evanston Northwestern HealthcareΣ
Kellogg Cancer Care Center
Evanston Hospital
Evanston
847-570-2110
{
Kellogg Cancer Care Center
Glenbrook Hospital
Glenbrook
847-657-5800
http://www.enh.org

Loyola University Medical Center
Oncology Institute Σ
Maywood
708-226-4357
*http://www.lumc.edu/research/
oncinst.htm*

Lutheran General Hospital Σ
Park Ridge
847-723-2210
*http://www.advocatehealth.com/sites/
hospitals/luth/index.html*

Indiana
Clarian Health Σ
Indiana University Medical Center
Indianapolis
317-274-5000
{
Methodist Hospital
Indianapolis
317-929-2000
http://www.clarian.com

Iowa

University of Iowa Hospitals and
Clinics Σ
Iowa City
319-356-2296
http://www.uihc.uiowa.edu

Kentucky

University of Kentucky HealthCare Σ
Lexington
606-323-5000
http://www.ukhealthcare.uky.edu

Louisiana

Ochsner Foundation Hospital Σ
New Orleans
504-842-3000
http://www.ochsner.org

Maryland

Greater Baltimore Medical Center Σ
Baltimore
410-828-2000
http://www.gbmc.org

Johns Hopkins Oncology Center ** Σ
Baltimore
410-955-5000
http://www.med.jhu.edu/cancerctr

Massachusetts

Brigham and Women's Hospital Σ
Boston
617-732-5500
http://www.partners.org/bwh/
home.html

Dana-Farber Cancer Institute ** Σ
Boston
617-632-3476
http://www.dfci.harvard.edu

Massachusetts General Hospital Σ
Boston
617-726-2000
http://cancer.mgh.harvard.edu

Michigan

University of Michigan
Comprehensive Cancer Center ** Σ
Ann Arbor
800-865-1125/734-936-9583
http://www.cancer.med.umich.edu

Josephine Ford Cancer Center Σ
Henry Ford Hospital
Detroit
800-653-6568/313-876-2600
http://henryfordhealth.org

Harper Hospital Σ
Detroit Medical Center
Detroit
313-745-8040
http://www.phypc.med.wayne.edu/er/
harper.htm

Barbara Ann Karmanos Cancer
Institute **
Detroit
313-833-0710
http://www.karmanos.org

William Beaumont Hospital Σ
Royal Oak
248-551-5000
http://www.beaumont.edu

Minnesota

University of Minnesota
Cancer Center ** Σ
Minneapolis
612-626-3000
http://www.cancer.umn.edu

Mayo Clinic Cancer Center * Σ
Rochester
507-284-4137
http://www.mayo.edu/
cancercenter.index.html

Missouri

Ellis Fischel Cancer Center Σ
University of Missouri Health
Sciences Center
Columbia
573-882-4141
http://www.muhealth.org/~ellisfischel

Barnes-Jewish Hospital Σ
St. Louis
314-747-3000
http://www.bjc.org/bjh.html

Nebraska
UNMC Epply Cancer Center Σ
Omaha
402-559-4090
http://www.unmc.edu/cancercenter

New Hampshire
**Norris Cotton Cancer Center ** Σ
Dartmouth-Hitchcock Medical Center
Lebanon
603-650-5527
http://NCCC.hitchcock.org

New Jersey
The Cancer Institute of New Jersey *
Robert Wood Johnson Medical School
New Brunswick
732-235-2465
http://130.219.231.104

New York
**Albert Einstein Comprehensive
Cancer Center ****
Montifiore Medical Center
Bronx
718-920-4826
http://www.ca.aecom.yu.edu

**Roswell Park Cancer Institute ** Σ
Buffalo
800-767-9355/716-845-2000
http://rpci.med.buffalo.edu

**Herbert Irving Comprehensive
Cancer Center ** Σ
Columbia University
New York
212-305-8610
http://www.ccc.columbia.edu

Kaplan Cancer Center **
New York University Medical
Center
New York
212-263-6485
http://kccc-www.med.nyu.edu

**Memorial Sloan-Kettering Cancer
Center ** Σ
New York
212-639-2000
http://www.mskcc.org

Mount Sinai Medical Center Σ
New York
212-241-6500
http://www.mountsinai.org

**The New York Hospital-Cornell
Medical Center** Σ
New York
212-746-5454
http://surgery.med.cornell.edu

University of Rochester Cancer Center *
Rochester
800-462-6763/716-275-4911
*http://www.urmc.rochester.edu/
strong/cancer/cancerpg.htm*

North Carolina
**UNC Lineberger Comprehensive
Cancer Center ** Σ
University of North Carolina School
of Medicine
Chapel Hill
919-966-3036/919-966-1101
http://www.med.unc.edu

**Duke Comprehensive Cancer
Center ** Σ
Durham
919-684-3377
http://www.canctr.mc.duke.edu

**Comprehensive Cancer Center of
Wake Forest University ** Σ
Wake Forest University Medical Center
Winston-Salem
336-716-4464
http://bgsm.edu/cancer

North Dakota
MeritCare Health System Roger Maris Cancer Center Σ
Fargo
800-511-6161/701-234-6161
http://www.meritcare.com

Ohio
University of Cincinnati Medical Center Σ
Cincinnati
513-558-1000
http://medcenter.uc.edu

Cleveland Clinic Cancer Center Σ
Cleveland
216-444-2200
http://www.ccf.org/cc

University Hospitals Ireland Cancer Center ** Σ
Cleveland
216-844-1000
http://www.uhhs.com/uhc/cancer

Arthur G. James Cancer Hospital and Research Institute ** Σ
Ohio State University
Columbus
800-293-5066/614-293-5066
http://www.cancer.med.ohio-state.edu

Kettering Medical Center Σ
Kettering
937-298-4331
http://www.ketthealth.com

The Toledo Hospital Σ
Toledo
419-471-4000
http://www.promedica.org/hosp/tth.asp

Oklahoma
University Hospital Σ
Oklahoma City
405-271-4700

Oregon
Oregon Cancer Center * Σ
Oregon Health Sciences University
Portland
503-494-1617
http://www.ohsu.edu

Pennsylvania
Penn State Geisinger Cancer Center Σ
Hershey
717-531-8521
http://www.collmed.psu.edu/cancer

Fox Chase Cancer Center ** Σ
Philadelphia
215-728-2570
http://www.fccc.edu

Kimmel Cancer Center * Σ
Thomas Jefferson University
Philadelphia
215-955-6000
http://www.kcc.tju.edu

University of Pennsylvania Cancer Center ** Σ
Philadelphia
800-383-8722/215-662-6364
http://cancer.med.upenn.edu/upcc

Allegheny General Hospital Σ
Pittsburgh
877-284-2000/412-359-3131
http://www.allhealth.edu

University of Pittsburgh Cancer Institute ** Σ
Pittsburgh
800-237-4724
http://www.pci.upmc.edu

Rhode Island
Roger Williams Medical Center Σ
Providence
401-456-2000
http://www.rwmc.com

Tennessee
St. Jude Children's Research Hospital *
Memphis
901-495-3300
http://www.stjude.org
Treats children only

Vanderbilt Cancer Center * Σ
Vanderbilt University
Nashville
615-322-6053
http://www.mc.vanderbilt.edu/vumc/cancer.html

Texas
Baylor University Medical Center Σ
Dallas
214-820-0111
http://www.Baylordallas.edu/BUMC

University of Texas M. D. Anderson
Cancer Center ** Σ
Houston
800-392-1611/713-792-6161
http://www.mdanderson.org

San Antonio Cancer Institute **
San Antonio
210-616-5798
http://www.ccc.saci.org

Scott and White Hospital and Clinic Σ
Temple
254-724-2111
http://www.sw.org

Utah
Huntsman Cancer Institute *
University of Utah
Salt Lake City
877-585-0303/801-585-0303
http://www.hci.utah.edu

Vermont
Vermont Cancer Center **
University of Vermont College of
Medicine
Burlington
802-656-4414
*http://www.vtmednet.org/vcc/
index.org*

Virginia
University of Virginia Cancer
Center * Σ
Charlottesville
804-924-5004
*http://www.med.virginia.edu/
medcntr/cancer/home.html*

Inova Fairfax Hospital Σ
Falls Church
703-698-1110
http://www.inova.com/fh/index.html

Massey Cancer Center *
Virginia Commonwealth University
Richmond
804-828-5116
http://views.vcu.edu/mcc

Washington
Fred Hutchinson Cancer Research
Center **
Seattle
206-667-5000
http://www.fhcrc.org

University of Washington Medical
Center Σ
Seattle
206-548-3300
*http://www.washington.edu/
medical/uwmc*

Wisconsin
University of Wisconsin
Comprehensive Cancer Center ** Σ
Madison
608-263-8091
*http://www.medsch.wisc.edu/
cancer/homepage.html*

tals and large community hospitals that boast many of the same services—including multidisciplinary treatment planning and clinical studies—only perhaps scaled down in terms of size and availability.

Some Definitions, Please

Exactly what is a community hospital? And how does an academic institution differ from a teaching hospital? The definitions are imprecise, to say the least, and growing increasingly fuzzy as state-of-the-art centers branch out into the community by launching satellite programs at smaller hospitals, for reasons of economics as much as altruism.

Academic Medical Center—a large hospital, usually located on or near the campus of a major university, with its own medical school program. For example, Georgetown University School of Medicine is part of Georgetown University Medical Center, home to the Lombardi Cancer Center. Other hallmarks of an academic institution generally include a full-time house staff and extensive basic laboratory research as well as clinical studies. Why should a patient be concerned about a facility's commitment to lab research? Dr. David Johnson contends that outstanding research and outstanding patient care go hand in hand.

"When you have high-quality patient-focused research and excellent laboratory research," he says, "you tend to attract first-rate, highly dedicated clinicians. If I'm dedicated to good patient care, I want to work with the best scientists in the world, who have the brilliance to come up with new treatments and approaches."

Teaching Hospital—a term typically applied to hospitals that are affiliated with medical schools. They can be large or small. Inova Fairfax Hospital, a teaching hospital in Falls Church, Virginia, has more beds than Georgetown University Medical Center, conducts clinical trials, and was rated by *U.S. News & World Report* as one of the top cancer-treatment facilities in the country. Unlike an academic center, however, it has no basic research program and no full-time house staff. The hospital's eighteen hundred physicians, all in private practice, share the teaching load with the faculty from Georgetown University School of Medicine.

The Three Tiers of Cancer-Treatment Facilities
1. NCI clinical cancer centers and comprehensive cancer centers and large non-NCI academic medical centers
2. Teaching hospitals and large community hospitals able to offer comprehensive diagnostic and treatment services, including clinical studies
3. Smaller community hospitals and freestanding facilities that offer limited diagnostic and treatment services and minimal or no access to clinical studies

Community Hospital—any hospital where the emphasis is solely on patient care: no medical students, no laboratory research. Four in five U.S. hospitals fall into this broad category. They vary widely in size and services. According to Dr. Larry White, president of the Association of Community Cancer Centers, "More than 80 percent of the cancer patients in this country are treated in the community setting."

Freestanding Facility—an outpatient office or clinic in a nonhospital setting. A group practice may consist of practitioners in the same medical specialty—say, a group medical-oncology facility—or multiple disciplines, like medical oncology and radiation oncology. Rarely, though, will you find a freestanding facility staffed by specialists in all three of the major cancer modalities: chemotherapy, radiotherapy, and surgical oncology.

Not every patient will benefit significantly from undergoing treatment at such high-caliber facilities as Buffalo's Roswell Park Cancer Institute or Chicago's Rush-Presbyterian St. Luke's Medical Center. In cases where effective standard therapy exists and no serious complications are anticipated, a person might fare equally well at a community-hospital cancer program or a freestanding clinic. One example would be someone with a localized tumor of the upper throat, which is often treatable with external-beam radiation alone. But head and neck cancer patients have a 30 percent chance of developing second malignancies in the same area. At a research-oriented center, they could possibly participate in a clinical trial studying chemopreventive agents to help reduce the odds of a future cancer.

As for men and women with advanced disease who wish to explore all possible avenues, a state-of-the-art institution almost certainly offers their best hope. Dr. Brian Kimes, associate director of the National Cancer Institute's Cancer Centers Program, puts it bluntly: "People at a serious stage of cancer have little chance of being cured under standard protocols."

How Many Patients with Your Form of Cancer Does the Facility See per Year?

Not to belabor the body-as-car analogy, but if something went wrong with your transmission, you probably wouldn't entrust your car to the general mechanic at the corner gas station who handles oil changes and other routine maintenance. You'd bring it to a specialist, someone who repairs transmissions regularly and has encountered most mechanical problems. Similarly, in determining where to go for cancer therapy, what you're looking for above all else is clinical experience. As Dr. Fred Appelbaum of Seattle's Fred Hutchinson Cancer Research Center emphasizes, "It's called the *practice* of medicine."

A wall full of framed diplomas doesn't tell you a physician's experience in diagnosing and treating your disease. The way to find out is to ask, "How many people with my type of cancer have you treated in the last year?" If the answer is two or three, we'd suggest you continue your search.

"You want to see a doctor who thinks about the disease on a daily basis," advises Dr. Vincent DeVita, whose subspecialty is cancers of the lymphatic system. "And you don't think about it on a daily basis if you treat three cases a year." The numbers vary, of course, depending on whether you have a common or rare form of cancer, but ideally you want an oncologist who treats dozens, if not hundreds, of patients like you every year. Consider that Dr. John Marshall, my oncologist, estimates that he annually diagnoses 100 to 150 cases of colon cancer alone.

> ## A Word About Mortality Rates
>
> One of the yardsticks for assessing the level of care at a cancer-treatment facility is to inquire about its ratio of deaths per number of patients. For instance, in clinical trials studying bone-marrow transplantation in women with breast cancer, the national mortality rate is 5 percent. "If you go to a center where it's 15 percent, you might want to think twice," cautions Dr. Kenneth Meehan, acting director of the BMT program at the Lombardi Cancer Center. Bear in mind, though, that because top-rated cancer institutions are often a last resort for many patients with advanced disease or for those who've been declared terminal, their mortality rates may actually be higher than those of less accomplished facilities.

In cancer care, bigger is often better. Without question there are small-town general oncologists well versed in treating tumors of the prostate, lung, breast, and other frequently occurring cancers. As a general rule, though, institutions with sizable cancer-patient populations possess superior experience across the board: in cancer surgery, managing side effects and complications, diagnosis and staging, and so on. Greater experience is usually synonymous with greater expertise, which in any of these areas can markedly improve not only your prospects for survival but your quality of life during treatment.

Why Surgical Expertise Is So Important

Cancer surgery, still the definitive treatment for most cancers, can be complex, even life-threatening, as when a tumor has wrapped itself around a major blood vessel. "People with cancer want to go to a surgeon who does these procedures regularly," stresses Dr. Charles Fuchs, a medical oncologist at Dana-Farber Cancer Institute. For as studies have shown consistently, "in experienced hands, the rates of mortality and complications can be reasonably low."

A 1998 study from Memorial Sloan-Kettering Cancer Center compared the surgical mortality rates at medical centers that treated many people with cancer versus those that treated relatively few. In all, the researchers reviewed statistics on more than five thousand elderly patients who'd undergone one of five particularly complex operations over a nine-year period. They found that the percentages of patients who did not survive these operations were two to five times higher at the hospitals with low caseloads than at the more experienced centers:

Operation	Mortality rate (patients who died up to thirty days after surgery)	
	Low-Volume Hospital	High-Volume Hospital
Esophagectomy (resection of the esophagus)	17.3%	3.4%
Pancreatectomy (resection of the pancreas)	12.9%	5.5%
Hepatic resection (resection of the liver)	5.4%	1.7%
Pelvic exenteration (partial resection of the pelvic organs	3.7%	1.5%
Pneumonectomy (resection of a lung)	No significant difference	

Reducing your risk of serious surgery-related complications is just one reason for seeking a surgical oncologist with a wealth of experience. Other potential advantages include:

• A more aggressive approach to proceeding with complicated surgeries. "There are many patients who've been able to have their tumors resected at a big hospital after a small hospital had told them they were inoperable," says general surgeon Dr. Charles Yeo, director of the pancreas-cancer center at Johns Hopkins. Though he is referring to pancreatic resection specifically, Dr. Yeo could be talking about any number of exacting procedures when he adds, "A doctor who performs this operation only once a year is more likely to say, 'I can't take this out,' whereas when you do it once a week you're much more determined about trying to remove the tumor."

• **Mastery of surgical techniques that can preserve form and function,** such as nerve-sparing radical prostatectomy to excise the prostate gland through an incision in the lower abdomen. This method, pioneered in the 1980s by Dr. Patrick Walsh, also of Johns Hopkins, considerably improves a man's chances of retaining sexual potency once he's recovered. Nerve-sparing prostatectomy is widely practiced today. But Dr. Walsh's success rate for men in their fifties is 5 to 25 percent higher than the national average. Is this worth a trip to Baltimore? It's up to each patient—not to mention his health insurer—to decide.

Experience is no less important in reconstructive surgery, which may be necessary in a number of situations—perhaps in constructing a new throat, or grafting skin over the site where a melanoma was excised, or rebuilding a breast following mastectomy. Even when the object of surgery is cosmetic rather than therapeutic, as with breast reconstruction, a poorly performed procedure can inflict lasting emotional and psychological damage. "Every surgeon in the country fancies himself a breast surgeon," observes Dr. David Johnson. "As someone who sees the results, believe me, they ain't all the same." Granted, experience is no guarantee of a physician's competence. But for the consumer with little or no medical background, which describes most of us, it is our most reliable barometer.

Why Expertise in Managing Side Effects and Complications Is So Important

Your medical team's ability to anticipate and control side effects and complications affects more than your immediate health and comfort. It can influence whether or not you receive the optimum level of treatment. In a national Gallup survey of approximately fifteen hundred men and women who were receiving chemotherapy, nearly half had their medication delayed at some point due to adverse side effects. Among the culprits that most often force a postponement of treatment: abnormally low counts of white blood cells, and to a lesser degree, red blood cells and blood platelet cells; mucositis, an inflammation of the digestive tract that can make eating painfully difficult; and other gastrointestinal disorders such as profuse vomiting and diarrhea.

At large centers that emphasize cancer care, says Yale's DeVita, "it's the normal standard of practice to be able to get people past these kinds of complications; we tend to go straight through a treatment protocol. But in the general-practice community, there is a greater tendency to modify dosing because they're not necessarily staffed adequately to manage complications that might occur. So when they give a dose of chemotherapy, and the patient's bone marrow does not recover as fast as they would like, instead of going ahead—as we often will do—and being vigilant to take care of whatever complications develop, they may wait, which reduces the dose intensity.

"A lot of doctors will say they gave the full dose," he points out. "But when you look at the patient's records, you find they gave the full dose perhaps a month apart rather than three weeks apart," as per the standard protocol. "That results in a 25 percent reduction of the intensity of that particular dose, because the week off counts as if you didn't give any therapy."

Insufficient supportive care can preclude patients getting state-of-the-art cancer treatment in surgery and radiotherapy too. In order to resect a tumor in the lowermost segment of the throat, for example, the surgeon frequently must excise not only that portion of the throat but all or part of the adjoining larynx, which results in impaired speech and swallowing. During the lengthy procedure, doctors also create an airway directly into the windpipe and restore swallowing by building a new throat with tissue transplanted from another part of the body.

"These are often very involved operations," says Dr. Randal Weber, director of the head and neck cancer center at Philadelphia's University of Pennsylvania Cancer Center. "I don't mean this as an indictment of the community-hospital system, because in some areas they do the surgery quite well. But there's a tendency not to offer aggressive therapy on account of the potential problems with speech and swallowing, and so patients don't always get the best initial modality of treatment. And if they fail that, the chances of saving them are quite poor."

When faced with laryngeal cancer, progressive centers typically make every effort to offer alternatives to laryngectomy. According to Dr. William Richtsmeier, chief of otolaryngology head and neck surgery at Duke Comprehensive Cancer Center, "Even for advanced-stage disease, we still salvage a large number of patients without having to operate." The standard treatment there consists of simultaneous chemotherapy and hyperfractionated irradiation, in which radiation is given twice a day. Small nonacademic hospitals are less likely to pursue this intensive approach, he says, "because managing the potential side effects takes more of an effort on the part of the oncologist."

Does the Facility Offer Pain-Management and Palliative-Care Services?

Palliative medicine to ease pain and other symptoms and side effects of disease and its treatment "is still an evolving field," says Dr. Jane Ingham, director of the palliative-care program at the Lombardi Cancer Center. Aside from Lombardi, Memorial Sloan-Kettering, and other institutions at the forefront of cancer therapy, few hospitals have established departments dedicated exclusively to palliative care.

But physicians are increasingly recognizing the importance of effective symptom control in enhancing a cancer patient's quality of life, and not only in the context of terminal illness. "For instance," says Dr. Ingham, "early in the disease, when a person is going through chemotherapy, the palliative-care service might be involved in helping to alleviate nausea or the pain from mucositis."

See "Pain Management" in Chapter Eight, "Take Control: Managing Symptoms, Side Effects, and Complications."

Does the Facility Offer Access to Clinical Trials and to Advanced Techniques and Technologies?

In order of priority, says Dr. Marc Lippman, director of the Lombardi Cancer Center, "the resources that a physician is able to bring to the table" are every bit as important as his or her clinical expertise—perhaps even more so. By resources, we mean experimental therapies, not to mention modern equipment and the latest techniques for the detection and treatment of cancer as well as managing its complications. On all counts, here again NCI-designated centers and large university hospitals often hold an advantage.

"It is wrong to imagine that there aren't wonderful doctors in community practice every bit as caring and competent as those in academic life," stresses Dr. Lippman. "On the other hand, at one time if a person with colon cancer failed fluorouracil," then the standard post-surgical chemotherapy for that disease, "there would have been no treatment in the community as good as what he could have received here, simply because it wasn't available."

Options. That's what I wanted first and foremost from a treatment center. Perhaps it took on added significance because in the wake of a cancer diagnosis life's possibilities no longer seem so limitless. Even if you ultimately decide to undergo a conventional protocol, you'll have the comfort of knowing that you were afforded all available treatment choices. Dr. John Marshall, whose patients usually come to him after having been diagnosed at other hospitals, reflects, "I don't know how many times patients have said to me, 'No one told me any of this! The doctor just said, "This is a bad situation, this is what you should do, and we'll start tomorrow.""'"

Finding State-of-the-Art Cancer Care in Community Centers

CCOP, CGOP, CRG

If you're considering a community cancer center for your treatment, add the following to your list of questions about its features: "Do you belong to CCOP? CGOP? CRG?" All are abbreviations for outreach programs designed to bring experimental therapies to a wider segment of the population.

CCOP (Community Clinical Oncology Program) and *CGOP* (Cooperative Group Outreach Program) were established by the National Cancer Institute to enable community hospitals and even private oncology practices to enter patients in its federally funded Clinical Trials Cooperative Group Program. (To qualify for CCOP, a facility must enroll at least fifty patients in NCI studies; there is no minimum requirement to become a CGOP.)

There are nine major groups, each made up of NCI centers, academic institutions, CCOPs, and CGOPs. All told, the Cooperative Group Program involves fourteen hundred facilities and places twenty thousand new cancer patients in large-scale multicenter investigational studies every year. While the program allows community cancer centers to be more competitive in terms of offering cutting-edge therapies, NCI's Dr. Rick Ungerleider points out that large research-based institutions still afford access to a broader range of promising treatments, and earlier in the FDA approval process, too, "before they are put into the general pool of community hospitals."

The third set of initials mentioned above, *CRG*, stands for Collaborative Research Group, a program of the Association of Community Cancer Centers. The ACCC represents some five hundred community cancer centers and private cancer clinics. Its Collaborative Research Group serves as a coordinating body, linking qualified ACCC member facilities with clinical trials being sponsored by pharmaceutical and biotechnology companies.

To find out if a community cancer center or private oncology practice is a member of CCOP, call the Cancer Information Service: 800-422-6237.

To find out if a community cancer center or private oncology practice is a member of CRG, call the Association of Community Cancer Centers: 301-984-9496.

Hospital Outreach Programs

An encouraging trend in cancer medicine has been the formation of satellite programs and affiliate networks, in which a center of excellence exports its staff and/or experimental protocols to smaller neighboring facilities. Memorial Sloan-Kettering opened branches at several New York and New Jersey hospitals, where patients see doctors on the Sloan-Kettering faculty and where chemotherapy and radiotherapy are delivered by Sloan-Kettering personnel.

Tennessee's Vanderbilt Cancer Center developed an affiliate network for sharing its clinical trials regionally while still maintaining a high level of quality control. As Dr. David Johnson explains, "We didn't want to send out cancer protocols to physicians we weren't familiar with, or whose facilities we didn't have 100 percent confidence in. So we set up stringent criteria for joining the program. A center has to be a full-service facility, its physicians have to be board-certified, the pathology labs and radiation-oncology units have to meet the minimum standards of the College of American Pathologists and the American College of Radiology, and so on. In short, it has to have the features that we feel are important for delivering high-quality care.

"When a hospital requests membership, we visit the site," he continues. "If it passes muster, it becomes part of the network, and we permit it to take part in clinical trials that patients in the area normally would have had to drive to Nashville to receive. Today we're set up in every metropolitan area in Tennessee." Similar outreach programs are springing up across the United States, an appealing option for patients who can't or don't wish to undergo treatment at a major cancer institution, whatever the reason.

Does the Facility Practice a Multidisciplinary Approach to Cancer Treatment?

"Medicine is a complex field," says Dr. DeVita. "Most of it consists of opinions." Given that more and more cancers call for multimodality protocols, we *want* to hear the viewpoints of experts in surgery, chemotherapy, radiotherapy, and other disciplines. Obviously, you can go about this by soliciting second opinions from individual practitioners. Our suggestion, though, is to arrange a consultation at a multidisciplinary cancer facility, where a panel of specialists reviews your case and forms a consensus on a recommended plan of treatment. Besides cutting down on the number of appointments, it eliminates the potential for confusion. "I think people find it very frustrating to confer with several doctors and come away with conflicting opinions," comments Dr. Christine Berg, Lombardi's director of the breast radiation-therapy program.

The process at Lombardi is representative of what you would find at most university centers that practice multidisciplinary cancer care, which is virtually all of them. In addition to weekly "tumor-board" conferences, where cases are bandied about and, as Dr. Marshall puts it, "it's open season for anyone to critique or comment on what I'm doing for a particular patient," there are weekly meetings dedicated to specific types of cancer: colorectal, lung, gynecologic, urologic, breast.

"First one member of the team evaluates the patient," explains Dr. Berg. Next the case is discussed by the entire group, typically consisting of a surgical oncologist, medical oncologist, radiation oncologist, pathologist, and oncology nurse. A psychologist, oncology social worker, and/or nutritionist may also attend the conferences. "Then," she says, "as a group we share our recommendation with the patient and family, and answer any questions they may have."

General tumor boards at community cancer centers meet anywhere from once a week to once every three months. Holding regular subspecialty tumor-board meetings "is not typical for a lot of community hospitals," says Dr. Nicholas Robert, a medical oncologist and chairman of education and research at Inova Fairfax Hospital, one of the rare nonacademic hospitals that does.

The obvious question—why don't all medical facilities adopt the multidisciplinary-team structure?—has an equally obvious answer: It's more time-consuming and less cost-effective. "But it's darn cost-effective for the patient, I'll tell you that," says Dr. David Johnson, who speaks from his experience as both physician and patient. When he was diagnosed with lymphoma in 1989, the doctor's case was brought up before his colleagues on the tumor board at the Vanderbilt Cancer Center, just like any other patient's.

Other Advantages of Multidisciplinary Cancer Care

More opinions, more options. Physicians are not invulnerable to professional myopia. Therefore, a doctor may overlook a form of cancer therapy that might in fact prove beneficial. Dr. DeVita recounts a disturbing conversation he once had with a radiation oncologist who'd neglected to refer a person with lung cancer to a medical oncologist, despite its having been well established that this type of tumor responds best to a combination of radiotherapy and chemotherapy.

"The patient was irradiated, didn't receive chemotherapy, and the cancer recurred, as you would expect," recalls Dr. DeVita. "Received more radiation; the cancer recurred. More radiation; another recurrence. Finally, after the fifth go-round, we were asked to see the patient, who at this point had no chance. I politely asked the doctor, 'Why wasn't he administered chemotherapy with the radiotherapy?'

"He looked at me and said, '*I don't believe in chemotherapy.*' Not 'I don't believe chemotherapy is appropriate for this patient.' He meant he didn't believe in the entire field." While this particular doctor's arrogance was atypical in the extreme, for a patient not to be offered appropriate multimodality therapy occurs more often than we would like to imagine—not because information is being withheld, but because the physician is unfamiliar with combined-modality protocols.

"Breast cancer is a classic example," says Dr. DeVita. Three-fourths of women with stage I or II breast cancer are candidates for breast-conservation surgery, better known as lumpectomy, which is followed by six weeks of outpatient radiation therapy. Instead of a mastectomy to remove the entire breast, only the cancerous tissue is taken out. The two approaches are equally effective.

Yet in a major study of nearly eighteen thousand patients with early-stage breast cancer, more than half of those who were eligible for the less invasive operation lost their breast to mastectomy unnecessarily. Furthermore, although age is not supposed to influence a doctor's decision, fifty-year-old women were 11 percent more likely than forty-year-olds to have mastectomies performed; sixty-year-old women, 22 percent more likely; seventy-year-old women 33 percent more likely; and so on.

Most breast-cancer patients, Dr. DeVita continues, are first seen by a surgeon. "Unless the surgeon is part of a team, a woman may well get a mastectomy, when a lumpectomy and radiation might be indicated." It's simply easier for a breast surgeon who belongs to a multidisciplinary facility to be aware of all forms of breast-cancer treatment. The same study—conducted jointly by the American College of Surgeons, the American College of Radiology, and the College of American Pathologists—found that of the patients who opted for breast-sparing surgery, almost one in four never received the postoperative radiation, which is crucial to the treatment's success. In half the cases, the surgeon *never recommended it.*

"The surgeon, the radiotherapist, the medical oncologist—none of us can do it alone," says Dr. Larry Norton of Memorial Sloan-Kettering. "The attending surgeons here know when hormone therapy is indicated, just as I know which surgical procedure is appropriate, even though I can't perform the operation. We share a common knowledge base, and that comes about from working together for a long time and discussing cases together."

Regular communication among the members of your medical team. "Having ten doctors doesn't mean that you've got a *team* of doctors," points out Dr. Jane Ingham. "They've got to talk to one another." In the multidisciplinary setting, your physicians, nurses, and other team members interact constantly, which improves the continuity of care and tightens the safety net for catching relatively minor problems before they mushroom into major ones.

For instance, a person with cancer might not feel like eating for a number of reasons: a sore throat from radiation therapy; a metallic taste in the mouth due to chemotherapy; chronic diarrhea. But appetite loss can also signal depression. The staff dietitian is as likely to intercept the problem as the staff psychologist, says Susan Sloan, a clinical dietitian at the Lombardi Cancer Center. "It's not like I focus solely on food and the psychologist focuses only on depression. We're all aware of these symptoms being very much intertwined, and everyone tries to work together, saying, 'Have you noticed Mr. Smith isn't eating?' So although depression may in fact be the major issue, it may be detected through my counseling the person on his diet."

A cohesive, long-range care plan. For some cancers, the growing use of chemotherapy and radiotherapy prior to surgery has multiplied the number of possible treatment sequences. For one patient with stage III rectal cancer, the first stop may be the operating room, after which he receives chemotherapy and radiotherapy. Another patient with the same disease, same stage, may travel the reverse course: neoadjuvant chemotherapy and radiation therapy; surgery to resect the tumor; then additional chemotherapy, this time adjuvantly.

The most efficient way to coordinate multimodality therapy is for the various specialists to be involved from the get-go, says Dr. DeVita, returning to his example of breast conservation. "A lumpectomy is a simple surgical procedure, and certainly any general surgeon could do it. However, radiation therapy of the breast is tricky: We can't irradiate very large breasts, for example. On the other hand, we don't want to perform a lumpectomy on very small breasts, because the cosmetic effect is almost the same as a mastectomy. So if the surgeon is going to have a radiotherapist irradiate, he or she should be part of the initial planning."

Furthermore, adjuvant chemotherapy, hormone therapy, or a combination of the two "is almost always added," says Dr. DeVita. "Therefore, there has to be a medical oncologist involved. Logistically, it's very complex, and you have to map out the sequence of events in advance. Many times, doctors in private practice pull this together one step at a time.

"Some do it extremely well," he hastens to add, "but it's much easier to do at a large cancer center," where multidisciplinary treatment planning is standard practice except perhaps in cases that clearly warrant a single type of therapy.

Does the Center Have a Laboratory, Imaging and Other Testing Facilities On-Site?

It's not something we like to dwell on, but cancer and its treatment can leave you feeling downright awful at times: weak, nauseous, exhausted. I know that when I was undergoing outpatient chemotherapy, I appreciated being at a large medical center like Georgetown, where I had access to every conceivable testing procedure all under one roof.

The first morning of each monthly cycle, I could have my blood drawn right there instead of having had to drive to another lab the day before. Or when Dr. Woolley sent me for X rays during my initial visit, I merely had to take the elevator downstairs to the radiology suite. If a battery of tests was ordered, I didn't have to schedule appointments at multiple facilities, and a nurse made all the arrangements. I'd arrive at eight in the morning and bustle from one procedure to the next as if on a presidential whistle-stop campaign two days before Election Day. Besides saving considerable time, such "one-stop shopping" is bound to minimize stress, the last thing you need when you have cancer. For some patients, the added trips for tests may necessitate lining up transportation and child care as well as taking time off from work.

But increasingly, insurance companies—managed-care plans in particular—are offsetting the advantages of going to a full-service hospital. Maureen Sawchuk, nursing coordinator of the Lombardi Cancer Center, sees more and more of her chemotherapy patients being ordered by third-party payers to have their blood counts and other routine tests performed elsewhere. In a 1996 survey of more than three hundred medical oncologists, approximately one in three reported that their managed-care patients must frequently travel long distances or to multiple locations for treatment.

"Many patients can no longer come in and get their blood drawn and have treatment all on the same day," she says. "It now takes days to get this done. We spend so much time trying to help people understand where they can receive certain aspects of their care. Only *this* facility can do your MRI. You have to get your EKG done *here.* The rules change every week, and no payer does it exactly the same way. It's enormously fatiguing for patients." Chapter Ten contains strategies for maximizing your medical-insurance coverage and for challenging rejected claims. Unfortunately, consumers whose policies dictate that only certain health-care providers can carry out medical tests have little clout when it comes to convincing insurers to make exceptions.

See "Insurance Issues," in Chapter Ten, "Getting Help When You Need It."

Does the Facility Offer Other Patient Services: Psycho-oncology, Social Work, Nutrition, Rehabilitation, Chaplain/Pastoral Care?

Quality cancer care goes beyond simply ridding the body of malignant cells. It includes treating the patient as a whole—psychologically, spiritually, nutritionally—as well as addressing the impact of the crisis on family members. You will find that for the most part large centers specializing in cancer treatment offer more than small hospitals do in the way of patient support services, which generate less income for the institution.

For instance, New York's Memorial Sloan-Kettering Cancer Center, the first hospital in the country to establish a psychiatry service for people with cancer and their loved ones, runs a Post-Treatment Resource Program for cancer survivors. PTRP provides educational seminars and workshops, support groups, individual and family counseling, and practical advice on insurance and employment issues. Not all patients feel the need to participate in such "extracurricular" activities, and that's fine. But if you are so inclined, how convenient it is to have these resources made available by your treatment facility.

Patient Support Services: What They Do, How They Can Be of Help

Department of Psycho-oncology—made up of mental-health professionals who specialize in addressing the social and emotional effects of having cancer. They provide talk therapy, teach patients visualization and other stress-reduction techniques, and treat anxiety and depression medically, if necessary.

Department of Clinical Social Work—Early on in your treatment, get to know the hospital social worker. An invaluable source of information, she can refer you to available services in your community (examples: free transportation to and from medical appointments; homemaker and chore-maintenance services; limited financial aid) as well as help you with everything from disputing rejected insurance claims to applying for federal entitlement programs to offering short-term counseling. The social worker also serves as facilitator at meetings of hospital patient support groups and is responsible for coordinating your discharge plan from the hospital. Will you require home health care temporarily? It's her job to determine your family's needs and assist you in making the necessary provisions.

Chaplain/Pastoral Care—In a hospital setting, the term "chaplain" is nondenominational. The department of pastoral care at Georgetown University Medical Center includes several priests, ministers, and rabbis, each formally trained in clinical pastoral education. All hospitalized patients receive a visit from a staff cleric within forty-eight hours of admittance, although they are by no means obligated to receive pastoral counseling. Incidentally, the patient determines whether or not these bedside conversations touch on religious or spiritual concerns. One person may derive great solace from reading Bible passages with a priest, while another may wish only for a sympathetic ear and a comforting presence while she pours out her fears.

See Chapter Nine, "Don't Neglect Your Emotional Health."

Nutrition Service—In facilities that practice multidisciplinary cancer care, the staff nutritionist is considered part of the health-care team, and proper nourishment is considered an integral component of therapy. All cancer patients should be able to request a consultation with a nutritionist for tips on how to keep up their appetite during treatment and to maximize the nutritional value of the foods they do eat.

Rehabilitation Service—*Speech and language therapy* should be routine for patients who must undergo a laryngectomy or operation to remove part of the tongue, as may sometimes be necessary in treating cancers of the head and neck. At Duke Comprehensive Cancer Center, says Dr. William Richtsmeier, "the rehabilitation team includes not only the physicians involved but a speech therapist, a swallowing therapist, a social worker, and a support group in which patients get to talk to other people who've had laryngectomies." Other cancers may call for *physical therapy, occupational therapy,* or *pulmonary rehabilitation.*

Going to a Large Cancer Center: A Couple More Pros, a Few Cons

---

By now the advantages of seeking a second-opinion consultation or treatment at a large facility specializing in cancer should be fairly evident. The drawbacks are mainly matters of ambiance, not the caliber of care. Still, it's up to each patient to decide which qualities are most important to him or her.

First the Cons . . .

A bias toward aggressive treatment—sometimes overly so. Academic institutions depend on research grants from the government and private industry for a good portion of their funding. Conspiracy theorists will be disappointed, but I do not believe that the financial incentive for accruing patients drives doctors' decisions about which patients enter clinical trials. If anything, it's the commitment to furthering medical science that occasionally clouds a physician's judgment and causes him to encourage a terminally ill patient to undergo an experimental therapy that undoubtedly will not benefit her and, in fact, stands a good chance of adversely affecting her quality of life.

"There is probably some basis for the perception that an academic center is much more likely to take treatment further than a nonacademic center," Dr. Marshall concedes, "although I don't think it's fair to say that we treat patients like guinea pigs. What sometimes happens is that if a patient insists on forging on with treatment, the doctor will often go along with the decision instead of saying, 'No, it's really time to stop.' " On the other hand, he recalls many times when a desperately ill patient expressed interest in joining a clinical trial, "and the nurses would say, 'This isn't right,' " prompting a discussion among the medical team as to whether or not the study was appropriate for someone so sick.

On this issue, the bottom line for patients—and for their loved ones—is that no one should be pressured into signing up for a clinical trial. The decision to participate, or not to, should always be a personal one.

A less patient-friendly atmosphere (or so they say). Driving me home from my first visit to Lombardi, Valerie began to weep.

"Why are you crying?" I asked.

"The hospital just seemed so big, cold, and impersonal," she replied. "It upsets me that you have to go there." Since I didn't feel that way at all, her reaction took me by surprise. Granted, the Georgetown University Medical Center is an imposing complex of buildings. But the interior of the cancer center isn't antiseptic at all. To the contrary, it's warm and reassuring, the waiting area painted in soothing tones and decorated with plants. There's even valet parking.

At first you might feel intimidated by all the activity at a large institution. Setting foot in the Pasquerilla Healthcare Center on my way to the Lombardi wing was like entering a Metrorail subway station at rush hour, with people bustling to and fro. By my third visit, though, I felt completely at home.

A seemingly endless procession of doctors. Such is the routine at a teaching hospital, where in addition to an *attending physician,* you are seen by M.D.'s at various rungs on the training ladder. Dr. Woolley su-

---

TABLE 5.2   **The Medical Hierarchy: A Scorecard**

Attending Physician

The senior doctor responsible for overseeing and coordinating your cancer care is called the attending physician. While often a medical oncologist, he or she could also be a surgical oncologist, for cancers treated surgically; a radiation oncologist; or an oncologist diagnostician, a physician who diagnoses cancer and perhaps specializes in cancer prevention but does not treat the disease. Your attending usually brings in other specialists as needed. In a group practice, you may have multiple attendings, but ultimately one doctor is in charge of managing your case.

M.D.'s Under the Attending Physician's Supervision

Interns ➡	Residents ➡	Fellows
Medical school graduates who are apprenticing at a hospital for a minimum of one year in order to receive their license to practice medicine. Any order they write must be reviewed or cosigned by the attending physician or the chief resident.	Licensed physicians who have completed their internship and are studying a speciality, such as surgery or gynecology, typically for two years	Doctors who have completed their residency and are studying a sub-speciality, such as surgical oncology or gynecologic oncology, typically for three years

pervised two *fellows:* Dr. Marshall and Dr. Chitra Rajagopal. When I had to be hospitalized following my second cycle of chemotherapy, I probably saw more of them on a daily basis than I did Dr. Woolley. *Residents* and *interns* also took part in my care.

One aspect of an academic facility that patients may find offputting is the repetition of medical histories and bedside exams—which are sometimes conducted before a small audience of inquisitive young doctors. On the other hand, the added visits and extra pairs of eyes might lead to having a complication picked up earlier rather than later.

Now Some More Pros . . .

Despite Valerie's initial misgivings about the size of the Georgetown campus, both of us felt a sense of security there that we hadn't felt at the community hospital. As she puts it, "For the doctors and nurses who work at Lombardi, cancer is their 'business.' "

One of the criticisms sometimes leveled at large medical institutions is that they function too much like "factories." While I don't fully agree, I considered that to be an asset, to tell you the truth, not a liability. For as Dr. Marc Lippman observes candidly, "In the setting of a bone-marrow transplantation, for instance, you *want* to be a cookie on a conveyor belt. You just want to be 'stamped out' at a medical center where every complication has been seen and dealt with before."

I also liked the idea of going to a cancer center adjoining a major medical facility like Georgetown. Bear in mind that a person's cancer may have to be treated against the backdrop of cardiovascular disease, kidney failure, diabetes, a concurrent primary tumor in another organ, or some other preexisting condition that complicates the course of therapy. In a large medical center, the oncologist overseeing your care has access to a wide spectrum of specialists.

"The richness of the environment benefits the patients," says Dr. Marshall, offering an example: "I have a colon-cancer patient who also has prostate cancer, which is tricky to treat. I know I should focus on the colon, but if I give this patient therapy for the tumor in the prostate, he won't be eligible for some colon-cancer-related clinical trials, and he's run out of standard options. Here I can walk next door and run ideas past an expert in prostate cancer."

I disagree with the factory metaphor because the word connotes a lack of caring among the staff. I found the doctors and nurses at Lombardi exceptionally friendly and compassionate, despite the grueling demands of their work. Interestingly, did you know that physicians in academia generally earn less than their colleagues in private practice? They usually receive a flat salary, with minimal or no bonus programs contingent on the number of patients they see. "I think people in academia are hesitant to say it," says Dr. David Johnson of Vanderbilt, "but there are fewer reasons for an academic institution to do things inappropriately."

This is how satisfied I was with my experience at Lombardi: I've since turned the place into my personal HMO, with Dr. Marshall as my primary-care physician. I have all of my health care handled through the oncology department. If I have so much as a cold, I call the oncology department for a referral to a Georgetown doctor and go there.

Resources: How to Find Quality Cancer Care Locally

With nearly 90 percent of cancer therapy conducted on an outpatient basis, the importance of receiving treatment close to home—whenever possible—shouldn't be underestimated. As we examined earlier in this chapter, many times protocols can be planned at major institutions, then delegated to local oncologists, including some phase III clinical trials. The following resources can help steer you to a quality cancer facility near you:

Cancer Information Service—(800-422-6237) This free service of the National Cancer Institute directs callers to NCI-designated sites as well as to cancer programs peer-approved by the American College of Surgeons (ACS) (see below). Peer approval, in which doctors from outside an institution review a hospital's standards, science, and so forth, doesn't by itself ensure first-rate care. "But," says Dr. Lippman, "since patients rarely have the ability or the opportunity to gauge the quality of medical care, you have a greater guarantee if you're seen by a group of doctors in an institution that's already been peer-reviewed and has been proven to be good." Dr. Lippman likens the rigorous peer-review process required to receive an NCI designation or an ACS certification to a seal of approval.

The Commission on Cancer of the American College of Surgeons—(312-649-7081) Established by the American College of Surgeons in 1922, the Commission on Cancer (COC) approves cancer programs in all kinds of centers, from NCI-designated comprehensive cancer centers to freestanding clinics. As of 2000, it had approved more than 1,450 or about 20 percent of the acute-care facilities in the United States. But participation is voluntary, and so a number of renowned institutions do not have COC accreditation—among them several NCI facilities—although they undoubtedly meet the approval criteria.

Standards vary according to the type of facility, but all must offer some degree of multidisciplinary care, either on the premises or by referral elsewhere. Other prerequisites for approval may include regular tumor-board conferences and clinical research, again depending on which of nine categories the facility falls under (see table 5.3). You can find out if a center you're considering is approved and the category it belongs to by calling the ACS's Chicago headquarters or by visiting its Web site: *http://www.facs.org*.

Association of Community Cancer Centers—(301-984-9496) Membership in the ACCC is also voluntary. Although the association's more than five hundred participating facilities constitute only 10 percent of U.S. acute-care hospitals, they provide care for about 40 per-

TABLE 5.3   The Commission on Cancer's Categories of Approved Cancer Programs

Category	Available General Services Include	Does It Practice Multi-disciplinary Care?	Frequency of Tumor-Board Conferences	Does It Offer Access to Clinical Studies?
NCI-designated Comprehensive Cancer Program (NCIP)	Provides the full range of diagnostic and treatment services onsite	Yes	At least weekly	Yes
Teaching Hospital Cancer Program (THCP)	Provides the full range of diagnostic and treatment services on-site or through referral	Yes	At least weekly	Yes
Community Hospital Comprehensive Cancer Program (COMP)	Provides the full range of diagnostic and treatment services on-site or through referral	Yes	At least weekly	Yes, if the program sees at least 750 new patients per year; optional if less
Community Hospital Cancer Program (CHCP)	Provides the full range of diagnostic and treatment services, but often through referral elsewhere	Yes	Twice monthly or monthly	Limited
Hospital Associate Cancer Program (HACP)	This program, which sees 100 or fewer new cases per year, provides a limited range of diagnostic and treatment services on-site and other services through referral.	Yes	Monthly	Optional
Integrated Cancer Program (ICP)	Provides one treatment modality on-site, but the facility forms a partnership with a hospital to offer the full range of diagnostic and treatment services	Yes, through the associated hospital	Depends on the requirements for the associated hospital	

Category	Available General Services Include	Does It Practice Multi-disciplinary Care?	Frequency of Tumor-Board Conferences	Does It Offer Access to Clinical Studies?
Freestanding Cancer Center Program (FCCP)	Provides two treatment modalities on-site and the full range of diagnostic and treatment services through referral	Yes	Weekly	Optional
Affiliate Hospital Cancer Program (ACP)	Provides limited access to services on-site, but the facility forms a partnership with a sponsoring hospital to offer the full range of diagnostic and treatment services	Yes	4 to 6 per year	Optional
Managed Care Organization (MCO)	Provides or refers patients to medical staff with the major specialty boards	Yes	Requirements are specific to the hospital category	

cent of all cancer patients. The ACCC differs from the Commission on Cancer in that it is not an accreditation organization. While it encourages members to offer multidisciplinary care, clinical trials, and so on, these are not required standards.

To learn if a community cancer center belongs to the ACCC, call the association in Rockville, Maryland, or drop into its excellent Web site *(http://assoc-cancer-ctrs.org)*, which details the size and features of each facility, and lists key contacts in surgical oncology, medical oncology, and other departments.

If You Want to Learn About a Particular Physician

- Ask your library if it has *The Directory of Physicians in the United States* or the *Official American Board of Medical Specialties Directory of Board Certified Medical Specialists.* Each of these hefty reference books lists physicians' areas of specialization, where they practice, and additional helpful information. The American Board of Medical Specialties (ABMS), the organization that represents the twenty-four approved medical-specialty boards in the United States, sponsors both a toll-free number and a Web site for confirming whether or not a physician is board certified.

Call 800-776-2378 or drop into the on-line Certified Doctor Verification Service at *http://www.certifieddoctor.org.*

- AMA Physician Select, a free on-line service of the American Medical Association (*http://www.ama-assn.org/aps/amagh.htm*), provides vital information on virtually every licensed physician in the United States: more than 650,000 in all.

> **Medical Terms You're Likely to Hear**
>
> **Board certified:** Board certification tells you that a physician has passed rigorous exams in one or more specialties. For instance, a radiologist may specialize in radiation oncology and subspecialize in nuclear radiology. Medical oncology is a subspecialty of internal medicine. No subspecialty exists for surgical oncology.

- Cancer-center Web sites, such as those listed in table 5.1, often contain brief profiles—and even photos—of staff physicians and nurses.

How to Arrange an Independent, Multidisciplinary Second Opinion

Why an independent second opinion? As in any profession, doctors may gravitate toward colleagues who hold similar attitudes on treatment. Thus, contends Dr. Vincent DeVita, if a physician opposes postoperative chemotherapy for early-stage breast cancer, "he's more likely to refer his patients to someone who thinks the same way and will support his recommendation." His advice for patients is to maximize their odds of finding a cancer doctor "who's not hooked into the same line of thought." To do this, we suggest contacting one of the centers listed in table 5.1, or calling the Cancer Information Service, which refers only to multidisciplinary facilities.

Cancer centers understand that time is of the essence for men and women diagnosed with cancer. They make every effort to schedule a consultation within two weeks or so, if not sooner. In some instances, though, a specialist who's been recommended to you, perhaps by a doctor or a satisfied patient, may be on vacation or otherwise unavailable within a reasonable time frame. In that event, a staff physician will be assigned to your case.

Who Makes the Arrangements?

Your doctor can make the initial contact for you, as well as arrange for your medical records to be sent to the referral center. But some patients choose to handle this personally. "One of the misconceptions among patients," says Dr. Marshall, "is that you can't get into an NCI cancer center or a university hospital without a referral from a doctor, when in fact access to academic physicians has never been easier." Most institutions have set up patient-referral lines specifically for routing callers to an appropriate doctor.

A Second Opinion by Phone or Fax? Forget It

Few oncologists will make a treatment recommendation without examining a patient themselves. Not only is it time-consuming, explains Dr. Larry Norton of Memorial Sloan-Kettering ("I get six inches of faxes pouring in unannounced every day"), "it eliminates an extremely important part of the decision-making process, which is the patient's expertise about her own life, her personality, her goals."

Obtaining Medical Records

If obtaining medical records should fall to you or a loved one, call the consulting doctor's office and ask his assistant to send you a list of the medical records that will be needed. Typically, you will be asked for pathology slides and reports, films, and any and all written records. Medical reports are kept in the referring physician's office and/or the hospital's department of medical records. To obtain slides and films, contact the hospital's department of pathology and department of radiology, respectively.

Questions to Ask . . . the Office Receiving Your Medical Records

- Which records do you need in advance of my appointment? Which records can I bring with me?

- Are duplicates of X-ray films acceptable? Ask the person to specify, if possible, which films, because the cost of having copies made can range from several dollars to more than $100 each. *Never* send original films or slides through the mail; have them hand-delivered only.

Questions to Ask . . . the Hospital Releasing Your Medical Records

- Can I authorize the release of records, films, and slides over the phone? Is a letter necessary, and if so, must it be notarized?

- Can you send copies of films directly to my consulting doctor, or do I have to pick them up? Find out how the records will be delivered (messenger? Federal Express?) and when. Then relay this information to the consulting physician's office.

> **Mammograms: Original Films Only**
>
> According to Dr. Rebecca Zuurbier, director of breast imaging at the Lombardi Cancer Center, women seeking a second opinion regarding a mass in the breast should always request the original mammograms. "Copy films are usually worthless," she says, "and a waste of your money."

Be forewarned: Expect the new center to insist on conducting some of its own tests. No sooner had I met Dr. Woolley than the oncology research nurse, Barbara Lewis, informed me she was going to send me downstairs for X rays.

I remember becoming a little testy. "X rays? I must have been X-rayed fifteen times in the last few weeks! They've X-rayed every inch of me!"

"I know," she said sympathetically, "but we need to have our own."

"It's not a moneymaking scheme," asserts nurse Maureen Sawchuk, who perhaps has heard this suspicion voiced more than once by annoyed patients. Yes, you did have X rays taken two weeks ago, but with certain tumors, a great deal of cancer activity can occur in that short amount of time. What's more, the referring facility might have misinterpreted the pathology slides, or the referral institution might have superior imaging equipment, and so on.

MONEY MATTERS

Will Your Insurance Pay for a Second Opinion?

"We are seeing a health-care system that will make getting second opinions more difficult," Dr. Lippman says ominously. However, some insurers *require* second opinions before they will consent to paying for treatment; others, including Medicare—and to a lesser extent, Medicaid—cover a second opinion if you request it. Managed-care policies, however, typically will not pay for second opinions from physicians outside their network of providers. A patient intent on consulting with physicians at a state-of-the-art institution must then bear the expense himself.

The cost can vary widely, explains Maureen Sawchuk, depending on the number of tests that must be ordered. At Lombardi, for instance, "the physician fees for a second opinion run from $250 to $300. If you have slides reviewed, that can add $300 to as much as $1,000," she says, "and having films reviewed can add several hundred dollars more." Be sure to ask upfront for an estimate of the costs, to eliminate an unpleasant surprise later on.

What If Your Primary Physician Resists Your Wish to Seek a Second Opinion or Treatment Elsewhere?

People are sometimes reluctant to pursue a second opinion for fear of offending their primary doctor. They worry that it might be construed as a vote of little confidence (which, in fact, it might very well be). Understandably, no one wants to insult the person charged with orchestrating his medical care.

> **Before Your First Visit to a Cancer Center**
>
> Most cancer centers publish brochures containing a map of the campus, directions, and parking instructions, to help acclimate new patients. You might also find this information posted on a facility's Web site.

The decision to change physicians, particularly midcourse, should not be taken lightly. It's preferable to maintain continuity of care. But should your expressing an interest in having your case reviewed elsewhere meet with even a hint of resistance or resentment, find a new primary doctor straightaway. Obtaining a second opinion is your right—and, you might remind your physician, strongly encouraged by the National Cancer Institute.

Fortunately, the majority of doctors will support your decision. Dr. Marshall says he routinely recommends treatment strategies to local oncologists after having seen their patients for a second-opinion consultation. "I find they're usually very open to our suggestions," he says. "They call regularly to keep me apprised of what's going on."

A Third Opinion? A Fourth?

Here's a possible scenario: A woman diagnosed with early-stage breast cancer goes to a multidisciplinary center for a second opinion. Her current oncologist has outlined a treatment plan consisting of lumpectomy and radiotherapy followed by long-term hormone therapy. The panel of experts, after reviewing her case, comes back with a different recommendation for postoperative therapy: hormone therapy plus six months of combination chemotherapy. Now what?

In making her decision, she might weigh the credentials and experience of the doctors involved. Let's say the first recommendation came from a medical oncologist in private practice (which doesn't discount the validity of his opinion); the second from a multimodality team of oncologists at a busy academic cancer center. Or she might consider obtaining a third opinion, to help sway her one way or the other. In politics we'd call that a swing vote. Of course, the additional consultation could generate yet *another* treatment strategy. But as oncologist Dr. Michael Hawkins of the Lombardi Cancer Center points out, "If you have a potentially curable malignancy, there usually are no more than one or two proven approaches to treatment, and physicians are extremely hesitant to stray from them. You should be too.

"On the other hand, a person whose cancer is no longer curable is suddenly faced with many more options," although, he adds, "sometimes that's the same thing as saying he's run out of proven options."

There are cancer patients who delay treatment while they endlessly collect opinions, ostensibly to help them reach a decision. Some may genuinely be confused by conflicting medical recommendations. But Dr. Marc Lippman suggests that when a patient seeks five, eight, *twenty* opinions, "and I've seen that," in reality there may be a subconscious motive at work which the person is not even aware of. He may be dashing from doctor to doctor "as a way to *avoid* having to make a decision."

You and Your Health-Care Team: A Partnership

I'd be the last person to discourage cancer patients from reading up on their disease and its treatment. But once you've settled on a facility and a team of doctors you trust, let them act as your consumer advocates, to interpret material for you. All too often, says Dr. Hawkins, "I've seen inquisitive patients go down the wrong path and start looking at research that is irrelevant to their situation. They frequently wind up susceptible to whoever has the flashiest Web site. There's nothing sadder than to get a phone call from somebody who is confused and trying to become medically sophisticated enough to make decisions themselves. It's usually not possible."

As Dr. David Johnson says, "It took me eight years of training to become an oncologist. You can't expect to learn what I know in the space of a few weeks—although I've had patients who've come close." Even if that were possible, adds Dr. Larry Norton, "a person can't make sound medical judgments about his own body. The best physicians put themselves in the hands of other good doctors when they get sick."

The purpose of this book is to give you tools you need to become an effective *advocate* for yourself, not to transform you into your own physician. An advocate is simply someone charged with getting a patient the services she needs, be it appropriate therapy, prompt symptom relief, or temporary home-nursing care. A patient can be her own advocate, but usually it's a family member, a friend, or a health-care professional such as a hospital social worker.

One common complaint you may hear from other patients is that they feel excluded from crucial medical decisions. "My doctors never tell me anything." To be fair, many seriously ill people willingly relinquish decision-making to their physician. Either explicitly or through their behavior, they send the message "Do whatever you think is best, Doc." Without question, that is their prerogative. My guess is that you, like me, are inclined to want to join the huddle rather than sit on the sidelines. Taking it upon yourself to learn about cancer sends a signal to your health-care providers that you intend to be involved in your medical care, something that I believe most doctors genuinely welcome.

"Patients have to recognize that they are an important part of the team and that their judgment is an important part of the decision-making process," says Dr. Norton. When determining treatment, "the correct decision is an equal mix of medicine, biology, and knowledge of a patient's life. The doctor may be an expert in medicine and biology," he says, "but the patient is the expert in her own life. We can't do it alone."

Tips for Communicating Effectively with the Medical Staff

For many patients, conversations with health-care professionals can be awkward and frustrating. That burning question from the day before seems to evaporate the moment they get their oncologist on the phone, only to rematerialize as soon as they hang up. Or they're too inundated with information, or too intimidated, to ask a physician to clarify something they didn't quite understand. Certainly, there are doctors and nurses whose interpersonal skills could stand polishing, but by and large the responsibility for building and maintaining a rapport with the staff lies with us. We think you'll find the following suggestions helpful.

• At the outset, tell your primary physician how much you wish to know about your condition as well as how you'd like to be informed. "It can be hard for a doctor to judge the amount of information a patient can handle," says Dr. Christine Berg. Your physician will be grateful to learn your preferences. Be specific. You might say, "I'm interested in knowing everything about my case and would appreciate your being candid with me. But whenever possible, I'd rather you tell me about major developments in person instead of over the phone."

• Arrange for someone to accompany you to medical appointments, to take notes and to serve as a second pair of ears. "That way," explains Maureen Sawchuk, "you can focus on your questions and talking to the doctor." Afterward, the two of you should compare your impressions of what you heard. During the first several months of treatment, when I was at my lowest, my memory seemed to be riddled with holes. Many times Valerie and I would be driving home from a consultation, and she would mention something one of my oncologists had said.

"He *did?*" I'd reply, dumbfounded. "I don't remember that." Fortunately, Valerie has an infallible memory and always took copious notes. What's more, by then she'd become fluent in medical terminology, the names of the medications I was taking, and so forth. She would recount the gist of the conversation for me.

A word to family and friends: Another way that concerned loved ones can be of help is to keep the doctor apprised of changes in the patient's condition. People who are ill may not fully let on how they're feeling. Physicians value the caregiver's observations; after all, you see the sick person on a regular, if not daily, basis. My second cycle of chemotherapy left me terribly weak, racked with diarrhea, and dehydrated. Yet I downplayed the side effects, attributing them to the cumulative effect of treatment. Valerie, however, sensed that this was potentially serious. Unbeknownst to me, she got on the phone to Barbara Lewis, my oncology nurse, and described my condition. Barbara advised her to drive me to the hospital at once. I wound up being admitted for eight days.

• **Keep a notebook in which to jot down questions for the doctor as they occur to you**. Also maintain a daily log of your symptoms and any other information that could conceivably prove helpful.

See table 8.1, "Simple Symptoms Chart," in Chapter Eight, "Take Control: Managing Symptoms, Side Effects, and Complications."

• **Before appointments, mail or fax your doctor an update** describing any changes in your medical condition since your last visit. Include your questions. Besides saving time, this will help your physician be better prepared to address your concerns.

• **If you come across a newspaper article that might be relevant to your cancer, clip it out and share it with your physician.** "In a fast-moving field like cancer, even a super-specialist can't know every single thing," says Dr. Marshall. "Of the new developments I hear about, maybe one in four come from my patients. They read something and ask me about it. Then I read it and help interpret it for them."

• **To make certain that you understand the doctor correctly, restate what he said in your own words:** "So you're saying that the tumor in my lung is superficial enough that I might be a candidate for photodynamic therapy instead of surgery."

• **Ask your doctor to show you illustrations** of where your cancer is located, how upcoming tests and treatments are performed, and so forth. Many people find that being able to form a picture in their mind helps them to better understand unfamiliar concepts.

• **If you don't grasp something the doctor said, don't nod your head, pretending to understand. Ask him to repeat it.** No need to feel self-conscious or worry about sounding foolish. Oncologists routinely field the same question more than once from intelligent adults whose minds suddenly go blank due to illness, fatigue, stress, or the effect of medications. Having said that, it's not productive to ask scattershot questions that force the physician to repeatedly redirect the conversation. Dr. Berg makes an excellent point when she says, "Patients have responsibilities too. They need to focus." If you find that difficult to do, bring along a third party.

• **Consider tape-recording consultations,** so that you can listen to the doctor's exact words—several times, if necessary. Unless you're a court stenographer, it's not uncommon to review your hastily scrawled notes at home and barely be able to make sense out of what is written. But before you pull out a tape recorder, ask the doctor for permission, as a courtesy. In these litigious times, you don't want to risk being marked as an adversarial patient. All you have to say is: "This is a lot of information for me to absorb. Do you mind if I tape-recorded our discussion?" Few physicians will deny your request. Most of the time, says nursing coordinator Sawchuk, "the doctors get so engrossed in the conversation with the patient, they forget the tape recorder is even there."

• **Confine important questions to health-care professionals who are well acquainted with your case.** Doctors, nurses, and technicians can speak out of turn on occasion, causing patients needless anxiety and distress. Tempting as it may be, resist the impulse to grill the radiology nurse performing an ultrasound exam about what she sees on the monitor (she's not supposed to say). Likewise, refrain from asking an unfamiliar resident questions concerning pivotal treatment-related decisions—for instance, "Am I going to need chemotherapy?"

• **Establish a rapport with a nurse in your doctor's office, and call *her* with routine questions.** Realistically, you're not going to reach your physician every time you call. He may be in surgery all day, making rounds at the hospital—whatever. "In our experience," says Maureen Sawchuk, "90 percent of patients' questions can be answered by a nurse. It's not a matter of the nurse trying to keep patients away from the doctor," she emphasizes, "but we're usually able to get back to the patient in a more timely manner than the doctor can."

What to Do If You Feel a Health-Care Provider Has Mishandled a Situation

With patients' and family members' nerves often wound tighter than a spool of thread during a medical crisis, a lapse in communication or difference of opinion with a member of the health-care team is all but inevitable. If the perceived transgression is relatively minor and appears to be an isolated incident, you might choose to let it go. Like everyone else, doctors and nurses can have an off day. But lingering dissatisfaction on your part or potentially serious miscues by the staff should be brought to the attention of either the offending party or your primary physician.

From my years in politics, I learned the value of diplomacy in resolving conflicts. Whether you're trying to sway votes on Capitol Hill or persuade a doctor that the dosage of pain medication is inadequate, the goal is not to *be right* but to achieve the desired outcome without needlessly alienating the other person. The skills outlined here apply to advocating not only with the health-care team but with the array of people you'll encounter (often over the phone) when faced with a life-threatening illness: from the hospital billing department to social service agencies to the insurance company, and so on.

• **Don't put off addressing a problem** so long that resentment begins to simmer or the urgency fades. On the other hand, give yourself sufficient time to compose yourself, to avoid saying or writing something in anger that you'll regret later.

• **If you're easily intimidated or flustered, commit your thoughts to paper,** listing your grievances in order of priority.

• **Avoid using accusatory language,** which is likely to put the other person on the defensive. Make "I" statements instead of "you" statements; for example, *"It upset me when I* left a message with your office and no one returned my call for forty-eight hours."

• **Be assertive, but not belligerent.** Not all patients navigate these waters gracefully. It goes without saying that you should refrain from raising your voice, affecting a harsh or sarcastic tone, and speaking disrespectfully.

• **Give examples to substantiate your claims.** Blurting "Your nurse is incompetent!" isn't going to improve the situation. Instead you explain, "Nurse Smith promised me that she would have you call in a prescription by the end of the day, but she never followed through, and I went the whole night without antinausea medication."

• **Don't dredge up old business.** Stick to the issue at hand.

• **Propose a solution to the problem.** You're unhappy with your doctor's chronic lateness in returning phone calls? Ask, "If I have a routine question that needs answering, and you're not available, is there someone else in your office I can speak to?"

• **If treatment takes place in a medical center, consider appealing to the department of social work.** One of a hospital social worker's many duties is to intervene in disputes and help bridge communication gaps between patients, family, and staff members, when necessary.

What Do You Look for in an Oncologist?

In our fantasies, we all hope for one doctor with the lifesaving surgical skill of a Dr. Michael DeBakey, the reassuring bedside manner of a Florence Nightingale, the infinite wisdom of television's kindly Dr. Marcus Welby. And don't forget house calls on a moment's notice and pro bono fees.

In reality, what you look for in an oncologist may depend on the role he is expected to fill in treatment. If I have colon cancer that has spread to the liver, and Dr. Jones is the only surgeon in the region who is experienced in performing hepatic resection surgery, I may be willing to overlook a lack of warmth or an overly paternalistic manner. Once the surgery is over, he essentially recedes from the picture, aside from several postoperative examinations. Yet I would not accept the same behavior from my primary oncologist, with whom I may have a relationship for years to come and will be relying upon to help me make crucial decisions about my cancer treatment.

Physicians' personalities and styles differ. Some become emotionally involved with their patients, while others come across as aloof, which is not to say they are uncaring. Neither way is right or wrong, but you will undoubtedly find that you enjoy a more natural chemistry with one doctor than with another.

You needn't adore your doctor. It is imperative, though, that you feel the two of you are working in partnership and share the same goals for treatment. "I would ask the doctor, 'What is your treatment philosophy?'" advises Dr. Lippman, a breast-cancer specialist. "I see women who say, 'I want every last milligram of drug, I want to push this to the limit, I really want to give myself every extra quarter of a percent edge for survival.' Then there are other women who say, 'I'm extremely concerned about side effects; I don't want to be treated too harshly.' That has to match up with the doctor's philosophy."

While there are instances in which a patient's preference determines the path to be followed, more often than not "a lot of what happens in treatment truly depends on the interest of the physician," says Dr. Lippman. "That is the only explanation for the fact that although breast conservation is the preferred option for at least 80 percent of American women with breast cancer, mastectomies are still performed two-thirds of the time."

Valid Reasons for Changing Oncologists

When you and your oncologist can't agree on the same approach to treatment, it's time to find a new cancer specialist. Other valid reasons for making a change include:

• **The doctor seems unjustifiably pessimistic about the benefit of further treatment,** when your research suggests that legitimate options are still open. However, there are cases where every avenue that could reasonably be expected to extend life—with quality—has been traveled, and the physician's assessment is indeed realistic. How do you know the difference? One way is to keep yourself informed about the disease.

• **The doctor discourages you from investigating other cancer therapies,** whether conventional or outside traditional medicine. I should be able to hand my oncologist an article downloaded off a dubious Web site touting the anticancer properties of transmission fluid mixed with raspberry Jell-O and still receive a thoughtful review of the material and an explanation of why or why not she believes it has any scientific merit.

• **You feel the doctor doesn't listen to you.** A physician isn't obliged to hold your hand and nod while you pour out your anxieties. Although a sympathetic ear is greatly appreciated, you can always request a referral to a mental-health professional or hospital chaplain to tend to your emotional well-being. But a patient should never feel uncomfortable asking questions relating to his health. Should you ever find yourself avoiding calling the doctor for fear that you'll be brushed aside, talked down to, or barked at, a change is in order.

"Patients need more than mere transmitters of information and deliverers of technology," says Dr. Lippman. "Medicine would be a much easier job if that were the case, but also a far less rewarding one. People need a *physician*. And the sicker you are, the more you need to feel that your doctor is there to see you through. It's a very complicated contract that has changed little in centuries."

• **You feel, for whatever reason, that your confidence in the doctor has been irreparably damaged.** After the foul-up on the operating table, I had no faith in the previous hospital to cure my cancer. Whether that hunch was rooted in fact or not was immaterial: It was how I felt. All that mattered was that I knew I wanted to be treated somewhere else.

At the Lombardi Cancer Center, Valerie and I enjoyed an excellent rapport with Dr. Woolley and Dr. Marshall. Dr. Marshall, the younger of the two, tended to be a little more casual and open to discussion. Both men, though, were extremely approachable. The nurses were marvelous as well, patiently taking time to answer all of my questions—well, *almost* all of my questions. They always seemed to neatly sidestep the one I wanted answered most: *Am I going to live?* You never do get them to give you an unequivocal yes.

Chapter Six

State of the Art:

Your Treatment Options

Selecting a treatment facility is one of the two most critical decisions you will make. The other is deciding, with your medical team, on the course of therapy. Either choice may influence the other, as when the decision to enter an investigational study leads a patient to a particular medical center.

This chapter presents state-of-the-art standard and experimental treatment strategies for each of the twenty-five most common cancers, by stage. All are adapted from the National Cancer Institute's treatment statements for health professionals, which are researched and prepared by a board of cancer specialists and updated monthly. Anyone can obtain the comprehensive, lengthy reports through the NCI's Physician Data Query (PDQ) database (see box on page 285). However, the PDQ statements are highly technical and dense with medical jargon. The institute also publishes concise treatment statements geared strictly to patients. While these offer a broad overview of how a specific cancer is treated, they might be most helpful as background material for interested family and friends. When investigating your own treatment options, you really want more in-depth information.

We've distilled for you the PDQ treatment statements in easy-to-understand language. We've also incorporated for each form of cancer a renowned specialist's perspective on therapy. Before you turn to the pages about your type and stage of disease, please understand that these are neither recipes nor recommendations. Several considerations may shape your treatment plan, including your age, general health, and a previous history of cancer treatment.

Where there's a choice of strategies, your personal preference can also come into play. "For example," says Dr. Larry Norton of Memorial Sloan-Kettering Cancer Center in New York, "conserving the breast is important for a lot of women with breast cancer, but it's not a priority for other women." Even though mastectomy and breast-sparing surgery followed by radiotherapy yield virtually identical survival rates, some women patients feel they will never rest easy unless the entire cancerous organ is removed. Dr. Norton recalls one candidate for breast-sparing surgery who chose mastectomy for reasons that had nothing to do with her health or psychological well-being: The six weeks of radiation, she explained, would force her to miss her daughter's school graduation, and so the woman opted for the more extensive operation.

A cancer center, too, may lean toward a certain modality or technique in situations where two or more approaches are believed to be equally effective, or, conversely, where no single regimen has stepped to the fore. Such is the case with surgery and radiation as treatments for localized tumors of the middle portion of the throat, or oropharynx. According to surgeon Dr. Randal Weber of the University of Pennsylvania Cancer Center in Philadelphia, "If you went to the M. D. Anderson Cancer Center, where I used to practice, you'd probably be irradiated, whereas the Mayo Clinic tends to be a stronger proponent of surgery for oropharyngeal cancer. There is no strong consensus," he says, to recommend one over the other. Often the facility's preference reflects its greater experience with that method.

When standard therapy has proved ineffective, or when none exists, an oncologist

---

How to Access PDQ Treatment Information

- **By phone: Call the Cancer Information Service at 800-422-6237.**

- **Via fax machine: Using the telephone for your fax machine, call CancerFax at 301-402-5874 and follow the recorded instructions.**

- **Via the Internet: Visit CancerNet at** *http://cancernet.nci.nih.gov.*

may devise a treatment strategy that is experimental but not part of a formal clinical trial. "Sometimes a physician must take his best educated guess to try to benefit a patient," explains Dr. Barnett Kramer of the National Cancer Institute. "That is part of the art of practicing medicine."

How to Use This Information

Familiarizing yourself with the available therapies will help foster discussion between you and your oncologist and aid you in asking pertinent questions. Suppose you'd been diagnosed with early-stage oropharyngeal cancer, and your doctor was presenting surgery as the sole means of treatment. After reading this chapter's section on treatment for cancer of the throat, you would know to ask about the less invasive alternative:

"I've been doing some reading on my own [and here you hand the doctor the material in question], and I see that some people with my kind of throat cancer fare well with radiotherapy instead of surgery. Do you have any experience in giving radiation as primary treatment? What can you tell me about it?" The physician's answer might prompt you to solicit another opinion, or perhaps expand your treatment team to include a radiotherapist—or perhaps find another doctor.

Note: In the "Treatment Options" boxed material throughout this chapter, the "braces" connecting two or more treatment options indicate that these treatments are used in conjunction with, or following, one another.

Questions to Ask . . . Before Consenting to Any Treatment

- What are my treatment options?
- What are the advantages and disadvantages of each?
- What is the treatment plan you recommend, and why?
- What is the goal of this treatment?
    To cure the cancer?
    To reduce the size of the tumor so that it can be treated by other means?
    To keep me comfortable?
    To prevent new symptoms from developing?

- Would a clinical trial be appropriate for me?

  See "What Are Clinical Trials?" in Chapter Four, "How Cancer Is Treated."

- Will I need to be hospitalized at any point during treatment, and if so, for how long? If an extended inpatient stay in an out-of-town hospital should be necessary—say, for a bone-marrow transplantation—ask that facility's department of social work for assistance in locating low-cost temporary housing nearby for loved ones.

- Will I receive all or part of my therapy as an outpatient?

- How long will treatment last?

- What are the possible short-term and long-term complications of the treatment(s) I will require, and how would these be managed?

  See Chapter Seven, "What You Can Expect During Treatment."

- Will I be able to go to work and participate in my normal daily activities?

- How often will I need to come in for follow-up visits?

- What is the treatment likely to cost?

Treatment Strategies for Each of the 25 Most Common Types of Cancer

Cancer of the Prostate

Overview

TREATMENTS FOR PROSTATE CANCER THAT HAS NOT METASTASIZED

Observation

Because prostate tumors usually grow slowly, the most appropriate course of action at any stage may be to delay therapy until the cancer begins to produce symptoms or perhaps to forgo therapy altogether. A pair of studies found that patients treated surgically or

PROSTATE CANCER/Treatment Options

STAGE I PROSTATE CANCER

The cancer produces no symptoms, cannot be felt during a digital rectal exam, and cannot be seen on an imaging study. It is usually discovered accidentally, as when surgery is performed to treat benign prostatic hyperplasia. Five percent or less of the tissue removed contains cancer that is well-differentiated in appearance or grade.

- Observation • *or*
- External-beam radiation therapy • *or*
- Radical prostatectomy, to remove the prostate gland and surrounding tissue, *with* pelvic lymph-node dissection • *alone or followed by*
- External-beam radiation therapy

Under Investigation #1
- Internal radiation therapy • *alone or in addition to*
- Pelvic lymph-node dissection

Under Investigation #2
- Cryosurgery
- ◆ Ask your doctor about any clinical trials that might benefit you.

STAGE II PROSTATE CANCER

(1) The cancer produces no symptoms, cannot be felt during a digital rectal exam, and cannot be seen on an imaging exam. It is usually discovered accidentally, as when surgery is performed to treat benign prostatic hyperplasia. Five percent or less of the tissue removed contains cancer that is moderately differentiated or poorly differentiated in grade. *Or:* (2) The cancer produces no symptoms, cannot be felt during a digital rectal exam, and cannot be seen on an imaging exam. It is usually discovered accidentally, as when surgery is performed to treat benign prostatic hyperplasia. More than 5 percent of the tissue removed contains cancer of any grade. *Or:* (3) The cancer produces no symptoms, cannot be felt during a digital rectal exam, and cannot be seen on an imaging exam. It is discovered by way of a needle biopsy, after an elevated PSA blood test. Any grade. *Or:* (4) The cancer produces no symptoms, cannot be felt during a digital rectal exam, and cannot be seen on an imaging exam. Any grade. *Or:* (5) The cancer, which is confined to the prostate, produces no symptoms, cannot be felt during a digital rectal exam, and cannot be seen on an imaging exam. It is discovered in one or both lobes of the prostate by way of a needle biopsy, after an elevated PSA blood test. Any grade. *Or:* (6) The cancer has extended into the capsule covering the prostate. Any grade.

- Observation • *or*

- External-beam radiation therapy • *or*

{
- Radical prostatectomy, *with* pelvic lymph-node dissection • *possibly followed by*

- External-beam radiation therapy

Under Investigation #1

- Internal radiation therapy • *alone or in addition to*

- Pelvic lymph-node dissection

Under Investigation #2

- Cryosurgery

♦ Ask your doctor about any clinical trials that might benefit you.

STAGE III PROSTATE CANCER

The cancer has extended through the capsule covering the prostate. Any grade.

- Observation • *or*

- External-beam radiation therapy, either to treat the cancer or to relieve symptoms • *or*

{
- Radical prostatectomy, *with* pelvic lymph-node dissection • *possibly followed by*

- External-beam radiation therapy

Under Investigation

- Internal radiation therapy • *alone or in addition to*

- Pelvic lymph-node dissection

♦ Ask your doctor about any clinical trials that might benefit you.

If the cancer is inoperable or unlikely to benefit from radiation:

- Transurethral resection of the prostate (TURP) to surgically cut out prostatic tissue, to relieve symptoms

- Hormonal therapy, frequently consisting of estrogen, or leuprolide or goserelin plus flutamide

STAGE IV PROSTATE CANCER

(1) The cancer has spread to nearby organs such as the neck of the bladder, external sphincter, rectum, surrounding muscle, or the pelvic wall. Any grade. *Or:* (2) The cancer has spread to the regional lymph nodes. Any grade. *Or:* (3) The cancer has spread to one or more distant organs.

- Observation

Or:
- Hormonal therapy, frequently consisting of estrogen, or leuprolide or goserelin plus flutamide

Or:
- Bilateral orchiectomy, to remove the testicles · *alone or with*
- Hormonal therapy, frequently consisting of flutamide or nilutamide

Or:
- External-beam radiation therapy, to relieve symptoms · *or*
- Transurethral resection, to relieve symptoms

If the cancer has not metastasized to distant organs:
- External-beam radiation therapy, to treat the cancer · *with or without*
- Hormonal therapy

Under Investigation
- Radical prostatectomy, *with* bilateral orchiectomy

If the cancer has been resistant to hormonal therapy:
- Chemotherapy
- ◆ Ask your doctor about any clinical trials that might benefit you.

See treatment options for metastases of the bone, liver, and lung.

RECURRENT PROSTATE CANCER

Your therapy will depend on how you were treated initially.
- External-beam radiation therapy, to relieve symptoms such as bone pain · *with or without*
- Internal radiation therapy

If you previously had a radical prostatectomy and the cancer has recurred in a small area:
- External-beam radiation therapy

If the cancer recurs elsewhere in the body:
- Hormonal therapy, frequently consisting of estrogen, or leuprolide or goserelin plus flutamide

Under Investigation
- Chemotherapy · *or*
- Immunotherapy
- ◆ Ask your doctor about any clinical trials that might benefit you.

with radiotherapy lived sixteen years from the time of diagnosis—approximately the same amount of time as those who'd only been observed by their doctors. "Watchful waiting," as it's called, might be the most sensible choice for a seventy-five-year-old man with a preexisting heart condition and a localized prostate tumor that is not causing pain or difficulty urinating. At the University of Alabama at Birmingham Cancer Center, patients who choose surveillance are seen "every three months for the first year," says Dr. Donald Urban, a urologic oncologist there. "After that, we see them about once every six months." Some physicians believe in administering hormonal therapy (see page 345) to decelerate the disease's progression.

Surgery

"In academic centers," says Dr. Urban, "we tend not to offer or encourage men over seventy to have surgical treatment, though some centers might extend that to age seventy-two, depending on the person's physiologic age."

Radical prostatectomy to remove the prostate affords men with localized cancer their best hope for a cure, even if their tumor is aggressive. Eighty-five percent of all patients to undergo the procedure live a minimum of ten years. Why, then, are doctors cautious about going this route? Any major operation carries some degree of risk, but prostatectomy can cause permanent incontinence and frequently results in irreversible impotence. A man may consider these complications unacceptable, especially given the alternatives to surgery—not to mention the reasonable expectation for years of good health with no therapy whatsoever.

There are three types of prostatectomies. The impotence rate from standard radical prostatectomy is between 65 and 90 percent. Excising the gland through the perineum has the greatest likelihood of costing a man his potency, although this method is safest for obese patients or those suffering from heart and lung problems; retropubic prostatectomy is the preferable method for large tumors.

In the early 1980s, Dr. Patrick Walsh of Johns Hopkins Oncology Center in Baltimore developed a nerve-sparing technique that in his hands is reputed to preserve potency for 75 percent of men in their fifties,

---

PROSTATE CANCER/ Surgical Procedures

Radical prostatectomy: surgical removal of the prostate and surrounding tissue. The incision is made either through the lower abdomen *(retropubic prostatectomy)* or, in a *perineal prostatectomy*, through the *perineum,* the area between the scrotum and the anus. Average hospital stay: 3–5 days

Transurethral resection of the prostate (TURP): surgical removal of prostatic tissue to relieve symptoms. Here the surgeon passes a flexible *cystoscope* up through the urethra and into the prostate. An electrified wire loop is inserted through the scope and used to cut away the tumor or nonmalignant tissue that is obstructing the flow of urine. Average hospital stay: 2–3 days

Bilateral orchiectomy: surgical removal of the testicles, through a small incision in the front of the scrotum. Average hospital stay: 1 day

60 percent of men in their sixties, and 25 percent of men in their seventies. Two bundles of erectile nerves run along either side of the prostate. In this operation, the surgeon severs the nerves only where they meet the gland, while maintaining the connection to the penis. Bear in mind, though, that Dr. Walsh is perhaps the top urologic surgeon in the country. The American Cancer Society puts the success rate for *bilateral nerve-sparing retropubic prostatectomy* slightly lower: 70 to 75 percent for men under age sixty; 50 to 60 percent for men aged sixty to seventy; and 20 to 30 percent for men seventy and older. "It's hard to predict what the outcome is going to be," Dr. Urban observes. "It takes time and recovery from surgery to see how a patient does."

If either set of nerves and adjoining blood vessels must be removed, a man's chances of maintaining the ability to have an erection are roughly 40 percent. Some surgeons will not perform a *unilateral* nerve-sparing procedure: Should one neurovascular bundle contain cancer cells—a finding that can be determined only during the operation—they will excise its counterpart, as a precaution.

"The nerve-sparing approach is best offered to younger men who have very early localized cancers," says Dr. Urban, noting that the surgery sometimes compromises a cure by leaving behind traces of disease. He emphasizes that even with the loss of the erectile nerves, men can continue to experience orgasm. "The penis doesn't emit ejaculation fluid," he explains, "but the sensation is still intact." According to the doctor, "I think the prospect of possibly becoming incontinent upsets patients more than the idea of impotence."

See "Cancer and Sexuality" in Chapter Eight, "Take Control: Managing Symptoms, Side Effects, and Complications."

Radical prostatectomy leaves roughly one in twenty men without urinary control. Another one in five must contend with long-term *stress incontinence:* A sneeze, a cough, a laugh, or a sudden movement may induce minor wetting. Following the operation, which involves reattaching the urethra tube to the bladder, virtually all patients can expect to be incontinent for three to four months, on average. The University of Alabama Cancer Center has been experimenting with biofeedback training and teaching patients exercises to strengthen the pelvic-floor muscles prior to surgery, says Dr. Urban, in an attempt to shorten the period of incontinence. For patients who do not regain full urinary control, there are now several promising surgical and nonsurgical techniques to alleviate stress incontinence.

Should a tumor extend through the prostate's fibrous *capsule* to infiltrate neighboring lymph nodes or scatter to distant sites (both stage IV), prostatectomy is no longer a viable option. One advantage of the retropubic approach is that it enables your surgeon to biopsy the nodes in the pelvic area (*pelvic lymphadenectomy*). If no evidence of nodal disease is found, the prostate is removed right then and there. Even when a frozen section confirms metastasis, some doctors will proceed with the prostatectomy, on the grounds that it is still beneficial to reduce the body's total tumor burden.

The perineal route, however, doesn't allow access to the lymph nodes. To accomplish this, the surgeon must make one or more incisions in the abdomen and sample nodes conventionally or through a laparoscope. The customary practice among surgeons is *not* to perform a two-step procedure. Consequently, men who require a surgical biopsy because their doctors suspect possible nodal involvement face the possibility of having to undergo two separate operations, with the perineal prostatectomy slated for a later date.

According to the National Cancer Institute, there is mounting evidence that a pelvic lymph-node biopsy probably isn't necessary for a man with a PSA below 20 and low-grade disease, especially if the tumor was detected by ultrasonography and not by digital rectal exam. A British study observed that the Gleason biopsy score seems to be a relatively accurate indicator of whether or not the lymph nodes are involved. One hundred sixty-six men with stage I or II prostate cancer underwent radical prostatectomies. The risk of nodal metastasis was 2 percent for patients whose Gleason score was 5. At 6, the risk rose to 13 percent; and at 8, to 23 percent.

See "Incontinence" in Appendix A for the names of organizations that offer information and support to people who are incontinent.

Radiation Therapy

For men who want to avoid the operating room or for those whose health rules out major surgery, external-beam radiotherapy is an appealing alternative. As a treatment for stage I and stage II prostate tumors, it boasts the same ten-year outcomes as radical prostatectomy, but with a lower complication rate. Irradiating the gland, says Dr.

Urban, renders 30 to 50 percent of patients impotent, while the threat of incontinence stands at less than 5 percent.

But radiation can bring about bothersome side effects not generally associated with surgery. The prostate sometimes swells during treatment, inhibiting the flow of urine. Or the high-energy rays may irritate the rectum, in what is called *radiation proctitis,* characterized by painful bowel movements, burning, bleeding, and diarrhea. Both conditions are temporary, thankfully, and usually go away on their own. To prevent acute urinary obstruction due to an enlarged prostate, your urologist may instruct you on how to relieve your bladder by inserting a flexible plastic catheter into your urethra.

If you're considering radiotherapy, ask your doctor about *three-dimensional conformal radiation* and *seed-implant therapy,* two exciting innovations that are most likely to be available at a state-of-the-art cancer center. In three-dimensional radiation, explains radiation oncologist Dr. Christine Berg of the Lombardi Cancer Center, "we use a CT scanner and a computer to conform the radiation field precisely to the shape of the prostate and give a higher dose than conventional external-beam radiation therapy." A study comparing the two forms of radiotherapy found that conformal radiation not only caused fewer symptoms, but those that did arise were significantly milder. The new method of delivery also appears to produce superior results in terms of prolonging remission.

Seed-implant therapy is internal radiation. With the patient unconscious or anesthetized from the waist down, the doctor inserts a needle containing a tiny radioactive pellet through the perineum and into the prostate, where it emits a continuous dose of radiation for several days before eventually becoming inert. In all, anywhere from several dozen to more than one hundred seeds are injected this way. Implant radiation, best reserved for small tumors, "can minimize side effects," says Dr. Berg, "because it doesn't affect the surrounding tissue." Incontinence is rarely a concern, and the risk of impotency is the lowest (10 to 30 percent) of any method of prostate-cancer treatment.

The Informed Patient:
When Might Radiation Therapy Not Be Appropriate?

"Contraindication" is the medical term for a condition that precludes a certain type of treatment. When a tumor is blocking the urethra, giving rise to urinary problems, radiotherapy may not be suitable, cautions Dr. Urban. Normally, if symptoms worsen, the next step would be a transurethral resection (see page 347) to open up the narrow urethral channel. "But it's very problematic to go to surgery with a patient who has had radiation," he explains, "because resecting the prostate following radiation has a greater incidence of complications such as incontinence and bleeding. Therefore, many radiotherapists are concerned about irradiating someone with preexisting obstructive-voiding symptoms." This is a matter that should be discussed with your doctor.

Postsurgical Treatments

"Fully half of all patients operated on for prostate cancer," says Dr. Urban, "will have positive surgical margins or capsular penetration," meaning that they may not be totally cancer free. Again, because prostate tumors develop slowly, you and your physician may adopt the wait-and-see approach. Another strategy, for all localized tumors, is to follow prostatectomy with radiotherapy. Researchers are hoping that large-scale clinical trials comparing postoperative observation and radiation will conclusively answer which protocol is most effective.

Dr. Urban's preference (and remember what we said before about physicians having their professional biases) is not to resort to pelvic irradiation as a matter of course. "First of all," he explains, "I try to select for surgery patients with early disease, who are most likely not going to have positive surgical margins and capsular penetration. Sometimes, despite those efforts, there are patients who do have capsular penetration or involvement of the seminal vesicles. Depending on how their PSA [prostate specific antigen level] progresses after surgery, we might elect to do additional therapy. But I favor hormonal therapy over radiation for those patients."

TREATMENTS FOR ADVANCED PROSTATE CANCER

Hormonal Therapy

At stage IV, the cancer has disseminated, typically to the lymph nodes, or to the bone, liver, and/or lung. Hormonal therapy, while not a cure, can stem the cancer's spread, often for a period of years. It may also be employed as an adjuvant to local treatment and as a palliative measure to shrink a tumor that is causing pain or encroaching on the urethra. The purpose of *hormonal ablation therapy* is to halt the testicles' production of testosterone, which incites prostate-tumor cells to

---

**PROSTATE CANCER/
Drug Therapy**

*First-line therapy frequently
consists of:*
- **estrogen (H)**

- **leuprolide (H) or goserelin +
  flutamide (H)**

*Other drugs that may be used
include:*
- **prednisone (H)**
- **estramustine**
- **nilutamide (H)**
- **ketoconazole***
- **bicalutamide (H)**
- **mitoxantrone**
- **cisplatin**
- **cyclophosphamide**
- **doxorubicin**

(H) = hormonal agent

*Ketoconazole, an antifungal, has testos-
terone-lowering properties.

---

grow. "Ablation" means "to eradicate," whether by surgical or chemical means.

Orchiectomy—"Orchiectomy," says Dr. Urban, "is considered the gold standard for hormonal ablation therapy." The operation, typically performed as same-day surgery, removes the testicles from the scrotum. "There are techniques for removing only the hormone-secreting portion of the testicle and leaving something in the scrotum. But in traditional orchiectomy, we take out everything."

Drug Therapy (Medical Castration)—The major unwanted effect of all hormonal therapies is that not only do they usually result in impotence, but turning off testosterone can shift one's sex drive into low gear. Yet another side effect may play havoc with a man's sexual identity: He may experience hot flashes, the same hormonal phenomenon that's experienced by menopausal women. Because orchiectomy is most effective at shutting down the body's manufacturing of testosterone, it tends to have the greatest bearing on sexuality. Now add to this the loss of one's testicles. Many men simply will not hear of surgical castration.

Three types of drugs achieve essentially the same end, but each operates in a different manner. *LHRH agonists* work in a roundabout way to block production of *luteinizing hormone-releasing hormone.* As the name implies, LHRH triggers a gland at the base of the brain to secrete *luteinizing hormone,* which in turn stimulates testosterone production.

Diethylstilbestrol (DES) is a synthetic *estrogen,* the main female sex hormone, that acts similarly upon another gland to bar release of LHRH. DES, the first chemical alternative to orchiectomy, has fallen out of favor somewhat, says Dr. Urban, "because it is associated with a higher incidence of complications, such as blood clots and congestive heart disease."

The testicles discharge about 95 percent of the body's testosterone, an *androgen;* the adrenal glands atop the kidneys serve as the production site of the remaining 5 percent. In order to effect a maximum androgen blockade, therapy is generally rounded out with an *antiandrogen* medication, which stops male hormones from reaching malignant cancer cells. Thus the possible combinations are an antiandrogen drug plus (1) orchiectomy, (2) an LHRH agonist, or (3) DES. However, the results of a 1999 study may lower the profile of maximal-androgen-blockade (MAB) therapy in prostate cancer. Italian researchers gave one group of men with advanced prostate cancer the antiandrogen drug bicalutamide (brand name: Casodex); another group received a different antiandrogen and an LHRH agonist. Three years later, the outcomes were all but indistinguishable in terms of PSA level and longevity. But the bicalutamide-only group had fewer complaints about diminished sex drive and erection problems, and overall enjoyed a higher quality of life.

> **MONEY MATTERS**
> **Insurance Coverage of Surgical and Medical Castration**
>
> Some men choose orchiectomy because it is the least involved and least expensive method of hormonal ablation. LHRH agonists must be given by injection once a month in the physician's office, at a cost of about $300 per shot. Diethylstilbestrol (brand name: Stilphostrol), an oral agent, costs less, which, says Dr. Urban, may eventually bring it back in favor. Antiandrogens, oral medications taken one to three times a day, also cost around $300 a month. According to Dr. Urban, "Medicare covers the injections but not the pills."

Prostate-cancer cells are not uniformly sensitive to testosterone. Those that are can be kept in check indefinitely by depriving them of the hormone. Other cells are moderately dependent on testosterone. But a third type of cell is oblivious to the presence or absence of testosterone and continues to multiply. Over time, the hormone-independent cells begin to dominate, and the tumor resumes growing. The proportion of these various cells differs from one patient to another.

Still, hormonal therapy is highly effective, with an average response time of three years. "Some patients," says Dr. Urban, "have lived for five years—even ten years—from the time of orchiectomy or hormonal ablation therapy."

Surgery (Palliative Treatment)

Transurethral resection of the prostate is traditionally used to remedy benign prostatic hyperplasia. "In cancer," says Dr. Urban, "TURP would be performed for a patient who either was diagnosed late in the course of the disease and didn't respond to medical therapy, or who chose watchful waiting and then had progressive local disease that caused bladder-outlet obstruction." It is strictly a palliative treatment for relieving pain and restoring normal urine flow. Two potential complications you should be aware of: Roughly one in twenty men who undergo the so-called Roto-Rooter operation experience partial impotence or incontinence. As many as nine in ten are left with what's called *retrograde ejaculation,* in which the semen discharges into the bladder instead of through the urethra and out the penis. This is rarely an issue for men with prostate cancer, who at this stage of their lives are usually enjoying their grandkids and not looking to father any more children.

OTHER THERAPIES THAT MAY BE USED IN THE TREATMENT OF PROSTATE CANCER

Cryosurgery (investigational)—The once-high enthusiasm for destroying cancerous prostate tissue using cold-tipped probes has waned. The profile of a patient eligible for cryotherapy would be someone who has a small, localized tumor that did not respond to radiation therapy and who cannot withstand other treatments.

Cryotherapy is minimally invasive: The urologist, relying on transrectal ultrasound to guide him, makes several tiny incisions in the perineum, places flexible catheter tubes in the prostate and the seminal vesicles, then inserts three to five cryoprobes and freezes the tumor. It is still unclear just how well this treatment manages prostate cancer. What's more, few medical centers offer cryosurgery, which is rarely covered by insurance.

Chemotherapy (investigational)—A number of anticancer agents have been tested in clinical studies, but according to Dr. Urban, "to date, chemotherapy has not been shown to be effective."

Drug Therapy—The same types of medications used to shrink enlarged prostates in men with benign prostatic hyperplasia may be given for symptomatic relief. These include finasteride (brand name: Proscar), tamsulosin (Flomax), terazosin (Hytrin), and doxazosin (Cardura).

◆ *Ask your doctor about these and any other investigational therapies that might benefit you.*

Cancer of the Breast

Overview

TREATMENTS FOR BREAST CANCER THAT HAS NOT METASTASIZED

Surgery with or without Radiation

Lumpectomy, Mastectomy, Axillary-Node Dissection—About two in three breast-cancer patients are diagnosed with the tumor limited to the breast. Most should be given the choice of a mastectomy or *breast-conservation therapy* (BCT) to eradicate the disease locally. A mastectomy removes the whole breast as well as some—rarely all—of the lymph nodes under the arm, which a pathologist examines for cancer. The breast-sparing approach consists of surgery to excise only the tumor and a rim of normal tissue, a lymph-node dissection, and then approximately six weeks of external-beam radiotherapy to the breast. One or two weeks after radiation ends, patients usually return for an additional five to ten days of outpatient *electron-beam radiation.* The highly concentrated "booster" dose can also be delivered directly to the tumor by surgically implanting radioactive seeds into the breast and leaving them there for two or three days.

Since 1990, the National Cancer Institute has recommended breast conservation as "an appropriate therapy for the majority of women with stage I or stage II breast cancer." Yet two in three breast-cancer patients undergo the more disfiguring operation, and in some regions of the country the rate is as high as four in five. Why? Some surgeons' outdated attitudes toward multimodality therapy may partly account for this. Another explanation would be the misconception on the part of many patients that having a mastectomy enhances their prospects for survival.

As Dr. Larry Norton stresses to patients at Memorial Sloan-Kettering Cancer Center in New York, "For suitable candidates, breast conservation does not compromise their cure rate at all. There may be reasons why a woman chooses mastectomy"—as one in five do, despite being eligible for BCT—"but increasing her chances of being cured should not be one of them." When making this decision, women should know that no mastectomy ever removes one hundred percent of the breast. If the tumor recurred locally, it would grow in the chest and require a second surgery.

BREAST CANCER/
Surgical Procedures

Lumpectomy: surgical removal of the tumor and a border of healthy breast tissue. If the cancer is invasive, the surgeon usually excises some of the lymph nodes under the arm. This procedure, an *axillary node dissection,* also accompanies mastectomy. It is occasionally performed as a separate operation. Average hospital stay:

- **Lumpectomy, 1 day**

- **With axillary node dissection, 2–4 days**

Partial/segmental mastectomy: surgical removal of the cancer, a wedge of normal tissue around it, and the lining over the chest muscle below the tumor. Usually some underarm lymph nodes are taken out. Average hospital stay: 1–2 days

Total/simple mastectomy: surgical removal of the entire breast and usually a few underarm lymph nodes. Average hospital stay: 1–3 days

Modified radical mastectomy: surgical removal of the breast, many underarm lymph nodes, the lining over the chest muscles, and sometimes the smaller of the two chest muscles. This procedure has replaced radical mastectomy as the most common operation for breast cancer. Average hospital stay: 2–4 days

Radical mastectomy: surgical removal of the breast, chest muscles, all of the underarm lymph nodes, and some additional fat and skin in patients whose cancer has spread to the chest muscles. Also called the Halsted radical, after the surgeon who developed it. Average hospital stay: 2–4 days

If you've been diagnosed with ductal carcinoma in situ (DCIS): Mastectomy alone cures 98 percent of ductal carcinomas in situ. "However," says Dr. Norton, "there is increasing evidence that for many patients lumpectomy plus irradiation is an adequate treatment." At the present time, it has yet to be established which is the superior strategy. The factors that may guide your doctor's decision in recommending one operation over the other are the same as for early-stage invasive disease. Because noninvasive tumors do not metastasize, with rare exception "removing the axillary lymph nodes under the arm is not indicated," says Dr. Norton.

Mastectomy or *excision to clear margins* (the term preferred over "lumpectomy") followed by radiation therapy marks the end of treatment for ductal carcinoma in situ, although oncologists are looking at the possible benefits of prescribing the oral hormonal agent tamoxifen (brand name: Novaldex) to women who underwent the less extensive surgery.

A 1999 investigational study from the National Surgical Adjuvant Breast and Bowel Project (NSABP), one of the National Cancer Institute's cooperative groups for clinical trials, divided approximately eighteen hundred women with DCIS into two groups. All the women underwent lumpectomy and radiotherapy, but the experimental protocol added tamoxifen, to be taken twice a day for five years.

Over that time, the rate of invasive breast cancer among the patients treated with tamoxifen was nearly half (43 percent) that of the participants who did not receive hormonal therapy. The survival rate, though,

BREAST CANCER/Treatment Options

DUCTAL CARCINOMA IN SITU

The cancer is isolated within the breast duct and has not infiltrated other parts of the breast.

- Total mastectomy, to surgically remove the whole breast, *with or without* lymph-node dissection under the arm • *or*

{
- Lumpectomy, to surgically remove the cancerous tissue and a margin of normal tissue, *with or without* lymph-node dissection under the arm • *followed by*

- External-beam radiation therapy
}

Under Investigation

- Lumpectomy, *with or without* lymph-node dissection under the arm • *followed by*

- External-beam radiation therapy • *with or without*

- Hormonal therapy, consisting of tamoxifen

◆ Ask your doctor about any clinical trials that might benefit you.

STAGE I BREAST CANCER

The cancer measures no larger than 2 centimeters (3/4 inch) and has not spread outside the breast.

{
- Lumpectomy, *with* lymph-node dissection under the arm • *or*

- Partial mastectomy, to surgically remove part of the breast, *with* lymph-node dissection under the arm • *followed by*

- External-beam radiation therapy
}

Or:

- Total mastectomy, *with* lymph-node dissection under the arm • *or*

- Modified radical mastectomy, to surgically remove the whole breast plus the lining over the chest muscles and sometimes part of the chest muscles, *with* lymph-node dissection under the arm

Systemic Therapy

If the cancer is estrogen-receptor (ER) negative:

- Chemotherapy, frequently consisting of a regimen such as CMF, CA, or CMF (see "Drug Therapy" box)

If the cancer is ER positive:

- Hormonal therapy, consisting of tamoxifen

Under Investigation #1

- Chemotherapy *and* hormonal therapy, for selected women considered to be at inordinate risk of a recurrence

Under Investigation #2

- No chemotherapy or hormonal therapy, for selected women considered to be at reduced risk of a recurrence

Under Investigation #3

If the cancer is ER positive and you are premenopausal:

- Ovarian ablation, to prevent the ovaries from functioning, through (1) bilateral oophorectomy, to surgically remove the ovaries, (2) external-beam radiation therapy, or (3) hormonal therapy, frequently consisting of goserelin or another LHRH agonist

Under Investigation #4

- Chemotherapy, possibly consisting of CMF, given before surgery in the hopes of shrinking the tumor sufficiently to allow for breast-conservation surgery

◆ Ask your doctor about any clinical trials that might benefit you.

STAGE II BREAST CANCER

IIA: The cancer measures between 2 and 5 centimeters ($3/4$ inch to 2 inches); or the cancer is no larger than 2 centimeters but involves the axillary lymph nodes located under the arm.

IIB: The cancer measures between 2 and 5 centimeters and has spread to the underarm lymph nodes; or the cancer is larger than 5 centimeters but has not spread to the underarm lymph nodes.

- Lumpectomy, *with* lymph-node dissection under the arm • *or*
- Partial mastectomy, *with* lymph-node dissection under the arm • *followed by*

- External-beam radiation therapy

Or:

- Total mastectomy, *with* lymph-node dissection under the arm

Systemic Therapy

If no cancer was found in the lymph nodes and the tumor is ER negative:

- Chemotherapy, frequently consisting of CA, CMF, or another regimen

If no cancer was found in the lymph nodes and the tumor is ER positive:

- Hormonal therapy, consisting of tamoxifen

If no cancer was found in the lymph nodes and the tumor is ER positive but considered large:

- Chemotherapy, frequently consisting of CA, CMF, or another regimen

If cancer was found in the lymph nodes and the tumor is ER positive:

- Hormonal therapy, consisting of tamoxifen • *alone or with*

- Chemotherapy, frequently consisting of CA, CMF, or another regimen

If cancer was found in the lymph nodes and the tumor is ER negative:

- Chemotherapy, frequently consisting of CA, CMF, or another regimen

Under Investigation #1

- Chemotherapy, possibly consisting of CMF, given before surgery in the hopes of shrinking the tumor sufficiently to allow for breast-conservation therapy

Under Investigation #2

For patients with cancer in four or more lymph nodes:
- High-dose chemotherapy · *followed by*

- Autologous bone-marrow transplantation

◆ Ask your doctor about any clinical trials that might benefit you.

STAGE IIIA BREAST CANCER

The cancer is smaller than 5 centimeters and has spread to the lymph nodes under the arm, and the lymph nodes are attached to each other or to other structures; or the cancer measures larger than 5 centimeters and has spread to the underarm lymph nodes.

- Modified radical mastectomy, *with* lymph-node dissection under the arm · *or*

- Radical mastectomy, to surgically remove the whole breast and the chest muscles, *with* lymph-node dissection under the arm · *followed by*

- External-beam radiation therapy · *followed by*

- Chemotherapy, frequently consisting of CMF, CA, or CAF, or a regimen containing the hormone prednisone, such as CMFP or CMFVP

◆ In cases where the cancer is difficult to remove surgically, chemotherapy may be given preoperatively.

Under Investigation #1

- Preoperative chemotherapy · *followed by*

- Lumpectomy, *with* lymph-node dissection under the arm · *or*
- Partial mastectomy, *with* lymph-node dissection under the arm

Under Investigation #2

- High-dose chemotherapy · *followed by*

- Autologous bone-marrow or peripheral-blood stem-cell transplantation

◆ Ask your doctor about any clinical trials that might benefit you.

STAGE IIIB BREAST CANCER (INOPERABLE DISEASE)

The cancer has spread to nearby tissues, such as the skin or the chest wall, including the ribs and chest muscles; or the cancer has spread to lymph nodes inside the chest wall along the breastbone.

◆ Inflammatory breast cancer is treated similarly to stage IIIB and stage IV breast cancers.

- Fine-needle aspiration biopsy · *or*
- Surgical biopsy · *followed by*

- Chemotherapy, frequently consisting of CMF or another regimen • *or*
- Hormonal therapy, consisting of tamoxifen • *followed by*

(1) If the cancer responded well to chemotherapy:
- Mastectomy, *with* lymph-node dissection • *and/or*
- External-beam radiation therapy

(2) If the cancer responded poorly to chemotherapy:
- External-beam radiation therapy, to relieve symptoms

Under Investigation #1
- High-dose chemotherapy • *followed by*
- Autologous bone-marrow or peripheral-blood stem-cell transplantation

Under Investigation #2
- New chemotherapy drugs and immunologic agents
- ◆ Ask your doctor about any clinical trials that might benefit you.

STAGE IV BREAST CANCER

The cancer has metastasized to other organs of the body or to the skin and lymph nodes inside the neck, near the collarbone.
- Surgical biopsy, to determine tumor type and its levels of ER and PR (progesterone) receptors • *followed by*

{
- External-beam radiation therapy • *or*
- Mastectomy, to relieve symptoms

Or:
If the cancer has not spread to a large organ, is ER and PR positive, and you are pre-menopausal:
- Hormonal therapy, frequently consisting of tamoxifen • *or*
- Bilateral oophorectomy

If the cancer has spread to a large organ, or is ER and PR negative:
- Chemotherapy, frequently consisting of one of the following regimens: CMF, CAF, CA, CMFP, or CMFVP

If the tumor is HER-2 positive:
- Immunotherapy, consisting of trastuzumab, alone or in combination with paclitaxel

Under Investigation #1
- High-dose chemotherapy • *followed by*
- Autologous bone-marrow or peripheral-blood stem-cell transplantation

Under Investigation #2
- New chemotherapy drugs and immunologic agents
- ◆ Ask your doctor about any clinical trials that might benefit you.

See treatment options for metastases of the bone, brain, liver, and lung.

RECURRENT OR RESISTANT (REFRACTORY) BREAST CANCER

Your therapy will depend on how you were treated initially.

If the cancer has recurred in the breast or any large organs:
- Surgery, to resect the tumor(s) • *and/or*

- External-beam radiation therapy

If the cancer has not recurred in a large organ, or if it is limited to one large organ and is minimal; and the tumor is ER and PR positive (or your hormone-receptor status is unknown); and you do not have symptoms:
- Hormonal therapy, consisting of tamoxifen

Or, for premenopausal women only:
- Ovarian ablation, through bilateral oophorectomy *or* hormonal therapy, frequently consisting of goserelin or another LHRH agonist

If the cancer responded to initial hormonal therapy:
- Hormonal therapy not used previously, including tamoxifen, letrozole, progestins, androgens, or anastrozole

Or, for premenopausal women only:
- Ovarian ablation, through bilateral oophorectomy *or* hormonal therapy, frequently consisting of goserelin or another LHRH agonist

If the cancer has recurred in a large organ and is ER and PR negative:
- Chemotherapy, frequently consisting of one of the following regimens: CMF, CAF, or CA

◆ If you previously received an anthracycline drug such as doxorubicin, you may be given paclitaxel, docetaxel, vinorelbine, or another drug.

If the cancer did not respond to chemotherapy and is HER-2 positive:
- Immunotherapy, consisting of trastuzumab

Under Investigation #1
- New chemotherapy drugs, hormonal drugs, and immunologic agents

Under Investigation #2
- High-dose chemotherapy • *followed by*

- Autologous bone-marrow transplantation

Under Investigation #3
- Hyperthermia • *with*

- External-beam radiation therapy

◆ Ask your doctor about any clinical trials that might benefit you.

was uniformly excellent for the two groups: At the end of the five years, 97 percent of the women were alive.

Other patient trials are trying to determine whether or not some DCIS patients can bypass the radiation portion of breast-conservation therapy. Based on a 1999 study from the University of Southern California School of Medicine, that decision may be contingent upon the size of the surgical margin.

USC researchers tracked 133 subjects, none of whom took radiation. They found that when the surgeon was able to remove a border of healthy tissue 10 millimeters (.04 inch) wide, the odds that the patient would still be free of breast cancer eight years later were a comforting 96 percent. But if the perimeter measured less than 1 millimeter (.004 inch), the patient faced a fifty-fifty chance of a recurrence. Radiation reduced the risk of relapse substantially, but only to 30 percent. The researchers concluded that wide, clear surgical margins rendered additional radiation of little benefit. But they also emphasized that follow-up treatments cannot compensate for inadequate surgery.

If you've been diagnosed with early-stage breast cancer: When deciding between mastectomy and breast-conservation therapy, two major considerations are (1) the tumor's cell type and (2) the likelihood that the surgeon will be able to achieve sufficient clear margins around the tumor site. These factors are interrelated. Four in five breast cancers are ductal carcinomas. But another type, infiltrating lobular carcinoma, poses a formidable challenge. At the H. Lee Moffitt Cancer Center and Research Institute in Tampa, Florida, fewer than half the attempted lumpectomies of invasive lobular cancers were successful.

Tumor volume in relation to the size of the breast is also an issue. From a cosmetic standpoint, a woman with small breasts might be more satisfied with the results of a mastectomy and reconstructive surgery.

At Memorial Sloan-Kettering and other major centers, women with operable stage III disease may still be eligible for breast conservation. At this point, the cancer is said to be "locally advanced," having invaded the underarm lymph nodes on the corresponding side of the body. If the cancer is diagnosed as beyond surgery, you may be given chemotherapy in an attempt to render the disease operable. Some clinical researchers, says Dr. Norton, "are looking at whether or not we can conserve the breast in that situation. Except in very special circumstances, right now mastectomy is the definitive surgery because the attempts at breast conservation in that setting have been disappointing, with a very high rate of local recurrence."

Axillary-Node Dissection—Whether or not breast cancer has invaded the underarm lymph nodes may be the single most crucial piece of information for planning treatment—as well as for predicting its probable long-term success. The axillary nodes under the arm (*axilla*) are divided into three groups: Level I nodes lie beneath the armpit; level II nodes, in the armpit itself; and level III nodes, in front of the shoulder. Virtually all women with invasive breast cancer face some degree of axillary-node surgery. "A standard dissection," says breast surgeon Dr. Marie Pennanen, "consists of sampling the level I and level II nodes." In all, about fifteen nodes are taken out through a separate incision in the fold of the armpit, although the number can vary from as few as four to more than thirty. If these nodes test negative for cancer, the odds that the disease has infiltrated level III are less than 1 percent. A *complete axillary dissection*—removing all three levels—excises roughly two dozen nodes.

Traumatic as it is to lose all or part of a breast, some of the most severe aftereffects result from the node dissection. The loss of muscle and lymphatic tissues in the arm on the side of the cancerous breast can saddle patients with weakness, numbness, and a painful swelling known as *lymphedema*.

> ## Factors That Unequivocally Rule Out Lumpectomy with Radiation
>
> - **Prior radiation therapy to the breast or chest**
> - **Being in the first or second trimester of pregnancy**
> - **Diffuse suspicious-looking *microcalcifications*. Breast tumors contain these particles of calcium. An X ray showing malignant microcalcifications scattered throughout the breast would indicate a large tumor.**
> - **A previous excisional biopsy—and perhaps even a reexcision—has not completely removed the cancer**
>
> ## Factors That *Might* Rule Out Lumpectomy with Radiation
>
> - **Two or more large, visible tumors in separate quadrants of the breast**
> - **A tumor that is large in comparison to the size of the breast**
> - **A history of diseases of the connective tissues, such as arthritis**

"A lot of research is going on questioning whether we can sample fewer nodes, or whether node dissection is necessary at all for every patient," says Dr. Norton. In one such study, doctors at the Moffitt Cancer Center employed a new technique to pinpoint the first node to receive drainage from the tumor. This pea-sized *sentinel* lymph node (SLN) is believed to reflect the disease status of the other nodes in the armpit. If a biopsy of the SLN reveals no tumor, its counterparts can also be expected to be cancer free. In the Moffitt Center trial, the sentinel nodes tested negative in 60 percent of the participants, thus sparing them from radical underarm surgery. Removing only one or two nodes considerably lowers the risk of lymphedema. It also greatly reduces one's hospital bill, by about $5,000.

When you're scouting around for a treatment facility, ask the doctor if the oncology team is experienced in sentinel-node *mapping*. It is not yet standard for breast cancer, says Dr. Douglas Reintgen of the Moffitt Center, "simply because not all surgeons have learned the technique yet." Dr. Reintgen and his colleagues combined two methods: During the definitive cancer operation, the tissue around the tumor was injected with a blue dye and then a radioactive agent. Both materials pick up the trail any malignant cells would follow from the tumor to the nodes under the arm. The doctor aims a Geiger-counter-like device at the patient's upper body and waits for the beep signaling that the tracer substances have reached the first node. Out it comes, in a simple surgical procedure, to be studied under the microscope. Other surgeons use only the blue-dye technique.

What Is Lymphedema?—Approximately two in five women with breast cancer will develop some degree of lymphedema as a complication of axillary-node dissection. The lymphatic channels in the arm carry lymph fluid back into the body's circulation. When the nodes and their connecting vessels are removed, Dr. Pennanen explains, "the fluid may not drain as efficiently and then accumulate in the tissue, producing swelling." In severe lymphedema, it's not unheard-of for a person's arm to balloon to twice its normal size. What's more, the deficient drainage predisposes the arm to serious infection.

Why does lymphedema occur in some patients and not others? The extent of the dissection is one factor; postsurgical radiation is another. Women who receive radiotherapy following a modified radical mastectomy, for example, have double the incidence of lymphedema as those treated without radiation. Obesity, too, elevates a person's risk. Lymphedema is highly treatable, especially when caught early. But for one in twenty breast-cancer patients, the condition is controllable but not curable, which is why practicing preventive measures is essential.

"There are two major things patients can do to avoid getting lymphedema or to reduce the symptoms," says Dr. Pennanen. "One is to protect the arm from injury. A cut, a burn, or an infection can cause swelling and overload the remaining lymphatic system, resulting in transient or even permanent lymphedema. The other is to exercise the arm, because that causes the muscles to act like a pump and help return that fluid to the central circulation."

See "Lymphedema" in Chapter Eight, "Take Control: Managing Symptoms, Side Effects, and Complications."

Breast-Reconstruction Surgery—Mastectomy leaves a lengthy horizontal scar and a flat chest. "Most women opt for breast reconstruction," says Dr. Norton, "but not all." Rather than undergo surgery, you might feel comfortable living with a single breast, or perhaps you'd prefer to wear an external *prosthesis*. Typically made of silicone or foam rubber, artificial breasts come in a wide variety of sizes, shapes, weights, and colors. At a greater cost, you can have one custom-made to better match the size and contour of your remaining breast. Some models adhere directly to the body with an adhesive glue, while others slip inside a sleeve in a specially designed brassiere. There are also clothing manufacturers that make bathing suits, lingerie, and other garments with hidden pockets for holding the prosthesis. Your surgeon, a nurse, or one of the patient organizations listed under "Breast Cancer" in Appendix A should be familiar with some of these companies.

> **MONEY MATTERS**
>
> Both Medicare and Medicaid pay for breast prostheses, as do the great majority of private insurance policies.

Breast prostheses are sold at surgical supplies stores, corsetieres, and through catalogs. Before you go shopping, you might want to make an appointment at your local division of the American Cancer Society (800-227-2345), where a volunteer can show you the different types available and explain the pros and cons of each. For patients who cannot afford them, the ACS also provides breast prostheses free of charge.

Reconstruction surgery entails fashioning an artificial breast, using either synthetic implants or tissue transferred from another part of the body. In the past, it was widely believed that undergoing breast reconstruction at the same time as the mastectomy might prevent doctors from detecting a recurrence of the cancer, and so women were frequently advised to wait two years before having the operation. We now know that these fears are unfounded and that there are several *benefits* to immediate breast reconstruction. For one thing, you go through a single general anesthesia and surgical recovery, saving $5,000 to $10,000 in hospital fees.

The most significant advantage, though, is the improved appearance. In most cases, the combined mastectomy-reconstruction makes it possible for the breast surgeon and the plastic surgeon to collaborate on an innovative technique called *skin-sparing mastectomy.* The aim, explains Dr. Pennanen, "is to preserve as much of the normal skin as possible, by making more complicated incisions instead of the conventional elliptical incision." Sparing the uninvolved breast tissue not only results in a near-perfect match with the other breast in terms of color and texture but also aids the plastic surgeon in molding the reconstructed mound.

When selecting a plastic surgeon, the two main qualities you're looking for are a lengthy track record in breast reconstruction and a low complication rate. "You want to make sure you're in skilled hands," Dr. Norton stresses, offering an example of why.

"Let's say you're going to require chemotherapy. You don't want it delayed because of complications related to the reconstruction. It's tragic when we see a woman who is at inordinate risk for a systemic recurrence have to wait three, four, or six months before she can receive treatment. Saving your life has got to be the primary goal."

There are two main types of breast reconstruction:

Saline or Silicone Implants—Breast implants, small balloonlike sacs that contain either a saltwater solution or a silicone gel, are surgically inserted under the chest muscle to create a mound. In 1992, the federal Food and Drug Administration imposed severe restrictions on the use of the silicone-filled devices, by far the more popular of the two. This followed years of complaints that as many as one in three silicone implants eventually leaked or ruptured, releasing the gel into the body. Since then, only women requiring implants for medical reasons—reconstruction following mastectomy being one of them—may receive them, and then only if they participate in a long-term research study.

Breast Implant Info from the FDA

Call the FDA for a recorded update on breast implants or to obtain a free copy of its publication "Breast Implants: An Information Update": 800-532-4440.

Saline implants can also break, but their contents are harmless. Ironically, the salt water is encased in silicone. "No material is 100 percent safe," says Dr. Scott Spear, chief of plastic surgery at Georgetown University Medical Center. "But a silicone envelope is the safest one we know of."

If you are small-breasted, implants alone may be sufficient. Most women, though, need an additional step: *tissue expansion.* In order for the chest muscle and skin to accommodate a larger implant, the surgeon first places an inflatable sac beneath the chest wall. Over the next two to six months, patients pay numerous visits to the physician's office so that saline can be injected into the tissue expander. This gradually stretches the tissue to twice the desired breast size. Then, in a separate operation, the expander is replaced with the permanent prosthesis, creating a more natural breast appearance.

Autogenous Breast Reconstruction—A breast fashioned from a flap of the patient's own tissue produces the best results, both cosmetically and in terms of maintaining more sensation. The transplant site used most often is the lower abdomen.

More complicated than implant reconstruction, "flap surgery" requires four to five days of hospitalization, as opposed to one to three days. It is also the more expensive procedure—initially, that is. In the long run, implants prove to be more costly because of their high rate of subsequent complications.

In a study conducted by the Mayo Clinic, nearly one in four women who received breast implants suffered at least one complication serious enough to warrant further surgery within five years. Researchers there also found that mastectomy patients were three times as likely to develop surgical complications as women who'd undergone the operation for cosmetic reasons, due to tissue damage caused by the cancer treatment. The most common problem by far is what's called *capsular contracture,* in which surrounding scar tissue hardens and compresses the implant, making it feel rigid and painful. To correct this, the scar tissue may have to be surgically reduced or removed, or the implant replaced or possibly taken out.

Either type of reconstruction is carried out in two or three stages. Six to twelve months after the initial operation, the plastic surgeon can create a nipple from additional tissue. Any modifications that might be necessary would also be done at that time. "When we make a breast out of abdominal tissue," explains Dr. Spear, "we anticipate having to change the shape and size and adjust scars. It's unusual for the reconstruction to turn out perfectly in the first step." Step three consists of coloring the nipple and simulating an areola, using a technique not unlike tattooing.

It's important for anyone contemplating breast reconstruction to understand that plastic surgery has its limitations. While the completed artificial breast will appear natural (to what extent depends on several factors, including the surgeon's expertise and the size of the tumor) and feel normal to the touch, it will not have the same sensation as before.

You may decide plastic surgery isn't the right choice for you. Many women who have gone this route, however, find that breast reconstruction has helped enhance their feelings of femininity and sexuality, and has better enabled them to shed the identity of "cancer patient." Georgetown University Medical Center's department of psychiatry interviewed more than seventy women following reconstruction surgery. More than four in five credited the operation with playing a major part in their recovery from cancer.

MONEY MATTERS

Insurance Coverage for Breast-Reconstruction Surgery

With rare exception, all forms of insurance cover basic breast reconstruction for cancer patients. "Where the arguments tend to arise," explains Dr. Spear, "is when we go to steps two and three. If we're reconstructing the nipple, some insurers will actually question the need for it or the need for coloring the nipple and areola. They'll contend that these are cosmetic procedures.

"Our position," he says, "is that if we're going to construct a breast, it should *look like* a breast. Most of the time the insurance companies eventually cave in, but there are times when they don't."

Another area of contention involves breast reduction for women with extremely large breasts. "We may recognize that it's foolish to try to make a breast that big," says Dr. Spear, "and so we'll propose reducing the size of the healthy breast. There the insurance companies may say, 'That's not necessary; there's no cancer on the other side.' We get into an argument again, about how we feel it is necessary in order to do a reasonable construction. Those are battles sometimes, and we don't always win."

See "Insurance Issues" in Chapter Ten, "Getting Help When You Need It."

Chemotherapy and/or Hormonal Therapy and/or Immunochemotherapy

When carcinoma of the breast has migrated to the lymph nodes, doctors incorporate chemotherapy or hormonal therapy—and sometimes both—into the treatment plan, typically after surgery. In 1988, the National Cancer Institute began recommending that oncologists also consider adjuvant therapy for the 50 percent of breast-cancer patients said to have "node-negative" disease, nearly one-third of whom will see their tumor return if mastectomy or breast conservation is not followed by systemic treatment.

For stage I breast cancer, which measures less than an inch and hasn't infiltrated any lymph nodes, the standard practice is to prescribe hormonal therapy for malignancies found to contain estrogen receptors, and chemotherapy for ER-negative cancers. An ER-positive tumor depends on this female sex hormone to grow and therefore responds to an estrogen-blocking drug such as tamoxifen.

At stage II, planning treatment grows more complicated. For instance, most node-negative, ER-positive patients would probably be offered tamoxifen. "In a lot of cases," says Dr. Norton, "we might say to a woman, 'With tamoxifen, your risk of a recurrence will be so low that chemotherapy would add very little.'" Given tamoxifen's far milder side effects, in this example "it would clearly be the way to go."

But if a patient were at above-average risk—perhaps due to a family history of breast cancer—her oncologist might recommend hormonal therapy *and* chemotherapy, for stage II and possibly even stage I disease. The National Surgical Adjuvant Breast and Bowel Project conducted a major study at hospitals in the United States and Canada to determine whether chemotherapy plus tamoxifen provided an advantage over tamoxifen alone in treating node-negative, ER-positive early-stage breast cancer. More than two thousand patients took part.

The results were striking: After five years, the disease-free survival rate was 4 percent higher for the women who received tamoxifen and chemotherapy *(91 percent to 87 percent)*, leading the authors to conclude that patients with early-stage invasive breast cancer should be offered chemotherapy "regardless of age, lymph-node status, tumor size, or estrogen-receptor status."

As with many cancers, tumor size is usually the foremost predictor of whether or not breast cancer will come out of remission, followed closely by nodal status, cell type, and the grade of the tumor. In breast cancer, there are still other meaningful *prognostic indicators.* Any or all can influence which type of postoperative treatment you receive.

Hormone Receptivity—A high level of estrogen receptors opens the door to the possibility of hormonal therapy and is also a favorable sign, because ER-positive tumors behave less aggressively. Two-thirds of all breast-cancer patients will have significant estrogen-receptor levels, and about two in three will test positive for progesterone receptors as well.

HER-2 Gene Level—Normally, each of our cells holds two copies of a gene called HER-2. But in one-third of breast-cancer patients, it over-

If You're . . .			Probable Treatment
Premenopausal	Node positive	ER positive	Chemotherapy *or* Combination systemic therapy
Postmenopausal	Node positive	ER positive	Hormonal therapy *or* Combination systemic therapy
Premenopausal	Node negative or positive	ER negative	Chemotherapy
Postmenopausal	Node negative or positive	ER negative	Chemotherapy
If the Tumor Is Small and You're . . .			
Premenopausal	Node negative	ER positive	Hormonal therapy
Postmenopausal	Node negative	ER positive	Hormonal therapy
If the Tumor Is Large and You're . . .			
Premenopausal	Node negative	ER positive	Chemotherapy *or* Combination systemic therapy
Postmenopausal	Node negative	ER positive	Hormonal therapy *or* Combination systemic therapy

multiplies, spurring tumor growth and greatly increasing the chance of a recurrence. Overexpression of HER-2 calls for treatment with the monoclonal-antibody therapy trastuzumab (Herceptin).

Nuclear Grade and DNA Content—In forming a profile of the cancer, the oncologist may also study its genetic material. *Nuclear* grade, expressed on a scale of 1 to 3, differs from *tumor* grade in that it describes the rate at which cancer cells divide rather than their appearance. Thus a nuclear grade of 3 denotes a rapidly proliferating and malignant tumor. *Flow cytometry,* a technique for evaluating nuclear grade, can also measure the breast cancer cells' DNA content. This, too, yields useful information, for aggressive tumors have a higher percentage of cells with abnormal amounts of DNA.

Menopause and Breast-Cancer Treatment—Whether or not you've reached menopause may determine the type of systemic treatment recommended. A postmenopausal woman whose breast cancer involves the lymph nodes and tests positive for hormone receptors would usually be put on tamoxifen, while a premenopausal woman with the same tumor characteristics would receive cytotoxic chemotherapy, in order to preserve her ability to bear children. Combination systemic therapy seems to benefit patients who are past menopause more than those who are not, but oncologists do sometimes order both types of agents for premenopausal women, as long as their tumors are ER positive.

In breast cancer, adjuvant therapy can dramatically reduce the odds of the tumor coming back. Yet more than a decade after the NCI alerted cancer doctors to the curative potential of postoperative drug therapy, fewer than half of all women with localized breast cancer were receiving either. Statistically speaking, a number of them probably would have benefited from systemic treatment, though not all. If a patient has favorable prognostic features—a small, well-differentiated node-negative tumor, successfully removed, with adequate margins; a normal HER-2 gene count; and so on—her outlook is already excellent. "In that case," says Dr. Norton, "the patient has to decide if it is worth it" to incur the possible side effects of therapy.

Women aged seventy or older appear not to gain from postoperative chemotherapy. There's also a question as to whether or not elderly patients who undergo a lumpectomy should be subjected to lymph-

---

**BREAST CANCER/
Drug Therapy**

*First-line therapy frequently
consists of one of the following
drugs, hormones, or drug regimens:*

- **tamoxifen (H)**

- **CMF: cyclophosphamide +
  methotrexate + fluorouracil**

- **CA: cyclophosphamide +
  doxorubicin**

- **CAF: cyclophosphamide +
  doxorubicin + fluorouracil**

- **CEF: cyclophosphamide +
  epirubicin + fluorouracil**

- **CMFP: cyclophosphamide +
  methotrexate + fluorouracil +
  prednisone (H)**

- **CMFVP: cyclophosphamide +
  methotrexate + fluorouracil +
  vincristine + prednisone (H)**

- **paclitaxel + trastuzumab (I)**

- **methotrexate + fluorouracil +
  leucovorin**

- **doxorubicin followed by CMF**

*Other drugs or hormones that
may be used include:*

- **goserelin (H)**

- **progestins (H)**

- **pamidronate (B)**

- **anastrozole (H)**

- **paclitaxel**

- **docetaxel**

- **vinorelbine**

- **androgens (H)**

- **aminoglutethimide (H)**

- **letrozole (H)**

- **thiotepa**

- **estrogens (H)**

(cont.)

---

node dissection and radiotherapy. Ordinarily, tamoxifen is offered following surgery.

Chemotherapy—Chemotherapy for breast cancer revolves primarily around cyclophosphamide (Cytoxan), which is administered along with other agents. The typical course of drug therapy lasts three to six months. The three most frequently used combinations, CA, CMF, and CAF, "are totally equivalent in terms of cure rates," says Dr. Norton. "Some doctors lean toward one or the other." For patients deemed at higher risk—say, those with four or more cancerous lymph nodes—"it has become almost standard to use something called the Buzoni regimen, which is Adriamycin [doxorubicin] followed by CMF.

"But in any event," Dr. Norton continues, "we're moving beyond CMF toward more effective chemotherapies involving doxorubicin or Taxol [paclitaxel], or both."

Until the mid-1990s, the conventional sequence after breast-conservation surgery was radiation followed by chemotherapy. "Now," says Dr. Pennanen, "patients who are at a substantial risk for a systemic recurrence frequently have chemotherapy as the second step, with radiation coming last." The switch was prompted by several studies that suggested that deferring chemotherapy slightly increases the odds that the cancer will return elsewhere in the body. Other clinical trials, meanwhile, demonstrated that radiation could be delayed for up to seven months after surgery without adding to the possibility of a local recurrence. As Dr. Pennanen points out, "we're more concerned about metastasis" because a locally recurrent breast tumor is more readily treatable than a metastatic tumor. Your oncologist may recommend what has been referred to as the "sandwich" strategy: postoperative chemo, then radiation, then the remaining cycles of chemo.

Administering anticancer drugs prior to breast surgery doesn't appear to improve patients' long-term prognosis. But in another NSABP study, 68 percent of women who received neoadjuvant chemotherapy were then able to undergo lumpectomies, compared to 60 percent of those in the adjuvant-chemo group. More than one in four of the participants in the preoperative-chemo group had originally been scheduled for a mastectomy, but the cytotoxic agents shrank the tumor so much that a lumpectomy could be performed instead.

• **testolactone**
• **toremifene (H)**
• **trastuzumab (I)**
• **capecitabine**
• **cisplatin**
• **dexamethasone (H)**
• **leuprolide**
• **lomustine**
• **melphalan**
• **mitomycin**
• **vinblastine**
(B) = bone-resorption inhibitor   **(H) = hormonal agent**   **(I) = immunologic agent**

Hormonal Therapy—Unlike chemotherapy, tamoxifen isn't commenced until after the completion of radiation. The oral estrogen blocker produces a response in about three-fourths of all estrogen-sensitive tumors. Of these, two in three will also test positive for receptors to progesterone, the other female hormone secreted by the ovaries.

Tamoxifen, most effective when administered for five years, protects against a second cancer in the opposite breast. Its health benefits may extend to the cardiovascular and skeletal systems as well, because it is believed to lower blood cholesterol and maintain the density of the bones. Possible complications such as hot flashes, erratic menstrual periods, nausea, and weight gain tend to be of less concern to most women than the possibility that the drug can double or triple their risk of endometrial cancer. Even so, it's important to remember that the incidence of cancer of the uterine lining is very low: two to three in one thousand with tamoxifen, up from one in one thousand—or about the same risk associated with taking hormone replacement therapy to relieve the symptoms of menopause.

While you're on tamoxifen, notify your doctor of any unusual vaginal bleeding, a potential early warning sign of endometrial cancer.

Tamoxifen does not shut down estrogen production outright; it prohibits tumor cells from feeding on the female sex hormone. One strategy for premenopausal women is to undergo a *bilateral oophorectomy* to remove the still-functioning ovaries. This effectively starves the tumor. Ovarian failure can also be induced by irradiating the glands or by administering a type of drug known as *luteinizing hormone-releasing hormone* (LHRH) *agonists*, which inhibit the brain from secreting a hormone that stimulates estrogen production.

Surgery and radiation bring on menopause immediately. The cessation of estrogen production is so abrupt and dramatic that the resulting symptoms are more severe than those usually seen during natural menopause, where estrogen levels drop off over many years. Although undeniably effective, ovarian ablation is performed only occasionally in the United States. The reason, explains Dr. Norton, is that most premenopausal breast-cancer patients are on the cusp of menopause. "Chemotherapy, in addition to killing cancer cells, will often end ovarian function in older premenopausal patients anyway, and so the issue of ablation therapy usually becomes moot."

TREATMENTS FOR ADVANCED AND RECURRENT BREAST CANCER

Breast cancer differs from most other tumors in that even after the disease has spread, says Dr. Norton, "there is a wide variety of treatments available." Standard options include chemotherapy or hormone therapy, and radiation, "all of which are effective." At this point, newer drugs enter the picture, among them paclitaxel, docetaxel (Taxotere), and toremifene (Fareston), a tamoxifen-like *antiestrogen* agent.

Women whose tumor comes back in the same location can be helped—and in select cases cured—by surgery, radiation, or a combination of the two. If you were treated initially with a lumpectomy plus radiotherapy, a mastectomy at this time can often grant you many more years. In one study of thirty such patients, half were still free of disease ten years later. Attaining a cure is less likely once the cancer has metastasized to other organs, but 10 to 20 percent of women with stage IV breast cancer do experience an extended complete remission.

On the investigational-therapy front, "there's a lot of very exciting research going on," says Dr. Norton. Clinical trials are testing the effectiveness of various cancer vaccines, gene therapies, immunotherapies, and high-dose chemotherapy with stem-cell support.

Immunotherapy—Trastuzumab (Herceptin), the first monoclonal-antibody therapy for breast cancer, was approved for treating stage IV tumors that contain too many copies of the aberrant HER-2 gene. The intravenous drug may be prescribed alone or with a chemotherapeutic agent, but not an anthracycline such as doxorubicin (Adriamycin). In patient tests, that combination sometimes caused damage to the heart muscle. The safest pairing to date appears to be with Taxol, although all patients taking Herceptin should regularly see a doctor for cardiac checkups.

OTHER THERAPIES THAT MAY BE USED IN THE TREATMENT OF BREAST CANCER

High-Dose Chemotherapy with Autologous Bone-Marrow or Peripheral-Blood Stem-Cell Transplantation (investigational)—More *autotransplants* (reinfusing patients with their own healthy bone marrow or stem cells) are carried out for breast cancer than for any other type of cancer, yet the costly and potentially risky procedure is still considered experimental in this setting. The treatment may be suggested for women who have four or more cancerous lymph nodes or a secondary tumor elsewhere in the body.

Being able to replenish the marrow—the body's factory for blood cells—allows for higher-than-normal doses of anticancer agents to be administered. Inevitably, this destroys not only the tumor cells but the marrow. Proponents of BMT in breast-cancer treatment had hoped that five sizable studies would establish its value once and for all. But when the collective results were made public in 1999, they raised more questions than they answered.

Only one of the clinical trials reported that high-dose chemotherapy with stem-cell support made a substantial difference in prolonging life. South African researchers tracked 154 women. Half received standard chemotherapy; the others were bombarded with heavy doses. After more than five years, 17 percent of the patients in the transplanted group had died versus 35 percent in the other group.

Why didn't the other four studies produce similar results? One reason may have been that the regimens given to the women

> **You Are Not Alone**
>
> Do you think that speaking with a woman who has been treated for breast cancer might help you to decide between breast-conservation therapy and mastectomy, or whether or not to go forward with breast-reconstruction surgery? If so, contact the American Cancer Society at 800-227-2345. Its Reach to Recovery program puts newly diagnosed patients in touch with breast-cancer survivors willing to share their experiences.

in the control groups were actually higher than what is normally administered. Dr. Norton also suspects, as do other cancer specialists, that several more years will have to pass before the benefits of high-dose chemotherapy over conventional-dose treatment become apparent.

> *See "Insurance Coverage for Cancer Treatments" in Chapter Ten, "Getting Help When You Need It," and "Cost and Controversy" under "Bone-Marrow Transplantation" in Chapter Four, "How Cancer Is Treated."*

◆ *Ask your doctor about this and any other investigational therapies that might benefit you.*

Cancer of the Lung

Overview

TREATMENTS FOR LUNG CANCER THAT HAS NOT
METASTASIZED

Non-small-cell and small-cell lung cancers call for different approaches. Small-cell lung cancer (SCLC) is treated medically, with radiotherapy added. Surgery, the principal strategy for non-small-cell lung cancer (NSCLC), rarely has a place in SCLC. "The only patients who would be operated on," says Dr. Kasi Sridhar of the Sylvester Comprehensive Cancer Center in Miami, "are those in whom we don't know the diagnosis prior to surgery or who have a small centrally located tumor with no lymph-node involvement."

Small-Cell Lung Cancer

Chemotherapy

"Small-cell lung cancer tends to respond extremely well to chemotherapy and radiotherapy," says Dr. Sridhar, a pulmonary oncologist. If the tumor is limited to the lung, which describes about four in ten people diagnosed with small-cell carcinoma, "this is a potentially curable disease."

Radiation Therapy

Once the cancer is in remission, your physician may recommend additional radiation to the brain, a frequent site of metastases from SCLC. According to a National Cancer Institute study of three hun-

---

LUNG CANCER/Treatment Options

Small-Cell Lung Cancer

LIMITED-STAGE SMALL-CELL LUNG CANCER

The cancer is confined to one lung and to neighboring lymph nodes.

- Chemotherapy, frequently consisting of various combinations of the following drugs: cisplatin, etoposide, vincristine • *followed by*

- External-beam radiation therapy • *with or without*

- Preventive external-beam radiation therapy to the brain

Or:
- Chemotherapy, frequently consisting of various combinations of the following drugs: cisplatin, etoposide, vincristine • *with or without*

- Preventive external-beam radiation therapy to the brain

Or, in selected patients:
- Wedge resection, to surgically remove a small portion of the lung • *or*

- Lobectomy, to surgically remove a section of the lung • *followed by*

- Chemotherapy, using two or more of the above-mentioned agents • *with or without*

- Preventive external-beam radiation therapy to the brain

Under Investigation

◆ Ask your doctor about any clinical trials that might benefit you.

EXTENSIVE-STAGE SMALL-CELL LUNG CANCER

The cancer has spread outside the lung to other tissues in the chest or to other sites in the body.

- Chemotherapy, frequently consisting of various combinations of two or more of the following drugs: cisplatin, etoposide, cyclophosphamide, doxorubicin, vincristine, carboplatin, ifosfamide • *alone or followed by*

- External-beam radiation therapy • *with or without*

- Preventive external-beam radiation therapy to the brain

Under Investigation

◆ Ask your doctor about any clinical trials that might benefit you.

See treatment options for metastases of the bone, liver, and lung.

RECURRENT SMALL-CELL LUNG CANCER

Your therapy will depend on how you were treated initially.

- Chemotherapy, frequently consisting of paclitaxel, topotecan, etoposide, or etoposide and cisplatin • *and/or*

- External-beam radiation therapy, to relieve symptoms

Non-Small-Cell Lung Cancer

NON-SMALL-CELL CARCINOMA IN SITU OF THE LUNG

The cancer is found in only a few layers of cells in a local area and has not penetrated the lung's top lining.

- Wedge resection *or* segmental resection, to surgically remove a small portion of the lung • *or*
- Photodynamic therapy

Under Investigation

◆ Ask your doctor about any clinical trials that might benefit you.

STAGE I NON-SMALL-CELL LUNG CANCER

The cancer is confined to the lung.

- Wedge or segmental resection • *or*
- Lobectomy • *or*
- External-beam radiation therapy • *or*
- Photodynamic therapy, to relieve symptoms

Under Investigation

- Chemotherapy following surgery
◆ Ask your doctor about any clinical trials that might benefit you.

STAGE II NON-SMALL-CELL LUNG CANCER

The cancer has spread to nearby lymph nodes.

- Wedge or segmental resection • *or*
- Lobectomy • *or*
- Pneumonectomy, to remove the entire lung • *alone or followed by one or more of the following experimental therapies:*

Under Investigation

- Postoperative chemotherapy, frequently consisting of cisplatin, doxorubicin, and cyclophosphamide • *or*
- Postoperative external-beam radiation therapy
◆ Ask your doctor about any clinical trials that might benefit you.

Or:

- External-beam radiation therapy

Or:

- Photodynamic therapy, to relieve symptoms

STAGE III NON-SMALL-CELL LUNG CANCER

The cancer has spread to the chest wall or the diaphragm; or to the lymph nodes in the mediastinum; or to the lymph nodes on the other side of the chest or in the neck.

If the cancer is operable (stage IIIA):

{
- Chemotherapy, frequently consisting of combinations of drugs such as cisplatin, doxorubicin, cyclophosphamide, gemcitabine, and/or other agents • *with or without*

- External-beam radiation therapy, given at the same time • *followed by*
}

- Wedge or segmental resection, lobectomy, or pneumonectomy

Or:

- Wedge or segmental resection, lobectomy, or pneumonectomy • *alone or followed by*

- Radiation therapy

Or:

- Radiation therapy

Or:

- Internal radiation therapy *and/or* laser therapy *and/or* photodynamic therapy, to shrink a tumor obstructing an airway

If the cancer is inoperable (stage IIIB):

- Chemotherapy, frequently consisting of combinations of drugs such as cisplatin, vincristine, doxorubicin, cyclophosphamide, gemcitabine, and/or other agents • *plus*

- External-beam radiation therapy, given at the same time or afterward

Or:

- Radiation therapy • *or*

- Chemotherapy, frequently consisting of combinations of drugs such as cisplatin, vincristine, doxorubicin, cyclophosphamide, and/or other agents

Or:

- Internal radiation therapy *and/or* laser therapy *and/or* photodynamic therapy, to shrink a tumor obstructing an airway

STAGE IV NON-SMALL-CELL LUNG CANCER

The cancer has metastasized to other parts of the body.

- External-beam radiation therapy, to relieve symptoms • *and/or*

- Chemotherapy, frequently consisting of combinations of drugs such as cisplatin, vinblastine, mitomycin, vinorelbine, paclitaxel, and carboplatin

Or:

- Internal radiation therapy *and/or* laser therapy *and/or* photodynamic therapy, to shrink a tumor obstructing an airway

See treatment options for metastases of the brain, liver, lung, and bone.

RECURRENT NON-SMALL-CELL LUNG CANCER

Your therapy will depend on how you were treated initially.

- **External-beam radiation therapy, to relieve symptoms • *or***

- **Internal radiation therapy *and/or* laser therapy and/or photodynamic therapy, to shrink a tumor obstructing an airway • *or***

- **Chemotherapy, frequently consisting of docetaxel, paclitaxel, and/or other agents**

If the cancer has metastasized to the brain:
- **Stereotactic radiosurgery • *or***

- **Surgical resection of brain metastases**

LUNG CANCER/ Drug Therapy

Small-Cell Lung Cancer

First-line therapy frequently consists of:
- **EC: etoposide + cisplatin or carboplatin**

- **ECV: etoposide + cisplatin + vincristine**

- **CAV: cyclophosphamide + doxorubicin + vincristine**

- **CAE: cyclophosphamide + doxorubicin + etoposide**

- **ICE: ifosfamide + carboplatin + etoposide**

Other drugs or drug combinations that may be used include:
- **CEV: cyclophosphamide + etoposide + vincristine**

- **cyclophosphamide + methotrexate + lomustine with or without vincristine**

- **etoposide alone**

- **teniposide alone**

- **topotecan**

- **paclitaxel**

- **yttrium-90 radiolabeled carcinoembryonic-antigen antibody (I)**

(I) = immunotherapy

dred patients, *prophylactic cranial irradiation* (PCI) can lower a person's chances of developing a secondary tumor of the central nervous system by more than half.

Non-Small-Cell Lung Cancer

Surgery or Radiation Therapy

"In the studies that are available, patients who are operated on have a better rate of survival than those who are irradiated," notes Dr. Sridhar. "Unless there are contraindications for surgery, or the person refuses to have it, one should go for the operation." Among the situations that can thwart plans for lung-resection surgery are:

- A heart attack in the preceding three months

- A tumor in the opposite lung

- Malignant *pleural effusion,* a pooling of cancer-contaminated fluid in the pleural space between the membranes that encase each lung

- Dissemination of the cancer to sites outside of the chest

Another consideration is whether or not the patient can be expected to withstand the loss of lung tissue. Advanced age, however, does not necessarily determine someone's suitability for surgery. "We have eighty-five-year-olds who go through lung surgery with no major complications," says Dr. Sridhar. "Nevertheless, the older the patient, the more apt we are to go nonsurgical."

Types of Lung-Cancer Surgery—Lobectomy with lymph-node dissection is the standard minimal surgery for lung cancer. A wedge or segmental resection would be performed in situations where the doctor is looking to relieve symptoms rather than effect a cure. "We might also be forced to go to a wedge resection because a patient's lung capacity is so poor from smoking that he can't tolerate the more extensive surgery," says Dr. Sridhar. (Many people with lung cancer suffer from chronic obstructive pulmonary disease too.)

LUNG CANCER/ Surgical Procedures
Wedge resection/segmental resection: surgical removal of a small portion of the lung. Average hospital stay: 7 days; 3–5 days if done by way of video surgery, or *thoracoscopy*
Lobectomy: the standard surgery for lung tumors, in which a section, or lobe, is taken out. The left lung has two lobes; the right lung, three. A *bilobectomy* removes two lobes of the right lung. Average hospital stay: 7 days
Pneumonectomy: surgical removal of the entire lung. Average hospital stay: 7 days

---

The Informed Patient
Advantages and Disadvantages of Video Surgery (Thoracoscopy)

In the traditional operation to remove all or part of a lung, the thoracic surgeon makes a six-to-ten-inch incision around the side of the chest and spreads the ribs apart. Video thoracoscopy, a less invasive technique for wedge resections as well as lobectomies, requires several small incisions, none longer than two inches. Surgery takes place through these portals in the chest, and patients leave the hospital in about half the time.

The downside to thoracoscopy is that it affords limited exposure to the lung, says Dr. Sridhar, who compares the procedure to "looking through a telescope; you're able to inspect only one part at a time." Accordingly, the chances of the cancer recurring are higher following video surgery than following formal surgery. It may, however, be an option for tumors situated on the surface of the lung.

Doctors usually refrain from ordering the most debilitating lung-cancer operation, pneumonectomy, "unless they believe there is a good chance of curing the cancer," Dr. Sridhar says, because going through life with a single lung places a person at heightened risk for a number of potentially life-threatening complications. The Sylvester Comprehensive Cancer Center and other institutions are experimenting with delivering chemotherapy first, says Dr. Sridhar, "in an effort to reduce the amount of tissue that needs to be sacrificed, so that the patient can have a lobectomy rather than a pneumonectomy."

Recuperating from Lung Surgery—The recovery from any of these surgeries averages six weeks, although one in ten patients continue to feel pain at the incision site longer. Your surgeon may recommend a respiratory therapist to teach you special breathing exercises and techniques for coughing effectively so that secretions from the lung don't accumulate in the air passages.

Radiation Therapy

External-beam radiotherapy, delivered over six weeks, robs patients of some degree of lung function. This is a permanent condition, as is the mild difficulty in swallowing that afflicts approximately one in twenty patients. One setting where radiation might hold an edge over surgery, says Dr. Sridhar, is if the tumor is embedded deep within the lung of a person with poor respiratory function. Irradiating the cancer will spare at least some of the surrounding tissue, he explains, whereas the surgical option "may necessitate removing the entire lung."

For free referrals to
pulmonary-rehabilitation
programs, contact:

American Association of
Cardiovascular and Pulmonary
Rehabilitation
7611 Elmwood Avenue, Suite 201
Middleton, WI 53562
608-831-6989
http://www.aacvpr.org

Chemotherapy

"The major advance in treatment for non-small-cell lung cancer is the recognition that stage III NSCLC is sensitive to chemotherapy," says Dr. Sridhar. "I now have survivors of ten years or longer who at the time of diagnosis were told they had just weeks to live." A study conducted by the Hoag Cancer Center in Newport Beach, California, followed two groups of patients with stage III NSCLC: one treated with chemotherapy and radiation, the other with radiation alone. After five years, one in six members of the dual-therapy arm were still alive— nearly three times as many as in the radiation-only group.

For operable stage III non-small-cell lung cancer (stage IIIA), "the majority opinion today is to give chemotherapy, or chemo and radiotherapy, followed by surgery." For inoperable patients (stage IIIB), state-of-the-art treatment consists of chemotherapy followed by radiation, or the two treatments administered simultaneously. The cornerstone of drug therapy for lung cancer is cisplatin (brand name: Platinol), often in combination with vinblastine (Velban). Another popular pairing, cisplatin and vinorelbine (Navelbine), is preferred by some patients because it is less likely to make their hair fall out.

Patients diagnosed with clinical stage II disease on the basis of imaging exams are frequently found to have stage III NSCLC at the time of surgery and therefore would also be candidates for chemotherapy. In stage I disease, however, the evidence of benefit isn't compelling enough to warrant administering such toxic chemicals.

TREATMENTS FOR ADVANCED LUNG CANCER

LUNG CANCER/ Drug Therapy

Non-Small-Cell Lung Cancer
A variety of drugs and combinations of drugs may be used:
- **cisplatin + vinblastine**
- **cisplatin + doxorubicin + cyclophosphamide**
- **cisplatin + paclitaxel**
- **cisplatin + gemcitabine**
- **mitomycin**
- **vinorelbine**
- **carboplatin**
- **docetaxel**
- **topotecan**
- **irinotecan**
- **ifosfamide**
- **porfimer (PS)**

(PS) = photosensitizer

Nearly half of all people with lung cancer are diagnosed with metastatic disease. Chemotherapy, radiotherapy, and surgery may be used individually or together to prolong life and to ease symptoms such as pain, belabored breathing, chronic coughing, and spitting up blood due to bleeding in the respiratory tract.

In some instances, treatment can add years to patients' lives. For example, lung-cancer cells that break off from the primary tumor often form a secondary tumor in the brain. "Most physicians consider this situation hopeless," observes Dr. Sridhar. "But with the judicious use of surgery and chemotherapy, we now have some patients with metastatic lung cancers of the brain living for many years."

An isolated secondary lesion in the brain ("which is not uncommon") is potentially curable. "If treated properly with chemotherapy and surgery," says Dr. Sridhar, "about 20 percent of the patients will be alive in five years." The same combination of therapies can cure a comparable percentage of patients whose tumor has spread to a single site beyond the chest.

The palette of chemotherapeutic agents expands to possibly include paclitaxel (Taxol), docetaxel (Taxotere), topotecan (Hycamtin), and others. If the cancer reemerges, "patients who had a dramatic response to first-line therapy are more likely to respond to second-line chemotherapy than those who did not." One potential complication for men and women with recurrent or resistant (refractory) non-small-cell lung cancer, he notes, "is the unfortunate fact that more and more insurance companies are refusing to pay for second-line treatment."

See "Insurance Issues" in Chapter Ten, "Getting Help When You Need It."

OTHER THERAPIES THAT MAY BE USED IN THE TREATMENT OF LUNG CANCER

Photodynamic Therapy—PDT may be used palliatively to reduce the size of a tumor that is obstructing one of the lung's airways. The procedure is also approved for treating *microinvasive* NSCLC in cases where surgery and radiotherapy have been ruled out. "Microinvasive" describes in situ carcinoma that has made microscopic inroads into neighboring tissue.

See "Photodynamic Therapy" in Chapter Four, "How Cancer Is Treated."

Stereotactic Radiosurgery (investigational)—Stereotactic radiosurgery plays a minor role in metastatic lung cancer of the brain, partly because so few medical centers own the prohibitively expensive "gamma knife" machine that bombards tumors with pencil-thin beams of high-dose radiation. At the University of Miami's Sylvester Comprehensive Cancer Center, a leading proponent of this technique, "the gamma knife has proved extremely effective in treating brain lesions that are small in number [no more than three] and in size [each no more than 1¼ inches]," says Dr. Sridhar.

See "Stereotactic Radiosurgery" in treatment options for (adult) cancers of the brain, page 508.

Internal Radiation Therapy (palliative treatment)—Most lung tumors grow in the bronchial tubes that deliver oxygen and take away carbon dioxide. The obstruction of an airway can give rise to *postobstructive pneumonia,* in which secretions build up, making it difficult for patients to catch their breath. Until the dangerous condition is brought under control, chemotherapy cannot be given.

Endobronchial radiation, performed using sedation, delivers radiation directly to the tumor through a thin catheter that is fed down the throat and the windpipe. "It is highly effective for relieving the pneumonia," says Dr. Sridhar, "which then allows us to give the chemotherapy."

Endobronchial Stenting (palliative treatment)—Another way to open up a blocked airway endoscopically is for the physician to laser out or burn out *(fulgurate)* a portion of the tumor. With the patient unconscious, a cylinder-like *stent* is passed through a bronchoscope and placed in position, creating a tunnel through the obstruction.

◆ *Ask your doctor about these and any other investigational therapies that might benefit you.*

Cancer of the Colon or Rectum

Overview

TREATMENTS FOR COLORECTAL CANCER THAT HAS NOT METASTASIZED

Surgery

Endoscopic Surgical Procedures—Most colon cancers arise from adenomatous polyps on the intestine's inner lining. The tiny masses, which can also form in the rectum, are usually discovered and removed while in a benign state. Sometimes, though, the biopsy will reveal that the polyps harbor noninvasive cancer.

Endoscopic surgery involving no incision (polypectomy, electrofulguration, or local excision) is often sufficient for eradicating small polyps. However, large lesions that cannot be removed safely this way require abdominal surgery.

Colon Resection (Colectomy)—"In the most common operation for colon cancer, the surgeon removes the cancer and the surrounding normal colon," explains Dr. Peter Rosen, director of the solid-oncology program at the Jonsson Comprehensive Cancer Center in Los Angeles.

COLORECTAL CANCER/Surgical Procedures

Polypectomy: a technique for removing colorectal polyps without cutting into the abdomen. A flexible scope is inserted in the anus and up the bowel. The physician then passes a wire snare through the scope and around the polyp. Generating an electrical current through the loop cuts the polyp and cauterizes the area.
Average hospital stay: 1 day

Electrofulguration: a type of electrosurgery that destroys cancerous tissue with heat generated by a high-frequency current.
Average hospital stay: 1 day

Local excision: A tube is placed in the colon or rectum through the anus and the cancer cut out.
Average hospital stay: 1–2 days

Bowel resection: surgical removal of the large intestine or, more typically, a section of it, with the severed ends sutured together. The surgeon also dissects area lymph nodes, which are sent to pathology for analysis. If the bowel must be excised or the healthy sections cannot be reconnected, an artificial opening, or *stoma,* for eliminating solid waste must be surgically created in the lower abdomen. This is called a *colostomy.*
Average hospital stay: 7–10 days

Pelvic exenteration: If the cancer has invaded the bladder, uterus, vagina, or prostate, the diseased organ is removed at the same time as the cancer in the bowel.

"He also takes out the *mesentery*—the fatty connective tissue that holds the colon in place—and anywhere from ten to thirty adjacent lymph nodes, to stage the disease."

In both cancer of the colon and cancer of the rectum, a finding of positive lymph nodes classifies the tumor as stage III. The number of affected nodes is a significant piece of information, for patients who have one to three involved lymph nodes, as I did, tend to fare considerably better than those with four or more.

Some surgeons are now performing *laparoscopic* colon surgery. The advantages of this technique include smaller scars, a shorter hospitalization, and a quicker convalescence than from open surgery. But is it as effective?

"On this issue, there are as many opinions as there are doctors," says Dr. Rosen. "Adherents of standard colectomy feel that you can remove a much larger segment of the bowel and its surrounding contents that way, and that you can better stage the rest of the abdomen. Then there are others who believe equally fervently that the laparoscopic approach serves the purpose just as well."

The twisted colon that forced me to undergo a second operation one week after my colectomy was the exception rather than the rule. According to Dr. Rosen, the recuperation from conventional surgery is generally free of serious complications. "Within a month, most patients are beginning to gain back weight, feel stronger, and doing well overall." Unlike what happens when part of the stomach is surgically removed, you shouldn't have to make any major dietary adjustments. Depending on how large a segment of intestine was taken out, the lone noticeable difference may be more frequent bowel movements.

COLORECTAL CANCER/Treatment Options

Colon Cancer

CARCINOMA IN SITU OF THE COLON

Cancer cells exist in the innermost lining of the colon.

- Polypectomy, to surgically remove the cancer endoscopically, with or without electrofulguration • *or*
- Local excision, to surgically remove the cancer endoscopically • *or*
- Bowel resection, to surgically remove a larger portion of the colon

STAGE I COLON CANCER (DUKES A)

The cancer has spread beyond the inner lining to the second or third layer and involves the wall of the colon.

- Bowel resection

STAGE II COLON CANCER (DUKES B)

The cancer has spread outside the colon to nearby tissue.

- Bowel resection

Under Investigation

- Bowel resection • *followed by*
- Immunochemotherapy, frequently consisting of fluorouracil and levamisole • *or*
- Chemotherapy, frequently consisting of fluorouracil and leucovorin • *or*
- External-beam radiation therapy
- ◆ Ask your doctor about any clinical trials that might benefit you.

STAGE III COLON CANCER (DUKES C)

The cancer involves nearby lymph nodes.

- Bowel resection • *followed by*
- Chemotherapy, frequently consisting of fluorouracil and levamisole • *or*
- Immunochemotherapy, frequently consisting of levamisole and fluorouracil

Under Investigation

- Bowel resection • *followed by one or more of the following therapies:*
- Chemotherapy, frequently consisting of fluorouracil and leucovorin
- Immunochemotherapy, frequently consisting of fluorouracil and levamisole
- External-beam radiation therapy
- Immunologic therapy such as monoclonal-antibody therapy
- ◆ Ask your doctor about any clinical trials that might benefit you.

STAGE IV COLON CANCER (DUKES D)

The cancer has spread to other parts of the body.

- **Surgery, to remove metastases in other organs such as the liver, lung, or ovary •** *or*

- **External-beam radiation therapy, to relieve symptoms •** *or*

- **Chemotherapy, frequently consisting of one or more of the following drugs—fluorouracil, levamisole, leucovorin, irinotecan, methotrexate—to relieve symptoms**

If the cancer is blocking the bowel:

- **Bowel resection, to remove the obstruction •** *or*

- **Bypass surgery, to create an alternate route around the blockage**

Under Investigation

- **New chemotherapy drugs and immunologic agents**

◆ Ask your doctor about any clinical trials that might benefit you.

See treatment options for metastases of the bone, brain, liver, and lung.

RECURRENT COLON CANCER

Your therapy will depend on the treatment you received initially.

- **Chemotherapy, frequently consisting of one or more of the following drugs—fluorouracil, levamisole, leucovorin, irinotecan, methotrexate—to relieve symptoms •** *or*

- **External-beam radiation therapy, to relieve symptoms**

If the cancer has recurred in only one part of the body:

- **Surgery, to remove the cancer**

Under Investigation

- **New chemotherapy drugs and immunologic agents**

◆ Ask your doctor about any clinical trials that might benefit you.

Rectal Cancer

CARCINOMA IN SITU OF THE RECTUM

Cancer cells exist in the innermost lining of the rectum.

- **Local excision •** *or*

- **Polypectomy, with or without electrofulguration •** *or*

- **Electrofulguration •** *or*

- **Bowel resection •** *or*

- **External-beam** *or* **internal radiation therapy**

STAGE I RECTAL CANCER (DUKES A)

The cancer has spread beyond the inner lining to the second or third layer and involves the wall of the rectum.

- Bowel resection

Or:

{
- External-beam radiation therapy · *with or without*
- Chemotherapy, frequently consisting of fluorouracil · *followed by*
- Bowel resection

Or:

- Internal radiation therapy

Or, in selected patients:

- Electrofulguration

STAGE II RECTAL CANCER (DUKES B)

The cancer has spread outside the rectum to nearby tissue.

- Bowel resection · *followed by*
- Chemotherapy, frequently consisting of fluorouracil, alone or in combination with leucovorin

Or:

{
- External-beam radiation therapy · *with or without*
- Chemotherapy, frequently consisting of fluorouracil, alone or in combination with leucovorin · *followed by*
- Bowel resection · *followed by*
- Chemotherapy

Or:

- External-beam radiation therapy administered during bowel resection

If the cancer has spread to neighboring organs, such as the bladder, uterus, vagina, or prostate:

{
- Bowel resection · *plus*
- Pelvic exenteration, to surgically remove any organ(s) affected by the cancer · *followed by*

{
- Chemotherapy, frequently consisting of fluorouracil, alone or in combination with leucovorin · *plus*
- External-beam radiation therapy

STAGE III RECTAL CANCER (DUKES C)

The cancer involves nearby lymph nodes.

- Bowel resection · *followed by*
- Chemoradiation, frequently consisting of fluorouracil, alone or in combination with leucovorin

Or:
- **External-beam radiation therapy** • *or*
- **Chemoradiation, frequently consisting of fluorouracil, alone or in combination with leucovorin** • *followed by*
- **Bowel resection** • *followed by*
- **Chemotherapy**

Or:
- **External-beam radiation therapy given during surgery**

Or:
- **Chemoradiation, frequently consisting of fluorouracil, alone or in combination with leucovorin, to relieve symptoms**

If the cancer has spread to neighboring organs, such as the bladder, uterus, vagina, ovary, or prostate:
- **Bowel resection** • *plus*
- **Pelvic exenteration** • *followed by*
- **Chemotherapy, frequently consisting of fluorouracil, alone or in combination with leucovorin** • *plus*
- **External-beam radiation therapy**

STAGE IV RECTAL CANCER (DUKES D)

The cancer has spread to other parts of the body.
- **Surgery, to remove a secondary tumor in other organs such as the liver, lung, or ovary**

Or:
- **Chemoradiation, frequently consisting of fluorouracil, alone or in combination with other agents, to relieve symptoms**

If the cancer is blocking the rectum:
- **Bowel resection, to remove the obstruction** • *or*
- **Bypass surgery, to create an alternate route around the blockage**

Under Investigation
- **New chemotherapy drugs and immunologic agents**
- ◆ Ask your doctor about any clinical trials that might benefit you.

See treatment options for metastases of the brain, bone, liver, and lung.

RECURRENT RECTAL CANCER

- **External-beam radiation therapy, to relieve symptoms** • *with or without*
- **Chemoradiation, frequently consisting of fluorouracil, alone or with other agents, to relieve symptoms**

If the cancer has recurred in only one part of the body:
- Surgery, to remove the cancer

Under Investigation
- New chemotherapy drugs and immunologic agents

◆ Ask your doctor about any clinical trials that might benefit you.

Rectum Resection (Proctectomy)—Many patients, upon learning they have colorectal cancer, assume they will need to have a permanent colostomy: a surgically fashioned opening in the abdomen for the elimination of solid waste. In colon cancer, this can be avoided 99 percent of the time.

A tumor in the rectum presents a greater challenge for the surgeon, particularly if it's situated low in the tube, near the anus. "The difficulty," explains Dr. Rosen, "is that the rectum cannot be joined back together with the bowel. If we remove the rectum, in what's called an *abdominal-perineal resection*, there's nothing to attach it to. We seal off the anus, and the person must live with a colostomy.

"That doesn't pertain to all rectal cancers," he emphasizes. Overall only 15 percent of colorectal-cancer patients undergo colostomies. "By using modern stapling techniques, we can still connect the rectum to the colon after surgery, without the need for a colostomy." The medical term for this procedure is a *low anterior resection*, or LAR. Additionally, a skilled surgeon may be able to take one of two alternate routes to the rectum, going in through the anus (transanal) or through the buttocks (transcoccygeal). Neither technique is widely practiced, though, "because most of the cancers we are faced with are too large and too extensive for that approach," according to Dr. Rosen.

See "Ostomies" in Appendix A for the names of organizations that offer information and support to people with colostomies.

Radiation Therapy

Radiation has little place in colon cancer because the colon is a moving target, contracting and expanding as it nudges liquid waste from one end to the other. Conventional wisdom holds that the risk of irradiating surrounding organs outweighs the potential benefits, although the treatment is being studied in some patients.

By contrast, says Dr. Rosen, "the rectal area is 'fixed,' " and easily irradiated without damaging neighboring tissues. Men and women with stage II or III disease frequently receive radiation and chemotherapy following surgery. "Now we also have many protocols that involve *pre*operative radiation, sometimes with chemotherapy, in order to limit the amount of surgery by diminishing the amount of cancer that's present." If the tumor has perforated the rectal wall (stage II and beyond), drug therapy continues after proctectomy.

Pelvic radiotherapy can inflame the rectum, causing it to narrow. A less common complication of *radiation proctitis* is rectal bleeding. These and other symptoms often heal spontaneously, but should they persist, drug therapy, endoscopic laser treatment, or, as a last resort, surgery may be necessary.

See "Radiation Proctitis" in Chapter Seven, "What You Can Expect During Treatment."

Chemotherapy/Immunochemotherapy

Colon Cancer—"The use of chemotherapy after surgery for colon cancer hadn't been very successful until the late 1980s," says Dr. Rosen, "when several studies conducted in the United States and in Europe showed strongly that a combination of fluorouracil and levamisole had a significant effect on prolonging the duration of disease-free survival and enhancing overall survival."

Levamisole (brand name: Ergamisol) is something of an enigma among anticancer agents. Though often classified as an immune response modifier, "we don't know exactly how it works," says Dr. Rosen. It may not be a biologic at all. Around the time that I was diagnosed with cancer, in 1991, investigators were pairing fluorouracil (5-FU) with leucovorin, a drug that enhances the effect of the fluorouracil.

What was then an experimental treatment is now considered at least the equivalent of fluorouracil-levamisole, and may be more effective. In addition, patients complete the fluorouracil-leucovorin regimen in half the time: six months as opposed to twelve. In one survey of one hundred physicians who treated colon cancer, eighty said they put their patients on 5-FU and leucovorin, which is also known as Wellcovorin.

Either combination is considered standard adjuvant treatment for stage III colon cancer. Adjuvant therapy is generally not considered necessary for stage II disease, "because most patients are cured by surgery," explains Dr. Rosen. However, it may be appropriate for a small group of men and women whose cancer extends throughout the multiple layers of the bowel wall. "The conventional management is still observation following surgery," says Dr. Rosen, "but some oncologists, myself included, will look at the particulars of each case. If a patient is young and the tumor poorly differentiated, I tend to offer those patients adjuvant therapy."

Rectal Cancer—In rectal cancer, the same situation—a stage II tumor that pervades the entire thickness of the rectum—typically warrants postoperative chemotherapy and external-beam radiation therapy. The drugs of choice are either fluorouracil-leucovorin or 5-FU alone, delivered by *continuous infusion* during the approximately six weeks of radiotherapy.

TREATMENTS FOR ADVANCED
COLORECTAL CANCER

**COLORECTAL CANCER/
Drug Therapy**

Colon Cancer
First-line therapy frequently consists of:
- **fluorouracil + levamisole (I) or leucovorin**

Other drugs that may be used include:
- **irinotecan**
- **methotrexate**
- **floxuridine**
- **mitomycin**
- **lomustine**

Rectal Cancer
First-line therapy frequently consists of:
- **fluorouracil alone or + leucovorin**

(I) = immunologic agent

Surgery

Stage IV colorectal cancers travel most commonly to the liver and the lungs. A person with secondary colorectal cancer of the liver is considered operable so long as the liver bears no more than three metastatic lesions. Remarkably, one in five of these patients can be cured by *hepatic resection surgery,* even if they have relapsed. Surgery may also be performed to relieve symptoms; for example, to construct a detour around a tumor blocking the large intestine.

Chemotherapy (Palliative Treatment)

"Fluorouracil is the standard drug for stage IV colon or rectal cancer," says Dr. Rosen, "although there is controversy over how to best give the 5-FU: By injection? By continuous infusion? With or without leucovorin?" To date, no combination incorporating fluorouracil has surpassed 5-FU alone.

Similar questions surround irinotecan (Camptosar), introduced commercially in 1996, four decades after the development of fluorouracil. "It is a totally different compound than 5-FU," says Dr. Rosen, who took part in the clinical trials testing the *enzyme inhibitor* in patients. "We know it is active against colon cancer. Whether irinotecan is best used in combination with fluorouracil or separately is the subject of investigation."

OTHER THERAPIES THAT MAY BE USED IN THE TREATMENT OF COLORECTAL CANCER

Immunotherapy (investigational)—Monoclonal antibody 17-1A, the first *MOAB* approved for use anywhere, in Germany, is presently being assessed in the United States. According to one German study, antibody 17-1A (Panorex) improved the five-year survival rate among patients with stage III colon cancer by 30 percent. Other biologics under evaluation include alpha-interferon 2A (Roferon-A) and tumor vaccines.

◆ *Ask your doctor about these and any other investigational therapies that might benefit you.*

Hodgkin's Disease and Non-Hodgkin's Lymphomas

Overview

The strategies for treating Hodgkin's disease and non-Hodgkin's lymphomas are similar, usually consisting of radiotherapy and/or chemotherapy. But given the various factors that influence the direction of therapy—not to mention the more than ten different types of non-Hodgkin's lymphomas—we review the two cancers separately, to minimize confusion.

Hodgkin's Disease

TREATMENTS FOR HODGKIN'S DISEASE THAT HAS NOT METASTASIZED

Because Hodgkin's disease advances slowly, more than three in four patients can be cured. The treatment strategy depends on several considerations, beginning with the cancer's presentation. Patients whose initial symptoms included sheet-soaking night sweats, unexplained fever over 101 degrees, and a similarly mysterious weight loss of more than 10 percent over the previous six months are said to have "B symptom" Hodgkin's disease. For them, the primary treatment is generally drug therapy, regardless of stage.

HODGKIN'S DISEASE and NON-HODGKIN'S LYMPHOMAS/ Treatment Options

Hodgkin's Disease

Each stage of Hodgkin's disease is divided into A or B, with B indicating that a patient has experienced these symptoms: (1) weight loss exceeding 10 percent of normal body weight in the previous six months, (2) fever, and (3) night sweats.

STAGE I HODGKIN'S DISEASE

The cancer is found in only one region of lymph nodes or in only one area or organ outside of the lymph nodes.

Stage IA

If the cancer is above the diaphragm and does not involve a large part of the chest:

- External-beam radiation therapy

Or:

- Chemotherapy, frequently consisting of one of the following regimens: ABVD, VBM (see "Drug Therapy" box) • *alone or followed by*
- External-beam radiation therapy

If the cancer is above the diaphragm and involves a large part of the chest:

- External-beam radiation therapy • *plus*
- Chemotherapy, frequently consisting of one of the following regimens: ABVD, MOPP/ABV, MOPP/ABVD

Or:

- External-beam radiation therapy

If the cancer is below the diaphragm:

- Chemotherapy, frequently consisting of ABVD • *alone or followed by*
- External-beam radiation therapy

Stage IB

- Chemotherapy, frequently consisting of ABVD • *alone or followed by*
- External-beam radiation therapy

STAGE II HODGKIN'S DISEASE

The cancer is found in two or more lymph nodes on the same side of the diaphragm; or the cancer is found in only one area or organ outside of the lymph nodes and in the surrounding nodes, and other lymph nodes on the same side of the diaphragm may also have cancer.

Stage IIA

If the cancer is above the diaphragm and does not involve a large part of the chest:

- **External-beam radiation therapy** · *with or without*
- **Chemotherapy, frequently consisting of one of the following regimens: ABVD, VBM**

If the cancer is above the diaphragm and involves a large part of the chest:

- **External-beam radiation therapy** · *with or without*
- **Chemotherapy, frequently consisting of one of the following regimens: ABVD, MOPP/ABV, MOPP/ABVD**

If the cancer is below the diaphragm:
- **Chemotherapy, frequently consisting of ABVD** · *alone or followed by*
- **External-beam radiation therapy**

Or:
- **External-beam radiation therapy alone**

Stage IIB

- **Chemotherapy, frequently consisting of ABVD** · *alone or followed by*
- **External-beam radiation therapy**

STAGE III HODGKIN'S DISEASE

The cancer is found in lymph-node regions on both sides of the diaphragm and may also have spread to an area or organ near the lymph-node areas and/or to the spleen.

Stage IIIA

If the cancer does not involve a large part of the chest:

- **Chemotherapy, frequently consisting of one of the following regimens: ABVD, MOPP/ABV, MOPP/ABVD** · *alone or followed by*
- **External-beam radiation therapy**

Or:
- **External-beam radiation therapy alone**

If the cancer involves a large part of the chest:
- **Chemotherapy, frequently consisting of one of the following regimens: ABVD, MOPP/ABV, MOPP/ABVD** · *followed by*
- **External-beam radiation therapy**

Stage IIIB

- **Chemotherapy, frequently consisting of one of the following regimens: ABVD, MOPP/ABV, MOPP/ABVD** · *alone or followed by*
- **External-beam radiation therapy**

STAGE IV HODGKIN'S DISEASE

The cancer has spread in more than one spot to an organ or organs outside the lymphatic system, and cancer cells may or may not be found in lymph nodes near these organs; or the cancer has spread to only one organ outside the lymphatic system but involves lymph nodes far away from that organ.

- Chemotherapy, frequently consisting of one of the following regimens: ABVD, MOPP/ABV, MOPP/ABVD, MOP-BAP • *alone or followed by*

- External-beam radiation therapy

Under Investigation

- High-dose chemotherapy • *followed by*

- Autologous peripheral-blood stem-cell transplantation or bone-marrow transplantation

- ◆ Ask your doctor about any clinical trials that might benefit you.

RECURRENT HODGKIN'S DISEASE

Your therapy will depend on how you were treated initially.

If you previously received radiation therapy alone:
- Chemotherapy

If you previously received chemotherapy alone and the cancer comes back only in the lymph nodes:
- External-beam radiation therapy • *alone or followed by*
- Chemotherapy

If the cancer recurs in more than one area:
- Chemotherapy • *or one or more of the following experimental therapies:*

Under Investigation

- High-dose chemotherapy • *with or without*

- Total-body irradiation • *in preparation for*

- Autologous peripheral-blood stem-cell transplantation or bone-marrow transplantation

- ◆ Ask your doctor about any clinical trials that might benefit you.

Non-Hodgkin's Lymphomas

Low-Grade (Indolent) Lymphomas Include:	High-Grade (Aggressive) Lymphomas Include:
Follicular small cleaved-cell lymphoma	Diffuse mixed-cell lymphoma
Follicular mixed-cell lymphoma	Diffuse large-cell lymphoma
Follicular large-cell lymphoma	Immunoblastic large-cell lymphoma
Diffuse small cleaved-cell lymphoma	Lymphoblastic lymphoma
Small lymphocytic lymphoma	Diffuse small noncleaved-cell lymphoma and Burkitt's lymphoma
Cutaneous T-cell lymphoma	

STAGE I AND CONTIGUOUS STAGE II NON-HODGKIN'S LYMPHOMAS

I: The cancer is found in only one region of lymph nodes or in only one area or organ outside of the lymph nodes.

II: The cancer is found in two or more lymph nodes on the same side of the diaphragm; or the cancer is found in only one area or organ outside of the lymph nodes and in the lymph nodes around it, and other lymph nodes on the same side of the diaphragm may also have cancer.

Medical Terms You're Likely to Hear

Contiguous: This term, which applies solely to stage II non-Hodgkin's lymphomas, denotes that the areas of cancerous lymph nodes are located next to each other. In *noncontiguous* stage II, the positive nodes aren't adjacent to each other but are on the same side of the diaphragm.

Low-Grade (Indolent) Lymphomas
- **External-beam radiation therapy**

If you cannot undergo radiation therapy:
- **Chemotherapy, frequently consisting of CHOP (see "Drug Therapy" box) or another regimen • *or***
- **Observation**
- **Photopheresis, to relieve skin-related symptoms of cutaneous T-cell lymphoma (CTCL), at any stage**

Under Investigation
- Chemotherapy, frequently consisting of CHOP • *plus*
- External-beam radiation therapy
- ◆ Ask your doctor about any clinical trials that might benefit you.

High-Grade (Aggressive) Lymphomas
- Chemotherapy, frequently consisting of CHOP or another regimen • *and/or*
- External-beam radiation therapy

NONCONTIGUOUS STAGE II, STAGE III, AND STAGE IV NON-HODGKIN'S LYMPHOMAS

II: The cancer is found in two or more lymph nodes on the same side of the diaphragm; or the cancer is found in only one area or organ outside of the lymph nodes and in the lymph nodes around it, and other lymph nodes on the same side of the diaphragm may also have cancer.

III: The cancer is found in lymph-node regions on both sides of the diaphragm and may also have spread to an area or organ near the lymph-node areas and/or to the spleen.

IV: The cancer has spread in more than one spot to an organ or organs outside the lymphatic system, and cancer cells may or may not be found in lymph nodes near these organs; or the cancer has spread to only one organ outside the lymphatic system but involves lymph nodes far away from that organ.

Low-Grade (Indolent) Lymphomas

- **Observation** • *or*

- **Chemotherapy, frequently consisting of CHOP, C(M)OPP, CVP, or one or more of the following drugs: fludarabine, cladribine, cyclophosphamide, chlorambucil**

If low-grade follicular non-Hodgkin's lymphoma fails to respond to standard therapy:

- **Immunotherapy, consisting of rituximab, a monoclonal antibody** • *or*

- **Immunotherapy, consisting of denileukin diftitox, an immunotoxin, to relieve symptoms**

Under Investigation #1

- **High-dose chemotherapy** • *with or without*

- **Total-body irradiation** • *in preparation for*

- **Autologous peripheral-blood stem-cell transplantation or bone-marrow transplantation *or* allogeneic bone-marrow transplantation**

Under Investigation #2

- **Immunochemotherapy, frequently consisting of interferon in combination with one or more anticancer drugs**

◆ **Ask your doctor about any clinical trials that might benefit you.**

High-Grade (Aggressive) Lymphomas

- **Chemotherapy, frequently consisting of CHOP or another regimen** • *alone or with*

{
- **Intrathecal chemotherapy, frequently consisting of methotrexate, injected into the cerebrospinal fluid (CNS prophylaxis)** • *and/or*

- **External-beam radiation therapy**

Under Investigation

- **High-dose chemotherapy** • *with or without*

- **Total-body irradiation** • *in preparation for*

- **Autologous peripheral-blood stem-cell transplantation or bone-marrow transplantation *or* allogeneic bone-marrow transplantation**

◆ **Ask your doctor about any clinical trials that might benefit you.**

Lymphoblastic Lymphoma

- **Chemotherapy, frequently consisting of CHOP or another regimen** • *plus*

{
- **Intrathecal chemotherapy, frequently consisting of methotrexate, injected into the cerebrospinal fluid (CNS prophylaxis)** • *with or without*

- **External-beam radiation therapy to areas containing large amounts of cancer**

Under Investigation

- High-dose chemotherapy · *with or without*
- Total-body irradiation · *in preparation for*
- Autologous peripheral-blood stem-cell transplantation or bone-marrow transplantation *or* allogeneic bone-marrow transplantation
- ◆ Ask your doctor about any clinical trials that might benefit you.

Diffuse Small Noncleaved-Cell Lymphoma and Burkitt's Lymphoma

- Chemotherapy, frequently consisting of CHOP or another regimen · *plus*
- Intrathecal chemotherapy, frequently consisting of methotrexate, injected into the cerebrospinal fluid (CNS prophylaxis)

Under Investigation

- High-dose chemotherapy · *with or without*
- Total-body irradiation · *in preparation for*
- Autologous peripheral-blood stem-cell transplantation or bone-marrow transplantation
- ◆ Ask your doctor about any clinical trials that might benefit you.

See treatment options for metastases of the bone, brain, liver, and lung.

RECURRENT NON-HODGKIN'S LYMPHOMAS

Your therapy will depend on how you were treated initially.

Low-Grade (Indolent) Lymphomas

- Chemotherapy, frequently consisting of cyclophosphamide, vincristine, prednisone, fludarabine, cladribine, used singly or in combination, to relieve symptoms · *and/or*
- External-beam radiation therapy

Or:
- Immunotherapy, frequently consisting of rituximab · *or*
- Immunotherapy, consisting of denileukin diftitox, an immunotoxin, to relieve symptoms

Under Investigation

- High-dose chemotherapy · *with or without*
- Total-body irradiation · *in preparation for*
- Autologous peripheral-blood stem-cell or bone-marrow transplantation *or* allogeneic bone-marrow transplantation
- Other immunologic agents
- ◆ Ask your doctor about any clinical trials that might benefit you.

High-Grade (Aggressive) Lymphomas

- High-dose chemotherapy · *with or without*
- Total-body irradiation · *in preparation for*

- **Autologous peripheral-blood stem-cell or bone-marrow transplantation *or* allogeneic bone-marrow transplantation**

Under Investigation

- **Immunotherapy**

◆ Ask your doctor about any clinical trials that might benefit you.

In the absence of these features, the cancer is classified as Hodgkin's disease "A." The tumor's stage, size, and location all enter into the treatment decision. Generally, limited early-stage (IA and IIA) tumors above the diaphragm call for radiation, possibly in conjunction with chemotherapy, while the opposite approach would be taken for cancerous lymph nodes below the diaphragm. There are exceptions, however. According to Dr. Paul Carbone of the University of Wisconsin Comprehensive Cancer Center, "A person could have stage II Hodgkin's disease with two malignant nodes in the neck, and radiation might be the primary treatment. But when someone has a large stage II mass in the mediastinum [the chest compartment], most physicians would probably use the combination of chemotherapy and radiotherapy."

Stage III disease afflicts nodes above and below the diaphragm, and possibly the spleen or a neighboring organ. At this point, chemotherapy emerges as the principal form of treatment. It may be administered alone or with radiotherapy, particularly if the chest contains a massive tumor, or "bulky disease."

Radiation Therapy

External-beam radiation alone achieves cure rates in the vicinity of 90 percent for stage IA Hodgkin's disease and 80 percent for stage IIA. The lymph nodes are interspersed along the body's channels of lymphatic vessels, with clusters located in the neck, armpits, abdomen, and pelvic region. In lymphoma, the high-energy X rays are most effective when trained not only on the tumor but on the surrounding area, or *field:*

Medical Terms You're Likely to Hear

Bulky disease: in Hodgkin's disease, a mass measuring 4 inches, or one that occupies more than one-third of the chest cavity.

---

1. The *mantle field* encompasses the neck, armpits, and chest. The term alludes to the shape of the treatment area, which resembles a cloak draped about the shoulders.

2. The *abdominal field* includes both the spleen and the *para-aortic* nodes in the upper abdomen.
3. The pelvic nodes make up the third field.

HODGKIN'S DISEASE/ Drug Therapy

First-line therapy frequently consists of one of the following regimens:

- ABVD: doxorubicin + bleomycin + vinblastine + dacarbazine

- MOPP/ABV: mechlorethamine + vincristine + procarbazine + prednisone (H) + doxorubicin + bleomycin + vinblastine

- MOPP/ABVD: mechlorethamine + vincristine + procarbazine + prednisone (H) *alternating with* doxorubicin + bleomycin + vinblastine + dacarbazine

- VBM: vinblastine + bleomycin + methotrexate

- MOP-BAP: mechlorethamine + vincristine + prednisone (H) + bleomycin + doxorubicin + procarbazine

Other drugs used may include:

- dexamethasone (H)

- etoposide

- lomustine

(H) = hormonal agent

Depending on the dimensions and location of the mass, one, two, or all three fields may be irradiated. Radiation to the mantle field and the abdominal field is called *subtotal nodal irradiation,* while blanketing the entire trunk is referred to as *total nodal irradiation.*

Chemotherapy

Some of the chemotherapeutic regimens used against Hodgkin's disease involve as many as seven or eight different agents. Of all those tried, the most effective and least toxic is ABVD: doxorubicin (brand name: Adriamycin), bleomycin (Blenoxane), vinblastine (Velban), and dacarbazine (DTIC-Dome).

Non-Hodgkin's Lymphomas

TREATMENTS FOR NON-HODGKIN'S LYMPHOMA THAT HAS NOT METASTASIZED

Non-Hodgkin's lymphomas are far less predictable than Hodgkin's disease and are more likely to spread beyond the lymph nodes. Even stage I tumors can form in the lymph tissue of organs that are not part of the lymphatic system, such as the liver, lung, skin, and bone.

Observation

With indolent lymphomas that have yet to produce symptoms, it is not unusual for treatment to be deferred until the disease becomes symptomatic. This is true at any stage. Dr. Carbone tells of one patient who was three years postdiagnosis and had yet to be treated. "He has malignant lymph nodes in both armpits," he says, "but they have remained stable. He works in construction full-time. Another patient has had lymphoma probably for ten years, but he's never required any specific therapy either."

Dr. Carbone observes that patients can find it unsettling to be told they have cancer but aren't going to be treated. "Once they realize that their condition isn't changing," he says, "they tend to feel confident." When "watchful waiting" is the agreed-upon approach, initially Dr. Carbone will examine patients every three months, "just to monitor the disease's progression. If the tumor is slow-growing, I may see them every six months and get a CT scan once a year."

Radiation Therapy

In non-Hodgkin's lymphomas, unlike in Hodgkin's disease, radiotherapy is usually administered to only one side of the diaphragm. The first site to be irradiated is typically the mantle field: neck, underarms, and chest. If discovered at an early stage, low-grade lymphomas can frequently be cured by radiation alone.

Chemotherapy

Radiotherapy had long been the sole treatment for stage I and contiguous stage II high-grade lymphomas too, until a pair of large multicenter studies, published in the mid-1990s, demonstrated the value of adding chemotherapy. In both trials, all participants were given the four-drug regimen acronymed CHOP: cyclophosphamide (Cytoxan), doxorubicin, vincristine (Oncovin), and the steroid prednisone (Deltasone). The two control groups underwent no further therapy, while the two study groups received radiation. After four years in the first study and six years in the second, the survival rates stood at 87 percent and 73 percent for the combined-therapy arms, versus 75 percent and 58 percent for the single-modality arms. According to the National Cancer Institute, chemo supplemented by external-beam radiation is without question the "preferred option" for early-stage aggressive non-Hodgkin's lymphoma.

TREATMENTS FOR ADVANCED HODGKIN'S DISEASE AND NON-HODGKIN'S LYMPHOMAS

Chemotherapy

In advanced Hodgkin's disease and high-grade non-Hodgkin's lymphoma (NHL), oncologists generally rely on the same drug regimens

NON-HODGKIN'S LYMPHOMAS/Drug Therapy

First-line therapy frequently consists of one or more of the following drugs or drug combinations:

- CHOP: cyclophosphamide + doxorubicin + vincristine + prednisone (H)

- CVP: cyclophosphamide + vincristine + prednisone (H)

- C(M)OPP: cyclophosphamide + vincristine + procarbazine + prednisone (H)

- fludarabine

- cladribine

- cyclophosphamide

- chlorambucil

Other drugs or drug combinations used may include:

- MACOP-B: methotrexate + leucovorin + doxorubicin + cyclophosphamide + vincristine + prednisone (H) + bleomycin

- m-BACOD: methotrexate + bleomycin + doxorubicin + cyclophosphamide + vincristine + dexamethasone (H)

- ProMACE-CytaBOM: prednisone (H) + doxorubicin + cyclophosphamide + etoposide *followed by* cytarabine + bleomycin + vincristine + methotrexate

- interferon (I)

- rituximab (I)

- carmustine

- ifosfamide   *(cont.)*

used in early-stage disease: ABVD and CHOP, respectively. The conventional chemotherapeutic agents for low-grade lymphomas include fludarabine (Fludara) or cladribine (Leustatin), from the *antimetabolite* family; cyclophosphamide or chlorambucil (Leukeran), a pair of oral *alkylating agents;* or any of several combinations incorporating cyclophosphamide, vincristine, and prednisone.

Radiation therapy may be added.

Intrathecal Chemotherapy (CNS Prophylaxis)—More than half of all cases of NHL are advanced at the time of diagnosis. Having one of the aggressive forms heightens the possibility of developing a secondary tumor of the central nervous system in the future. The lifetime risk is 20 to 30 percent for men and women with any of three especially virulent high-grade lymphatic cancers: lymphoblastic lymphoma, diffuse small noncleaved-cell lymphoma, and Burkitt's lymphoma.

Under these circumstances, says Dr. Paul Moots, a neurologic oncologist at the Vanderbilt Cancer Center in Nashville, "it is standard practice to treat the brain and spinal cord as part of induction chemotherapy, whether there's any demonstrable metastasis present or not. The cancer is there," emphasizes Dr. Moots (who on that basis objects to the term *prophylactic,* or preventive, therapy), "but it is in a stage where it is not yet clinically apparent."

CNS prophylaxis would also be recommended in the event that the lymphoma has migrated to the testicles, the sinuses, or—depending upon your doctor's point of view (there's some controversy here)—the bone marrow. The chemotherapy, often methotrexate, is injected directly into the cerebrospinal fluid that surrounds the brain and spinal cord, with the needle placed between two vertebrae in the lower spine.

• **vinblastine**
• **mechlorethamine**
• **teniposide**
• **thiotepa**
• **denileukin diftitox (I)**
• **methoxsalen (PS)**
(H) = hormonal agent (I) = immunologic agent (PS) = photosensitizer

RECURRENT HODGKIN'S DISEASE AND NON-HODGKIN'S LYMPHOMAS

High-Dose Chemotherapy and Autologous Peripheral-Blood Stem-Cell or Bone-Marrow Transplantation *or* Allogeneic Bone-Marrow Transplantation

Clinical trials have yet to ascertain the value of barraging advanced-stage lymphomas with intensive chemotherapy, then replacing the ravaged bone marrow with healthy marrow from the patient (autologous) or a donor (allogeneic). However, it is the favored form of treatment when high-grade non-Hodgkin's lymphoma has come out of remission. The National Cancer Institute estimates that as many as four in ten relapsed patients who undergo high-dose chemotherapy followed by transplantation will live disease free for a lengthy period of time.

Autotransplantation, and to a lesser extent, allogenic transplantation, are certainly options for recurrent Hodgkin's disease and low-grade NHL, although the outlook tends to be brighter for these patients without resorting to such drastic measures. The ten-year survival rate from combination chemotherapy approaches 80 percent for people with relapsed Hodgkin's. And indolent non-Hodgkin's lymphomas are unique among cancers in that should they return, they often respond well to retreatment.

Another unusual characteristic of recurrent NHL is that the cell type can sometimes change from aggressive to indolent, and vice versa. This *histologic conversion* occurs most frequently with low-grade lymphoma in the bone marrow and high-grade lymphoma in the lymph nodes. The relapsed cancer is treated according to its current incarnation.

OTHER THERAPIES THAT MAY BE USED IN THE TREATMENT OF NON-HODGKIN'S LYMPHOMAS

Immunotherapy (standard)/**Immunochemotherapy** (investigational)— Clinical trials evaluating the effectiveness of combining chemotherapy and the *immune response modifier* interferon for advanced low-grade lymphomas have produced "a mixed bag in terms of results," says Dr. Carbone. Far more promising is the introduction of rituximab, the first *monoclonal antibody* to win approval from the federal Food and Drug Administration for treating cancer—specifically, any of the three follicular low-grade NHLs when other therapies fail.

Rituximab, known commercially as Rituxan, is a "naked" antibody—that is, it doesn't need to be coupled to a radioactive substance to wipe out cancer cells. In clinical trials, the genetically engineered antibody was given to 166 patients with advanced low-grade non-Hodgkin's lymphoma. All had previously undergone chemotherapy without success. Half the volunteers saw their tumors shrink by at least 50 percent; six went into complete remission. A 1999 study coordinated by Buffalo's Roswell Park Cancer Institute assessed the effectiveness of Rituxan and the four-drug chemo regimen known as CHOP. Of forty patients, all but two experienced a full response (55 percent) or a partial response (40 percent). Adding to Rituxan's appeal is the fact that the four infusions can be completed within three weeks, as compared to the four to six months necessary for delivering chemotherapy.

Rituximab was soon joined by a second immunotherapy for a chemo-resistant non-Hodgkin's lymphoma: denileukin diftitox (Ontak). The *immunotoxin* may be ordered for certain patients with a rare, slow-growing disease called *cutaneous T-cell lymphoma*, or CTCL. Its signature is unsightly patches of scaly brownish-black skin that if left untreated can blanket the body and face. Eventually the plaques turn malignant. They itch like mad, are prone to infection, and can tunnel under the skin to attack internal organs.

Scientists discovered that three in five CTCL tumors have receptors on their surfaces for the natural immune protein interleukin-2. Ontak is produced in the laboratory by fusing material from the diphtheria toxin to IL-2. When infused into the patient's bloodstream, the interleukin escorts the toxin to its intended target.

The company that manufactured and marketed the innovative therapy tested it in seventy-one patients, all of whom had failed standard chemotherapy. (Wouldn't it be more accurate to say that standard chemotherapy had failed them?) Thirty percent of the tumors shrank by a minimum of 50 percent, while 10 percent of the lesions vanished entirely.

Photopheresis (palliative treatment)—Photopheresis, another palliative therapy for cutaneous T-cell lymphoma, can best be described as a cross between photodynamic therapy and immunotherapy, only it takes place outside the body. T cells are a type of white blood cell. In CTCL, a mutation occurs, and abnormal T cells begin to proliferate out of control.

Here is how photopheresis works. First, a catheter needle is placed in the patient's arm, and a portion of the blood is routed into a special machine. The unit culls out the white cells and sends the rest of the blood back to the arm. Next a light-activated drug called methoxsalen (Uvadex) is injected into the machine. This *psoralen,* a family of natural compounds found in certain vegetables and fruits, infiltrates the nucleus of the white blood cells and attaches itself to the DNA within. Previously, patients took the Uvadex orally, and at a higher dose, but the injection method exposes more cells to the agent.

When ultraviolet light is aimed at the white cells, the methoxsalen tightens its grip on the DNA. This prevents the cell from reproducing. The treated cells are then returned to the patient. Based on laboratory tests, it is believed that photopheresis may also reprogram cells that in turn stimulate an immune response against cancerous T cells. In a trio of studies, 28 to 54 percent of patients with CTCL responded to the treatment within six months, and their skin condition improved dramatically.

♦ *Ask your doctor about these and any other investigational therapies that might benefit you.*

Cancer of the Bladder

Overview

TREATMENTS FOR BLADDER CANCER THAT HAS NOT METASTASIZED

Surgery

Transurethral Resection with Fulguration—Seventy to 80 percent of bladder tumors are superficial at the time of diagnosis, meaning that the disease is either on the surface of the organ's inner lining (carcinoma in situ) or has penetrated the lining (stage I) but not the bladder's muscular wall. Most can be treated without having to remove the bladder, and the five-year survival rate approaches 95 percent.

In a transurethral resection, the surgeon inserts a flexible cystoscope through the urethra and into the bladder. An electrified wire

BLADDER CANCER/Treatment Options

CARCINOMA IN SITU OF THE BLADDER

The cancer is found only on the bladder's inner lining.
- **Transurethral resection with fulguration** · *alone or followed by*

{
- **Intravesical immunotherapy, consisting of Bacillus Calmette-Guérin (BCG) or alpha-interferon** · *or*

- **Intravesical chemotherapy, frequently consisting of thiotepa, doxorubicin, mitomycin, or valrubicin**

Under Investigation #1
- **Photodynamic therapy**

Under Investigation #2
- **Intravesical immunotherapy, consisting of alpha-interferon** · *or*

- **Immunochemotherapy, consisting of mitomycin and interferon**

♦ **Ask your doctor about any clinical trials that might benefit you.**

STAGE I BLADDER CANCER

The cancer has spread a little deeper into the inner lining.
- **Transurethral resection with fulguration** · *alone or with*

{
- **Intravesical immunotherapy, consisting of BCG** · *or*

- **Intravesical chemotherapy, frequently consisting of thiotepa, doxorubicin, or mitomycin**

Or:
- **Segmental cystectomy, to surgically remove the cancerous portion of the bladder** · *or*

- **Radical cystectomy, to surgically remove the bladder, prostate, and seminal vesicles in men; and the bladder, uterus, ovaries, fallopian tubes, urethra, and part of the vagina in women**

Or:
- **Internal radiation therapy** · *with or without*

- **External-beam radiation therapy**

Under Investigation
- **Intravesical chemotherapy** *alone*

♦ **Ask your doctor about any clinical trials that might benefit you.**

STAGE II BLADDER CANCER

The cancer has spread to the inner half of the bladder's muscular wall.
- **Radical cystectomy, *with or without* pelvic lymph-node dissection** · *with or without*

- **External-beam radiation therapy, given prior to surgery**

Or:
- **External-beam radiation therapy** • *and/or*
- **Internal radiation therapy**

Or, in selected patients:
- **Transurethral resection with fulguration** • *or*
- **Segmental cystectomy**

Under Investigation

{
- **Transurethral resection** • *or*
- **Segmental cystectomy** • *followed by*
}

- **Chemotherapy, frequently consisting of various combinations of drugs, such as methotrexate, cisplatin, and vinblastine, with or without doxorubicin** • *followed by*
- **Chemoradiation**

Or:

{
- **Transurethral resection** • *or*
- **Segmental cystectomy** • *preceded or followed by*
}

- **Chemotherapy, frequently consisting of various combinations of drugs, such as methotrexate, cisplatin, and vinblastine, with or without doxorubicin**

- ◆ **Ask your doctor about any clinical trials that might benefit you.**

STAGE III BLADDER CANCER

The cancer has spread throughout the muscular wall and/or to the layer of tissue surrounding the bladder.
- **Radical cystectomy, *with or without* pelvic lymph-node dissection** • *or*

{
- **External-beam radiation therapy** • *with or without*
- **Internal radiation therapy**
}

Or:
- **External-beam radiation therapy** • *with*
- **Chemotherapy, frequently consisting of cisplatin**

Or, in selected patients:
- **Segmental cystectomy** • *or*
- **Internal radiation therapy**

Under Investigation
- **Chemotherapy, given before or after surgery, or at the same time as radiation therapy**

- ◆ **Ask your doctor about any clinical trials that might benefit you.**

STAGE IV BLADDER CANCER

The cancer has spread to the nearby reproductive organs or to area lymph nodes and may also have metastasized to distant sites in the body.

If no regional lymph nodes or distant organs are affected:
- Radical cystectomy

If the cancer has spread to one or more lymph nodes:
- External-beam radiation therapy · *alone or with*
- Chemotherapy, frequently consisting of various combinations of drugs, such as methotrexate, cisplatin, and vinblastine, with or without doxorubicin

Or:
- Cystectomy to surgically remove the bladder, to relieve symptoms · *or*
- Urinary-diversion surgery, to relieve symptoms · *alone or with*
- Chemotherapy, frequently consisting of various combinations of drugs, such as methotrexate, cisplatin, and vinblastine, with or without doxorubicin, to relieve symptoms

Under Investigation
- Chemotherapy, given before or after surgery, or at the same time as radiation therapy
- ◆ Ask your doctor about any clinical trials that might benefit you.

If the cancer has spread to distant sites:
- External-beam radiation therapy, to relieve symptoms · *or*
- Cystectomy or urinary-diversion surgery, to relieve symptoms

Or:
- Chemotherapy, frequently consisting of various combinations of drugs, including carboplatin, paclitaxel, gemcitabine, and methotrexate, cisplatin, and vinblastine, with or without doxorubicin, to relieve symptoms · *alone or following*
- External-beam radiation therapy, to relieve symptoms · *or*
- Cystectomy or urinary-diversion surgery, to relieve symptoms

Under Investigation
- Other chemotherapy drugs
- ◆ Ask your doctor about any clinical trials that might benefit you.

See treatment options for lung metastases.

RECURRENT BLADDER CANCER

Your therapy will depend on how you were treated initially.

If the cancer recurs only in the bladder:
- Intravesical immunotherapy, consisting of BCG · *or*
- Intravesical chemotherapy, frequently consisting of thiotepa, doxorubicin, or mitomycin

> *Or:*
> - Transurethral resection with fulguration • *followed by*
> { - Intravesical immunotherapy, consisting of BCG • *or*
> - Intravesical chemotherapy, frequently consisting of thiotepa, doxorubicin, or mitomycin
>
> *Or:*
> - External-beam radiation therapy • *or*
> - Cystectomy
>
> *If the cancer recurs locally and you previously had your bladder removed:*
> - Chemotherapy, frequently consisting of M-VAC (see "Drug Therapy" box)
>
> *If the cancer recurs in other organs:*
> - Chemotherapy, frequently consisting of M-VAC • *and/or*
> - Cystectomy or urinary-diversion surgery, to relieve symptoms

loop is then passed through the scope. "The wire 'heats up' and cuts the tumor off the bladder wall," explains Dr. Michael Cooper of Duke University Medical Center. "At the same time, it coagulates the site, to prevent bleeding."

Cystectomy—Even when the cancer has invaded the bladder muscle, three in four patients will reach the five-year postdiagnosis milestone. Segmental cystectomy to take out only the diseased bladder and a margin of healthy tissue is rarely applicable because of the tumor's propensity for growing in multiple areas of the organ.

Most patients undergo radical cystectomy. In women, this extensive operation entails taking out the bladder and the reproductive organs, thus bringing on instant menopause. In male patients, the surgeon excises the bladder, seminal vesicles, and the prostate, which results in impotence. If preserving sexual function is important to you, look for a surgeon experienced in *nerve-sparing radical cystoprostatectomy.* The technique isn't practiced widely but appears to be effective. Baltimore's Johns Hopkins Oncology

---

BLADDER CANCER/ Surgical Procedures

Transurethral resection (TUR) with fulguration: surgical removal of the tumor through a flexible *cystoscope.*
Average hospital stay: 2–3 days

Cystectomy: surgical removal of the bladder. A *segmental cystectomy* resects only the cancerous section of the bladder. Far more common is a *radical cystectomy,* which removes the bladder as well as surrounding organs. The pelvic lymph nodes, too, may be taken out.
Average hospital stay:

- Radical cystectomy, 7–10 days
- Cystectomy, 3 days
- Segmental cystectomy, 7 days

**BLADDER CANCER/
Drug Therapy**

*First-line therapy often consists
of one of the following:*
- **Bacillus Calmette-Guérin (I)**

- **thiotepa**

- **mitomycin**

- **doxorubicin**

*Others drugs or drug combina-
tions used may include:*
- **M-VAC: methotrexate +
  vinblastine + doxorubicin +
  cisplatin**

- **CMV: cisplatin +
  methotrexate + vinblastine**

- **carboplatin**

- **paclitaxel**

- **ifosfamide**

- **gemcitabine**

- **valrubicin**

- **bleomycin**

- **cyclophosphamide**

- **fluorouracil**

- **alpha-interferon (I)**

(I) = immunologic agent

Center, a leader in nerve-sparing prostate surgery, assessed the outcome of seventy-six such operations, performed over a six-year period in the 1980s. More than three in five of the men retained their potency, and the researchers concluded that nerve-sparing cystoprostatectomy in no way compromised cancer control.

Should the bulb-shaped receptacle have to be taken out, the surgeon constructs an alternate route for urine to exit the body. In a *urostomy,* Dr. Cooper explains, "the two ureter tubes that transport urine from the kidneys to the bladder are implanted into a small loop of small intestine, which is then brought out through the abdominal wall." A soft-plastic external pouch, worn on the abdomen, attaches to the protruding opening, or *stoma,* and collects the urine. In Dr. Cooper's experience, "most patients adapt well."

If the idea of having to live with an ostomy bag doesn't appeal to you, inquire about a *continent urostomy.* Here the surgeon uses a segment of intestine to fashion a new pouch for storing urine. To relieve themselves, patients insert a catheter tube through a small opening in the lower abdomen or the belly button. Some men and women may be able to undergo a variation of this in which the artificial bladder is connected to the urethra, facilitating normal urination.

New approaches that allow for bladder-sparing surgery by incorporating systemic chemotherapy and radiation therapy are being evaluated in patient studies. Among the sequences that have been investigated are the following:

1. transurethral resection → chemo → chemo and radiation
2. chemo → radiation and chemo → conservative surgery → chemo

Some clinical trials have reported survival rates comparable to that achieved with aggressive surgery.

♦ *Ask your oncologist if you might be a candidate for bladder preservation.*

See "Sexual Problems" in Chapter Eight, "Take Control: Managing Symptoms, Side Effects, and Complications," and "Ostomies" in Appendix A for the names of organizations that offer information and support to people with urostomies.

Intravesical Immunotherapy or Chemotherapy

Once bladder cancer has occurred, even if it is superficial, the organ's entire inner lining is at risk for a future cancer. Therefore, after the urologist removes all the tumor he can see through the cystoscope, the patient is asked to return for drug treatment to reduce the likelihood of new malignancies developing. One or more drugs is instilled directly into the bladder through a catheter tube. "We then clamp the tube for a period of time," says Dr. Cooper, "so that the drug remains in contact with the bladder lining."

The medication used most often for *intravesical* chemotherapy, Bacillus Calmette-Guérin, or BCG, is considered an immunologic agent, though not in the usual sense. "It's an antituberculous vaccine," explains Dr. Cooper, director of Duke's experimental-therapeutics program. Rather than initiating an immune response specifically against the cancer, "BCG acts as an irritant to provoke a general inflammatory response within the bladder wall." The tumor cells, caught in the cross fire of this cellular skirmish, are destroyed along with other types of cells.

Several chemotherapy drugs have been used for superficial bladder cancer, "but studies suggest that BCG is actually our most effective agent," says Dr. Cooper. It is typically administered once a week over the course of six to eight weeks. According to a study conducted at West Virginia University's Robert C. Byrd Health Science Center, the benefit from BCG improves significantly if three additional weekly treatments are given after three months; and higher still if the three doses are repeated every six months.

Despite a long-term survival rate exceeding 90 percent, drug therapy for carcinoma in situ of the bladder is not a permanent cure, Dr. Cooper stresses. One study tracked patients who'd been treated for superficial bladder cancer. Twenty years or more after therapy, four in five of the tumors came back. Fortunately, recurrences tend to be local. To preserve the bladder, the cancer is cut out endoscopically (transurethral resection with fulguration), after which patients receive BCG. In theory, this can be repeated an unlimited number of times. "Some people," notes Dr. Cooper, "keep on experiencing superficial recurrences and eventually decide to have their bladder taken out. But most patients prefer to keep their bladder if at all possible."

Radiation Therapy with or without Chemotherapy

Radiotherapy is an option for people who are considered poor surgical risks or who are adamant about not having their bladder removed. "Most physicians rely solely on external-beam radiation," says Dr. Cooper, who previously practiced at the Vermont Cancer Center. That may be augmented by *interstitial radiation:* the implantation of a radioisotope directly into the tumor through thin plastic tubes. Although the advantage of adding the drug cisplatin (brand name: Platinol) hasn't been widely studied, it does appear to improve the odds of avoiding a recurrence in the bladder.

TREATMENTS FOR ADVANCED BLADDER CANCER

Metastasis to other sites rules out surgery, unless cystectomy or urinary-diversion surgery is necessary because of a tumor blocking the flow of urine. According to Dr. Cooper, the most promising advances in the treatment of this disease have been in the area of chemotherapy. The conventional regimen of methotrexate, vinblastine (Velbane), doxorubicin (Adriamycin), and cisplatin, or M-VAC, "is highly toxic," says Dr. Cooper, who no longer uses it. "We now have single agents and combinations of drugs, like cisplatin or carboplatin [Paraplatin] given with paclitaxel [Taxol], which are far better tolerated than M-VAC and seem to be just as effective if not more so." Drug therapy for stage IV bladder cancer is curative in only a small percentage of patients and is generally intended to ease symptoms.

OTHER THERAPIES THAT MAY BE USED IN THE TREATMENT OF BLADDER CANCER

Immunotherapy/Immunochemotherapy—Interferon alfa-2a (Roferon-A) has been tested, both alone and combined with chemotherapy, as a second-tier treatment for superficial bladder cancers that fail to respond to BCG therapy.

Photodynamic Therapy (PDT) (investigational)—Destroying superficial tumors with PDT has proved reasonably successful, but its place in bladder cancer has yet to be determined. Furthermore, few medical centers currently practice the technique.

See "Photodynamic Therapy" in Chapter Four, "How Cancer Is Treated."

♦ *Ask your doctor about these and any other investigational therapies that might benefit you.*

Melanoma

Overview

TREATMENTS FOR MELANOMA THAT HAS NOT METASTASIZED

Surgery

Surgery alone is the sole standard therapy for the majority of melanomas. If you've been diagnosed with a noninvasive lesion (melanoma in situ), chances are that the excisional biopsy to remove the questionable mass for pathologic analysis is all the treatment you'll need.

The current trend in dermatology is to biopsy as little surrounding tissue as possible, on the grounds that the growth might be benign. Patients whose cancer has penetrated the skin will usually have to return to the office for a second procedure to widen the border around the site of the excavated tumor.

How wide that margin will be depends on the melanoma's thickness, because the deeper the invasion into the skin, the closer the cancer comes to the vessels that carry blood and lymph fluid throughout the body. "Years ago it was thought that taking a very large margin improved survival," says Dr. Allan Oseroff of the Roswell Park Cancer Institute. "More and more, the feeling is that even if malignant cells have migrated a short distance from the primary lesion, excising a huge amount of tissue increases the morbid-

> **MELANOMA/ Surgical Procedures**
>
> **Conservative reexcision:** surgery to remove any remaining melanoma, plus a margin of surrounding skin. Average hospital stay: outpatient procedure
>
> **Wide excision/reexcision surgery:** surgery to remove the entire melanoma, along with a wider perimeter of tissue. Or it may be performed after the excisional biopsy for the purpose of extending the margin. Average hospital stay: outpatient procedure

MELANOMA/Treatment Options

MELANOMA IN SITU

The cancer exists only in the outer layer of the skin, the epidermis.
- **Excisional biopsy**

STAGE I MELANOMA

The cancer, found in the epidermis and/or the upper part of the dermis, measures less than 1.5 millimeters thick (¹/₁₆ inch).
- **Conservative reexcision following biopsy, to remove any residual cancer along with a rim of normal surrounding tissue •** *or*
- **Wide surgical excision, to remove the melanoma along with a wider rim of normal surrounding tissue**

STAGE II MELANOMA

The cancer, measuring 1.5 millimeters to 4 millimeters (less than ¹/₆ inch) in thickness, has spread to the lower part of the dermis.
- **Wide surgical excision,** *with or without* **lymph-node dissection**

Under Investigation #1
- **Postoperative chemotherapy, possibly consisting of dacarbazine or any of a number of drugs**

Under Investigation #2
- **Postoperative immunotherapy, possibly consisting of high-dose alpha-interferon**

Under Investigation #3
If the melanoma is in the extremities:
- **Postoperative chemotherapy, administered directly into the affected arm or leg (isolated arterial perfusion or intra-arterial infusion)**
- ◆ **Ask your doctor about any clinical trials that might benefit you.**

STAGE III MELANOMA

The cancer measures more than 4 millimeters in thickness; or (2) the cancer has spread to the body tissue below the skin; or (3) the cancer has spawned "satellite" tumors within one inch of the original tumor; or (4) the cancer has spread to nearby lymph nodes, or satellite tumors have developed between the primary tumor and area lymph nodes.

- **Wide surgical excision,** *with or without* **lymph-node dissection • alone or followed by**
- **Immunotherapy, frequently consisting of high-dose interferon**

Under Investigation #1
- **Postoperative chemotherapy, possibly consisting of dacarbazine or any of a number of drugs**

Under Investigation #2
- Postoperative immunotherapy, possibly consisting of levamisole

Under Investigation #3
If the melanoma is in the extremities:
- Postoperative isolated arterial perfusion chemotherapy or intra-arterial infusion chemotherapy

◆ Ask your doctor about any clinical trials that might benefit you.

STAGE IV MELANOMA
The cancer has spread to other organs or to distant lymph nodes.
- Surgery to remove distant metastases, to relieve symptoms *and/or*
- External-beam radiation therapy or internal radiation therapy, to relieve symptoms

Under Investigation #1
- Immunotherapy, frequently consisting of alpha-interferon or interleukin-2; or Bacillus Calmette-Guérin (BCG), injected directly into the cancerous lesions

Under Investigation #2
- Chemotherapy, possibly consisting of dacarbazine or any of a number of drugs

◆ Ask your doctor about any clinical trials that might benefit you.

See treatment options for metastases of the bone, brain, and lung.

RECURRENT MELANOMA
Your therapy will depend on how you were treated initially.

- Surgery to remove the melanoma, to relieve symptoms • *and/or*
- External-beam radiation therapy *or* internal radiation therapy, to relieve symptoms

Under Investigation #1
- New chemotherapy drugs and immunologic agents

Under Investigation #2
If the melanoma recurs in the extremities:
- Isolated arterial perfusion chemotherapy or intra-arterial infusion chemotherapy

◆ Ask your doctor about any clinical trials that might benefit you.

ity of the procedure but doesn't contribute much to the ultimate outcome." Morbidity, in this instance, refers to disfigurement from the operation.

"So for thin melanomas—those measuring less than 1 millimeter in thickness—where the overall prognosis is quite good, the current recommendations are to take a margin of about 1 centimeter, or less than half an inch." This procedure is referred to as a conservative reexcision. Tumors with a depth of roughly 1 millimeter or more call for wider margins. Wide-excision surgery may be performed after the pathology report confirms that the mass is indeed cancerous. Or, in instances where the lesion is clearly a sizable melanoma, says Dr. Oseroff, "we might decide to do a single procedure rather than two." In other words, biopsy and definitive surgery in one.

Wide margins range anywhere from 2 centimeters (¾ inch) to 5 centimeters (2 inches). Remember, that's not 2 inches in diameter, but 2 inches out from the tumor, on all sides. Fortunately, notes Dr. Oseroff, "over the years, the excisions have become less wide than they used to be." For intermediate melanomas, 1 to 4 millimeters deep, a border of 2 centimeters may well be sufficient.

A pair of clinical trials compared the results in two groups of men and women with intermediate melanomas. One had 2-centimeter margins taken; the other, 4-centimeter margins. After six years, the rates of local recurrence, metastasis, and overall survival were virtually identical, with one dramatic difference: Nearly half the patients with the more radical surgery required a *skin graft* to close the incision, whereas among the patients who had lesser margins taken, plastic surgery was necessary in only one in ten cases.

The standard recommendation for stage III melanomas greater than 4 millimeters in depth is to cut out 4 to 5 centimeters of surrounding tissue.

Reconstructive Surgery—"Sometimes when you make a large hole in the skin," says Dr. Oseroff, "you can't always draw the edges together without causing a lot of puckering and distortions." A skin graft, almost always carried out at the same time as the excision, fills the defect with tissue transplanted from another part of the body. If you elect to undergo reconstructive surgery as a separate procedure— also done on an outpatient basis, using local anesthesia—it must take place within a few days, because grafting skin becomes progressively more difficult once the wound has begun to heal. Dr. Oseroff describes the operation as "relatively uncomplicated." Nevertheless, he encourages patients to make sure that their plastic surgeon is experienced in skin repair following the removal of a melanoma.

Whether or not you will need a skin graft depends not only on the tumor's size but on its location, explains Dr. Oseroff. "If the melanoma is on the back, shoulder, or other areas where we can easily move the skin when closing the wound, there's no need for a graft. But if it's on the lower leg, which doesn't have much extra skin, then even a conservative reexcision may require a graft."

Biopsying and Removing the Regional Lymph Nodes—When melanoma has infiltrated nearby lymph nodes (stage III), the surgeon removes the nodes in the region, with the intent of achieving a cure. Tumors up to 1.5 millimeters thick (stage I) don't justify a precautionary lymph-node dissection, says Dr. Oseroff, because the outlook is so encouraging, with a five-year survival rate of 95 percent. "Therefore, it's unlikely that taking out the nodes would do anything other than to cause problems."

The great debate in melanoma concerns the value of sampling lymph nodes when presented with stage II melanomas, which can be as shallow as 1.5 millimeters or as deep as 4 millimeters. "Because melanomas occur in random areas of the body, it's not always clear which set of lymph nodes the tumor feeds," says Dr. Oseroff. In addition, a clinical exam can sometimes miss a melanoma that has spread to nearby lymph nodes.

One of the major breakthroughs in melanoma was the advent of *sentinel-node mapping* in the early 1990s. This technique to pinpoint the sentinel lymph node (SLN)—the first node or nodes to receive drainage from the tumor—has been used experimentally in breast cancer, but at state-of-the-art centers it is now standard in melanoma.

During wide-excision surgery, the surgeon injects a blue dye and a radioactive tracer agent into the melanoma. A handheld probe then tracks the path of the mapping agent. The first node reached is designated the sentinel node, which is immediately biopsied and examined under the microscope. When lymph-node mapping and SLN biopsy are preceded by a nuclear-medicine scan called *lymphoscintigraphy,* the ability to identify the draining lymph node nears 100 percent. Preoperative lymphoscintigraphy, says Dr. Douglas Reintgen of the H. Lee Moffitt Cancer Center and Research Institute, "tells us which regional nodal basins are at risk for metastatic disease."

If the SLN tests negative for melanoma, both doctor and patient can rest reasonably assured that the other nodes in that area are also cancer free. Dr. Reintgen and his colleagues at the Moffitt Cancer Center conducted a clinical trial of fifty-six men and women with stage I or II melanoma. Lymphoscintigraphy, lymphatic mapping, and sentinel-node biopsy revealed thirteen to have nodal involvement. As part of the study, all the participants underwent a complete regional lymph-node dissection. Then those specimens were sent off to the pathology department. Of the forty-three patients whose sentinel nodes were negative, not one was found to have melanoma in any of the non-SLN lymph nodes.

Other medical institutions have reported a "false negative" rate of less than 4 percent, which, while slightly higher, should inspire confidence in the procedure.

This early study prompted the Moffitt Center to change its standard of practice. In a follow-up trial of 404 melanoma patients, lymphadenectomy was recommended only to the 47 whose SLN biopsies came back positive. Not only did the other 357 avoid the additional surgery, but after five years, a mere 3 had experienced a recurrence in the regional lymph nodes.

Immunotherapy or Chemotherapy

Systemic treatment following surgery is considered standard only for melanomas that have spread to the nodes, although people with large stage II tumors may be encouraged to enroll in an investigational study.

A number of drugs have been tried, but according to Dr. Oseroff, "there is no clear winner." Reponse rates—the percentage of patients whose tumor size is reduced by at least half—hover in the range of 15 to 25 percent.

Compared to most other cancers, melanoma is unusually sensitive to drugs that manipulate the body's immune system. Interferon alfa-2B (brand name: Intron-A), in high doses, has exhibited the most vigorous assault against this cancer. However, it is often kept on the sidelines as a backup for chemotherapy, the reason being that prior chemotherapy does not compromise interferon's anticancer activity. Then, too, the high doses bring about severe side effects, frequently forcing delays in treatment and a reduction in dosage. Oncologists are currently evaluating the effectiveness of a less toxic regimen of interferon. Levamisole (Ergamisol), believed to be an immune response modifier, has also shown promise as a systemic therapy for melanoma patients who are at inordinate risk for a recurrence.

Among chemotherapeutic agents, dacarbazine (DTIC-Dome) has

been the drug of choice since the 1960s. About one in twenty patients taking dacarbazine can expect a complete remission. Preliminary studies indicate that the drug works best when paired with other anticancer medicines, among them cisplatin (Platinol), vinblastine (Velban), and vincristine (Oncovin).

TREATMENTS FOR ADVANCED MELANOMA

Surgery or Radiation Therapy (Palliative Treatment)

Metastatic melanoma typically disseminates to the lungs, digestive tract, bones, brain, or to lymph nodes far away from the primary tumor. Surgically removing the secondary cancers does not effect a cure, but the degree of symptom relief and an improved quality of life can be "substantial," says Dr. Oseroff.

One study specifically looked at the propriety of surgery for men and women with operable stage IV melanoma. Whereas an untreated metastatic brain lesion can bring about death "relatively quickly," according to Dr. Oseroff, participants who volunteered for brain surgery saw their lives extended eight months, on average. The survival after excision of abdominal metastases was also eight months; lung metastases, nine months; and distant skin and lymph-node metastases, fifteen months. Sixteen percent of the patients lived for two years or longer. "In situations where melanoma produces symptoms, which it often does," says Dr. Oseroff, "surgery is certainly indicated."

The success of the operation hinges on such factors as the cancer's location and the number of metastases. For instance, excising a lesion in the brain tends to be more problematic than removing a melanoma in the lung. And, in general, the outcome is more favorable when a person has a solitary tumor rather than metastases in multiple sites. We emphasize these points because unless the surgeon can resect the entire cancer, the patient stands to gain little benefit at great potential risk. As another study noted, unsuccessful procedures often resulted in lengthy hospitalizations,

---

MELANOMA/Drug Therapy

No standard drug therapy currently exists for treating melanoma. Agents that may be used include:

- dacarbazine
- alpha-interferon (I)
- interleukin-2 (I)
- levamisole (I)
- carmustine
- lomustine
- cisplatin
- tamoxifen (H)
- Bacillus Calmette-Guérin (I)
- melphalan
- vincristine
- vinblastine
- dactinomycin

(H) = hormonal agent

(I) = immunologic agent

with some of the patients spending more than half their remaining time in the hospital.

One alternative to surgery is radiotherapy, delivered externally or internally. "Many of these metastatic lesions are responsive to radiation," says Dr. Oseroff. Furthermore, "in many cases, the morbidity from radiation therapy is far less than from surgery."

Immunotherapy, Chemotherapy, and Immunochemotherapy

Advanced melanoma is resistant to most standard chemotherapy. Here combination therapy incorporating dacarbazine has not produced results superior to that from carbazine alone. Similarly, interferon alfa-2A (Roferon-A) administered in conjunction with interleukin-2 (Proleukin) appears to be no more effective than either immunologic agent by itself. But when physicians at Chicago's Lutheran General Hospital gave eighty-three metastatic melanoma patients alternating doses of dacarbazine-based chemotherapy *and* alfa-2 and IL-2, the overall response rate was among the highest ever reported: 55 percent. One in seven patients had full remissions. The experimental regimen extended the participants' lives by more than a year, on average, which was also unusually long.

Immunotherapy is also used as a local treatment to shrink secondary malignancies of the skin or the subcutaneous tissue beneath it. Injecting the *immunostimulant* Bacillus Calmette-Guérin directly into the tumor stirs up what Dr. Oseroff describes as "an enormous inflammatory reaction that can wipe out the melanoma." Employing BCG as a system-wide treatment—injecting it below the skin in an attempt to rev up the body's entire immune system—"doesn't really work, although there are some doctors who believe in it strongly," he says. "The primary use comes in direct lesion-by-lesion treatment."

OTHER THERAPIES THAT MAY BE USED IN THE TREATMENT OF MELANOMA

Isolated Arterial Perfusion/Intra-arterial Infusion (investigational)—More than half of all melanomas occur in an arm or leg. Isolated arterial perfusion, also known as *isolated limb perfusion* (ILP), enables oncologists to deliver high doses of chemotherapy that would otherwise be toxic or potentially deadly if administered systemically.

First, circulation to the extremity is temporarily cut off by applying a tourniquet. Then the physician inserts a needle catheter into a blood vessel. The withdrawn blood is run though a special machine that adds both oxygen and the anticancer drug(s). Then it is pumped back into the main artery that feeds the arm or leg. Melphalan (Alkeran), used for this purpose since the 1960s, expressly targets melanoma cells. Heating the blood slightly *(hyperthermia)* seems to enhance its effect. The treatment typically lasts sixty to ninety minutes, after which the chemotherapy is flushed from the limb and the tourniquet is removed, reestablishing normal blood flow.

A clinical trial conducted in Germany compared two groups suffering from melanoma of the extremities. Following wide-excision surgery and lymph-node dissection, half the patients received isolated limb perfusion chemotherapy. Nearly six years later, twenty-six of the fifty-four subjects treated with surgery alone had relapsed, as compared to only six of the fifty-three members of the perfusion group.

Clinical researchers at the National Cancer Institute augmented the melphalan with two immunologics: tumor necrosis factor (TNF) and gamma-interferon. Melphalan alone induces a complete response—meaning no evidence of cancer can be detected—as much as 60 percent of the time. The triple combination exceeded that by 20 percentage points.

A similar technique, intra-arterial infusion, calls for infusing the medicine into the major artery supplying the limb, as opposed to treating the blood externally and then returning it to the body. Another difference is that dacarbazine and cisplatin are typically used in place of melphalan.

♦ *Ask your doctor about this and any other investigational therapies that might benefit you.*

Cancer of the Uterus (Endometrial Cancer)

Overview

TREATMENTS FOR ENDOMETRIAL CANCER THAT HAS NOT
METASTASIZED

Surgery

Three in four cases of endometrial cancer are detected when the
disease is confined to the uterus and are highly curable through total
hysterectomy and bilateral salpingo-oophorectomy. "A lot of women
refer to it as a 'complete' hysterectomy," notes Dr. Michael Hogan, "because it involves taking out the entire uterine body, including the
cervix, plus the ovaries and the fallopian tubes."

The operation is typically recommended to postmenopausal
women diagnosed with atypical uterine hyperplasia, a precancerous
condition that can progress to invasive disease if not treated. A woman
who wishes to forgo hysterectomy or who is a poor surgical candidate
would be offered an oral progesterone-like drug such as hydroxyprogesterone (brand name: Prodrox), medroxyprogesterone (Depo-
Provera), or megestrol (Megace).

If you choose hormonal therapy (discussed in detail under "Treatments for Advanced Endometrial Cancer"), it's important to first undergo a dilatation and curettage (D&C), in which the cervix is dilated
and a spoon-shaped curette used to scrape tissue from the inner wall of
the uterus. "The purpose of the D&C is to exclude the possibility of
an invasive cancer," explains Dr. Hogan. "About one-fourth of postmenopausal patients with atypical hyperplasia will have a concurrent
endometrial carcinoma." Hormonal therapy, he says, reverses most
uterine hyperplasias.

Lymph-Node Dissection—A spread to the lymph nodes in the
pelvis and abdomen would put the cancer at stage III. It is currently
standard procedure to sample nodes during surgery, Dr. Hogan notes,
"because if we don't have any information about the lymph nodes, we
can't accurately stage the patient." However, there is some controversy
over whether or not all patients with stage I disease require a lymph-
node dissection. Many cancer centers base their decision on the depth
of incursion into the uterine wall (the myometrium) and the differentiation, or grade, of the tumor.

ENDOMETRIAL CANCER/Treatment Options

ATYPICAL UTERINE HYPERPLASIA

A precancerous condition in which an overproliferation of normal cells causes the inner lining of the uterus to thicken.
- Total hysterectomy, to surgically remove the uterus and cervix; and bilateral salpingo-oophorectomy, to surgically remove both ovaries and fallopian tubes • *or*
- Hormonal therapy, frequently consisting of hydroxyprogesterone, medroxyprogesterone, or megestrol

STAGE I ENDOMETRIAL CANCER

The cancer is limited to the uterus.
- Total hysterectomy and bilateral salpingo-oophorectomy, *with* lymph-node dissection • *alone or followed by*
  - External-beam radiation therapy • *and/or*
  - Internal radiation therapy

Or:
- External-beam radiation therapy • *and/or*
- Internal radiation therapy

STAGE II ENDOMETRIAL CANCER

IIA: The cancer has spread to the glandular tissue in the area where the uterus narrows into the cervix.
- Total hysterectomy and bilateral salpingo-oophorectomy, *with* lymph-node biopsy • *alone or followed by*
  - External-beam radiation therapy • *and/or*
  - Internal radiation therapy

Or:
- External-beam radiation therapy • *and/or*
- Internal radiation therapy

IIB: The cancer has spread deeper into the tissue of the cervix.
- Total hysterectomy and bilateral salpingo-oophorectomy, *with* lymph-node dissection • *followed by*
  - External-beam radiation therapy • *and/or*
  - Internal radiation therapy

Or:
  - External-beam radiation therapy • *and/or*
  - Internal radiation therapy • *followed by*
- Total hysterectomy and bilateral salpingo-oophorectomy, *with* lymph-node dissection

Or:
- Radical hysterectomy, to surgically remove the uterus, cervix, both

ovaries and fallopian tubes, and part of the vagina, *with* lymph-node dissection

STAGE III ENDOMETRIAL CANCER

The cancer has invaded other tissues outside the uterus but remains within the pelvis.

- **Total hysterectomy and bilateral salpingo-oophorectomy or radical hysterectomy,** *with* **lymph-node dissection** · *alone or followed by*
- **External-beam radiation therapy**

If the cancer is inoperable:
- **External-beam radiation therapy** · *plus*
- **Internal radiation therapy**

Or:
- **Hormonal therapy, frequently consisting of hydroxyprogesterone, medroxyprogesterone, or megestrol**

STAGE IV ENDOMETRIAL CANCER

The cancer has metastasized beyond the pelvis, to other parts of the body, or to the lining of the bladder or the rectum.
- **Hormonal therapy, frequently consisting of hydroxyprogesterone, medroxyprogesterone, or megestrol**

Or:
- **External-beam radiation therapy** · *plus*
- **Internal radiation therapy**

Under Investigation
- **Chemotherapy, frequently consisting of doxorubicin, alone or in combination with other agents**
- ◆ **Ask your doctor about any clinical trials that might benefit you.**

RECURRENT ENDOMETRIAL CANCER

Your therapy will depend on which treatment was used initially.

- **Hormonal therapy, frequently consisting of hydroxyprogesterone, medroxyprogesterone, megestrol, or tamoxifen** · *or*
- **External-beam radiation therapy**

Under Investigation
- **Chemotherapy, frequently consisting of doxorubicin, alone or in combination with other agents**
- ◆ **Ask your doctor about any clinical trials that might benefit you.**

Grade, established prior to surgery by way of an endometrial biopsy or a D&C, expresses the normalcy and abnormalcy of the cells' appearance under the microscope. Tumor depth, though, can be determined only by excising the uterus and performing a frozen-section biopsy during the operation. A high grade (3, on a scale of 1 to 3) and deep myometrial invasion in particular are frequent harbingers of lymph-node involvement. Someone with a grade 1 tumor limited to the endometrial lining (stage IA) has less than a 5 percent chance that the cancer will spread to the nodes. In contrast, the risk multiplies two to fifteen times for a grade 3 tumor that has grown at least halfway into the myometrium (stage IC).

According to Dr. Hogan, a high-grade tumor warrants a lymph-node dissection, regardless of its depth. It's the same situation as when a surgeon would want to harvest some nodes in the pelvis and abdomen if a stage I

ENDOMETRIAL CANCER/ Surgical Procedures

Total hysterectomy: surgical removal of the uterus and cervix, plus both ovaries and fallopian tubes *(bilateral salpingo-oophorectomy).* Some lymph nodes in the pelvis and abdomen may also be taken out and examined for evidence of cancer. Average hospital stay:

- **Abdominal hysterectomy, 3–7 days**
- **Laparoscopic hysterectomy, 1–2 days**

Radical hysterectomy: surgical removal of the uterus, cervix, fallopian tubes, ovaries, part of the vagina, and area lymph nodes. Average hospital stay: **4–5 days**

---

malignancy of any grade was found to be deeply invasive. "But most doctors would say that patients with superficial grade I or grade II endometrial cancer do not need to have a lymph-node dissection.

"We might also take into account the size of the tumor," he continues. "Some physicians feel that if the lesion is larger than 2 centimeters [¾ inch], it has a greater chance of being deeply invasive, and therefore we would go ahead and sample the nodes." Once the cancer has extended into the cervix, lymphadenectomy becomes a foregone conclusion.

Laparoscopic Hysterectomy—Conventional abdominal hysterectomy leaves a five-inch vertical scar from just below the belly button to the pubic bone; or, if you opt for a "bikini incision," from side to side. Laparoscopic hysterectomy, first performed in 1988, requires three or four small incisions no more than half an inch long. A viewing instrument is inserted through an incision in the navel. The surgeon then severs the uterus, tubes, and ovaries and takes them out through one of the other incisions. If necessary, the lymph-node dissection can also be done this way.

This minimally invasive procedure causes far less discomfort for patients, the majority of whom go home the same day. At most, you can expect a hospital stay of forty-eight hours. The recuperation is considerably shorter as well: one to two weeks versus the six-to-eight-week convalescence associated with standard hysterectomy.

Some 600,000 women in the United States undergo hysterectomies every year, mainly for noncancerous conditions such as benign fibroid tumors, abnormal bleeding, and endometriosis. Consequently, a number of community hospitals offer the laparoscopic alternative. But as Dr. Hogan points out, "the ability to do the hysterectomy *and* the staging laparoscopically, which includes node dissection, is more likely to be found at cancer centers."

Radical Hysterectomy—Doctors generally try to avoid the most extensive form of hysterectomy, which additionally removes the upper portion of the vagina. At stages II and III, when the cancer involves the cervix, the usual strategy consists of total hysterectomy plus pelvic radiotherapy. "The only time we might perform a radical hysterectomy," says Dr. Hogan, "is when a patient has associated bowel disease or some other condition that makes radiation therapy too risky."

Radiation Therapy

Obesity predisposes women to cardiovascular disease, diabetes, and other disorders that may preclude surgery. In this instance, radiation serves as primary therapy. The survival rates, while not quite as high as those associated with surgery, are heartening. In one study of patients with stage I endometrial cancer, approximately eight in ten who received external and/or internal radiotherapy were alive and free of cancer ten years later. Another situation that calls for definitive radiation therapy is a stage III tumor that has spread to the pelvic wall, at which point the cancer is declared inoperable.

Pelvic radiation routinely follows surgery for stage III tumors. In stage II disease, it may be administered before or after the total hysterectomy. "Radiation can be given in two basic ways," explains Dr. Hogan. "We may use external-beam radiation exclusively, or we may give part of the treatment externally and part internally." In *intracavitary* radiation, a capsule containing a radioactive substance is inserted into the vagina and implanted in the uterus, where it remains approximately two or three days. The method recommended is often a matter of preference on the part of the medical center or the radiation oncologist.

No studies have uncovered any distinct benefit to postsurgical radiation for people with stage I endometrial cancer. Nevertheless, says

Dr. Hogan, "most institutions will offer radiotherapy on a selective basis, depending on the findings of the operation. High-grade tumors, or those that are deeply penetrating, or those with both characteristics, would require some form of postoperative irradiation." Other cases—like an intermediate-grade tumor that involves less than 50 percent of the muscular uterine wall (stage IB)—are less clear-cut. "If you talk to five doctors at five different institutions," Dr. Hogan observes, "you're likely to get five different postsurgical treatment plans."

TREATMENTS FOR ADVANCED ENDOMETRIAL CANCER

Hormonal Therapy (Palliative Treatment)

Endometrial cancer, like breast cancer, depends on the female sex hormone estrogen in order to grow. When the primary tumor has metastasized to or recurred in the lungs or another distant organ, patients are usually given a synthesized form of progesterone, estrogen's partner in reproduction. These oral drugs suppress estrogen levels.

Progestational agents are more likely to exert an effect on endometrial tumors that contain detectable levels of progesterone and estrogen receptors. Your progesterone-receptor (PR) status is determined from the biopsy. To give you a striking example from a clinical trial, 115 women with advanced endometrial cancer were put on progesterone. Seventy-five percent of the PR-positive group responded to treatment, as compared to just 7 percent of the PR-negative group. In place of progesterone, a physician might prescribe tamoxifen (Nolvadex), an antiestrogen.

> **ENDOMETRIAL CANCER/ Drug Therapy**
>
> *First-line hormonal therapy frequently consists of:*
> - medroxyprogesterone (H)
> - megestrol (H)
> - hydroxyprogesterone (H)
> - tamoxifen (H)
>
> *Other drugs that may be used include:*
> - doxorubicin
> - cisplatin
> - cyclophosphamide
> - fluorouracil
>
> (H) = hormonal agent

See "Why See a Gynecologic Oncologist?," page 529.

♦ *Hormonal therapy is an option in stage III disease for patients too ill to withstand either surgery or radiation.*

Radiation Therapy (Palliative Treatment)

When endometrial cancer spreads to or reemerges within the pelvic region, radiation is used to contain the tumor. If the cancer comes back in the vagina, patients who did not receive radiotherapy previously can occasionally be cured.

OTHER THERAPIES THAT MAY BE USED IN THE TREATMENT OF ENDOMETRIAL CANCER

Chemotherapy (investigational)—No standard chemotherapy currently exists for endometrial cancer. Hormonal therapy is usually offered as first-line treatment for metastatic tumors because its side effects are relatively mild. "Once the person showed signs of disease progression," says Dr. Hogan, "then we would go to a regimen of chemotherapy." Doxorubicin (Adriamycin) is the drug most often used, sometimes in combination with others.

> **Hormonal Therapy and Atypical Uterine Hyperplasia**
>
> Progesterone therapy can usually wrest control of the overly active cells in the inner lining and return them to normal. After three months, says Dr. Hogan, "we repeat the endometrial sampling, either by biopsy or D&C. If we see we've reversed the hyperplasia, from there on the patient can simply be followed."

"If you really get critical about it, there is no data to substantiate this," he points out. "But for disease that has spread outside the pelvis and is not surgically resectable for a cure, it makes sense that chemotherapy would benefit some patients and might even cure a very small percentage of them. Over the years, I've had some women with recurrent endometrial carcinoma who've gone into long-term remission, perhaps permanently."

◆ *Ask your doctor about this and any other investigational therapies that might benefit you.*

Leukemia

Overview

TREATMENTS FOR LEUKEMIA

The opening offensive against leukemia consists of drug therapy. While chemotherapeutic or immunologic agents can keep the disease at bay, often for a number of years, they rarely cure it. Whenever possible, the ultimate goal is to proceed to a bone-marrow transplant, which Dr. Fred Appelbaum considers the foremost advance in treating this disease.

"In 1974, when I first started in cancer medicine, chronic myeloid leukemia was incurable," says Dr. Appelbaum, head of clinical research at the Fred Hutchinson Cancer Research Center. "Now we're curing 70 to 80 percent of cases with marrow transplantation.

"Acute myeloid leukemia, too, was generally incurable, except in a small percentage of patients. Today, with allogeneic transplantation, 55 percent of them are cured, and the success rate appears similar in acute lymphocytic leukemia." BMT has less of a role in the fourth major type of leukemia, chronic lymphocytic leukemia, because CLL primarily afflicts men and women beyond the age where transplantation is considered a reasonable risk.

With leukemia, perhaps more so than with many other cancers, it is essential to find a medical facility that has experience in treating your disease. "Leukemia is a very complicated, high-tech area," observes Dr. Appelbaum. You want to be at a cutting-edge center where the focus from the get-go is on bone-marrow transplantation, if your overall condition and other factors allow. As Dr. Appelbaum points out, "time is of the essence, because seeking a donor takes time and effort, especially if the patient doesn't have a sibling with matching bone marrow."

Supportive care, in the form of transfusions of blood and blood products, and skill in preventing and managing complications are also crucial. Not only is the disease immunosuppressive, but the treatments themselves weaken the body's defenses against infections. "Much of the effort in intensive therapy—and particularly in transplantation—is directed at supporting patients so that they don't succumb to infection or bleeding along the way."

Chemotherapy

Acute Myeloid Leukemia—For many forms of cancer, chemotherapy is administered in three stages: induction, consolidation, then maintenance. In AML, however, few protocols include maintenance, in which a relatively low dose is given over a long period of time. Instead, once a complete remission has been achieved—usually in a matter of weeks, with cytarabine (brand name: Cy-

---

AML/Drug Therapy

First-line therapy frequently consists of:
- **cytarabine + daunorubicin with or without thioguanine or etoposide**
- **cytarabine + idarubicin**
- **mitoxantrone + etoposide**

Other drugs or drug combinations that may be used include:
- **cytarabine + mitoxantrone**
- **etoposide + cyclophosphamide**
- **asparaginase**
- **doxorubicin**
- **mercaptopurine**
- **fludarabine**
- **methotrexate**

LEUKEMIA/Treatment Options

Acute Myeloid Leukemia (AML)

UNTREATED AML

The blood and bone marrow contain excess white blood cells, and additional signs and symptoms of leukemia may be evident.

- Chemotherapy, frequently consisting of cytarabine and daunorubicin

Under Investigation
- New chemotherapy drugs
- Ask your doctor about any clinical trials that might benefit you.

AML IN REMISSION

Following treatment, the numbers of white cells and other blood cells in the blood and the bone marrow are normal, and there are no signs or symptoms of leukemia.

- Continued chemotherapy, frequently consisting of cytarabine and daunorubicin

Or:
- High-dose chemotherapy · *with or without*
- Total-body irradiation · *in preparation for*
- Allogeneic or autologous bone-marrow transplantation

Under Investigation #1
- New chemotherapy drugs

Under Investigation #2
- Allogeneic and autologous peripheral-blood stem-cell transplantation
- Ask your doctor about any clinical trials that might benefit you.

If the leukemia fails to go into remission:
- Allogeneic bone-marrow transplantation

RECURRENT AML

Your therapy will depend on how you were treated initially.

- Chemotherapy, frequently consisting of cytarabine and mitoxantrone or idarubicin, or other drug combinations

Or:
- High-dose chemotherapy · *with or without*
- Total-body irradiation · *in preparation for*
- Allogenic *or* autologous bone-marrow transplantation

Or:
- External-beam radiation therapy, to relieve symptoms

Under Investigation
- New chemotherapy drugs and drug combinations
- ◆ Ask your doctor about any clinical trials that might benefit you.

If the leukemia has affected the central nervous system:
- Chemotherapy, frequently consisting of cytarabine or methotrexate, injected into the cerebrospinal fluid (intrathecally)

See treatment options for brain metastases.

Acute Lymphocytic Leukemia (ALL)

UNTREATED ALL

The blood and bone marrow contain excess white blood cells, and other signs and symptoms of leukemia may be evident.

- Chemotherapy, frequently consisting of daunorubicin, vincristine, prednisone, and asparaginase or cyclophosphamide

To treat or prevent leukemia from infiltrating the central nervous system:
- Chemotherapy, frequently consisting of methotrexate, injected into the cerebrospinal fluid (intrathecally) · *alone or with*

{
- Systemic chemotherapy, frequently consisting of methotrexate · *or*
- External-beam cranial irradiation

Under Investigation
- New chemotherapy drugs and drug combinations
- ◆ Ask your doctor about any clinical trials that might benefit you.

ALL IN REMISSION

Following treatment, the numbers of white cells and other blood cells in the blood and the bone marrow are normal, and there are no signs or symptoms of leukemia.

- Continued chemotherapy, frequently consisting of daunorubicin, vincristine, prednisone, asparaginase, cyclophosphamide, and cytarabine

Or:
- High-dose chemotherapy · *with or without*
- Total-body irradiation · *in preparation for*
- Allogeneic bone-marrow transplantation

Under Investigation
- High-dose chemotherapy · *with or without*
- Total-body irradiation · *in preparation for*
- Autologous bone-marrow transplantation
- ◆ Ask your doctor about any clinical trials that might benefit you.

To treat or prevent leukemia from infiltrating the central nervous system:
- Intrathecal chemotherapy, frequently consisting of methotrexate · *alone or with*
- External-beam cranial irradiation

Or:
- Systemic chemotherapy, frequently consisting of methotrexate · *and*
- Intrathecal chemotherapy, frequently consisting of methotrexate

RECURRENT ALL

Your therapy will depend on how you were treated initially.

- External-beam radiation therapy, to relieve symptoms

Or:
- High-dose chemotherapy · *with or without*
- Total-body irradiation · *in preparation for*
- Allogeneic bone-marrow transplantation · *or one or more of the following experimental therapies:*

Under Investigation #1
- High-dose chemotherapy · *with or without*
- Total-body irradiation · *in preparation for*
- Autologous bone-marrow transplantation

Under Investigation #2
- New chemotherapy drugs and immunologic agents
- ◆ Ask your doctor about any clinical trials that might benefit you.

Chronic Lymphocytic Leukemia (CLL)

STAGE 0 CLL

The white-cell count is elevated, but no symptoms are evident.

If you have no symptoms:
- Observation

If you have symptoms:
- Chemotherapy, frequently consisting of fludarabine or chlorambucil

STAGE I CLL

The white-cell count is elevated; lymph nodes are swollen.

If you have no symptoms:
- Observation

If you have symptoms:
- External-beam radiation therapy, to relieve symptoms caused by a mass of cancer cells in a lymph node or the spleen · *or*
- Chemotherapy, frequently consisting of fludarabine, chlorambucil, or cyclophosphamide, with or without a corticosteroid such as prednisone

STAGE II CLL

The white-cell count is elevated; lymph nodes, the liver, and the spleen are swollen.

If you have no symptoms:
- Observation

If you have symptoms:
- Chemotherapy, frequently consisting of fludarabine, chlorambucil, or cyclophosphamide, with or without a corticosteroid such as prednisone · *or*
- External-beam radiation therapy to the spleen

Under Investigation
- Immunotherapy
- ◆ Ask your doctor about any clinical trials that might benefit you.

STAGE III CLL

The white-cell count is elevated, the red-cell count is abnormally low; lymph nodes, the liver, or the spleen may be swollen.

- Chemotherapy, frequently consisting of the following drugs, alone or in combination: chlorambucil, cyclophosphamide, prednisone, fludarabine, cladribine, pentostatin

If your leukemia brings on a condition called hypersplenism:
- Splenectomy, to surgically remove the spleen · *or*
- External-beam radiation therapy to the spleen · *or, in the event the above methods fail*
- Total-body irradiation

Under Investigation #1
- High-dose chemotherapy · *with or without*
- Total-body irradiation · *in preparation for*
- Allogeneic or autologous bone-marrow transplantation

Under Investigation #2
- Immunotherapy
- ◆ Ask your doctor about any clinical trials that might benefit you.

STAGE IV CLL

The white-cell count is elevated; the platelet count is abnormally low; the red-cell count may also be abnormally low; lymph nodes, the liver, or the spleen may be swollen.

- Chemotherapy, frequently consisting of the following drugs, alone or in combination: chlorambucil, cyclophosphamide, prednisone, fludarabine, cladribine, pentostatin

If your leukemia brings on a condition called hypersplenism:
- Splenectomy · *or*
- External-beam radiation therapy to the spleen · *or, in the event the above methods fail*
- Total-body irradiation

Under Investigation #1
- New chemotherapy drugs and immunologic agents

Under Investigation #2
- High-dose chemotherapy • *with or without*
- Total-body irradiation • *in preparation for*
- Allogeneic or autologous bone-marrow transplantation
- ◆ Ask your doctor about any clinical trials that might benefit you.

RECURRENT OR RESISTANT (REFRACTORY) CLL
Your therapy will depend on how you were treated initially.

- Chemotherapy, using either the same drug as before or a different one

Under Investigation #1
- New chemotherapy drugs

Under Investigation #2
- High-dose chemotherapy • *with or without*
- Total-body irradiation • *in preparation for*
- Allogeneic or autologous bone-marrow transplantation
- ◆ Ask your doctor about any clinical trials that might benefit you.

Chronic Myeloid Leukemia (CML)

CHRONIC PHASE CML
A few blast cells are found in the blood and bone marrow.

- Chemotherapy, frequently consisting of hydroxyurea • *and/or*
- Immunotherapy, frequently consisting of alpha-interferon

Or:
{
- Chemotherapy, frequently consisting of hydroxyurea • *and/or*
- Immunotherapy, frequently consisting of alpha-interferon • *followed by*
- High-dose chemotherapy • *with or without*
- Total-body irradiation • *in preparation for*
- Allogeneic bone-marrow transplantation

If your leukemia brings on a condition called hypersplenism:
- Splenectomy

Under Investigation
- Autologous bone-marrow or peripheral-blood stem-cell transplantation
- ◆ Ask your doctor about any clinical trials that might benefit you.

ACCELERATED PHASE CML
More blast cells appear in the blood, and there are fewer normal cells.

- Chemotherapy, frequently consisting of hydroxyurea, cytarabine, or busulfan • *and/or*

- Transfusions of blood or blood products, to relieve symptoms

Or:

- High-dose chemotherapy • *with or without*
- Total-body irradiation • *in preparation for*
- Allogeneic or autologous bone-marrow transplantation

BLASTIC PHASE CML

Blast cells make up more than 30 percent of the cells in the blood or bone marrow; tumors may arise in bones or lymph nodes.

- Chemotherapy, frequently consisting of drugs such as vincristine, prednisone, hydroxyurea, cytarabine, mitoxantrone, and doxorubicin or another anthracycline, alone or in combination

Or:

- High-dose chemotherapy • *with or without*
- Total-body irradiation • *in preparation for*
- Allogeneic or autologous bone-marrow transplantation

If the leukemia has produced tumors in the bone:
- External-beam radiation therapy

Under Investigation
- New chemotherapy drugs
- ◆ Ask your doctor about any clinical trials that might benefit you.

MENINGEAL PHASE CML

Leukemia is found in the cerebrospinal fluid.

- Chemotherapy, frequently consisting of methotrexate or cytarabine, injected into the cerebrospinal fluid (intrathecally) • *and/or*
- External-beam cranial irradiation

RECURRENT OR RESISTANT (REFRACTORY) CML

Your therapy will depend on how you were treated initially.

Under Investigation
- New combinations of chemotherapy drugs
- ◆ Ask your doctor about any clinical trials that might benefit you.

If you've relapsed following a bone-marrow transplant:
- Immunotherapy, frequently consisting of alpha-interferon • *and/or*
- Adoptive immunotherapy, in which white blood cells extracted from the donor bone marrow are infused into the patient • *and/or*
- A second bone-marrow transplant

tosar-U) and daunorubicin (Cerubidine)—the next step is either short-term, more intensive consolidation chemotherapy or preparation for a BMT.

Induction therapy, usually administered on an inpatient basis, is successful about two-thirds of the time. According to the National Cancer Institute, about one in four of those patients will live at least three years and may be cured through chemo alone. "A number of different recipes have been used for consolidation," says Dr. Appelbaum. "None has outclassed the rest, but the most common regimen is two, three, or four cycles of cytarabine alone or in combination with an anthracycline such as daunorubicin, like we use for induction."

Acute promyelocytic leukemia (APL), a subtype of acute myeloid leukemia, has been successfully treated with an exciting new oral drug called tretinoin (Vesinoid). This derivative of vitamin A induces leukemia cells to mature and function normally. Your oncologist may also call it ATRA, short for "All Trans-Retinoic Acid." Dr. Appelbaum calls it amazing.

"You take this pill and watch the disease go into a complete remission, with virtually no toxicity." The side effects are usually mild: headache, fever, weakness, fatigue. "ATRA alone does not cure the disease," Dr. Appelbaum stresses. "But it does get patients into a complete remission, and, if combined with chemotherapy, appears to increase the cure rate."

ALL/Drug Therapy

First-line therapy frequently consists of:
- **daunorubicin + vincristine + prednisone (H) + asparaginase or cyclophosphamide**
- **methotrexate**

Other drugs used may include:
- **cytarabine**
- **mercaptopurine**
- **asparaginase**
- **dexamethasone (H)**
- **doxorubicin**
- **pegasparagase**
- **teniposide**
- **thioguanine**

(H) = hormonal agent

Acute Lymphocytic Leukemia—Induction chemotherapy for ALL lasts four to six weeks and requires some hospitalization. The favored regimen consists of four drugs: daunorubicin, vincristine (Oncovin), prednisone (Deltasone), and either asparaginase (Elspar) or cyclophosphamide (Cytoxan).

Fifteen percent of adults with ALL develop leukemia of the central nervous system, a higher percentage than seen with the other three major leukemias. Systemic chemotherapy, delivered into the bloodstream, is largely ineffective against cancer cells that have taken refuge in the brain and spinal cord, because of the *blood-brain barrier.* This network of blood-vessel walls protects the central nervous system from viruses, toxins, and other harmful substances that circulate in the bloodstream. Unfortunately, it also prevents systemic chemotherapy from reaching the brain and spinal cord in adequate concentrations to exert much of an effect.

Therefore, once systemic induction therapy is completed, patients receive *intrathecal* injections of chemotherapy, usually methotrexate, into the *subarachnoid space* surrounding the spinal cord. The *cerebrospinal fluid* within this canal then smuggles the drug to its intended destination. Intrathecal chemotherapy, with or without cranial irradiation, may be necessary in other leukemias should cancer take hold there, but only acute lymphocytic leukemia calls for preventive treatment, or *CNS prophylaxis.*

Sixty to 80 percent of patients go into remission from this two-pronged attack. Next comes short-term consolidation—using different combinations of the same drugs as before, with the addition of cyclophosphamide and cytarabine—followed by long-term maintenance therapy. All told, chemotherapy is administered over a period of eighteen to thirty-six months, unless you undergo a bone-marrow transplantation during that time.

See "Chemotherapy" in treatment options for (adult) cancers of the brain, page 509.

Chronic Lymphocytic Leukemia—Although chemotherapy cannot be expected to cure chronic lymphocytic leukemia, "many patients live for five to seven years, and sometimes much longer," says Dr. Appelbaum. About one in ten exhibit no symptoms when the disease is detected—often accidentally during a routine blood test—and remain asymptomatic for as long as fifteen years. Until the cancer progresses, no therapy is necessary. In one in five cases, though, CLL advances rapidly, forcing the initiation of treatment soon after diagnosis.

Most men and women with chronic lymphocytic leukemia fall somewhere in between. Given that the vast majority are elderly and are therefore not candidates for bone-marrow transplantation, and given the indolent nature of the disease, oncologists generally follow a conservative course.

CLL/Drug Therapy

First-line therapy frequently consists of:
- fludarabine
- chlorambucil
- cyclophosphamide
- prednisone (H)

Other drugs used may include:
- cladribine
- pentostatin
- dexamethasone (H)
- mechlorethamine

(H) = hormonal agent

"For many years," says Dr. Appelbaum, "we used to start treatment with chlorambucil [Leukeran], which is a pill that is easily taken. "But a large study has suggested that a new drug called fludarabine [Fludara] may be a better first drug, and it has become the treatment of choice." *Corticosteroids* such as prednisone may be added to correct *autoimmune hemolytic anemia* and/or *thrombocytopenia*. All cancer patients are subject to abnormally low red-blood-cell and platelet counts due to the immunosuppressive effects of the disease or treatment. But here the body's immune system mistakes its own red cells and platelets for foreign bodies and destroys them faster than the impaired bone marrow can replace them. The National Cancer Institute advises that oncologists give the corticosteroids prior to chemotherapy, if possible, to control the faulty autoimmune response and normalize the blood-cell levels without having to transfuse the patient.

Chronic Myeloid Leukemia—Like CLL, chronic myeloid leukemia crowds out normal marrow cells gradually, and frequently takes its time before producing symptoms. The initial chronic phase can last from several months to several years; again, sometimes without clinical evidence of disease.

In contrast to chronic lymphocytic leukemia, where it's not unusual to delay treatment, "there's probably a stronger push to begin therapy early," says Dr. Appelbaum. "We have higher expectations of what we can achieve with treatment for CML."

Traditionally, oncologists have started patients on hydroxyurea (Hydrea), an oral anticancer medication. "With hydroxyurea we can easily control the white count for a period of three to four years."

Immunotherapy

Since the mid-1990s, "alpha-interferon has relegated hydroxyurea to second-tier therapy, in some physicians' minds," says Dr. Appelbaum.

Chronic myeloid leukemia differs from

CML/Drug Therapy

First-line therapy frequently consists of:
- alpha-interferon (I)
- hydroxyurea

Other drugs or drug combinations used may include:
- alpha-interferon (I) and cytarabine
- vincristine + prednisone (H)
- busulfan
- doxorubicin
- cyclophosphamide
- daunorubicin
- methotrexate
- mechlorethamine
- mercaptopurine
- thioguanine

(H) = hormonal agent
(I) = immunologic agent

most other leukemias in that it causes a specific genetic defect: the so-called Philadelphia chromosome, which is present in more than nine in ten patients' bone-marrow-biopsy specimens. "Hydroxyurea can control the white count, but it never makes the Philadelphia chromosome disappear," Dr. Appelbaum explains, "whereas interferon can make the chromosomal abnormality disappear in 15 to 20 percent of patients, sometimes for ten years or more. So for patients who are not going to be transplanted, there's been a move toward trying interferon." Patients give themselves daily subcutaneous injections of the immunologic agent for two to three years, although some researchers believe interferon therapy should continue indefinitely. The side effects from alpha-interferon (Intron-A, Roferon-A) tend to be more severe than from hydroxyurea, and therefore chemotherapy may be preferable when bone-marrow transplantation is a realistic goal.

Interferon may be combined with cytarabine if the levels of immature blast cells in the blood and bone marrow should rise, announcing the transition to accelerated phase CML. The next progression, to blastic phase CML, may come on over the course of a year or more. Or it may appear abruptly, in which case a patient is said to be in *blast crisis*. In this advanced stage of disease, blast cells occupy more than 30 percent of the blood and marrow, and may form tumors in the bone and lymph nodes. "At this point," says Dr. Appelbaum, "hydroxyurea no longer works; nor does most other chemotherapy."

During either the accelerated or the blastic phase, the cancer can spread to the cerebrospinal fluid that cushions the brain and spinal cord. Oncologists treat meningeal-phase chronic myeloid leukemia with intrathecal cytarabine or methotrexate, and possibly cranial irradiation.

See "Treatments for Advanced or Recurrent Leukemia," page 440.

Bone-Marrow Transplantation

Allogeneic BMT—If the cure rates from allogeneic bone-marrow transplantation are so encouraging, why don't all leukemia patients go straight from induction chemotherapy to allogeneic BMT? As we've pointed out, age and general health can preclude undergoing the procedure. The cutoff point is between ages fifty and sixty-five, depending on the type of leukemia, whether or not the healthy marrow comes from a sibling or a matched unrelated donor (MUD), and the policy of the transplant center. But even under optimal circumstances, allogeneic transplantation carries a great deal of risk.

We'll use acute myeloid leukemia as an example. Let's say the prospective transplant recipient is in first remission, which in many physicians' opinion is the ideal time for performing alloBMT, although others recommend waiting until the patient relapses or a second remission is achieved. In another fortuitous development, his brother's marrow turns out to be a perfect match, the odds of which are only one in four. Yet his chances of dying as a result of the transplantation are still 20 to 40 percent. In addition, BMT is prohibitively expensive and disrupts the lives of patients and their families for several months, if not longer.

All these factors must be considered when weighing the procedure's pros and cons as well as the available alternatives. This same patient stands at least a 15 percent chance of being cured with chemotherapy alone, so is marrow transplantation, with its cure rate of approximately 55 percent, worth the risk? What about when there is no matching sibling? The use of MUD marrow lowers the cure rate by nearly half and increases the incidence of treatment-related mortality significantly.

In chronic myeloid leukemia, though, chemotherapy can merely keep the disease at bay, albeit for several years, while as many as four in five CML patients who opt for transplantation are able to say that they beat cancer. "Patients are now out twenty-plus years with this approach," notes Dr. Appelbaum. Worldwide, the majority of matched-unrelated-donor marrow transplants are performed for chronic myeloid leukemia.

Autologous BMT—An autologous transplant, while safer than allogeneic BMT, isn't nearly as effective. Once donor marrow "takes" in the recipient's bones, barring rejection by the body, the white blood cells it pumps out perceive any lingering leukemia cells as intruders and attack. Autologous stem cells, harvested from the patient's own marrow during remission and then reinfused, do not produce this *graft-versus-leukemia effect.*

AutoBMT has demonstrated its greatest success against acute myeloid leukemia. When performed during first remission, the cure rates range from 35 to 50 percent. Its application in the other three major leukemias is less clear. Thus far, autologous BMT doesn't appear to offer an advantage over chemotherapy in terms of prolonging life.

Although graft failure and graft-versus-host disease are rare, autologous marrow transplantation is by no means free of risk. The high doses of chemotherapy leave patients severely immunocompromised and susceptible to infection until the marrow rebuilds itself. In AML, for example, 10 to 20 percent of autologous transplant recipients die of treatment-related complications. Still, this may be the best alternative when a suitable marrow donor cannot be found.

Food for Thought: Drug Therapy or Bone-Marrow Transplantation?—Whether or not to go forward with a marrow transplant is a daunting decision for both the patient and the medical team. On the one hand, BMT often holds the best hope for curing leukemia. On the other, the procedure is debilitating and can prove fatal. The crucial question is: Do the potential benefits of bone-marrow transplantation exceed its potential risks? Here are some facts and figures to consider and to discuss with your doctor:

Prognostic Factors, and How They May Influence Leukemia Treatment—The four major types of leukemia encompass a number of rare subtypes, each characterized by a distinctive chromosomal aberration that predicts how well or how poorly a patient can generally be expected to respond to standard therapy. The bone-marrow sample withdrawn during the initial biopsy undergoes *cytogenetic testing* in the laboratory, because the presence of a cellular defect can influence the direction treatment takes. (*Cytogenetics* is the branch of genetic medicine devoted to the study of chromosomes.)

The twenty-three pairs of chromosomes in a cell contain DNA, which is divided into tiny units called genes. A leukemia cell may be found to have unusually large or misshapen chromosomes. Or two of the threadlike structures may exchange pieces, and with them genetic information, in what is referred to as *translocation.* The Philadelphia chromosome that identifies chronic myeloid leukemia and is also observed in one in five adults with acute lymphocytic leukemia is distinguished by a swap of genetic material between one chromosome in pair 9 and one in pair 22.

Another type of alteration is called *inversion.* Here the middle portion of a chromosome breaks off, then rejoins the other two segments,

Acute Myeloid Leukemia (AML)

Is there an alternative to BMT?

- Approximately 15 percent of patients can be cured through chemotherapy alone. But the majority will relapse within five years.

What are the potential benefits of bone-marrow transplantation?

- The cure rates from alloBMT during first remission are:
  Using marrow from a matched sibling, 45 to 60 percent
  Using matched-unrelated-donor marrow, less than 35 percent
- The cure rate from alloBMT following relapse or during second remission is approximately 30 percent.
- The cure rate from autoBMT during first or second remission ranges from 35 to 50 percent.

What are the potential risks of bone-marrow transplantation?

- The percentage of treatment-related deaths from alloBMT are:
  20 to 40 percent if the marrow comes from a matched sibling
  Higher if a MUD transplant
- The percentage of treatment-related deaths from autoBMT ranges from 10 to 20 percent.

Acute Lymphocytic Leukemia (ALL)

Is there an alternative to BMT?

- Approximately 35 to 40 percent of patients can be cured through chemotherapy alone.

What are the potential benefits of bone-marrow transplantation?

- The cure rate from alloBMT during first remission is:
  Using marrow from a matched sibling, approximately 60 percent
- The cure rate from alloBMT following a relapse is 15 percent.
- The cure rate from autoBMT during first remission ranges from 20 to 40 percent.

What are the potential risks of bone-marrow transplantation?

- The percentage of treatment-related deaths from alloBMT is:
  20 to 40 percent if the marrow comes from a matched sibling
  Higher if a MUD transplant

Chronic Lymphocytic Leukemia (CLL)

Is there an alternative to BMT?

- There is no other curative treatment for CLL, although the disease frequently advances slowly, and drug therapy can add years to patients' lives.

What are the potential benefits and risks of bone-marrow transplantation?

- Only one in ten people with CLL are under fifty, the age at which BMT is deemed safe. Although the procedure is not commonly performed, it has cured some younger patients.

Chronic Myeloid Leukemia (CML)

Is there an alternative to BMT?

- There is no other curative treatment for CML, although the disease frequently advances slowly, and drug therapy can add years to patients' lives.

What are the potential benefits of bone-marrow transplantation?

- The cure rates from alloBMT during chronic-phase CML are:
  Using marrow from a matched sibling, 60 to 80 percent (the prognosis is most favorable if the procedure is carried out within one year of the diagnosis)
  Using matched-unrelated-donor marrow, 40 to 60 percent

- The odds for a cure from alloBMT fall drastically if the procedure is performed during accelerated-phase CML, and plummet to less than 10 percent if performed during blastic-phase CML.

- AutoBMT has not been shown to cure CML. But reinfusing patients' marrow during the accelerated phase will return 10 to 20 percent of them to chronic-phase CML for more than a year.

What are the potential risks of bone-marrow transplantation?

- The percentage of treatment-related deaths from alloBMT is:
  15 to 30 percent if the marrow comes from a matched sibling
  35 to 50 percent if a MUD transplant

Some of the data presented here were obtained from the statistical center of the International Bone Marrow Transplant Registry. The analysis has not been reviewed or approved by the advisory committee of the IBMTR.

---

but reversed, thus changing the linear order of the genes. In a *monosomic* cell, one pair of chromosomes is missing its twin, while a *trisomic* cell bears an extra chromosome.

This is not as complicated as it probably sounds. All a patient needs to know is whether he has one of these chromosomal abnormalities—which, incidentally, are caused by the cancer, not the other way around—and if so, its implications. Acute myeloid leukemia provides several examples.

A translocation between pairs 8 and 21 portends a favorable prognosis, as does an inversion of one of the chromosomes in pair 16. "These two subcategories of AML seem to do pretty well with chemotherapy alone and therefore may not benefit as much from

---

Chromosomal Abnormalities in AML

Favorable:
- Translocation of chromosomes 8 and 21; 15 and 17
- Inversion of chromosome 16

Unfavorable:
- Various abnormalities of chromosomes 5, 7, 8, or 11q23
- Translocation or inversion of chromosome 3
- Translocation of chromosomes 6 and 9; 9 and 22

---

bone-marrow transplantation," says Dr. Appelbaum. "So we might give patients the option of having chemotherapy first, then being transplanted in the event of a relapse."

But if the cytogenetic test revealed a translocation between chromosomes 6 and 9, or an inversion of chromosome 3, or any of several other flaws (see box), an oncologist might be more inclined to recommend BMT during first remission, since these genetic alterations are considered unfavorable prognostic indicators.

In acute lymphocytic leukemia, the discovery of the Philadelphia chromosome is associated with a poor response to treatment. (In CML, the *absence* of the telltale chromosome would mark a person as being at increased risk for a relapse.) Whereas chemotherapy is a sensible primary treatment for standard-risk ALL, the National Cancer Institute recommends allogeneic bone-marrow transplantation, whenever possible, for Ph-positive ALL and other high-risk subtypes.

Chromosomal Abnormalities in ALL

Unfavorable:
- Philadelphia chromosome
- Translocation of chromosomes 4 and 11; 2 and 8; 8 and 12; or 8 and 22

In addition to analyzing the leukemic cells' cytogenetic composition, tests are conducted to detect the production of certain antigens, oncogenes, and other substances. These markers, too, can impart important information that may affect the treatment plan.

TREATMENTS FOR ADVANCED OR RECURRENT LEUKEMIA

Acute Myeloid Leukemia—Roughly three in ten patients whose cancer reappears can be cured through allogeneic bone-marrow transplantation if it is carried out shortly after the recurrence—or once *re*induction therapy has put the leukemia into remission. In order to spare patients the toxicity of the drugs, some oncologists believe that it is preferable not to repeat the chemotherapy. BMT can also salvage cases that would otherwise be terminal: (1) following a second relapse, (2) a recurrence more than one year posttransplant, or (3) when induction chemotherapy fails. Remarkably, 10 to 20 percent of these patients will be cured.

Autografting is another option, provided that reinduction therapy succeeds in eradicating all detectable traces of the disease. The cure rate from autologous BMT in this setting is equivalent to that from autografting during a first remission: 35 to 50 percent.

Acute Lymphocytic Leukemia—In ALL, where chemotherapy stands a reasonable chance of effecting a cure, one strategy is to reserve allogeneic bone-marrow transplant for recurrent disease. First, though, reinduction chemotherapy must induce a second remission. If matching marrow from a sibling is available, the cure rate is 35 percent. A MUD transplant isn't out of the question, but the mortality rates are worrisome enough that instead the oncologist might recommend clinical trials of autoBMT, or new chemotherapies or immunotherapies.

Chronic Lymphocytic Leukemia—CLL is one of the rare cancers where the same drug or drugs can be employed a second time to halt the cancer's progression or to coax the disease back into remission following a relapse. "Retreatment with the same drug is often successful," says Dr. Appelbaum, "particularly if a couple of years have passed since the first treatment. If the interval is measured in a year or less, then we generally switch to new agents. A patient initially treated with fludarabine can be switched over to chlorambucil, or vice versa." Other agents that may come into play in advanced or recurrent CLL include cladribine (Leustatin) and pentostatin (Nipent).

Chronic Myeloid Leukemia—Once CML has progressed beyond the chronic phase, it becomes increasingly difficult to contain. In blastic phase, the cure rate for allogeneic bone-marrow transplantation falls to less than 10 percent. Autologous BMT cannot cure advanced CML, but it has been shown to revert the leukemia to the chronic phase, where the disease may remain stable for some time.

Advanced CML is usually resistant to chemotherapeutic agents. But some patients who have relapsed following alloBMT do respond to alpha-interferon. Another experimental tact that may be taken in this instance is adoptive immunotherapy, described below.

OTHER THERAPIES THAT MAY BE USED IN THE TREATMENT OF LEUKEMIA

Adoptive Immunotherapy (investigational, CML)—We've already noted that autologous BMT does not generate the crucial graft-versus-leukemia effect achieved with alloBMT. Instead of subjecting relapsed CML patients to a second transplant, a doctor may recommend adoptive immunotherapy as a method for obtaining a long-lasting remission.

The technique is surprisingly simple: The patient is infused with normal white blood cells taken from the marrow donor's blood. According to the International Bone Marrow Transplant Registry, about 80 percent of relapsed patients treated in this manner during the chronic phase went into remission. One drawback to adoptive immunotherapy is its extremely high incidence of graft-versus-host disease (GVHD), which of course can be fatal. However, a clinical trial performed at Memorial Sloan-Kettering Cancer Center in New York found that infusing smaller amounts of donor white cells significantly reduced the rate of GVHD. Nineteen of twenty-two participants experienced complete remissions. Of the nineteen, eight had been given low doses of white blood cells, while the other eleven had received high doses. Only one patient in the low-dose group developed GVHD, as compared to eight in the high-dose group.

Leukapheresis/Thrombapheresis (CML)—Though rarely applied, either or both of these procedures can be used to temporarily lower dangerously high levels of white blood cells (leukocytes) or platelets (thrombocytes). The patient's blood is circulated through a special processor that separates out the white cells and/or platelets before it is returned to the bloodstream.

Splenectomy (CLL, CML)—The spleen, situated in the upper abdomen, normally measures about five inches long. In chronic leukemia, the oblong-shaped organ frequently enlarges—sometimes enormously—as it accumulates leukemic cells, red blood cells, platelets, and transfused blood cells from the bloodstream.

Though surgery to remove the spleen is "pretty uncommon," according to Dr. Appelbaum, the operation may be necessary for someone whose spleen has become so distended that it is pressing against the stomach, making it difficult to eat, or against the diaphragm, interfering with breathing. Splenectomy is also sometimes used to manage hemolytic anemia or thrombocytopenia, in which the body destroys red blood cells and/or platelet cells, outpacing the bone marrow's ability to produce replacements.

**CLL and CML/
Surgical Procedures**

Splenectomy: surgery to remove the spleen.
Average hospital stay: 5–7 days

Radiation Therapy—In lieu of surgery, external-beam radiotherapy can reduce the size of the spleen and correct the blood disorders mentioned above. It, too, is rare in leukemia. Other applications would be to shrink masses in the lymph nodes—the result of a buildup of cancerous white blood cells—or to treat disease in the central nervous system. "Radiation has no impact on the overall management of leukemia," Dr. Appelbaum explains, "but it can help with a very local and specific problem."

♦ *Ask your doctor about these and any other investigational therapies that might benefit you.*

Cancer of the Kidney (Renal-Cell Carcinoma)

Overview

TREATMENTS FOR KIDNEY CANCER THAT HAS NOT METASTASIZED

Surgery

"If a kidney cancer appears at all resectable, an attempt will be made to remove it," observes Dr. Jim Mohler of the UNC Lineberger Comprehensive Cancer Center, "because there is no other effective treatment." Nearly half of all patients are diagnosed with local disease (stages I and II), which is frequently curable. At stage III, when the tumor involves either of two large veins—the *renal vein* and the inferior vena cava—surgery can still prolong life and bring about cures.

There are three types of kidney-cancer operations. The standard surgery is the most extensive, a radical nephrectomy. For stage I disease, there's some question as to whether or not a simple nephrectomy is equally effective. And should your tumor measure less than 4 centimeters (1½ inches), you may be able to undergo a kidney-sparing partial nephrectomy. Dr. Mohler was the first physician to perform the operation at UNC Lineberger. "As recently as the mid-1980s," he says, "the medical textbooks said that partial nephrectomy couldn't be done."

KIDNEY CANCER/ Surgical Procedures

Nephrectomy: surgical removal of part or all of the kidney. A *partial nephrectomy* excises only the cancerous portion of the kidney and a margin of healthy surrounding tissue, while a *simple nephrectomy* takes out the entire organ. In a *radical nephrectomy,* the surgeon removes the kidney, the adjacent *adrenal gland,* the surrounding fat, and *Gerota's fascia,* a filmy sac that envelops the kidney and its ureter tube. Five to twenty regional lymph nodes may be dissected as well. Average hospital stay: 5–7 days

KIDNEY CANCER/Treatment Options

STAGE I RENAL-CELL CARCINOMA

> **T1:** The cancer measures less than 2.5 centimeters (1 inch) and is confined to the kidney.
>
> **T2:** The cancer measures more than 2.5 centimeters but is still confined to the kidney.

- Radical nephrectomy, to surgically remove the kidney and the surrounding tissue, *with or without* lymph-node dissection • *or*

- Simple nephrectomy, to surgically remove only the kidney • *or, in selected patients*

- Partial nephrectomy, to surgically remove the cancerous portion of the kidney

If the tumor is inoperable:

- External-beam radiation therapy, to relieve symptoms • *or*

- Arterial embolization, to relieve symptoms

Under Investigation

◆ Ask your doctor about any clinical trials that might benefit you.

STAGE II RENAL-CELL CARCINOMA

The cancer has spread to the fat around the kidney but not beyond the organ's capsule.

- Radical nephrectomy, *with or without* lymph-node dissection • *or, in selected patients*

- Simple nephrectomy • *or*

- Partial nephrectomy

If the tumor is inoperable:

- External-beam radiation therapy, to relieve symptoms • *or*

- Arterial embolization, to relieve symptoms

Under Investigation

◆ Ask your doctor about any clinical trials that might benefit you.

STAGE III RENAL-CELL CARCINOMA

The cancer involves the kidney's main blood vessel (the renal vein); or the vessel that carries the blood from the kidney to the heart (the inferior vena cava); or neighboring lymph nodes.

- Radical nephrectomy, *with* lymph-node dissection *and* removal of the tumor from involved blood vessels • *alone or preceded by*

- Arterial embolization

Or:

- Simple or radical nephrectomy, to relieve symptoms

If the tumor is inoperable:
- External-beam radiation therapy, to relieve symptoms · *or*
- Arterial embolization, to relieve symptoms

Under Investigation
- Radical nephrectomy, *with or without* lymph-node dissection · *followed by*
- Immunotherapy, frequently consisting of alpha-interferon
- ◆ Ask your doctor about any clinical trials that might benefit you.

STAGE IV RENAL-CELL CARCINOMA
The cancer has spread to nearby organs or to distant sites.
- Immunotherapy, frequently consisting of interleukin-2 or alpha-interferon

If the tumor has spread only to the area around the kidney:
- Radical nephrectomy

If the tumor has metastasized, but to a limited area:
- Radical nephrectomy · *plus*
- Surgical removal of the secondary tumor

Or:
- Simple nephrectomy, to relieve symptoms · *or*
- External-beam radiation therapy, to relieve symptoms · *or*
- Arterial embolization, to relieve symptoms

Under Investigation
- Nephrectomy, to remove as much of the cancerous kidney as possible · *followed by*
- Immunotherapy, frequently consisting of alpha-interferon or interleukin-2
- New chemotherapy drugs and immunologic agents
- ◆ Ask your doctor about any clinical trials that might benefit you.

See treatment options for metastases of the bone, brain, and lung.

RECURRENT RENAL-CELL CARCINOMA
Your therapy will depend on how you were treated initially.
- Immunotherapy, frequently consisting of interleukin-2 or alpha-interferon · *or*
- Chemotherapy, frequently consisting of vinblastine · *or*
- External-beam radiation therapy, to relieve symptoms

If you are diagnosed with cancer in both kidneys:
- Radical nephrectomy of one kidney · *and*
- Partial nephrectomy of the other

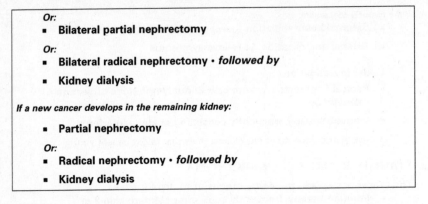

Besides tumor size, "the other generally accepted criterion for performing a partial nephrectomy is that the cancer not be centrally located and that the patient either has no kidney on the opposite side or suffers from impaired renal function, so that removal of that entire kidney would make him dependent on dialysis." In *hemodialysis,* administered three times a week in a hospital or dialysis clinic, a machine called a *dialyzer* carries out the kidneys' task of filtering the blood. Another method, *peritoneal dialysis,* performs the same function several times a day, but inside the person's body.

Most men and women with renal-cell carcinoma will not require dialysis, even if their cancerous kidney is removed, because its counterpart can more than compensate. *Synchronous bilateral neoplasms*—simultaneous tumors in both the left and the right kidneys—account for only about one in thirty cases.

"Typically, what we do is perform a partial nephrectomy on the kidney bearing the smallest tumor," explains Dr. Mohler. "Then if all goes well, we do a radical nephrectomy on the other side. But if for some reason we're unable to do a partial and have to completely remove the first kidney, we can still try to do a partial nephrectomy on the kidney with the larger tumor, to keep the person from having to go on dialysis." A double partial nephrectomy is applicable when both cancers are local and smaller than four centimeters. You may hear this referred to as a stage I, T1 tumor.

Another one in thirty patients treated for renal-cell cancer will subsequently develop a second malignancy (a separate tumor, *not* a metastasis) in the healthy twin. In this situation, which would also include anyone who'd lost a kidney to other, noncancerous forms of renal disease, early detection is crucial. The doctor's ability to perform a partial nephrectomy is all that stands between the patient and the need for permanent dialysis.

♦ *If you appear to meet the critaeria for a partial nephrectomy but are told the surgery can't be done, we'd recommend seeking a second opinion at a facility experienced in this operation.*

At stage II and beyond, radical nephrectomy is the only surgery that would be considered. Stage III renal-cell carcinoma includes tumors that grow into the renal vein or the vena cava, the large blood vessel that carries blood from the lower part of the body to the heart.* According to Dr. Mohler, "Provided the cancer in the blood vessels is below the heart, these patients do just as well as if they didn't have a tumor in the vessels at all." The radical nephrectomy is expanded to take out the entire renal vein and part of the vena cava as well as the regional lymph nodes.

> **Is Kidney Transplantation an Option?**
>
> The answer is rarely. As Dr. Mohler explains, "The transplant guidelines require that a patient with a favorable cancer needs to go two years without any evidence of a recurrence in order to qualify for a transplantation. If you have an unfavorable cancer, meaning stage II or higher, then you have to go five years before you can be transplanted.
>
> "So, yes, it has a role, but first you have to prove you're cured of your cancer."

Stage III also encompasses people who are node positive, a finding that is typically discovered during surgery. Although cures are still possible through radical nephrectomy and node dissection, with the discovery of nodal involvement, the five-year survival rate drops precipitously. "Patients would then be considered for experimental treatment," says Dr. Mohler, "such as immunotherapy."

TREATMENTS FOR ADVANCED KIDNEY CANCER

Immunotherapy (Palliative Treatment)

Renal-cell carcinoma, along with malignant melanoma, is one of the cancers most sensitive to immunomodulation. Even so, cautions Dr. Mohler, in kidney cancer immunotherapy has yet to distinguish itself as anything beyond "a minor advance."

The number of patients who respond is on the order of one in five—hardly extraordinary, but about twice that from chemotherapy, which as of now has not earned a place in kidney-cancer treatment. "When they do respond to immunotherapy," he says, "the responses

---

*Under another staging system for kidney cancer, this would be classified as stage II disease.

are often dramatic, although cures are very rare." Interleukin-2 (brand name: Proleukin) appears to hold slightly more promise than interferon alfa-2A (Roferon-A), producing long-lasting remissions in 5 percent of the people receiving it. But the high doses that have been used to date are extremely toxic. In one study of more than 250 men and women with metastatic renal-cell carcinoma, 4 percent died of treatment-related side effects. More recent research has indicated that lower doses of IL-2 can be effective as well as more tolerable.

**KIDNEY CANCER/
Drug Therapy**

*First-line therapy frequently
consists of:*
- **interleukin-2 (I)**
- **alpha-interferon (I)**

*Other agents that may be used
include:*
- **lomustine**
- **vinblastine**

(I) = immunologic agent

Interleukin-2 and interferon are just two of the many compounds being evaluated at cancer centers around the country for advanced kidney cancer. "There are all kinds of cutting-edge therapies available," Dr. Mohler observes. Clinical trials have been or are testing therapies incorporating *monoclonal antibodies, LAK cells, TIL cells,* various immune-system stimulants, and immunotherapy-chemotherapy regimens, as well as gene therapy.

See "Immunotherapy" in Chapter Four, "How Cancer Is Treated."

Surgery (Palliative Treatment)

Stage IV renal-cell carcinoma is generally considered inoperable. For patients who still have their cancerous kidney intact, drug therapy may shrink secondary lesions, but the systemic treatment rarely exerts an effect on the primary tumor. Surgery to take out the kidney and the distant metastases may be indicated in selected cases where the original tumor has migrated to a single organ or a limited number of sites. Otherwise, says Dr. Mohler, "it's rare nowadays that we can't control the local tumor with either radiation or arterial embolization."

Surgery and Immunotherapy (Investigational)

The kidney-cancer program at Los Angeles's Jonsson Cancer Center takes an unusually aggressive approach to treating metastatic renal-cell carcinoma. Based on its impressive results, reported in 1999, other medical centers may soon be following in UCLA's footsteps.

The study tracked thirty-one patients with kidney cancer that had spread to the lung, liver, bone, and other parts of the body. Few hospitals would have considered performing a surgery as complicated as radical nephrectomy. But Jonsson's department of urologic oncology went ahead and operated, on the premise that removing as much tumor as possible would help to level the playing field when it came time to initiate a harsh regimen of immunotherapy.

Many of the thirty-one men and women had been given six months or less to live before they sought a second opinion at UCLA. After eighteen months, one in four were still alive, and about half of the survivors with low-grade tumors or secondary cancers of the lung could look forward to reaching the five-year mark. Ordinarily, perhaps 15 percent of patients with stage IV disease live that long.

OTHER THERAPIES THAT MAY BE USED IN THE TREATMENT OF KIDNEY CANCER

Radiation Therapy (palliative treatment)—External-beam radiotherapy may be used to relieve symptoms in patients unable to undergo surgery.

Arterial Embolization (palliative treatment)—This technique for starving tumors of oxygen and nutrients by blocking their blood supply was once looked to as a potential cure for kidney cancer, but enthusiasm has all but faded, says Dr. Mohler. Arterial embolization has also been employed preoperatively to shrink large tumors and facilitate their removal. "But a well-conducted study has shown that it does not do that.

"The only reason that I would use arterial embolization," he continues, "is to stop life-threatening bleeding in somebody who has an unresectable cancer and no evidence of metastatic disease." The rarely performed procedure, which entails injecting a foreign substance into the targeted artery, "is extremely painful."

See "Arterial Embolization" in Chapter Four, "How Cancer Is Treated."

> **Spontaneous Regression: The Case of the Vanishing Tumor**
>
> Kidney cancer is one of the rare tumors that sometimes regress on their own, without any therapy. In one study, this was the case for five out of seventy-three participants. The reduction in size is usually temporary, however.

Hormonal Therapy (investigational)—In your research, you may come across material touting the benefits of hormonal therapy. Because kidney cancers have been found to contain high levels of progesterone receptors, progestational agents were once considered promising. But as with arterial embolization, hormonal therapy, too, has since been discounted in kidney cancer, except perhaps as a palliative measure.

◆ *Ask your doctor about these and any other investigational therapies that might benefit you.*

Cancer of the Pancreas

Overview

TREATMENTS FOR OPERABLE PANCREATIC CANCER THAT HAS NOT METASTASIZED

Because conventional treatments are frequently no match for cancer of the pancreas, you may want to consider participating in a clinical trial, whatever your stage of disease. That having been said, "not everyone who has pancreatic cancer is going to die of it," emphasizes Dr. Charles Yeo of the Johns Hopkins University School of Medicine. Cures are possible, particularly if you're among the one in five patients whose tumor has been staged as *T*1, which means that it is confined to the pancreas, with no involvement of the lymph nodes or spread to distant organs.

Surgery
The pancreas secretes the hormone insulin as well as several vital digestive enzymes. To take out the entire gland in a total or regional pancreatectomy leaves patients dependent on daily insulin injections and oral enzyme supplements.

Whenever possible, doctors look to preserve organ function by removing only part of it. With three-fourths of all pancreatic cancers occurring in the head of the wing-shaped gland, the most common operation is the Whipple procedure. Named after the surgeon who popularized it in the 1930s, the Whipple procedure consists of resecting the head and neck—or about one-third—of the pancreas, as well as the duodenum, the portion of the small intestine that joins to the stomach. Similarly, distal pancreatectomy, for tumors in the tail or body, leaves 30 to 70 percent of the pancreas intact.

In pancreatic cancer, stage I includes tumors that have grown into the duodenum, the bile duct, or surrounding tissues. The bile duct, a thin conduit that carries bile fluid from the liver and gallbladder to the small intestine, "runs smack through the head of the pancreas," explains Dr. Yeo, "so for the cancer to extend to the bile duct is the norm." A person with this tumor, designated *T2*, is still an "ideal candidate for Whipple surgery."

At a prominent cancer center such as Johns Hopkins, nine in ten patients undergo the Whipple procedure. According to Dr. Yeo, a local tumor warrants total pancreatectomy only in the rare event that it is *multicentric*, or extends across the whole organ. Unfortunately, total pancreatectomy sometimes becomes necessary when the less extensive operation is performed by a surgeon with limited experience in pancreatic resection.

"Some patients," says Dr. Yeo, "will undergo the Whipple procedure, then a week or two later develop a leak where the pancreas was sewn to the small intestine. The surgeon then has to go back in and remove the remainder of the gland in order to save the patient's life." In experienced hands, he says, such complications are rare. "But it definitely occurs more frequently when the Whipple operation is done only occasionally," which underlines the importance of seeking treatment at a medical facility practiced in pancreatic-cancer surgery.

The Informed Patient:
Why Expertise in Pancreatic Surgery Is Absolutely Essential

Any operation on the pancreas is potentially life-threatening. A 1997 study conducted by Johns Hopkins offers persuasive evidence that choosing a hospital where these surgeries are regularly performed can greatly enhance your odds of surviving the procedure.

PANCREATIC CANCER/Surgical Procedures

Whipple procedure (pancreatoduodenectomy): surgical removal of the head and neck of the pancreas, the duodenum, and some surrounding tissue.
Average hospital stay: 10–12 days

Total pancreatectomy: surgical removal of the whole pancreas as well as the duodenum, common bile duct, *gallbladder,* spleen, and most of the adjacent lymph nodes.
Average hospital stay: 12 days

Distal pancreatectomy: surgical removal of the body and tail of the pancreas, and usually the spleen as well. Only one in four pancreatic cancers grow in the body or tail.
Average hospital stay: 8 days

Regional pancreatectomy: surgical removal of the pancreas, adjacent lymph nodes, some of the blood vessels that supply the organ, and possibly the lower stomach.
Average hospital stay: 12–14 days

Biliary bypass surgery: procedure performed when an inoperable tumor is (1) blocking the duodenum, causing bile fluid to build up in the gallbladder, or (2) blocking the common bile duct that passes through the pancreas. If the former, the surgeon bypasses the cancer by connecting the bile duct to the *jejunum,* the section of the small intestine below the duodenum. In the latter situation, a catheter tube can be surgically implanted in the bile duct. The fluid then drains into a small external bag. A nerve block, to relieve pain, is performed during the operation.
Average hospital stay: 8 days

The study compared the outcomes of more than twelve hundred patients treated at one of four dozen Maryland hospitals: forty low-volume facilities; seven medium-volume centers; and Johns Hopkins, a high-volume institution, and the world's leading practitioner of pancreatic-cancer operations. The differences in the rates of surgery-related deaths among the three classes of hospitals tell you all you need to know:

At Johns Hopkins, less than 2 percent of patients to undergo curative surgery (Whipple procedure or total pancreatectomy) died in the hospital as a result of the operation. The in-hospital mortality rates for the same procedures were 6.9 percent at the medium-volume hospitals and 18.8 percent at the low-volume hospitals.

At Johns Hopkins, the in-hospital mortality rate from bypass surgeries to relieve symptoms of pancreatic cancer was 4.2 percent. The in-hospital mortality rates for the same procedures were 10.5 percent at the medium-volume hospitals and 15.3 percent at the low-volume hospitals.

A study of hospitals in New York State produced near-identical results.

Surgical expertise can add months or years to your life. It can even cure you. Nationally, 3 percent of men and women treated by the Whipple operation are alive five years later. The five-year survival rate at Hopkins is seven times that (21 percent), and higher still for other patients, depending on the characteristics of the cancer:

- 26 percent if the surgeon is able to obtain negative margins around the tumor site

- 28 percent if the tumor measures less than 3 centimeters (1¼ inches)

- 36 percent if no lymph nodes are involved

- 39 percent if the tumor cells are *diploid,* meaning they contain the normal twin sets of chromosomes

The significantly higher percentage of success stories partly reflects a willingness on the part of Hopkins physicians to resect pancreatic tumors that less experienced surgeons might declare inoperable. The philosophy, says Dr. Yeo, "is to try to resect every patient whenever possible."

Chemoradiation (Chemotherapy and Radiation Therapy)

Since the 1970s, the number of pancreatic-cancer patients who go on to live at least several years postdiagnosis has risen steadily, as has the average duration of survival. Contributing to these improved rates

PANCREATIC CANCER/Treatment Options

STAGE I PANCREATIC CANCER

> T1: The cancer is confined solely to the pancreas.

> T2: The cancer has extended to the portion of the small intestine that connects to the stomach (the duodenum), the bile duct, or other neighboring tissues.

- Whipple procedure (pancreatoduodenectomy), to surgically remove the head and neck of the pancreas, the duodenum, and some surrounding tissue • *or*

- Total pancreatectomy, to surgically remove the whole pancreas as well as the duodenum, common bile duct, gallbladder, spleen, and most of the adjacent lymph nodes • *or*

- Distal pancreatectomy, to surgically remove the body and tail of the pancreas and usually the spleen • *with or without*

- Chemotherapy, frequently consisting of fluorouracil, alone or in combination with leucovorin and/or mitomycin • *followed by*

- External-beam radiation therapy

Under Investigation

- External-beam radiation therapy • *or*

- Chemoradiation, frequently consisting of fluorouracil, alone or in combination with leucovorin and/or mitomycin, or gemcitabine, administered preoperatively, postoperatively, or intraoperatively, during surgery

◆ Ask your doctor about any clinical trials that might benefit you.

STAGE II PANCREATIC CANCER

The cancer has spread to adjacent organs, such as the stomach, spleen, or colon, but not to the lymph nodes.

- Whipple procedure • *or*

- Total pancreatectomy • *or*

- Distal pancreatectomy • *or*

- Regional pancreatectomy, to surgically remove the pancreas, adjacent lymph nodes, some of the blood vessels that supply the organ, and possibly the lower stomach • *with or without*

- Chemotherapy, frequently consisting of fluorouracil, alone or in combination with leucovorin and/or mitomycin • *followed by*

- External-beam radiation therapy

If the tumor is inoperable (rare):

- External-beam radiation therapy • *with or without*

- Chemotherapy, frequently consisting of one or more of the following drugs: fluorouracil, leucovorin, mitomycin, gemcitabine

To relieve obstruction of the bile duct:
- Biliary bypass surgery • *or*
- Biliary stent placement

Under Investigation #1
- Preoperative chemoradiation

Under Investigation #2
- Intraoperative external-beam or internal radiation therapy

Under Investigation #3
- Radiation therapy using radiosensitizing drugs to enhance the cancer cells' sensitivity

Under Investigation #4
- New chemotherapy drugs
- ◆ Ask your doctor about any clinical trials that might benefit you.

STAGE III PANCREATIC CANCER

The cancer involves the regional lymph nodes.
- Whipple procedure • *or*
- Total pancreatectomy • *or*
- Distal pancreatectomy • *or*
- Regional pancreatectomy • *with or without*
- Chemotherapy, frequently consisting of fluorouracil, alone or in combination with leucovorin and/or mitomycin • *followed by*
- External-beam radiation therapy

If the tumor is inoperable:
- External-beam radiation therapy • *with or without*
- Chemotherapy, frequently consisting of one or more of the following drugs: fluorouracil, leucovorin, mitomycin, gemcitabine

To relieve obstruction of the bile duct:
- Biliary bypass surgery • *or*
- Biliary stent placement

Under Investigation #1
- Preoperative irradiation

Under Investigation #2
- Intraoperative external-beam or internal radiation therapy

Under Investigation #3
- Radiation therapy using radiosensitizing drugs to enhance the cancer cells' sensitivity

Under Investigation #4
- New chemotherapy drugs

Under Investigation #5
- Chemoradiation, frequently consisting of one or more of the following drugs: fluorouracil, leucovorin, mitomycin, gemcitabine
◆ Ask your doctor about any clinical trials that might benefit you.

STAGE IV PANCREATIC CANCER

The cancer has metastasized to distant sites, most often the liver or lung.

- No further therapy • *or*
- Chemotherapy, frequently consisting of fluorouracil, gemcitabine, or other agents, to relieve symptoms

To relieve obstruction of the bile duct:
- Biliary bypass surgery • *or*
- Biliary stent placement

Under Investigation
- New chemotherapy drugs, immunologic agents, and cancer vaccines
◆ Ask your doctor about any clinical trials that might benefit you.

See treatment options for metastases of the liver and lung.

RECURRENT PANCREATIC CANCER

Your therapy will depend on how you were treated initially.

- No further therapy • *or*
- Chemotherapy, frequently consisting of fluorouracil, gemcitabine, or other agents, to relieve symptoms • *or*
- External-beam radiation therapy, to relieve symptoms

Under Investigation
- New chemotherapy drugs, immunologic agents, and cancer vaccines
◆ Ask your doctor about any clinical trials that might benefit you.

---

is the increasing practice of following surgery with chemotherapy and radiotherapy, which have been shown to slow the cancer's growth.

Another Johns Hopkins study tracked seventy-eight men and women with resectable pancreatic tumors. Fifty-six opted for adjuvant chemoradiation, while twenty-two declined further therapy. Two years later, thirty-five of the patients in the first group were still alive, whereas every participant in the no-treatment arm had died.

Once patients recover from surgery, they begin chemotherapy. Fluorouracil (5-FU) is typically the principal agent used, often in conjunction with leucovorin (brand name: Wellcovorin) and/or mitomycin (Mutamycin). Then the tumor bed and neighboring tissues receive external-beam radiation. Some research centers have experi-

---

**PANCREATIC
CANCER/Drug Therapy**

*First-line therapy often consists
of:*
- **fluorouracil, *with or without***
- **leucovorin, *and/or***
- **mitomycin**

Other drugs used may include:
- **dacarbazine**
- **gemcitabine**
- **yttrium-90 radiolabeled
  carcinoembryonic-antigen
  antibody (I)**

(I)=immunologic agent

---

mented with delivering external or internal radiation at the time of surgery, when the abdomen is open, but the results, says Dr. Yeo, "have not been universally favorable."

Preoperative Chemoradiation—By the time most pancreatic cancers are discovered, the disease has spread to the neighboring lymph nodes. Yet as long as the primary tumor remains restricted to the pancreas, the treatment plan is usually no different than if there were no nodal involvement: resection, chemotherapy, radiotherapy. According to Dr. Yeo, "Three-quarters of our patients who undergo the Whipple operation have positive regional lymph nodes."

Dr. Yeo describes another scenario that may call for giving chemo and radiation prior to surgery, in order to enhance the effectiveness of the operation. "Occasionally, we'll see a patient who presents with a large mass in the head of the pancreas and is found upon CT scan or staging laparoscopy to have cancerous lymph nodes situated outside the area that is removed during the Whipple procedure.

"In this case we have two options: We can either go ahead and do the Whipple operation, knowing that we're going to leave some positive nodes behind, and then give the patient postoperative chemo and radiation" (the likelihood of a cure, however, would be extremely slim) "or we can give the patient chemo and radiation up front in an effort to shrink the tumor and perhaps sterilize that nodal basin. Then, if the patient does well with that neoadjuvant therapy, in about three months she'd be a candidate for surgical resection."

TREATMENTS FOR INOPERABLE OR ADVANCED PANCREATIC CANCER

Surgery (Palliative Treatment)

In pancreatic cancer, stage II denotes that the tumor has invaded the stomach, spleen, colon, or adjacent large arteries or veins. According to Dr. Yeo, extension to the *aorta* or the *vena cava* renders the disease inoperable. "However, we can resect portions of the *portal vein* or the *superior mesenteric vein* if they should become involved. This makes the operation harder than a normal Whipple procedure, but it can be done."

When pancreatic cancer metastasizes (stage IV), it usually seeds secondary tumors in the liver. There is little point to operating on the primary cancer, explains Dr. Yeo, "because we'd be leaving behind billions of malignant cells in the liver." Tumors that spread to the nearby lymph nodes (stage III) are often beyond surgery too.

An operation may still be necessary to make patients more comfortable. If the tumor obstructs the bile duct, for example, the bile fluid builds up and enters the bloodstream, producing jaundice. The characteristic yellowing of the skin and whites of the eyes isn't terribly bothersome, but the intense itching, or *pruritus,* can be unbearable. What's more, untreated jaundice will eventually bring about fatal liver failure. Less frequently, the tumor pinches off the duodenum, interfering with eating and digestion.

Either problem can be corrected with surgery to circumvent the obstruction. In a *gastrojejunostomy,* the surgeon connects the stomach to the middle portion of the small intestine. Similarly, *biliary bypass surgery* reroutes the flow of bile by attaching the bile duct or gallbladder directly to the small intestine. Although the operation is effective, one in five patients will experience complications, and some will not survive. Biliary stent placement, a nonsurgical approach, is far less risky. However, the jaundice often recurs.

See "Biliary Stent Placement," page 458, and "Itching" under "Skin Disorders" in Chapter Eight, "Take Control: Managing Symptoms, Side Effects, and Complications."

Chemoradiation (Palliative Treatment)

Individually, chemotherapy or radiotherapy can ease pain and other symptoms of unresectable pancreatic cancer. Some studies indicate that when used in combination, they may prolong patients' lives. The standard agent at many state-of-the-art centers is a novel drug called gemcitabine (Gemzar).

"It's not a typical antitumor therapy in that it often doesn't seem to shrink cancer cells or induce a response we can see on X ray," explains Dr. Yeo. "Yet it has been shown to prolong life—and *quality of life*—in patients who have incurable pancreatic cancer." The drug, which is usually well tolerated, has proved effective in some men and women who did not respond to 5-FU.

OTHER THERAPIES THAT MAY BE USED IN THE TREATMENT OF PANCREATIC CANCER

Biliary Stent Placement (palliative treatment)—A stent, explains Dr. Yeo, is a small plastic or wire-mesh tube "that basically holds the tumor open and serves as a straw for the bile to travel through." There are two methods for inserting it in the bile duct, both nonsurgical.

In the *endoscopic* approach, the physician feeds a flexible viewing scope down the throat until it reaches the common bile duct, then passes the stent through the instrument and places it in position. This requires a topical anesthetic sprayed at the back of the throat and intravenous sedation. For *percutaneous* stent placement, patients are put to sleep and their right lower side numbed with local anesthetic. To give you an idea how small the stent is, it fits inside a needle, which the physician inserts through the skin and the liver and into the duct, using ultrasonography to guide him.

Although biliary stent placement is safer than the surgical method, you still want to have this procedure performed at a center with experience. In that same John Hopkins study cited earlier, the rate of deaths from stent placement was 1.6 percent at Hopkins, but about 10 percent at the hospitals that saw fewer pancreatic-cancer patients.

Celiac Block (palliative treatment)—There are several ways to control pain. In pancreatic cancer, one effective and long-lasting technique is to inject alcohol into the tangle of nerves serving the pancreas, thereby destroying them. A *celiac block* (also referred to as *chemical splanchnicectomy*) is often carried out at the same time as surgery to bypass an obstructive tumor in the abdomen. "The surgeon can actually hold the nerves in his hand and block them," says Dr. Yeo. A percutaneous celiac block accomplishes this without surgery, although "the results are not quite as good." Here the nerves are injected with a needle inserted through the back.

Immunotherapy/Tumor Vaccines (investigational)—For all the strides that have been made in treating pancreatic cancer, the malignancy remains one of the most forbidding carcinomas. Around the country, clinical trials are testing various forms of immunotherapies designed to incite patients' immune systems to attack the tumor. Being tested are vaccines, monoclonal antibodies, alpha-interferon, and interleukin-2, administered alone or in combination with chemotherapy.

With most cancers, unproven therapies are typically reserved for patients considered beyond cure. But at Johns Hopkins and other medical centers, immunotherapy is being offered as part of postoperative treatment, says Dr. Yeo, "in the hope that adding it to chemotherapy and radiation will achieve the best tumor kill."

◆ *Ask your doctor about these and any other investigational therapies that might benefit you.*

Cancer of the Ovary

Overview

TREATMENTS FOR OVARIAN CANCER THAT HAS NOT METASTASIZED

Surgery

Unless ovarian cancer has spread outside the abdomen or penetrated the surface of the liver (stage IV), the primary treatment is to surgically remove the female reproductive organs (total abdominal hysterectomy and bilateral salpingo-oophorectomy, with omentectomy and lymph-node dissection).

Most ovarian-cancer patients are past menopause. However, the disease can afflict women in their forties, thirties, even twenties. If the cancer is stage IA, grade 1, meaning that it involves only one ovary and is of low grade, fertility can often be preserved. "We limit our surgery to removing the cancerous ovary and the fallopian tube," explains Dr. Larry Copeland of the Arthur G. James Cancer Hospital and Research Institute. Low-grade ovarian cancer also goes by the name ovarian low-malignant-potential cancer and has an excellent outlook at any of its three stages. Nine in ten patients are still alive after twenty years.

Since it is not considered safe to biopsy

OVARIAN CANCER/ Surgical Procedures

Total abdominal hysterectomy and bilateral salpingo-oophorectomy, with omentectomy and lymph-node dissection: surgical removal of the uterus, both ovaries and fallopian tubes, and the omentum, an apron of fatty tissue that hangs from the stomach to the colon. Lymph nodes in the pelvis and abdomen are sampled and examined for cancer. If the tumor has spread to other organs, the surgeon cuts out as much of it as possible in what is referred to as *tumor debulking.* Average hospital stay: 3–5 days

Second-look laparotomy: exploratory surgery to look for evidence of any residual cancer following the completion of chemotherapy for stage III ovarian cancer. The surgeon carefully inspects the abdomen and pelvis, takes a number of tissue samples, and biopsies area lymph nodes. Average hospital stay: 3–5 days

OVARIAN CANCER/Treatment Options

Ovarian Epithelial Cancer

STAGE I OVARIAN CANCER

The cancer is confined to one ovary.

The cancer is found in both ovaries.

The cancer is found in one or both ovaries, but the tumor sits on the surface of the organ(s); or the tumor has ruptured the capsule(s) of the gland(s); or malignant cells are found in excess abdominal fluid known as ascites.

- Total abdominal hysterectomy and bilateral salpingo-oophorectomy, to surgically remove the uterus and both ovaries and fallopian tubes; *plus* omentectomy, to surgically remove the omentum tissue; *and* lymph-node dissection • *alone or followed by*

- Chemotherapy, frequently consisting of paclitaxel in combination with cisplatin or carboplatin • *or*

- Intraperitoneal radiation therapy, in which a radioactive liquid is injected into the peritoneum, the sac that lines the abdomen • *or*

- External-beam radiation therapy

Or:
- Unilateral salpingo-oophorectomy, to remove only the cancerous ovary and the attached fallopian tube

Under Investigation
- New methods of delivering chemotherapy

◆ Ask your doctor about any clinical trials that might benefit you.

STAGE II OVARIAN CANCER

The cancer is found in one or both ovaries and has spread to other body parts within the pelvis.

The cancer has infiltrated or metastasized to the uterus and/or the fallopian tubes.

The cancer has infiltrated other tissues within the pelvis.

The cancer is either stage IIA or stage IIB, but the tumor sits on the surface of the organ(s); or the tumor has ruptured the capsule(s) of the organ(s); or malignant cells are found in excess abdominal fluid known as ascites.

- Total abdominal hysterectomy and bilateral salpingo-oophorectomy, *with* omentectomy *and* lymph-node dissection *and* tumor debulking, to remove all or as much of the tumor as possible • *followed by*

{
- Chemotherapy, frequently consisting of paclitaxel in combination with cisplatin or carboplatin, or other drug combinations • *or*
- External-beam radiation therapy • *or*
- Intraperitoneal radiation therapy

Under Investigation #1
- New methods of delivering chemotherapy

Under Investigation #2
- High-dose chemotherapy • *followed by*
- Autologous bone-marrow transplantation

Under Investigation #3
- New chemotherapy drugs
- ◆ Ask your doctor about any clinical trials that might benefit you.

STAGE III OVARIAN CANCER

The cancer involves one or both ovaries and has spread to other body parts inside the abdomen, such as the surface of the liver or the intestines, and possibly the lymph nodes.

Microscopic amounts of the cancer are found on the surface of tissues in the abdomen.

None of the cancers found on the surface of tissues in the abdomen measures more than 2 centimeters (³/₄ inch).

One or more of the cancers found on the surface of the tissues in the abdomen measures 2 centimeters; or the cancer has spread to the lymph nodes.

- Total abdominal hysterectomy and bilateral salpingo-oophorectomy, *with* omentectomy *and* lymph-node dissection *and* tumor debulking • *followed by*
- Chemotherapy, frequently consisting of paclitaxel in combination with cisplatin or carboplatin, or other drug combinations • *possibly followed by*
- Second-look laparotomy, to inspect the abdomen and pelvis for evidence of remaining disease

Under Investigation
- Intraperitoneal chemotherapy, frequently consisting of paclitaxel and/or cisplatin
- ◆ Ask your doctor about any clinical trials that might benefit you.

STAGE IV OVARIAN CANCER

One or both ovaries contain cancer that has spread outside the abdomen or infiltrated the inside of the liver.

- Tumor-debulking surgery • *followed by*
- Chemotherapy, frequently consisting of paclitaxel in combination with cisplatin or carboplatin, or other drug combinations

See treatment options for liver metastases.

RECURRENT OR RESISTANT (REFRACTORY) OVARIAN CANCER

Your therapy will depend on how you were treated initially.

- Chemotherapy, frequently consisting of paclitaxel, cisplatin, or carboplatin, or a number of other drugs and drug combinations • *and/or*

- Surgery to relieve symptoms

Under Investigation #1
- New chemotherapy drugs and immunologic agents

Under Investigation #2
- High-dose chemotherapy • *followed by*

- Autologous bone-marrow transplantation

Under Investigation #3
- Surgery to remove as much of the tumor as possible

Under Investigation #4
- Intraperitoneal chemotherapy, frequently consisting of paclitaxel and/or cisplatin

◆ Ask your doctor about any clinical trials that might benefit you.

Ovarian Low-Malignant-Potential Tumor

STAGE I OVARIAN LOW-MALIGNANT-POTENTIAL TUMOR

- Total abdominal hysterectomy and bilateral salpingo-oophorectomy • *or*
- Unilateral salpingo-oophorectomy

STAGE II OVARIAN LOW-MALIGNANT-POTENTIAL TUMOR

- Total abdominal hysterectomy and bilateral salpingo-oophorectomy, *with* omentectomy *and* lymph-node dissection *and* tumor debulking • *with or without*

- Chemotherapy, frequently consisting of paclitaxel and cisplatin or carboplatin • *and/or*

- External-beam radiation therapy

STAGE III OVARIAN LOW-MALIGNANT-POTENTIAL TUMOR

- Total abdominal hysterectomy and bilateral salpingo-oophorectomy, *with* omentectomy *and* lymph-node dissection *and* tumor debulking • *with or without*

- Chemotherapy, frequently consisting of paclitaxel and cisplatin or carboplatin • *and/or*

- External-beam radiation therapy

part of a suspicious ovary, laparotomy is used to definitively diagnose, stage, and treat the disease, all in one procedure. It is a critical operation, one that the National Institutes of Health recommends be performed by an experienced gynecologic oncologist. These physicians are unique among cancer subspecialists in that they are trained in all three major treatment modalities: surgery, chemotherapy, and radiotherapy.

Upon surgery, three in four ovarian cancers will be found to have spread to other body parts within the pelvis (stage II), within the abdomen (stage III), or beyond the abdomen (stage IV), and therefore require some form of adjuvant therapy. According to Dr. Copeland, "Many doctors would classify even stage II ovarian cancer as advanced disease." But a number of women with localized (stage I) carcinoma can forgo further treatment, "depending upon the tumor's grade and cell type."

Stage/Grade/Cell Type	Adjuvant Therapy?
Stage IA, grade 1 (low-malignant-potential ovarian tumor) or grade 2 (intermediate grade)	Not necessary
Stage IB, grade 1 or grade 2	Not necessary
Stage IC, grade 1	Not necessary for some patients
Stage IC, grade 2	Probably necessary
Stage IA, IB, or IC, grade 3 (high grade)	Necessary
Stage I clear-cell carcinoma	Necessary
Stage II, III, IV LMP tumors	Rarely necessary

If you fall into one of the subcategories shown to benefit from postoperative therapy, you will be offered chemotherapy, external-beam radiation therapy, or intraperitoneal radiation. None has outshone the others in eradicating stage I ovarian cancer, although chemotherapy is the approach chosen most frequently.

Chemotherapy

Localized ovarian cancer calls for the same regimen as advanced disease. For many years, the first-line chemotherapy combined cisplatin (brand name: Platinol) or carboplatin (Paraplatin) with cyclophosphamide (Cytoxan). The latter drug has since been replaced by paclitaxel (Taxol), a naturally occurring compound that is extracted from the bark of the Pacific yew tree.

Taxol, approved for commercial use in 1992, has been hailed by some as the most important new chemotherapeutic agent in years.

OVARIAN CANCER/
Drug Therapy

First-line therapy frequently consists of:
- **TP: paclitaxel + cisplatin or carboplatin**

Other drugs or drug combinations that may be used include:
- **CP: cyclophosphamide + cisplatin**
- **CC: cyclophosphamide + carboplatin**
- **cisplatin or carboplatin**
- **topotecan**
- **ifosfamide**
- **altretamine**
- **fluorouracil + leucovorin**
- **etoposide**
- **chlorambucil**
- **doxorubicin**
- **melphalan**
- **thiotepa**
- **tamoxifen (H)**
- **chromic phosphate P-32 (R)**
- **yttrium-90 radiolabeled carcinoembryonic-antigen antibody (I)**

(H) = hormonal agent
(I) = immunologic agent
(R) = radiopharmaceutical

The way in which paclitaxel inhibits cancer development is unique: It causes the malignant cells to become so clogged with fiberlike structures that they cannot grow and divide.

"Taxol got its foot in the door by showing that it was effective in patients who had failed the old standard, cisplatin and cyclophosphamide," says Dr. Copeland. "The next step was to combine it with cisplatin and see how that compared to cisplatin-cyclophosphamide." In a large NCI-funded clinical trial conducted at more than forty major cancer centers, nearly three in four volunteers from the cisplatin-paclitaxel arm responded to the therapy, as compared to fewer than three in five of the women given cisplatin-cyclophosphamide. What's more, the median survival (the point at which half the patients had died and half were alive) for the Taxol-Platinol patients was thirty-eight months, versus twenty-four months for the other arm—a difference that Dr. Copeland calls "incredibly positive."

Additional clinical studies are seeking to determine whether or not three cycles of paclitaxel and carboplatin are as effective as six cycles for stage I and stage II ovarian cancers. Carboplatin impairs the bone marrow more than cisplatin does, but it is gentler on the kidneys and the central nervous system, and generally seems to be better tolerated by elderly patients.

Radiation Therapy

Postoperative radiotherapy is delivered in one of two ways: externally, to the abdomen and pelvic region, or internally. In the latter method, a liquid form of radioactive phosphorus (chromic phosphate P-32) is injected into the peritoneal membrane that lines the abdomen. *Intraperitoneal radiation* has fallen out of favor in the United States on account of its high complication rate. Total abdominal and pelvic radiation, too, is rarely used in place of chemotherapy for stage I ovarian cancer. It is used even less frequently for stage II disease.

TREATMENTS FOR ADVANCED OVARIAN CANCER

Surgery

Tumor Debulking—A malignant ovarian mass that has extended to other organs expands the mission of the laparotomy. In addition to excising the reproductive organs, the omentum, and the lymph nodes, the surgeon cuts out, or *debulks,* as much of the tumor as possible. The goal of this *cytoreductive surgery* is to eliminate every visible trace of cancer, although that's not always possible. If the tumor left behind measures 1 centimeter (not quite ½ inch) or less, it is called *optimal residual cancer;* larger tumors are referred to as *suboptimal residual cancers.* Dr. Copeland has been practicing gynecologic oncology since 1979. In that time, he says, "our surgical skills and our attitude have developed to where we tend to be much more aggressive about leaving no visible tumor in patients with advanced disease."

Second-Look Laparotomy (SLL)—As you might gather from its name, second-look laparotomy is repeat exploratory surgery for detecting any remaining disease following the completion of chemotherapy. Whether or not its value justifies subjecting patients to another major operation is one of the more hotly contested questions in cancer medicine.

It is generally accepted that SLL is not appropriate for women with stage I or stage II ovarian cancer, since fewer than one in ten will be found to have persistent disease at the time of the procedure. Nor is it recommended once the cancer has progressed to stage IV. The National Institutes of Health convened a panel of medical experts to suggest guidelines for the treatment and prevention of ovarian cancer. They concluded that second-look laparotomy should be done only in the setting of a clinical trial or in cases where the results could alter future treatment decisions.

The National Cancer Institute further recommends that before patients are scheduled for SLL, they undergo a physical exam, a CT scan, and a CA-125 tumor-marker blood test to reveal any evidence that the cancer has withstood the chemotherapy. Normally, the concentration of this protein in the blood is less than 35 units per milliliter. In recent studies, four in five women with elevated CA-125 levels were diagnosed with ovarian cancer. Another study lowered the bar to 20 units. Of the patients who tested within the 20-to-35 range, second-look laparotomy confirmed the presence of residual cancer in more than nine in ten. According to the NCI, a positive CA-125 tumor marker might provide sufficient information to render SLL unnecessary. However, the test isn't always reliable, whereas exploratory surgery is the most accurate method for discovering residual ovarian cancer.

See "Why See a Gynecologic Oncologist?," page 529.

Just what are the arguments for and against the controversial procedure?

"Critics point to the fact that we have no evidence that second-look surgery increases the probability of survival," says Dr. Copeland, who counts himself among the operation's proponents. "But no one disagrees that the results are of significant prognostic value. Women who have a negative second look are much more likely to have extended disease-free survival than women whose second look reveals visible tumor left behind.

"Neither finding is 100 percent accurate," he emphasizes. "A woman may be negative for cancer at the time of the second look, but the chance of a recurrence over the next five years can be as high as 50 percent." In the absence of a tumor, the patient might be spared additional chemotherapy, and with it the treatment's potential side effects. Or, given the disconcertingly high recurrence rate, her doctors might offer a short course of consolidation chemotherapy. Likewise, the discovery of a malignancy doesn't necessarily mark a patient as terminal. "There are women with visible disease at second look who go on to survive for more than five years," says Dr. Copeland. In this instance, having undergone SLL might prevent chemotherapy from being discontinued prematurely.

Whatever the results, another benefit of second-look laparotomy is psychological. In Dr. Copeland's experience, "many patients opt for second-look surgery just for planning their lives. They want to know whether they should buy that new house or whether they will need to make provisions for their children's care and upbringing, and so on."

TREATMENTS FOR RECURRENT OR REFRACTORY OVARIAN CANCER

Chemotherapy

Platinum-based chemotherapy regimens for ovarian cancer fail nearly half the time. Patients who responded to cisplatin or carboplatin and then relapsed six months or more after the initial treatment are said to be *platinum-sensitive.* They can be re-treated with either drug. The longer the duration of the remission, the greater the likelihood that they will respond the second time around.

When a regimen incorporating one of the platinums fails to induce a remission, or when the cancer recurs within six months, the oncologist must switch to another type of agent. Paclitaxel indisputably leads the pack, although other second-line therapies are available for women with *platinum-resistant* ovarian cancer. Some, like topotecan (Hycamtin), an *enzyme inhibitor,* are relatively new. Others have been used to treat other cancers. They include ifosfamide (IFEX), altretamine (Hexalen), etoposide (VePesid, VP-16), the *antiestrogen* tamoxifen (Nolvadex), and the combination of fluorouracil (5-FU) and leucovorin (Wellcovorin). The drugs "carry low toxicity," says Dr. Copeland, "so the quality of life can be preserved." And the response rates, while modest, "do allow patients to maintain some hope of therapeutic benefit."

Surgery

Like second-look laparotomy, a second operation to debulk a tumor that has recurred is controversial because there's no conclusive proof that it prolongs life. However, a study conducted at New York's Mount Sinai Medical Center found that the procedure, when successful, can in fact grant patients extra years.

One hundred women with progressive or recurrent ovarian cancer consented to tumor-reduction surgery. Twenty-two of these resections met the definition of optimal surgery, leaving behind disease measuring 1 centimeter or less in diameter. In another thirty-nine cases, surgeons were able to reduce the size of the cancer to less than 2 centimeters. The two groups were then followed. As of two years after the study ended, the length of survival for the women with the smaller residual cancers was three times that of the women who were suboptimally resected: twenty-seven months compared to nine months. Other studies have demonstrated extended survival only when the operation rids the body of all but microscopic disease.

OTHER THERAPIES THAT MAY BE USED IN THE TREATMENT
OF OVARIAN CANCER

The National Cancer Institute takes the position that clinical trials
should be considered at any stage of ovarian cancer.

Intraperitoneal Chemotherapy (investigational)—Intraperitoneal
chemotherapy injects concentrated doses of anticancer drugs directly
into the lining that encases the abdomen. Investigational studies using
paclitaxel, cisplatin, and other agents have produced encouraging results for this technique, which appears to be most suitable for women
whose cancer is limited to the abdominal cavity and the retroperitoneal
lymph nodes (stage IIIC).

**High-Dose Chemotherapy Followed by Autologous Bone-Marrow
Transplantation** (investigational)—Early-phase clinical trials have yet
to convince doctors that giving patients extremely high doses of
chemotherapy, then replacing the damaged bone marrow with their
own healthy marrow cells, offers enough of a benefit over conventional
chemotherapy to offset the risks inherent with BMT. Responses have
generally been measured in a matter of months, leading some experts to
believe that intraperitoneal chemotherapy may be a more effective and
certainly safer method of treating advanced ovarian cancer.

♦ *Ask your doctor about these and any other investigational therapies
that might benefit you.*

Cancer of the Stomach

Overview

TREATMENTS FOR STOMACH CANCER THAT
HAS NOT METASTASIZED

Surgery

Removing the whole stomach can interfere considerably with eating. Therefore, "total gastrectomy is avoided whenever possible," says
Dr. Harinder Garewal, a gastroenterology oncologist at the Arizona
Cancer Center. Two situations in early gastric cancer require a complete *gastrectomy:* (1) when the lesion is widespread *(diffuse)* throughout the stomach or (2) when a tumor in the central portion, or *body,*

STOMACH CANCER/Treatment Options

CARCINOMA IN SITU OF THE STOMACH

The cancer is found only in the innermost of the four layers of the stomach wall.

- Subtotal gastrectomy, to surgically remove part of the stomach, *with* lymph-node dissection • *or*
- Total gastrectomy, to surgically remove the entire stomach, *plus* part of the esophagus, *with* lymph-node dissection

STAGE I STOMACH CANCER

The cancer has infiltrated the second or third layers of the stomach wall but not the neighboring lymph nodes.

The cancer has spread to the second layer and to nearby lymph nodes.

- Subtotal gastrectomy, *with* lymph-node dissection • *or*
- Total gastrectomy, *with* lymph-node dissection

STAGE II STOMACH CANCER

(1) The cancer is in the second layer of the stomach wall and has spread to lymph nodes farther away from the tumor; or (2) the cancer is in the third layer and has spread to nearby lymph nodes; or (3) the cancer extends through all four layers but has not invaded lymph nodes or other organs.

- Subtotal gastrectomy, *with* lymph-node dissection • *or*
- Total gastrectomy, *with* lymph-node dissection • *with or without one or more of the following experimental therapies:*

Under Investigation
- Chemotherapy, frequently consisting of fluorouracil • *and/or*
- External-beam radiation therapy
- ◆ Ask your doctor about any clinical trials that might benefit you.

STAGE III STOMACH CANCER

(1) The cancer has reached the third layer of the stomach wall and has spread to lymph nodes farther away from the tumor; or (2) the cancer extends through all four layers and has spread to lymph nodes either very close to the tumor or farther away; or (3) the cancer is in all four layers and has spread to nearby tissues but may or may not have spread to neighboring lymph nodes.

- Subtotal gastrectomy, *with* lymph-node dissection • *or*
- Total gastrectomy, *with* lymph-node dissection • *with or without one or more of the following experimental therapies:*

Under Investigation

- Chemotherapy, frequently consisting of fluorouracil • *and/or*
- External-beam radiation therapy
- ◆ Ask your doctor about any clinical trials that might benefit you.

STAGE IV STOMACH CANCER

The cancer has spread to nearby tissues and to lymph nodes farther away from the tumor or has metastasized to other parts of the body.

- Surgical resection of the stomach, to relieve symptoms • *or*
- Chemotherapy, frequently consisting of fluorouracil, alone or in combination with other drugs, to relieve symptoms
- ◆ Ask your doctor about any clinical trials that might benefit you.

See treatment options for metastases of the liver and lung.

RECURRENT STOMACH CANCER

Your therapy will depend on how you were treated initially.

- Chemotherapy, frequently consisting of fluorouracil, alone or in combination with other drugs, to relieve symptoms • *or*
- Endoscopic electrosurgery or laser surgery, to relieve symptoms

Under Investigation

- New chemotherapy drugs and immunologic agents
- ◆ Ask your doctor about any clinical trials that might benefit you.

of the organ grows too close to either the cardia or the *pylorus.* The cardia is the area surrounding the upper opening, which receives food and liquid from the esophagus. The pylorus is where the churned-up contents idle before the wavelike contractions known as peristalsis pass it on to the small intestine.

Gastric cancer cannot be staged definitively until the time of surgery. Thus, while surgeons are able to give their patients a general idea of what will take place, says Dr. Garewal, "some decisions may need to be made during the operation." For example, a tumor that proves to be too large to resect without having to take out the entire stomach has usually spread. With dim prospects for a cure and in the interest of preserving the patient's quality of life, the surgeon would almost certainly not perform a total gastrectomy.

The conservative approach would also apply if a frozen-section biopsy performed during the operation revealed extensive lymph-node involvement. The majority of men and women diagnosed with stomach cancer will be found to have some degree of nodal disease. In the

TNM staging system (explained in Chapter Three) for gastric carcinoma, $N1$ denotes that the cancer is confined to the *perigastric* lymph nodes in the immediate vicinity of the primary lesion. Even at stage III, when the tumor has penetrated all four layers of the stomach wall and may also have invaded the spleen, the liver, or other neighboring organs, up to 15 percent of patients classified as having $N1$ nodal involvement can be cured through surgery. But if the cancer has metastasized to perigastric nodes farther away or to other regional lymph nodes—putting the nodal status at $N2$—"surgery would not be curative," says Dr. Garewal, thus ruling out total gastrectomy.

Subtotal gastrectomy leaves behind anywhere from 15 to 50 percent of the stomach. The size and site of the cancer dictate the magnitude of the surgery. The stomach tapers somewhat at both ends. From a surgeon's standpoint, the preferable location for a tumor is "the body of the stomach, where there is plenty of tissue. That is easier to resect than a cancer situated at the junction of the stomach and the esophagus, or down below, at the junction of the stomach and the small intestine."

If the tumor forms in the cardia, many surgeons will resort to a total gastrectomy rather than attempt a proximal subtotal gastrectomy, says Dr. Todd Heniford, a surgeon at the Cleveland Clinic Foundation in Ohio, "because hooking up the esophagus to the lower stomach doesn't work very well." A sizable resection of the bottom portion of the J poses less of a problem. It may preclude sewing the stomach remnant to the duodenum, explains Dr. Heniford. "But attaching the upper stomach to a loop of the *jejunum,* the middle segment of the small intestine, works equally well."

STOMACH CANCER/ Surgical Procedures

Gastrectomy: surgery to remove all *(total gastrectomy)* or part *(subtotal gastrectomy)* of the stomach. A *distal* subtotal gastrectomy takes out the lower portion of the J-shaped sac, then joins the remaining stomach to the small bowel. In a *proximal* subtotal gastrectomy, the surgeon removes the upper stomach as well as the lower esophagus, then sews the gullet to the stomach.

A total gastrectomy, besides taking out the whole stomach, involves excising part of the esophagus, which is then connected directly to the small intestine. Occasionally, the surgeon may remove the spleen. All three procedures call for resecting parts of nearby tissues and organs and dissecting the regional lymph nodes.

Average hospital stay: 4–7 days

Medical Terms You're Likely to Hear

Gastroduodenostomy: connecting what remains of the stomach to the duodenum; also referred to as a *Billroth I* (Theodor Billroth being the surgeon who first performed the operation in the 1880s).

Gastrojejunostomy (Billroth II): connecting what remains of the stomach to the jejunum.

Laparoscopic Gastrectomy—Since 1992, a small number of hospitals have been offering minimally invasive *laparoscopic gastrectomy,* mainly for ulcers of the upper digestive tract but also as a curative measure for gastric carcinoma in situ and stage I malignant tumors. The procedure is more common in Japan, which has one of the world's highest death rates from stomach cancer. Men and women there are routinely screened for the disease, so in situ lesions are picked up far more frequently than in the United States. Oftentimes they can be treated through a *limited gastrectomy.* Since little stomach tissue is taken out, no *anastomosis* (connecting one organ to another) is necessary. This operation, like subtotal and total gastrectomy, lends itself to the laparoscopic technique.

When the goal of surgery is palliative—perhaps to halt tumor bleeding or to remove a lesion that is interfering with digestion—laparoscopic gastrectomy can be performed at any stage. What a difference this is from open surgery. Instead of one large incision being made along the abdomen, three or four tiny incisions are made, including one in the belly button. The procedure reduces hospitalization by more than half, with most patients going home within twenty-four to forty-eight hours. It also pares recovery time from weeks to days. If you think you meet the criteria for laparoscopic gastrectomy, you might want to call around to major medical centers in your area and ask if they have experience in this high-tech, minimally invasive surgery.

How Will Stomach Surgery Affect Your Eating?—The stomach needs several days to heal sufficiently before you can eat. While you're recuperating, you will be fed through a vein in the chest. This is called *parenteral nutrition.* Eventually, liquids are introduced by mouth; next come soft foods, then solid foods.

Since subtotal or total gastrectomy leaves you with a smaller receptacle for food, it's common to experience increased heartburn and regurgitation and to feel full after only a few bites. Naturally, you will have to make adjustments in how and what you eat. A nurse or hospital dietitian will map out a special diet for you. "Over time," says Dr. Garewal, "things tend to settle down," and many people are able to resume normal eating habits. In the rare cases where these changes are permanent, "most people get used to it and manage very well."

Dumping Syndrome—One frequent complication of gastrectomy is dumping syndrome. Normally, the stomach dispenses food to the small intestine at a controlled rate and in small increments. But with most or all of the stomach missing, the food spills into the intestine too rapidly.

In *late* dumping syndrome, the more common form, the small intestine's being forced to absorb larger amounts of food than normal drives up the concentration of sugar *(glucose)* in the circulation. In response, the pancreas releases excess *insulin,* the hormone that regulates the blood's glucose level. Two to three hours after eating, patients may feel weak from a drop in blood pressure. They may also develop other symptoms such as headache, sweating, anxiety, and/or tremors.

Early dumping syndrome can take place mere minutes after eating. Blood pressure decreases, while blood flow to the intestine increases. Symptoms include an irregular or rapid heartbeat, dizziness, shortness of breath, flushed skin, vomiting, abdominal cramps, and diarrhea.

The smaller the remaining stomach, the harsher the symptoms. Usually, they subside after three to twelve months, but in some patients the condition becomes chronic. Most men and women learn to control dumping syndrome dietarily—by eating more frequent, smaller meals instead of the customary three squares a day and by avoiding foods high in *carbohydrates,* which the body converts to sugar. They also learn to drink fluids between meals, not during meals. Anticholinergic drugs may be prescribed to block the dumping reflex, along with diarrhea medications and vitamin and mineral supplements.

See "Digestive Disorders" in Chapter Eight, "Take Control: Managing Symptoms, Side Effects, and Complications."

All patients who've undergone gastrectomy eventually become deficient in *vitamin B$_{12}$,* which is found in meat, seafood, and milk products. Regular vitamin B$_{12}$ injections will restore your normal levels.

Chemotherapy and/or Radiation

Surgery is the only proven curative treatment for stomach cancer. Nonetheless, the National Cancer Institute recommends clinical trials of postoperative chemotherapy and radiation for stage II or stage III gastric tumors that have spread to four or more lymph nodes. An important consideration, says Dr. Garewal, is the patient's overall condition. The combination of fluorouracil (5-FU) and external-beam radiation does bring about unwanted side effects. "But if a patient was

---

**STOMACH CANCER/
Drug Therapy**

*First-line therapy frequently
consists of:*
• fluorouracil

*Other drugs or drug combina-
tions that may be used include:*
• **FAM:** fluorouracil + doxorubicin + mitomycin

• **FAMTX:** fluorouracil + doxorubicin + high-dose
  methotrexate

• **FAP:** fluorouracil + doxorubicin + cisplatin

• **ELF:** etoposide + leucovorin +
  fluorouracil

• **FLAP:** fluorouracil + leucovorin + doxorubicin + cisplatin

• **carmustine**

---

in good health otherwise and could be expected to tolerate the treatment," Dr. Garewal adds, "I would offer it."

None of the many postsurgical strategies that have been tried through the years has been effective, a point Dr. Garewal readily acknowledges. Why, then, bother with additional therapy at all?

"The textbook answer is that adjuvant therapy doesn't offer any advantage. But we do know that it decreases the chances of local recurrence, which is not a trivial matter. Because if the cancer comes back in the area that was operated on, it is much more difficult to get a handle on.

"Unfortunately," he adds, "improved local control has not translated into a significant survival advantage, as it has in colon cancer. Death is usually from metastatic disease to the liver or the lung.

"This is a disease where if a new investigational drug became available, I would encourage participation in a research study."

TREATMENTS FOR ADVANCED STOMACH CANCER

Chemotherapy (Palliative Treatment)

The mainstay of drug therapy for stomach cancer, 5-FU, has been matched with a number of agents for relieving symptoms from metastatic disease. The tumor-response rates are poor, in the range of 20 percent.

"Whether or not to use chemotherapy varies from individual to individual," says Dr. Garewal. "If a patient is elderly, in the physiologic sense, with no symptoms from the cancer, I would suggest holding off. On the other hand, occasionally we've seen dramatic responses, so under the right circumstances, a treatment trial can be worth it." Some patients' symptoms diminish considerably, while others may go into a lasting remission.

"My usual approach is to explain to patients what the data is with the agents that are currently available and to point out that if we do decide to treat, I'll want to assess the tumor after perhaps two cycles. Are the drugs working or not? Is the tumor smaller or not? If yes, then we continue." FAM, the first multidrug regimen to demonstrate some benefit in recurrent gastric cancer, "is very well tolerated," says Dr. Garewal. It consists of 5-FU, doxorubicin (brand name: Adriamycin), and mitomycin (Mutamycin).

Surgery (Palliative Treatment)

Some studies have shown that surgery to stop bleeding or excise an obstructive tumor not only improves the quality of life but may extend it. If the cancer is in the cardia and is causing difficulty in swallowing *(dysphagia),* electrosurgery and laser surgery—performed through a flexible endoscope—offer alternatives to surgical resection. Instead of the lesion's being cut out, it is destroyed by intense heat from the electric current or the laser.

Cancer of the Liver

Overview

TREATMENTS FOR OPERABLE LIVER CANCER

Surgery

Few people with liver cancer will have a tumor that can be completely resected. Either the disease is scattered throughout the liver or has spread to other organs, or the cancer is limited to a single mass, but liver damage from hepatitis or cirrhosis has made surgery too risky.

If you are a candidate for a partial hepatectomy, be sure to choose a surgeon who performs "at least a couple of liver resections a month," advises Dr. Ted Lawrence, a liver-cancer specialist at the University of Michigan Comprehensive Cancer Center.

"It's important that this surgery be performed by a pro because the anatomy of the liver is complex. Patients can bleed significantly if the procedure isn't done properly." Normally, the liver regenerates; a person can lose three-quarters of the football-sized organ and still retain normal liver function. "But many liver-cancer patients have cirrhosis, which means that their liver won't regenerate. It takes a tremendous amount of clinical judg-

> **LIVER CANCER/ Surgical Procedures**
>
> **Partial hepatectomy:** surgical removal of the cancerous portion of the liver.
> Average hospital stay: 5–7 days
>
> **Liver transplantation:** surgical removal of the liver and replacement with a healthy liver transplanted from the body of a donor who is declared brain dead and has a compatible blood type.
> Average hospital stay: 21 days

LIVER CANCER/Treatment Options

LOCALIZED RESECTABLE PRIMARY LIVER CANCER

The cancer is found in one place in the liver and can be completely removed surgically.

- Partial hepatectomy, to surgically remove the cancerous portion of the liver *or*
- Liver transplantation

Under Investigation

- Regional (intra-arterial) or systemic chemotherapy following surgery, frequently consisting of cisplatin, doxorubicin, or floxuridine

◆ Ask your doctor about any clinical trials that might benefit you.

LOCALIZED UNRESECTABLE PRIMARY LIVER CANCER

The cancer is found in one place in the liver but cannot be totally removed.

◆ There is no standard treatment.

Under Investigation #1

- Regional (intra-arterial) chemotherapy, frequently consisting of cisplatin, doxorubicin, or floxuridine • *with or without*
- External-beam radiation therapy

Under Investigation #2

- Systemic chemotherapy, frequently consisting of cisplatin, doxorubicin, or floxuridine

Under Investigation #3

- Partial hepatectomy *or* cryosurgery • *followed by*
- Regional (intra-arterial) chemotherapy, frequently consisting of cisplatin, doxorubicin, or floxuridine • *alone or with*
- Hyperthermia • *or*
- External-beam radiation therapy, • *with or without* radiosensitizing agents

Under Investigation #4

- Alcohol ablation therapy

Under Investigation #5

- Cryosurgery

Under Investigation #6

- External-beam radiation therapy, *with or without* radiosensitizing agents

Under Investigation #7

- Liver transplantation

◆ Ask your doctor about any clinical trials that might benefit you.

ADVANCED PRIMARY LIVER CANCER

The cancer has spread throughout much of the liver or to other parts of the body.

- ◆ There is no standard treatment.

Under Investigation #1
- ▪ **Chemotherapy, frequently consisting of cisplatin, doxorubicin, or floxuridine •** *with or without*
- ▪ **External-beam radiation therapy,** *with or without* **radiosensitizing agents**
- ◆ Ask your doctor about any clinical trials that might benefit you.

See treatment options for metastases of the lung and bone.

RECURRENT PRIMARY LIVER CANCER

Your therapy will depend on how you were treated initially.

- ▪ **No further therapy •** *or, in selected cases*
- ▪ **A second partial hepatectomy**

Under Investigation
- ▪ **New chemotherapy drugs and immunologic agents**
- ◆ Ask your doctor about any clinical trials that might benefit you.

---

ment to know how much of the liver you can remove safely." When patients are selected carefully for surgery, 10 to 30 percent will go on to live at least five years.

Liver transplantation is rarely a realistic option. "Most transplant centers are not doing liver transplants for liver cancer. The problem," Dr. Lawrence explains, "is that except for all but the tiniest tumors, liver-cancer cells are circulating in the blood at all times, and so most patients will develop cancer in the transplanted liver." Only 3 percent of donor livers go to people with hepatic carcinoma.

LIVER CANCER/Drug Therapy

First-line therapy frequently consists of:
- doxorubicin
- cisplatin
- floxuridine

TREATMENTS FOR LOCALIZED INOPERABLE LIVER CANCER

Chemotherapy/Chemoembolization

Because liver cancer frequently comes out of remission, chemotherapy may be offered postoperatively, although to date no advantage has been shown.

As for unresectable liver cancer, there is no standard therapy, says

Dr. Lawrence. "A patient might receive recommendations ranging from observation to highly aggressive local therapy." Clinical trials have centered mainly around chemotherapy, sometimes following surgery when a patient has one large mass and small diffuse lesions. The surgeon cuts out the dominant cancer, then anticancer agents are given, either alone or in combination with radiation, to eradicate the rest of the disease. System-wide chemotherapy has not been found to be effective. However, some patients do respond to *intra-arterial* chemotherapy consisting of floxuridine (brand name: FUDR), cisplatin (Platinol), or doxorubicin (Adriamycin).

"The concept of intra-arterial chemotherapy is a very clever one," Dr. Lawrence notes. "The liver gets 80 percent of its blood from the portal vein and about 20 percent from the hepatic artery. But with tumors of the liver, roughly the opposite is true." Infusing chemotherapy directly into the hepatic artery delivers a high concentration of cancer-killing medicine to the tumor; the normal liver tissue, however, receives only a partial dose.

Infusing the drug floxuridine provides an added benefit. Cisplatin and doxorubicin are not well metabolized, or broken down, by the healthy liver, and so enough of the drug circulates through the bloodstream to produce the side effects associated with systemic chemotherapy. "But the normal liver does a very good job of metabolizing floxuridine," explains Dr. Lawrence. "Almost none of it gets into the rest of the body." Hepatic-artery infusion can be administered through a surgically implanted pump or, more commonly, a temporary catheter tube.

Chemoembolization follows a similar principle. An anticancer agent, usually doxorubicin, is injected directly into the hepatic artery, causing it to close off. This robs the tumor of its primary blood supply and traps the chemo right where it's needed. Embolization can shrink hepatic cancers and relieve pain, but the benefits are typically short-lived.

Radiation Therapy, Cryosurgery, Alcohol Ablation Therapy, and Hyperthermia

A number of other experimental approaches have been tested in inoperable patients. According to Dr. Lawrence, the two most common are external-beam radiation, often combined with intra-arterial chemotherapy, and cryosurgery. The results of *alcohol ablation*—injecting pure alcohol into the tumor, destroying it—"have not been quite as good as the other two," while hyperthermia is the least popular of these methods.

TREATMENTS FOR ADVANCED OR RECURRENT LIVER CANCER

Once the cancer has spread throughout the liver or elsewhere in the body, a patient is usually looking at little more than a few months to live. Clinical trials testing new chemotherapy drugs and immunologic agents *may* be able to relieve symptoms, but they can just as easily hasten death, particularly if someone has tenuous liver function. In that situation, Dr. Lawrence says candidly, "I usually try to discourage patients from pursuing treatment."

When liver cancer recurs, little can be offered in the way of therapy, with one exception: patients whose tumor grows in the same location as the cancer that was surgically removed. "A small number can have the lesion re-resected," says Dr. Lawrence, "and they may do well for a number of years."

◆ *Ask your doctor about any investigational therapies that might benefit you.*

Cancers of the Lip and Oral Cavity

Overview

TREATMENTS FOR ORAL CANCER THAT HAS NOT METASTASIZED

Surgery and radiotherapy are equally effective in treating early stage oral cancers; these are localized tumors measuring up to 1½ inches. According to Dr. Rocco Addante of the Norris Cotton Cancer Center, it's often the patient's decision as to which approach to take. Other times, he says, "the choice is dictated by the anticipated functional and cosmetic results." For a 1-inch lesion on the front (anterior) portion of the tongue, a physician would most likely recommend radiation, in order to preserve speech and the ability to swallow. Elsewhere in the oral cavity, the general rule is to operate on smaller lesions and irradiate larger ones.

Stage III disease is considered advanced. The tumor has either seeded a small secondary lesion in a lymph node on the same side of the body; or it may not have spread but exceeds 1½ inches in size (classification: *T3*). Most of these patients undergo combined surgery and radiation, like people with stage IV oral cancer. However, either treatment may suffice when a *T3* lesion is small and if no nodes or distant

ORAL CANCER/Treatment Options

ORAL CARCINOMA IN SITU

Cancer cells are present, but only in the first layer of cells that make up the lining of the oral cavity.

- Surgical excision, to remove the tumor and a margin of normal tissue • *or*
- Laser surgery • *or*
- Cryosurgery

Under Investigation
- Mohs' micrographic surgery
- ◆ Ask your doctor about any clinical trials that might benefit you.

STAGE I ORAL CANCER

The cancer measures no more than 2 centimeters (³/₄ inch) and has not spread to area lymph nodes.

- Surgical excision, *with or without* lymph-node dissection • *and/or*
- External-beam radiation therapy • *and/or*
- Internal radiation therapy

Under Investigation
- Mohs' micrographic surgery • *followed by*
- External-beam or internal radiation therapy
- ◆ Ask your doctor about any clinical trials that might benefit you.

Site	Standard Treatment Options			
	Surgery Alone	Radiation Alone	Surgery *or* Radiation	Surgery *plus* Radiation
Lip			■	
Tongue	■	■		■
Buccal mucosa			■	
Floor of the mouth			■	
Lower gums			■	
Retromolar trigone	■			■
Upper gums and hard palate	■			■

STAGE II ORAL CANCER

The cancer measures more than 2 centimeters but not more than 4 centimeters (1¹/₂ inches) and has not spread to area lymph nodes.

- Surgical excision, *with or without* lymph-node dissection · *and/or*
- External-beam radiation therapy · *and/or*
- Internal radiation therapy

Under Investigation
- Mohs' micrographic surgery · *followed by*
- External-beam or internal radiation therapy
- ◆ Ask your doctor about any clinical trials that might benefit you.

Site	Standard Treatment Options			
	Surgery Alone	Radiation Alone	Surgery *or* Radiation	Surgery *plus* Radiation
Lip			■	
Tongue		■		■
Buccal mucosa			■	■
Floor of the mouth			■	■
Lower gums			■	
Retromolar trigone			■	■
Upper gums and hard palate				■

STAGE III ORAL CANCER

The cancer measures more than 4 centimeters; or the cancer is any size but has spread to only one lymph node, measuring 3 centimeters (1¹/₄ inches) or less, on the same side of the neck.

- Surgical excision, *with or without* lymph-node dissection · *and/or*
- External-beam radiation therapy · *and/or*
- Internal radiation therapy

Under Investigation
- Chemotherapy given before or after other treatments, possibly consisting of cisplatin alone or in combination with other agents
- ◆ Ask your doctor about any clinical trials that might benefit you.

Site	Standard Treatment Options			
	Surgery Alone	Radiation Alone	Surgery *or* Radiation	Surgery *plus* Radiation
Lip		■		■
Tongue		■		■
Buccal mucosa			■	■
Floor of the mouth			■	
Lower gums				■
Retromolar trigone				■
Upper gums and hard palate		■		■

STAGE IV ORAL CANCER

(1) The cancer has spread to tissues around the lip (bone, tongue, skin of the neck) or the oral cavity (bone, deep muscles of the tongue, skin, or the sinuses on either side of the nose), and possibly to one or more area lymph nodes; or (2) the cancer is any size and has spread to a single lymph node, measuring more than 3 centimeters but not more than 6 centimeters (more than 2$\frac{1}{4}$ inches), on the same side of the neck; or to multiple lymph nodes, none more than 6 centimeters in size, on the same side of the neck; or to lymph nodes, none more than 6 centimeters in size, on the opposite side of the neck or on both sides of the neck; or (3) the cancer has spread to other parts of the body.

- Surgical resection, *with or without* lymph-node dissection · *and/or*
- External-beam radiation therapy · *and/or*
- Internal radiation therapy

Under Investigation
- Chemotherapy before or after other treatments, possibly consisting of cisplatin alone or in combination with other agents

◆ Ask your doctor about any clinical trials that might benefit you.

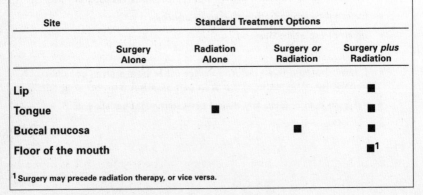

Site	Standard Treatment Options			
	Surgery Alone	Radiation Alone	Surgery *or* Radiation	Surgery *plus* Radiation
Lip				■
Tongue		■		■
Buccal mucosa			■	■
Floor of the mouth				■[1]

[1] Surgery may precede radiation therapy, or vice versa.

	Surgery Alone	Radiation Alone	Surgery *or* Radiation	Surgery *plus* Radiation
Lower gums			■	■
Retromolar trigone				■
Upper gums and hard palate				■

See treatment options for lung metastases.

RECURRENT ORAL CANCER

Your therapy will depend on how you were treated initially.

If surgery was performed initially:
- **Surgical resection • *and/or***
- **External-beam radiation therapy**

If you underwent radiation initially:
- **Surgical resection**

Under Investigation #1
- **Chemotherapy before or after other treatments, possibly consisting of cisplatin alone or in combination with other agents**

Under Investigation #2
- **Hyperthermia**

◆ **Ask your doctor about any clinical trials that might benefit you.**

sites are involved or if none of the involved lymph nodes measures more than ¾ inch.

Surgery

Some small oral cancers require no additional surgery beyond the excisional biopsy performed at diagnosis, as long as the surgeon is able to cut out a wide-enough rim of normal tissue. With larger tumors, this can pose a challenge. Achieving an adequate margin reduces the likelihood of a recurrence. But the physician also has to consider aesthetics. In the mouth, there is little flesh for the surgeon to work with. "If the lesion is on the cheek," says Dr. Addante, "we might remove less tissue, because the area is more difficult to close over.

"We may also have to tread carefully if the tumor grows too close to one of the many vital structures in the head and neck." Faced with a cancer infringing on one of the *carotid arteries* that carry blood to the brain, he further says that, "we might have to leave some tumor behind and incur a greater risk of a recurrence. The surgery can definitely be tricky, depending on its location."

**ORAL CANCER/
Surgical Procedures**

Surgical excision: surgery to remove the cancer and a margin of healthy tissue. Depending on the tumor's size and site, a more extensive operation may be necessary (see below).
Average hospital stay: 1–3 days

Glossectomy: surgery to remove the tongue. A *hemiglossectomy* takes out a portion of the tongue.

Hemimandibulectomy: surgery to remove the lower jaw *(mandible)* on one side of the mouth.

Laryngectomy: surgery to remove the voice box (larynx).

Neck dissection: surgery to remove the *cervical* lymph nodes in the neck. Whenever possible, the surgeon excises only the cancerous nodes plus a margin, but sometimes a *radical* neck dissection is necessary. This operation takes out a block of tissue on one side of the neck: from the collarbone up to the lower jaw, and from the front of the neck around to the back. The jugular vein, too, is removed.
Average hospital stay: 1–4 days

**Medical Terms You're
Likely to Hear**

Maxillofacial: pertaining to the upper jaw *(maxilla)* and the face.

Oral and maxillofacial surgeon: a surgeon who treats conditions and defects of the mouth, teeth, upper and lower jaw (mandible) and face.

Maxillofacial prosthodontist: a dentist specially trained in making artificial palates and other oral *prosthetic* devices.

In instances where the doctor successfully resects a localized lesion but the pathology report later reveals the margins to be inadequate or positive for cancer (the frozen-section biopsies performed tableside during the operation are not 100 percent accurate), the National Cancer Institute recommends adding radiation to the treatment plan.

Neck Dissection—The head and neck contain roughly one-third of the body's lymph nodes. When oral cancer metastasizes to the cervical nodes, it usually progresses down the same side of the neck. Nodal involvement calls for a radical or *modified-radical* neck dissection, performed during the operation to excise the primary tumor. This is usually followed by radiotherapy.

The more extensive of the two procedures becomes necessary if the cancer is found to have spread to the muscles and other tissue in the neck. Several vital nerves that pass through the neck may have to be sacrificed, among them the nerves responsible for movement of the neck, shoulder, lower lip, tongue, and diaphragm. Fortunately, the trend is toward the modified procedure, which preserves the neck muscle and jugular vein, as long as they are free of cancer.

Studies show that approximately 35 percent of *clinically* node-negative patients eventually relapse in the neck. "In other words, the physician won't feel any nodal involvement upon physical examination, and a CT scan of the neck will come back negative," explains Dr. Addante. "But the cancer is there microscopically, and it usually becomes clinically apparent within one year."

This has caused controversy over

whether or not to routinely subject early-stage oral-cancer patients to a limited neck dissection as a precaution. A less invasive alternative is to sterilize the neck with radiation postoperatively. "It is a difficult decision for a doctor to make," says Dr. Addante, "because there aren't any strong answers pointing one way or another." Among the determining factors would be the location, size, depth, and grade of the primary tumor. Cancers of the lip generally don't require elective neck treatment.

Reconstructive Surgery—Small tumors of the head and neck can usually be managed surgically without causing disfigurement or impairing speech and swallowing. An advanced lesion of the tongue may be so large, though, that part or all of the organ must be removed, and sometimes the larynx too. If the tumor invades the bones of the upper or lower jaw—as often occurs in oral cancer—it becomes necessary to resect the jaw.

Whereas most cancer operations involve internal organs, or external organs that are normally hidden beneath clothing, the results of head and neck surgery may be plainly visible or apparent once the person speaks. In the past, some patients would become virtual recluses following surgery to remove part of the jaw. But advances in reconstructive surgery, prosthetic devices, and rehabilitation therapy have improved appearance and function.

Reconstructive surgery harvests healthy bone or tissue from other parts of the body to fill the defect left by the tumor or to replace part of the lip, palate, tongue, or jaw. The most significant innovation has been *microvascular reconstruction,* in which the surgeon sews the blood vessels and nerves from the transferred tissue to the vessels and nerves in the head and neck. Conventional reconstruction is typically a separate three-stage procedure, so that up to two years may pass between the time the cancer is removed and reconstruction completed. The microvascular technique not only combines tumor excision and grafting into a single fourteen-to-eighteen-hour operation but also boasts a more natural appearance and function and quicker healing.

Will Treatment Affect Your Speech, Voice, or Swallowing?—Most cancer pa-

For free referrals to a certified speech-language pathologist in your area, contact:

American Speech-Language-Hearing Association
Action Center
10801 Rockville Pike
Rockville, MD 20852-3279
800-638-8255
http://www.asha.org

tients facing radical surgery of the tongue, jaw, or larynx are referred to a *speech-language pathologist* beforehand, but if no such consultation is offered, insist on one. In the event that you are unable to speak or swallow normally after the operation, it is the speech-language pathologist who will be in charge of your rehabilitation therapy. "We also work closely with the maxillofacial prosthodontist in constructing devices that assist in speech and swallowing," explains Dr. Cathy L. Lazarus, associate director of the voice, speech, and language service and swallowing center at Northwestern University Medical School in Chicago.

What degree of speech, voice, or swallowing impairment can you anticipate? That depends on the operation. A person who undergoes a total laryngectomy still swallows and articulates normally. But because her voice box has been taken out, she must be taught new ways of producing sound. Jaw resection rarely interferes with either speech or swallowing, so long as the tongue is preserved. It does, however, impair chewing.

See "Total Laryngectomy and Tracheostomy," page 544.

As for a partial glossectomy, says Dr. Addante, "a person can lose a sizable portion of the tongue and still retain very good function." When resecting a cancer situated in back *(posterior)*, the surgeon is often able to leave tissue on one side, so that the tongue remains intact from the base to the tip. "If that's the case," says Dr. Lazarus, "patients frequently can compensate well speech-wise and swallowing-wise."

An anterior excision taking off the front part of the tongue poses a bigger problem, she explains, "because the patients experience much more difficulty getting food through their mouth and into their throat." They can be fitted with a custom-made denturelike device called a *palatal drop*. The prosthesis "adds bulk to the upper palate, so the remaining tongue has something to come in contact with. It greatly improves both speech and swallowing." Rehabilitation therapy, consisting of several months of tongue and speech exercises, begins while patients are still in the hospital.

Surprisingly, people are able to undergo total glossectomies "and still be 100 percent intelligible," says Dr. Lazarus. "They compensate by figuring out how to shape their lips certain ways for the different sounds: one way for *p*'s and *b*'s; another for *t*'s and *d*'s." To approximate the back-tongue sounds of *k*'s and *g*'s, "they constrict the throat."

The major impact from a total glossectomy is on eating. With no tongue to press food against the teeth during chewing, "people are usually limited to liquids, because it's the easiest food to get through the oral cavity and into the throat." Some highly motivated patients will use the muscles in the floor of the mouth to mash thicker pureed or ground-up foods against their palatal prosthesis, but most find this too time-consuming and tiring.

For anyone with oral cancer, maintaining adequate nutrition can be an uphill battle—especially if surgery is followed by weeks of radiation therapy. "Some patients become severely malnourished," says Dr. Addante. Should that occur, your physician may recommend tube feedings, either as a temporary measure or as a permanent solution.

See "Tube Feedings" under "Appetite Loss (Anorexia)" in Chapter Eight, "Take Control: Managing Symptoms, Side Effects, and Complications."

Radiation Therapy

Radiotherapy can permanently eradicate roughly 85 percent of stage I and stage II oral cancers. For tumors of the tongue, floor, cheek, and lip, radioactive implants have been found to be superior to external-beam radiation. Frequently, the two methods are combined.

Although irradiation is noninvasive, severe complications can arise when the target area is the oral cavity and the neck. The radioactive rays often damage the taste buds and the salivary glands, as well as inflame and ulcerate the fragile lining of the mouth and throat. Because saliva helps to prevent tooth decay, a reduction in saliva production *(xerostomia)* can cause plaque to form on the teeth and quickly progress to cavities. Meticulous oral hygiene is essential when you're receiving radiation to the head and neck.

See "Oral Complications" in Chapter Eight, "Take Control: Managing Symptoms, Side Effects, and Complications."

What Is Trismus?—Both radiotherapy and surgery of the oral cavity can cause the connective tissues in the jaw to shrink, making it difficult to open your mouth. This is called *trismus.* If you can't fit three fingers in your mouth, trismus has probably set in. It can come on surprisingly quickly from radiation. "Some patients will complain that their jaw isn't opening well after just two or three days of treatment," says Dr. Lazarus. Fortunately, the condition is both preventable and sometimes reversible. The speech-language

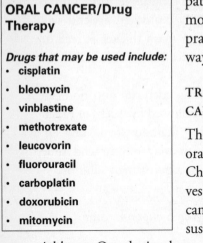

ORAL CANCER/Drug Therapy

Drugs that may be used include:
- cisplatin
- bleomycin
- vinblastine
- methotrexate
- leucovorin
- fluorouracil
- carboplatin
- doxorubicin
- mitomycin

pathologist can show you simple range-of-motion jaw-stretching exercises to begin practicing before radiotherapy gets under way.

TREATMENTS FOR ADVANCED ORAL CANCER

The majority of patients with stage III or IV oral cancer undergo surgery, then radiation. Chemotherapy may also be given on an investigational basis. It is theorized that in oral cancer the drugs "make the cancer cells more susceptible to the radiation," explains Dr. Addante. Oncologists have yet to determine the best way to integrate chemo and radiation. Nor has any agent thus far stood out as especially effective.

OTHER THERAPIES THAT MAY BE USED IN THE TREATMENT OF ORAL CANCER

Laser Surgery/Cryosurgery—Either nonincisional surgical procedure can be used for in situ lesions of the oral cavity.

Mohs' Micrographic Surgery (investigational)—This precise technique has been studied as a treatment for early-stage oral cancers. Mohs' micrographic surgery removes the tumor one thin layer at a time, after which the surgeon inspects the area through a microscope to make sure that no malignant cells remain.

Hyperthermia (investigational)—Killing cancer cells by heating the body has been employed experimentally for recurrent oral cancers.

Hyperfractionated Radiation Therapy (investigational)—Administering accelerated doses of external-beam radiation therapy has been tested against advanced lesions of the lip.

◆ *Ask your doctor about these and any other investigational therapies that might benefit you.*

Cancer of the Thyroid

Overview

TREATMENTS FOR THYROID CANCER THAT HAS NOT
METASTASIZED

All Types

Surgery

Four in five carcinomas of the thyroid are papillary or follicular.
For patients under forty-five years old, there are only two stages—localized and metastatic—as opposed to stages I, II, III, and IV for older
men and women.

When either of these well-differentiated thyroid cancers is confined
to the gland, a lobectomy, near-total thyroidectomy, or total thyroidectomy is performed. Lobectomy has a lower complication rate than
surgery to excise the whole thyroid, but approximately 5 to 10 percent of
patients will have a recurrence in the remaining lobe.

"Increasingly, we favor a total thyroidectomy over a subtotal thyroidectomy or lobectomy," says Dr. Colin Paul Spears, "because
there is a significant incidence of the cancer
arising in multiple sites of the thyroid at
once. That's something that is picked up only
on pathology"—in other words, after the tissue has been removed and examined under
the microscope. Nearly nine in ten papillary
and follicular tumors will be found to contain traces of disease in both lobes.

A lobectomy with isthmusectomy might
be recommended for a person under forty
with a small (*T*1) tumor measuring less than
1 centimeter, or just under $\frac{1}{2}$ inch. Most
other patients undergo total thyroidectomy.
If any lymph nodes in the neck feel swollen,
the surgeon will remove them. More than
half of all papillary tumors spread to the *cervical* nodes in the neck. While this is considered a possible harbinger of a future

---

**THYROID CANCER/
Surgical Procedures**

Lobectomy: surgery to remove
either of the thyroid's two lobes.
Also called a *hemithyroidectomy*.
The *isthmus,* the part that connects
the wing-shaped lobes, may also be
taken out, in an *isthmusectomy*.

Near-total thyroidectomy:
surgery to remove the lobe
containing the tumor, the isthmus,
and most of the opposite lobe. Also
called a *subtotal* thyroidectomy.

Total thyroidectomy: surgery to
remove the entire thyroid.
♦ Lymph nodes may be removed
during any of these surgeries.
Average hospital stay: 3–7 days

Tracheostomy: surgery to create
an opening in the windpipe, to
facilitate breathing.
Average hospital stay: 3–5 days

THYROID CANCER/Treatment Options

Papillary Thyroid Cancer

STAGE I PAPILLARY THYROID CANCER

The cancer is confined to one or both lobes of the thyroid.

{
- Total or near-total thyroidectomy, to surgically remove the thyroid · *or*
- Lobectomy, to surgically remove the side of the thyroid containing the cancer · *followed by*
- Thyroid hormone therapy *with or without*
- Radioiodine therapy

STAGE II PAPILLARY THYROID CANCER

If you are younger than forty-five years old: The cancer has spread beyond the thyroid.
If you are forty-five years old or older: The cancer remains confined to the thyroid and measures larger than 1 centimeter (about ½ inch).

- Total or near-total thyroidectomy *or* lobectomy, *with* lymph-node dissection · *followed by*
- Thyroid hormone therapy · *with or without*
- Radioiodine therapy

STAGE III PAPILLARY THYROID CANCER

The cancer, found in patients forty-five and older, is larger than 4 centimeters (1½ inches); or it has spread outside the thyroid but not outside the neck; or it has spread to the lymph nodes.

- Total or near-total thyroidectomy, *with* lymph-node dissection · *followed by*
- Thyroid hormone therapy · *with or without*
{
- Radioiodine therapy · *or*
- External-beam radiation therapy

STAGE IV PAPILLARY THYROID CANCER

The cancer, found in patients forty-five and older, has spread to other parts of the body.

- Radioiodine therapy

If the cancer is unresponsive to radioiodine therapy:
- External-beam radiation therapy · *or*
- Thyroid hormone therapy · *or the following experimental therapy:*

Under Investigation

- Chemotherapy, frequently consisting of doxorubicin, alone or in combination with cisplatin or carboplatin

◆ Ask your doctor about any clinical trials that might benefit you.

Follicular Thyroid Cancer

STAGE I FOLLICULAR THYROID CANCER

The cancer is confined to one or both lobes of the thyroid.

- Total or near-total thyroidectomy *or* lobectomy, *with* lymph-node dissection · *followed by*
- Thyroid hormone therapy · *and*
- Radioiodine therapy

STAGE II FOLLICULAR THYROID CANCER

If you are younger than forty-five years old: The cancer has spread beyond the thyroid.

If you are forty-five years old or older: The cancer remains confined to the thyroid and measures larger than 1 centimeter (about ¹/₂ inch).

- Total or near-total thyroidectomy *or* lobectomy, *with* lymph-node dissection · *followed by*
- Thyroid hormone therapy · *and*
- Radioiodine therapy

STAGE III FOLLICULAR THYROID CANCER

The cancer, found in patients forty-five and older, is larger than 4 centimeters (1¹/₂ inches); or it has spread outside the thyroid but not outside the neck; or it has spread to the lymph nodes.

- Total or near-total thyroidectomy, *with* lymph-node dissection · *followed by*
- Thyroid hormone therapy · *and*

{
- Radioiodine therapy · *or*
- External-beam radiation therapy
}

STAGE IV FOLLICULAR THYROID CANCER

The cancer, found in patients older than forty-five, has spread to other parts of the body.

- Radioiodine therapy

If the cancer is unresponsive to radioiodine therapy:
- External-beam radiation therapy · *or*
- Thyroid hormone therapy · *or the following experimental therapy:*

Under Investigation
- Chemotherapy, frequently consisting of doxorubicin, alone or in combination with cisplatin or carboplatin
◆ Ask your doctor about any clinical trials that might benefit you.

Medullary Thyroid Cancer

STAGE I MEDULLARY THYROID CANCER

The cancer measures less than 1 centimeter (about ¹/₂ inch).

- Total thyroidectomy, *with* lymph-node dissection · *followed by*
- Thyroid hormone therapy

STAGE II MEDULLARY THYROID CANCER

The cancer measures between 1 and 4 centimeters (1¹/₂ inches).

- Total thyroidectomy, *with* lymph-node dissection · *or* modified radical neck dissection · *followed by*
- Thyroid hormone therapy

STAGE III MEDULLARY THYROID CANCER

The cancer has spread to the lymph nodes.

- Total thyroidectomy, *with* modified radical neck dissection · *followed by*
- Thyroid hormone therapy

STAGE IV MEDULLARY THYROID CANCER

The cancer has spread to other parts of the body.

- Chemotherapy, frequently consisting of doxorubicin or paclitaxel, alone or in combination with cisplatin or carboplatin

Anaplastic Thyroid Cancer

There is no staging system for anaplastic cancer of the thyroid. All patients are considered to have stage IV disease.

If the cancer is operable:
- Total thyroidectomy · *with or without*
- Tracheostomy, to create an artificial opening in the windpipe · *followed by*
- Thyroid hormone therapy

If the cancer is inoperable:
- External-beam radiation therapy

If the cancer has metastasized:
- **Chemotherapy, frequently consisting of doxorubicin, paclitaxel, or docetaxel, alone or in combination with cisplatin or carboplatin**

See treatment options for metastases of the lung and bone.

RECURRENT THYROID CANCER

Your therapy will depend on how you were treated initially.

If the cancer comes back locally or in the regional lymph nodes:
- **Surgery • *with or without***
- **Radioiodine therapy**

If the cancer is unresponsive to radioiodine therapy:
- **External-beam radiation therapy, to relieve symptoms**

If the cancer comes back elsewhere in the body:
- **Chemotherapy, frequently consisting of doxorubicin, paclitaxel, or docetaxel, alone or in combination with cisplatin or carboplatin**

Or:
- **Surgery • *with or without***
- **Radioiodine therapy**

recurrence, it does not increase the chances of dying from the disease. Follicular tumors are far less likely to involve the lymphatic system.

All nonmetastatic medullary thyroid cancers warrant total thyroidectomy plus extensive lymph-node dissection, because the tumor frequently invades the cervical nodes (stage III). Typically, the physician takes out all the lymph nodes and fatty tissue in the middle area of the neck as well as on the side of the neck that contained the tumor.

Because it is an exacting procedure, be sure that your surgeon is practiced in thyroid-removal surgery. The nerves responsible for moving the vocal cords sit next to the thyroid. Damage to one vocal cord can cause hoarseness; damage to both seriously impedes speaking and breathing. This complication occurs less than 2 percent of the time, but studies show that the incidence rate is directly related to the surgeon's experience.

"The major risk of total thyroidectomy is damage to the adjacent parathyroid glands, which are difficult to identify during surgery," says Dr. Spears. The primary function of the *parathyroids* is to release a hormone that regulates the level of calcium in the blood. "If the parathyroid-gland tissue is not preserved, the patient will develop symptoms of low blood calcium." *Hypocalcemia* can bring about muscular twitching and cramping, convulsions, and abnormal heart rhythms.

Tracheostomy—Total thyroidectomy is rarely possible with anaplastic thyroid cancer. By the time the disease is detected, it has usually spread to the lung or affixed itself to vital structures in the neck. At diagnosis, one in four of these highly malignant tumors will have grown into the windpipe. A *tracheostomy* is often necessary in order to bypass the obstruction and restore breathing.

In this operation, the surgeon makes an incision through the neck and into the trachea. A curved *tracheostomy tube,* usually made of plastic, is then inserted into the hole, or *stoma*. From now on, the patient breathes through this opening instead of through the nose and mouth. If necessary, the trach (pronounced *trake*) tube can be connected to an oxygen tank or a mechanical ventilator.

The end of the trach that protrudes slightly from the neck often contains a small *cuff.* Inflating the cuff keeps the tube airtight in the windpipe. Some trachs have an inner *cannula* that slips inside the permanent outer tube, like a lining. Once the tracheostomy site heals, the stoma may be kept open with a smaller buttonlike device.

Should you need to undergo a tracheostomy, a nurse will show you and a family member or friend how to care for it and will send you home with instructions. The trach and surrounding skin must be cleaned at least once a day and the tube changed about once every week, to prevent infection.

Among the supplies you'll need to keep on hand is an electric suction device, available at most surgical supplies stores. Sometimes secretions from the lungs may become trapped in the airway, especially during the first few weeks after the tube is implanted. The aspirator tube is inserted in the trach for *no more than ten to fifteen seconds* at a time, because when you suction mucus, you're also sucking out oxygen. You can find a small battery-powered suction device to carry with you when you're away from home.

People with tracheostomies need to observe certain precautions, such as keeping water from getting into the tube. Consequently, they can no longer go swimming or take showers, although baths are permissible.

A tracheostomy may also affect your ability to speak. Unlike a person with a *laryngectomy,* you still have your voice box. But

---

For free referrals to a certified speech-language pathologist in your area, contact:

American Speech-Language-Hearing Association Action Center
10801 Rockville Pike
Rockville, MD 20852-3279
800-638-8255
http://www.asha.org

the air exhaled by the lungs gets diverted out the trach tube instead of continuing up the windpipe and through the vocal cords—generating sound—on its way out the mouth and nose. Trachs come in different widths. Smaller models may allow enough air to pass around the tube and vibrate the vocal cords. If yours fits snugly within the trachea, however, all of the exhaled air will exit out the stoma. Request a consultation with a *speech-language pathologist,* preferably before your operation. He or she can describe the various techniques and products available that enable people with tracheostomies to produce sound for speech:

- Hold a finger or place a cap over the tube for brief intervals.

- A type of trach called a *fenestrated* tube has an opening in front that when covered with a finger or by lowering the chin permits air to pass through the vocal cords.

- The *Passy-Muir tracheostomy speaking valve* fits on the end of a tracheostomy. The one-way valve allows air in but not out, thus forcing exhaled air around the tube and up past the vocal cords.

- An *electrolarynx* is a battery-powered handheld device that you place against your neck when speaking. It emits high-frequency vibrations, which you shape into words with your mouth and tongue. The technique is easy to learn, but the sound is robotic and monotonic.

- With a *Bivona talking tracheostomy tube,* an outside air source just above the cuff routes air through the vocal cords.

See "Total Laryngectomy and Tracheostomy," page 544.

Hormonal Therapy

All Types—Regardless of how much thyroid tissue is surgically removed, patients must take synthetic thyroid-hormone tablets for the rest of their lives. If the entire gland was excised, this is called *thyroid-hormone re-*

THYROID CANCER/ Drug Therapy

First-line hormonal therapy consists of:
- **levothyroxine (H)**

Other agents that may be used include:
- **doxorubicin**
- **cisplatin**
- **carboplatin**
- **paclitaxel**
- **docetaxel**
- **topotecan**
- **sodium iodide I-131 (R)**

(H) = hormonal agent
(R) = radiopharmaceutical

placement therapy; your body no longer produces the essential hormone and needs it supplemented with levothyroxine (T4) (brand names: Levothroid, Levoxyl, Synthroid).

But if a lobectomy or near-total thyroidectomy was performed, a higher-than-normal dose is given. This suppresses the pituitary gland's secretion of thyroid-stimulating hormone (TSH), which could spur the growth of any remaining tumor cells. The goal of *TSH-suppression therapy* is to virtually eliminate TSH from the bloodstream.

Papillary Thyroid Cancer and Follicular Thyroid Cancer

Radioiodine Therapy

Papillary and follicular thyroid cells are the only cells in the body to absorb iodine. They can be readily targeted for death by having patients swallow a small amount of radioactive iodine. Isotope I-131 is harmless to the body but lethal to thyroid cells, whether normal or cancerous. Your doctor may refer to this effective treatment as *I-131 ablation therapy.*

Compared to surgery alone, thyroidectomy and radioiodine therapy reduce the odds of the cancer coming back locally by about half. It is generally recommended at any stage of follicular thyroid cancer. With papillary thyroid cancer, candidates include patients aged forty-five or older and those with large or aggressive tumors or tumors that have spread to the lymph nodes or other areas. According to Dr. Spears, "Even with a relatively small thyroid malignancy and low risk factors, most medical centers now lean toward using thyroid ablation." The therapy is not used to treat medullary or anaplastic thyroid tumors because their cells do not collect iodine.

The treatment typically takes place about six weeks after surgery. Increasing the level of thyroid-stimulating hormone enhances the thyroid cells' uptake of the radioactive iodine. Therefore, about one to two weeks beforehand, your oncologist will take you off thyroid-hormone therapy in order to prompt the pituitary into flooding the circulation with TSH.

You will have to stay in the hospital for a few days while the radioactivity is at its peak. One of the appealing aspects of radioiodine therapy is that it has virtually no side effects. A number of patients lose their sense of taste, but this is usually temporary. An important point to remember: Ingesting the radioisotope in no way increases the risk of developing a new thyroid tumor or of passing on a genetic abnormality to one's offspring.

"For low-stage thyroid malignancies," says Dr. Spears, "a single thyroid-ablating dose may be enough." Sometimes, though, a second treatment using a higher dose of I-131 must be given roughly two months later to completely eradicate the remaining thyroid tissue. This time the isotope is infused intravenously. If necessary, radioiodine therapy can be repeated every six to twelve months.

Papillary Thyroid Cancer, Follicular Thyroid Cancer, and Anaplastic Thyroid Cancer

Radiation Therapy

If the radioiodine uptake is minimal, external-beam radiotherapy may be used to control localized papillary and follicular tumors. It is also part of the treatment for patients with inoperable anaplastic thyroid cancer.

TREATMENTS FOR ADVANCED THYROID CANCER

Papillary Thyroid Cancer and Follicular Thyroid Cancer

Radioiodine Therapy

The efficacy of I-131 extends to metastatic papillary and follicular lesions. Patients who were diagnosed with secondary thyroid carcinoma of the lung, the most frequent site of metastasis, have been cured with radioiodine therapy alone. "I don't know of any other cancer where you have an opportunity to get rid of metastatic disease with a single injection of a therapy," enthuses Dr. Spears.

Hormonal Therapy

Not all distant tumors will prove sensitive to radioactive iodine. One effective alternative is oral TSH-suppression therapy, using levothyroxine.

Radiation Therapy

As with nonmetastatic thyroid cancer, lesions that are unresponsive to I-131 may be given external-beam radiation therapy.

Medullary Thyroid Cancer and Anaplastic Thyroid Cancer

Chemotherapy

"Patients with metastatic disease that is beyond control by surgery and radiation should look to investigational therapies," says Dr. Spears, a medical oncologist. Researchers are currently experimenting with gene therapy and new chemotherapeutic agents. "If they are not eligible for a clinical trial, standard chemotherapy is a reasonable option." Doxorubicin (Adriamycin), the most commonly prescribed drug, can shrink tumors in about one in four patients; the combination of doxorubicin and cisplatin (Platinol) appears more powerful, particularly against anaplastic thyroid cancer.

TREATMENTS FOR RECURRENT THYROID CANCER

Ten to 30 percent of thyroid-cancer patients develop a recurrence, usually in the neck. A second operation can put half of them into remission again, after which radioiodine ablation may be used. If your cancer is detected during an I-131 scan, as opposed to a clinical exam, your outlook is excellent from radioiodine therapy alone. Approximately one in three recurrent papillary or follicular tumors will not concentrate the isotope, in which event radiation may be given. Chemotherapy is a consideration for cancers that recur in other areas of the body.

(Adult) Cancers of the Brain

Overview

Surgery

Surgery is the primary treatment for most brain tumors, so long as the patient is healthy enough to withstand the operation and the mass is accessible. Slow-growing astrocytomas and benign meningiomas are examples of lesions that often can be excised completely.

The majority of brain cancers, though, cannot be fully removed. Either they are rooted too deep within the brain or they are located too close to vital control centers to risk surgery that might injure the surrounding tissue and possibly impair speech, movement, or other neurologic functions. But even a partial resection is beneficial. *Debulking* the tumor reduces the pressure within the skull, relieving symptoms. It also leaves behind a less formidable adversary for subsequent irradiation or chemotherapy.

Craniotomy, once associated with high rates of mortality and neurologic deficits, "is now very well tolerated," says Dr. Michael L. Gruber, director of neuro-oncology at New York University Medical Center. Since the early 1990s, the average hospitalization has been halved from approximately eight days to three or four. The increased safety can be attributed partly to improved methods of controlling *cerebral edema,* a potentially fatal swelling of the brain. But Dr. Gruber points to technological innovations that have enhanced the surgeon's precision, so that the operation excises the maximum amount of cancer while sparing normal brain tissue.

But, because brain cancer is relatively rare, few hospitals are appointed with the elaborate and costly equipment necessary for performing such cutting-edge procedures as *stereotactic radiosurgery* or *intraoperative magnetic resonance imaging.* As of 1998, NYU Medical Center was one of just three dozen centers in the country to own a *gamma knife:* a stereotactic-radiosurgery device that costs $3 million and weighs twenty tons. "Unfortunately," says Dr. Gruber, "very few cancer centers have an interest in brain tumors. It is an extremely undersupported area of medicine." When deciding on a treatment facility, you should give equal weight to the expertise of the neurosurgeon and access to the surgical and radiographic techniques described on the following pages. More so than most other types of cancer, brain cancer demands that you may have to expand your search beyond your hometown or state.

Microsurgery—Today neurosurgeons routinely perform brain surgery with the help of a high-powered microscope for a magnified view of the operative area, or *field.*

Stereotaxy—Using computers to generate a three-dimensional image is called *stereotaxy.* The technique may be employed prior to or during surgery, to pinpoint the tumor's location as well as its position in relation to vital structures in the brain. It is particularly helpful for masses that are difficult to reach.

Stereotaxy begins with a presurgical CT scan or MRI scan—sometimes both. To keep your head perfectly still, a rigid frame is attached to your skull with several screws. The information from the imaging exam(s) is then fed into a computer, which creates a 3-D map of the surgical site. From this, the surgeon can simulate the operation on the computer and plan the safest route to the lesion.

BRAIN CANCERS/ Surgical Procedures

Craniotomy: surgical removal of a benign or malignant brain tumor. The neurosurgeon makes an incision in the scalp and peels back the tissue to reveal the skull. Next a special saw is used to cut out a plate of bone; imagine a trapdoor. Then the brain's tough outer membrane, the *dura mater,* is cut open, exposing the surface. After all or most of the mass is removed, the dura mater is sewn back together, the piece of skull sutured back into position, and the scalp closed. There are instances where the bone is *not* replaced; remarkably, the muscles in the back of the head are strong enough to adequately protect the brain. **Average hospital stay: 3–4 days**

BRAIN CANCERS/Treatment Options

Gliomas
SUBTYPE: *Astrocytomas*

WELL-DIFFERENTIATED ASTROCYTOMA (LOW GRADE)
- Craniotomy, to surgically remove or debulk as much cancer as possible · *alone or followed by*
- External-beam radiation therapy

Under Investigation
- Chemotherapy following surgery or radiation
- ◆ Ask your doctor about any clinical trials that might benefit you.

ANAPLASTIC ASTROCYTOMA (INTERMEDIATE GRADE)
- Craniotomy · *followed by*
- External-beam radiation therapy · *followed by*
- Chemotherapy, frequently consisting of procarbazine, lomustine, and vincristine

Or:
- Craniotomy · *followed by*
- Chemotherapy, consisting of carboplatin · *followed by*
- External-beam radiation therapy

If the cancer does not respond to first-line chemotherapy:
- Chemotherapy, consisting of temozolomide

Under Investigation #1
- New methods of delivering radiation therapy

Under Investigation #2
- New chemotherapy drugs and immunologic agents

Under Investigation #3
- Hyperthermia

Under Investigation #4
- Chemoradiation
- ◆ Ask your doctor about any clinical trials that might benefit you.

GLIOBLASTOMA MULTIFORME (HIGH GRADE)
- Craniotomy · *followed by*
- Chemotherapy, frequently consisting of one or more of the following drugs: carmustine, carboplatin, topotecan · *followed by*
- External-beam radiation therapy

Under Investigation #1
- New methods of delivering radiation therapy

Under Investigation #2
- New chemotherapy drugs and immunologic agents

Under Investigation #3
- Hyperthermia

Under Investigation #4
- Chemoradiation

◆ Ask your doctor about any clinical trials that might benefit you.

Surgery alone is the treatment of choice for low-grade astrocytoma. "It is unusual that we would recommend any other therapy," says Dr. Michael Gruber. Intermediate and high-grade astrocytomas, however, call for all three major modalities. In the past, the sequence consisted of surgery, radiation, then chemotherapy. Now high-dose chemotherapy typically follows the operation, with radiation given last.

The drugs procarbazine (brand name: Matulane), lomustine (CeeNU), and vincristine (Oncovin) have made up the standard regimen for anaplastic astrocytoma; carmustine (BiCNU), for glioblastoma multiforme. "That was the standard of care for perhaps thirty years," says Dr. Gruber. "But since the early 1990s, a number of newer agents have been used." Temozolomide (Temodar), an oral alkylating agent, was introduced in 1999 as a treatment for anaplastic astrocytoma that recurred or did not respond at all to frontline chemotherapy. It was the first new drug for this type of brain cancer in twenty years.

SUBTYPE: *Brain-Stem Gliomas*

- External-beam radiation therapy

If the cancer should recur:

Under Investigation
- New chemotherapy drugs and immunologic agents

◆ Ask your doctor about any clinical trials that might benefit you.

Tumors of the brain stem are considered inoperable. "The brain stem is a compact bundle of tissue that regulates heart function, blood pressure, breathing, and swallowing," explains Dr. Gruber. "To try to operate in this tiny area, the likelihood is great that the patient would wind up with significant impairment of his basic vital functions, including paralysis or needing a mechanical ventilator in order to breathe." External-beam irradiation is the only standard treatment.

SUBTYPE: *Ependymomas*

WELL-DIFFERENTIATED EPENDYMOMA (LOW GRADE)
- Craniotomy · *alone or followed by*
- External-beam radiation therapy

If a low-grade ependymoma should recur:

Under Investigation

- A second craniotomy • *with*
- External-beam radiation therapy, if not given previously • *or*
- Chemotherapy, possibly consisting of the following drugs or drug combinations: cisplatin, etoposide, cyclophosphamide, and vincristine; high-dose carboplatin; carmustine and cisplatin

♦ Ask your doctor about any clinical trials that might benefit you.

MALIGNANT EPENDYMOMA

- Craniotomy • *with*
- External-beam radiation therapy

If the cancer should spread to the spinal fluid:
- Craniospinal external-beam radiation therapy

Under Investigation
- Chemotherapy, given before, during, or after radiation, possibly consisting of the following drugs or drug combinations: cisplatin, etoposide, cyclophosphamide, and vincristine; high-dose carboplatin; carmustine and cisplatin

♦ Ask your doctor about any clinical trials that might benefit you.

If a malignant ependymoma should recur:

Under Investigation
- Chemotherapy, possibly consisting of the following drugs or drug combinations: cisplatin, etoposide, cyclophosphamide, and vincristine; high-dose carboplatin; carmustine and cisplatin

♦ Ask your doctor about any clinical trials that might benefit you.

Low-grade ependymomas, also referred to as benign, can often be resected completely, eliminating the need for radiation. With malignant ependymomas, however, radiation follows surgery. Irradiation of the spine may also be necessary, because these more aggressive tumors have a propensity for seeding the spinal fluid. Although many drugs have been employed against ependymomas on an experimental basis, "chemotherapy's role is not clear yet," says Dr. Gruber.

SUBTYPE: *Oligodendrogliomas*

WELL-DIFFERENTIATED OLIGODENDROGLIOMA (LOW GRADE)

- Craniotomy • *alone or followed by*
- External-beam radiation therapy

If the cancer cannot be completely resected:

Under Investigation

- Postsurgical external-beam radiation therapy • *with*
- Chemotherapy

◆ Ask your doctor about any clinical trials that might benefit you.

ANAPLASTIC OLIGODENDROGLIOMA

- Craniotomy • *followed by*
- External-beam radiation therapy • *with or without*
- Chemotherapy

Or:

- Craniotomy • *followed by*
- Chemotherapy, frequently consisting of procarbazine, carmustine, and vincristine • *followed by*
- External-beam radiation therapy

Or:

- Craniotomy • *followed by*
- High-dose chemotherapy, frequently including carboplatin • *followed by*
- Autologous bone-marrow transplantation • *or*
- External-beam radiation therapy

Under Investigation #1

- New methods of delivering radiation therapy

Under Investigation #2

- Hyperthermia

Under Investigation #3

- New chemotherapy drugs and immunologic agents

◆ Ask your doctor about any clinical trials that might benefit you.

Most oligodendrogliomas are low grade. Whether or not these tumors require postoperative radiation is a subject of debate. At NYU Medical Center, for instance, patients are treated with surgery alone. "There is absolutely no evidence that radiation is of benefit," asserts Dr. Gruber. Another institution may hold the opposite opinion. Whichever strategy your neuro-oncologist recommends, ask her to explain why she feels this is in your best interest and if she can show you any medical literature supporting this approach.

No such controversy exists regarding high-grade, or anaplastic, oligodendroglioma. Following surgery, says Dr. Gruber, "we treat with chemotherapy, then radiation. Oligo cells are highly sensitive to chemotherapy." Another tactic is high-dose chemotherapy with stem-cell rescue. The potent concentration of anticancer agents depletes the bone marrow, making it necessary for patients to receive an infusion of their own blood-forming cells.

SUBTYPE: *Mixed Gliomas*

- Craniotomy • *followed by*
- External-beam radiation therapy • *with or without*

- Chemotherapy, frequently consisting of procarbazine, lomustine, and vincristine

Or:
- Craniotomy • *followed by*
- Chemotherapy, frequently consisting of procarbazine, carmustine, and vincristine • *followed by*
- External-beam radiation therapy

Or:
- Craniotomy • *followed by*
- High-dose chemotherapy, frequently including carboplatin • *followed by*
- Autologous bone-marrow transplantation • *or*
- External-beam radiation therapy

Under Investigation #1
- New methods of delivering radiation therapy

Under Investigation #2
- Hyperthermia

Under Investigation #3
- New chemotherapy drugs and immunologic agents
- ◆ Ask your doctor about any clinical trials that might benefit you.

Mixed gliomas frequently contain high proportions of (1) astrocytes and oligodendrocytes, (2) astrocytes and ependymal cells, or (3) a combination of all three. The highest grade of cancer cell found in the tumor determines the direction of treatment.

Meningiomas

SUBTYPE: *Benign Meningiomas*

- Craniotomy • *alone or followed by*
- External-beam radiation therapy

SUBTYPE: *Malignant Meningiomas*

- Craniotomy • *followed by*
- External-beam radiation therapy

Under Investigation #1
- New methods of delivering radiation therapy

Under Investigation #2
- Hyperthermia

Under Investigation #3
- New chemotherapy drugs and immunologic agents
- ◆ Ask your doctor about any clinical trials that might benefit you.

Meningiomas are rarely malignant and are usually curable through surgery alone, unless the mass occupies an unreachable area of the brain. "In that setting," explains Dr. Gruber, "we'll perform as much surgery as we can, then use stereotactic radiosurgery to eradicate the rest of the tumor."

Craniopharyngioma

- Craniotomy · *alone or followed by*
- External-beam radiation therapy

Over the years, neurosurgeons have revised their thinking about how to best resect this often curable tumor. "In the old days," says Dr. Gruber, "the surgeon would do everything he could to remove every last cell, and, unfortunately, in many instances the patient would be left with serious neurological impairment." Today, he says, surgeons take a more conservative approach to craniopharyngiomas, "trying to cut out as much as they can safely, then irradiating the portion that can't be removed."

Adult Pineal Parenchymal Tumors

SUBTYPE: *Primitive Neuroectodermal Tumors (PNET)*

- Craniotomy · *followed by*
- External-beam radiation therapy · *with or without*
- Chemotherapy

Under Investigation #1
- New methods of delivering radiation therapy

Under Investigation #2
- Hyperthermia

Under Investigation #3
- New chemotherapy drugs and immunologic agents
- ◆ Ask your doctor about any clinical trials that might benefit you.

Pineal tumors are difficult to excise totally but are sensitive to radiotherapy. The conventional treatment for pineocytomas is surgery and external-beam radiation. For the faster-growing pineoblastomas, chemotherapy is added.

SUBTYPE: *Central Nervous System Germ-Cell Tumors*

Germinoma
- Chemotherapy, frequently consisting of etoposide and cisplatin, or high-dose carboplatin · *followed by*
- External-beam radiation therapy

Embryonal Carcinoma, Teratoma, Choriocarcinoma
- Craniotomy · *followed by*
- Chemotherapy, frequently consisting of various combinations of the following drugs: cisplatin, etoposide, bleomycin, carboplatin, and vincristine · *followed by*

- External-beam radiation therapy · *followed by*
- Chemotherapy

Germinoma, an extremely curable malignant tumor, is highly susceptible to chemotherapy. According to Dr. Gruber, most brain-tumor specialists treat it with high-dose carboplatin followed by irradiation. Because more than nine in ten patients will achieve a complete response from carboplatin, "it is possible to avoid radiation and cure patients with chemotherapy alone." Doctors at the Mayo Clinic discovered an equally effective but less toxic regimen: etoposide and cisplatin, administered at the conventional dosage, then low-dose radiation. The pair of drugs was given to seventeen patients. Nine had germinomas; eight had one of the nongerminoma forms of CNS germ-cell tumors. More than four years later, all seventeen were alive with no evidence of disease. Both PNET and germ-cell tumors may shed cells into the cerebrospinal fluid and require craniospinal radiotherapy.

Primary Central Nervous System Lymphoma

- External-beam radiation therapy

Or:
- Chemotherapy, possibly consisting of cyclophosphamide, doxorubicin, vincristine, and prednisone, or methotrexate with or without cytarabine · *alone or with*
- External-beam radiation therapy

Treating primary lymphoma of the central nervous system is often complicated by the fact that most people with this cancer have impaired immune systems. In those infected with the human immunodeficiency virus, it is one of the conditions that demarcate the passage from HIV-positive status to full-blown AIDS. By this point, the resistance to disease is so low that a diagnosis of CNS lymphoma "is usually a preterminal event," says Dr. Gruber. Yet organ-transplant recipients whose immunity is compromised from taking immunosuppressant medications can sometimes attain remission. "If we simply discontinue one of the immunosuppressant drugs, we may see the tumor in the brain disappear."

Although irradiation is still considered a standard treatment for this aggressive disease, around 1990 physicians began preceding it with drug therapy. "Now," says Dr. Gruber, "CNS lymphoma is frequently treated with chemotherapy alone," often in conjunction with blood-brain-barrier-disruption therapy. The average life expectancy for patients has quadrupled, "from about eleven months to close to four years. The advances in treatment for this disease have been amazing."

RECURRENT BRAIN CANCER

Your therapy will depend on how you were treated initially.
- Craniotomy · *alone or in conjunction with*
- Chemotherapy

Or:
- Chemotherapy alone

If radiation therapy was not given previously:
- **External-beam radiation therapy** • *alone or with*
- **Chemotherapy**

Or:
- **Internal radiation therapy**

Under Investigation
- **New chemotherapy drugs, new drug combinations, and new immunologic agents**

◆ **Ask your doctor about any clinical trials that might benefit you.**

When a brain lesion recurs, the possible treatment plans include a second surgery or stereotactic radiosurgery. Unlike conventional radiation, the gamma knife and similar devices can be used to eradicate lesions that were previously treated with radiotherapy. "Most patients who experience a recurrence," says Dr. Gruber, "are given chemotherapy." Certainly, he adds, this is a time to consider experimental protocols of new drugs or drug combinations. Realistically, the chance of a cure is remote, but "many patients can be given six to nine months of quality time."

In *stereotactic surgery,* the images are transmitted to a display unit on the surgical microscope and superimposed over the operative field. The doctor can then refer to them throughout. Once again your head will be secured within a frame, unless the hospital has what is called a *frameless navigational system.* Here the surgeon places a wandlike instrument against the brain as he is operating. The device superimposes its position on a computer monitor displaying a recent scan or three-dimensional image of the brain. Stereotactic surgery is less invasive than conventional craniotomy, requiring smaller incisions in the scalp, skull, and brain.

Intraoperative Magnetic Resonance Imaging—With an MRI machine serving as the operating table for brain-tumor excision, explains Dr. Gruber, "the surgeon is able to see what he is doing in 'real time.' " Other physicians use ultrasound imaging for the same purpose.

Evoked Potential Electrophysiological Mapping—During surgery, small electrodes are used to stimulate nerves and measure their electrical responses, or *evoked potential.* From establishing the function of specific nerves in each patient, the surgical team identifies the critical areas of the brain to avoid.

Functional Image-Guided Surgery—This technique follows a similar principle, except that it is carried out prior to the operation. During a special MRI scan, you are asked to perform certain repetitive tasks: tap your fingers, read a list of words, think about specific objects, and so on. The parts of the brain that govern these functions will demonstrate heightened activity, which the scan converts into an image. By merging this scan with a conventional MRI image outlining the tumor, the neurosurgeon now has a map to direct him to the mass and around sensitive areas.

Ultrasonic Aspiration—Bombarding the lesion with high-frequency sound waves from a handheld ultrasonic aspirator causes it to vibrate and break apart, while leaving nerves and blood vessels intact. At the same time, the instrument "vacuums" up the fragments of tumor tissue.

Laser Surgery—Lasers are often used with stereotactic localization to vaporize tumor cells in relatively inaccessible areas.

Radiation Therapy

Most brain lesions respond to external-beam radiotherapy. It is the definitive treatment for brain-stem gliomas and other brain cancers considered too risky to operate on. More typically, radiation is administered after surgery, to whittle down the residual tumor. The standard schedule is six weeks of daily treatment, with weekends off.

Clinical trials are testing new methods of delivery, including:

- The use of various drugs that either sensitize tumor cells to the effects of external-beam radiation, enhance the efficiency of the dose, or protect brain cells during irradiation treatments

- Giving radiation during surgery *(intraoperative radiotherapy)* in addition to afterward

- Using hyperthermia in conjunction with external-beam radiation therapy

- Interstitial radiation *(brachytherapy)*

Stereotactic Radiosurgery—The advantage of brachytherapy over external-beam radiation is that surgically implanting radioactive pellets into the tumor site delivers a lethal dose of radiation to the tumor but emits only minimal radiation to neighboring brain tissue. Still, it is an invasive procedure: A small hole must be made in the skull in which to place the radionuclides, which are subsequently withdrawn after six or seven days.

Stereotactic radiosurgery "accomplishes the same goal noninvasively," says Dr. Gruber, "and in a single procedure." Radiosurgery is not an operation at all but is, rather, a form of radiotherapy. Using the same computerized three-dimensional guidance as stereotactic surgery, one of several types of machines sends multiple narrow beams of high-dose radiation converging on the tumor from different angles.

The gamma knife, the first radiosurgery device to be developed, resembles an MRI scanner. You lie down on a portable table and are fitted with the halolike head frame described under "Stereotaxy." A scan is taken, and while you rest in a waiting area, the medical team plans the treatment.

Next you are repositioned on the table, with your head inside a large five-hundred-pound helmet containing 201 holes—one for each beam of gamma radiation emitted by the gamma knife. The couchlike platform draws you into the box-shaped machine, up to your shoulders. There is no discomfort and no noise. Some medical centers require that patients stay overnight for observation; others discharge them the same day.

The other types of machines used for radiosurgery are *adapted linear accelerators,* which direct arcs of radioactive rays at the tumor; and, the rarest of the three, *cyclotrons.* Days, weeks, or months may pass before the results of treatment become apparent, but typically most lesions stop growing soon afterward, then gradually shrink and disappear.

Stereotactic radiosurgery appears most effective for small primary and metastatic brain tumors that measure less than 4 centimeters (1½ inches) in diameter, and particularly for masses that are considered inoperable.

Chemotherapy

Anticancer agents play a central role in the treatment of oligodendrogliomas, primary CNS lymphoma, and CNS germ-cell tumors. But overall, chemotherapy has demonstrated limited effectiveness against brain cancer.

To begin with, many brain tumors are intrinsically resistant to the medicines used. The second obstacle is getting sufficient amounts of the drugs to the cancer. On the surface, this shouldn't pose a problem, since chemotherapy travels via the bloodstream, and fully one-quarter of the blood pumped by the heart is distributed throughout the brain tissue by an extensive network of arteries. But the brain is endowed with an elaborate security system of vessels and cells that filters out substances in the circulation, including anticancer drugs. Only salt, water, and vital nutrients are allowed through.

Oncologists have attempted a number of methods to cross this *blood-brain barrier.* Many of the therapies described below are experi-

BRAIN CANCERS/
Drug Therapy

First-line therapy frequently consists of:

Anaplastic Astrocytoma
- PCV: procarbazine + lomustine + vincristine

Glioblastoma Multiforme
- carmustine

Mixed Gliomas and Anaplastic Oligodendroglioma
- procarbazine + carmustine or lomustine + vincristine
- high-dose carboplatin

CNS Germ-Cell Tumors
- carboplatin
- cisplatin
- etoposide
- bleomycin
- vincristine

Primary CNS Lymphoma
- methotrexate
- cytarabine

Other drugs or drug combinations that may be used to treat brain cancers include:
- CHOP: cyclophosphamide + doxorubicin + vincristine + prednisone (H)
- Gliadel
- prednisone (H)
- prednisolone (H)
- dexamethasone (H)
- topotecan
- temozolomide

(H) = hormonal agent

mental and are not currently available at most medical facilities. Ask your neuro-oncologist if any of these techniques might be worth investigating for your type of brain cancer.

Interstitial Chemotherapy—One way to bypass the blood-brain barrier is to implant approximately eight dissolvable wafers impregnated with chemotherapy directly into the tumor bed. Gliadel, a dime-sized disc containing the drug carmustine (BiCNU), is an approved treatment for recurrent glioblastoma multiforme, the most malignant astrocytoma. Over the course of three weeks, it slowly delivers one thousand times the normal dose of carmustine to the affected area of the brain, but without the symptoms generally associated with systemic chemotherapy. While not a cure, Gliadel does add months, sometimes more, to patients' lives.

Implantable Infusion Pump—A pump surgically implanted in the skull infuses a steady stream of chemotherapy into the tumor for days or weeks.

Intra-arterial Chemotherapy—An anti-cancer agent administered intravenously becomes diluted by the time it travels through the veins, the heart, the lungs, back to the heart, into the arterial system, and, finally, into an artery leading to the brain. In intra-arterial chemotherapy, the drug is injected directly into one of those arteries, so that more of the chemical reaches its intended target.

Intrathecal Chemotherapy—The drugs are injected into the cerebrospinal fluid that bathes the outside of the brain and spinal cord. The needle is inserted in the central canal in the lower back, not unlike a lumbar puncture, or the patient has a small repository called an *Ommaya reservoir* surgically implanted beneath the scalp. The doctor or nurse administers the shot through the scalp and into the receptacle, which channels the chemo via a catheter tube to one of the cerebrum's canyonlike ventricles.

One drawback to intrathecal chemotherapy is that many of the agents that can be given intravenously are too toxic to be delivered into the cerebrospinal fluid. Another is that the fluid isn't able to distribute drugs any deeper than one or two millimeters into the brain.

Blood-Brain-Barrier Disruption—This therapy, developed by neurosurgeon Edward A. Neuwelt at Oregon Health Sciences University Hospital in Portland, outmaneuvers the blood-brain barrier into temporarily letting down its guard. It has been shown to be most effective in treating primary CNS lymphoma, even curing some patients.

The treatment is costly—in the neighborhood of $250,000—and physically rigorous. Each dose of chemotherapy must be administered in the operating room, under general anesthesia. A specially trained team of surgeons makes an incision in an artery in the groin and threads a flexible catheter up to one of the vessels that supply the brain. Next a sugar called mannitol is injected into the tube. For up to thirty minutes, the solution causes the cells lining the brain's capillaries to shrink and separate sufficiently for the antitumor drugs to slip through. Then the cells expand again, and the blood-brain barrier seals shut.

"High-dose chemotherapy increases the amount of chemotherapy in the blood only two- or threefold, whereas if you give chemotherapy directly into the artery *and* open the blood-brain barrier, the brain receives about one hundred times the normal dose," explains Dr. Neuwelt. "And it does this with far less risk than high-dose systemic chemotherapy, which wipes out the bone marrow." As of 1999, Oregon Health Sciences University Hospital was one of only five medical centers in the United States that performed the complicated procedure.

Conventional therapy for primary CNS lymphoma consists of methotrexate-based chemotherapy followed by radiation. Oregon Health Sciences University compared two groups of primary CNS lymphoma patients treated with chemotherapy by blood-brain-barrier delivery. One group additionally received radiotherapy, which can impair intellect or coordination. The results for both groups were superior to those for standard chemotherapy and radiotherapy. That includes the participants who forwent irradiation and therefore were unaffected cognitively.

Researchers are in the process of testing other substances to manipulate the blood-brain barrier and open the door for chemotherapeutic agents to reach cancers in the brain.

OTHER THERAPIES THAT MAY BE USED IN THE TREATMENT OF BRAIN CANCERS

Steroid Therapy/Shunt Surgery—It is not uncommon for a person with a brain tumor to develop swelling of the brain tissue, or edema. The mass itself may obstruct one of the ventricles, causing the cerebrospinal fluid to accumulate. This condition is known as hydrocephalus. When brain edema arises as a complication of craniotomy or radiation treatment, a short course of *steroid* medications may be prescribed. (These are not the *anabolic* steroids abused by athletes.) Two points to know in advance: Long-term steroid use frequently produces unwelcome side effects such as mood swings, water retention, and a voracious appetite. Second, the hormone must *never* be discontinued abruptly, but withdrawn slowly under a doctor's supervision.

Sometimes a *shunt* must be surgically implanted in a ventricle to divert the blocked fluid and relieve the attendant buildup of pressure within the skull *(increased intracranial pressure,* also known as IICP). The slender tube runs beneath the scalp down to either the abdominal cavity or, less commonly, one of the chambers of the heart. There the excess fluid drains and is absorbed.

A shunt may be removed after the craniotomy, or it may be left in place permanently. Your physician or nurse will review with you the warning signs of a shunt malfunction; the tube can become blocked, infected, or dislodged. Should any of these occur, it's important to notify your doctor immediately. The problem can then be corrected in a procedure called a shunt *revision.*

The average hospital stay is three to five days.

Seizure Medications—You may or may not experience seizures because of a brain lesion or following brain surgery. The location of the tumor greatly determines a patient's predisposition to convulsions. With *anticonvulsant medications,* however, most brain-tumor patients can go through life free of seizures.

A seizure is a spontaneous emission of electrical impulses from the brain cells. An episode is generally not dangerous by itself, unless of course a person loses consciousness while driving a car or operating heavy machinery. For that reason, patients may relinquish their driver's licenses temporarily, until a certain amount of time goes by without a seizure. This varies according to state.

Antiangiogenesis Therapy (investigational)—Several *angiogenesis inhibitors* are being tested against brain tumors, including thalidomide and TNP-470.

The Informed Patient:
The Benefits of Rehabilitation Therapy

Surgery, radiotherapy, and the tumor itself can all damage normal brain tissue, impairing the function(s) regulated by that part of the brain. Difficulty in speaking or finding the right words, personality and behavioral changes, poor concentration, loss of coordination—one or more of these are all possible effects of the disease or its treatment. Faster-growing tumors tend to produce multiple deficits, while a mass in one of the "silent" areas of the brain can bring about changes that are so subtle they may elude even the neurologist. Some of the disabilities improve with time or subside completely, but others, like short-term memory loss, may be permanent.

People with brain tumors often respond more dramatically to rehabilitation than do survivors of stroke or traumatic brain injury, because the effects of the tumor are usually milder. Yet they are less likely to receive timely referrals to therapy that could possibly help them regain lost abilities. "Doctors have been reluctant to make referrals," observes Dr. Mark Sherer, a neuropsychologist, "because the overall prognosis for primary malignant brain tumors has typically been viewed as grim."

We suggest taking the initiative and raising this issue with your primary oncologist and neurosurgeon before treatment commences so that you have a game plan in mind

---

Rehabilitation for Brain-Tumor Patients

Cognitive retraining: a technique of training one area of the brain to compensate for an area that has been damaged.

Occupational therapy: teaches patients new ways to perform the skills necessary for daily living, such as eating, dressing, and bathing.

Physical therapy: helps patients build up muscle strength and improve balance and coordination.

Speech and language pathology: assists patients who are experiencing difficulty with speech or swallowing.

Vocational rehabilitation: helps patients with disabilities return to work, be it to their former position or a new job. In addition to evaluating your skills and providing any necessary job-related training, the vocational counselors serve as liaisons between patients and employers.

TABLE 6.1 **Resources for Finding a Rehabilitation Program**

Patient Support Organizations

Contact these organizations for information on patient support groups in your area:

The Brain Tumor Society
124 Watertown St., Suite 3-H
Watertown, MA 02472
800-770-8287 or 617-924-9997
http://www.tbts.com

Cancer Information Service
800-422-6237

National Brain Tumor Foundation
414 Thirteenth St., Suite 700
Oakland, CA 94612
800-934-2873 or 510-839-9777
http://www.braintumor.org

These organizations may be able to refer you to rehabilitation facilities in your area:

Brain Injury Association
105 N. Alfred St.
Alexandria, VA 22314
800-444-6443 or 703-236-6000
http://www.biausa.org

National Rehabilitation Information Center
1010 Wayne Ave., Suite 800
Silver Spring, MD 20910
800-346-2742 or 301-562-2400
http://www.naric.com

National Stroke Association
96 Inverness Dr. E., Suite I
Englewood, CO 80112-5112
800-787-6537 or 303-649-9299
http://www.stroke.org

Accreditation/Certification Organizations

These two accreditation organizations can give you the names of accredited rehabilitation facilities near you. CARF requires a self-addressed stamped envelope. Inquiries to JCAHO can be made over the phone.

Commission on Accreditation of Rehabilitation Facilities
4891 E. Grant Rd.
Tucson, AZ 85712
520-325-1044
http://www.carf.org

Joint Commission on Accreditation of Healthcare Organizations
One Renaissance Blvd.
Oakbrook Terrace, IL 60181
630-792-5000
http://www.jcaho.org

Contact ASHA for referrals to certified speech-language pathologists *in your area.*

American Speech-Language-Hearing Association
Action Center
10801 Rockville Pike
Rockville, MD 20852-3279
800-638-8255
http://www.asha.org

should rehabilitation be appropriate for you. Ask, "When will be a good time for us to discuss a rehab consult?" Typically, the neuro-oncology team will want to wait several days after surgery or the completion of radiation or chemotherapy. Once the swelling of the brain abates, it becomes clearer which deficits were temporary complications of the edema and which need to be addressed through one or more forms of therapy.

New York University Medical Center has an entire facility devoted to rehabilitation medicine where brain-tumor patients with related disabilities are routinely evaluated and seen by appropriate specialists. Few hospitals, however, offer that caliber of rehabilitative care. And what if you'd had to travel to the institution that performed your surgery? Although NYU and other medical centers maintain apartments nearby for family and friends, it may be more practical for you to receive therapy closer to home.

These are all points to take up with the hospital *social worker, case manager,* or *discharge nurse,* all of whom regularly coordinate rehabilitation for patients who live out of town, even out of state. Should the task of finding a local rehab facility or individual practitioner fall to you or a member of your family, a good place to start is to ask your physician and other patients for recommendations. In addition, call around to the patient support organizations and accreditation agencies listed in table 6.1.

Not every brain-tumor patient will respond to rehabilitation. Those with moderate neurologic impairments appear to benefit most. The key to successful rehabilitation is to choose a program tailored to your specific needs. Bear in mind that many are geared toward stroke and head-injury patients—focusing on physical and occupational therapies—while brain-tumor patients are more likely to need cognitive retraining and vocational rehabilitation. Most brain-cancer survivors prefer outpatient programs. By the time rehabilitation begins, they have been out of the hospital for a while and are not eager to return if it's not necessary.

Questions to Ask . . . When Considering a Rehabilitation Program or Practitioner

- Does the program provide the services I need?

- Does the program match my abilities? Or is it too demanding or not demanding enough?

- If this is an outpatient program, does the facility provide transportation?

- Are family members encouraged to participate in rehabilitation sessions and to practice with me?

- What is the total cost of therapy, and how much can I expect private insurance, Medicare, or Medicaid to cover?

- Is the program accredited and state-licensed?

For accreditation information, contact either the Joint Commission on Accreditation of Healthcare Organizations or the Commission on Accreditation of Rehabilitation Facilities. To check if a program is state-licensed, call your state department of health; you'll find its number in the "State Government Offices" section of the phone book.

If you want to verify the credentials of an individual physical therapist, speech-language pathologist, and so on, contact your state's licensing board for that profession and give the person's name. The simplest way to find the telephone number is to call directory assistance in your state capital and request the listing for the licensing board for the profession you want to check on (occupational therapy, for instance).

Multiple Myeloma

Overview

TREATMENTS FOR MULTIPLE MYELOMA

Observation
Multiple myeloma usually isn't detected until the cancer is advanced. Some patients, though, are diagnosed with "smoldering" stage

MULTIPLE MYELOMA/Treatment Options

STAGE I MULTIPLE MYELOMA

Relatively few cancer cells have spread throughout the body; the blood contains normal amounts of red blood cells and calcium; no tumors are found in the bone; and the amount of M proteins in the blood or urine is very low.

If you do not have symptoms:
- **Observation**

If you have symptoms:
- **Chemotherapy, frequently consisting of melphalan and prednisone, or one of several other drug combinations •** *and*
- **External-beam irradiation, to relieve symptoms**

Under Investigation #1
- **High-dose chemotherapy, frequently consisting of melphalan, cyclophosphamide, or busulfan, alone or in combination •** *with or without*
- **Total-body irradiation •** *followed by*
- **Autologous peripheral-blood stem-cell transplantation** *or* **bone-marrow transplantation** *followed by*
- **Immunotherapy, consisting of alpha-interferon**

Under Investigation #2
- **New chemotherapy drugs, immunologic agents, and cancer vaccines**
- ◆ Ask your doctor about any clinical trials that might benefit you.

STAGE II MULTIPLE MYELOMA

A moderate number of cancer cells has spread throughout the body.

- **Chemotherapy, frequently consisting of melphalan and prednisone, or one of several other drug combinations •** *and*
- **External-beam irradiation, to relieve symptoms**

Under Investigation #1
- **High-dose chemotherapy, frequently consisting of melphalan, cyclophosphamide, or busulfan, alone or in combination •** *with or without*
- **Total-body irradiation •** *followed by*
- **Autologous peripheral-blood stem-cell transplantation** *or* **bone-marrow transplantation •** *followed by*
- **Immunotherapy, consisting of alpha-interferon •** *or*
- **Allogeneic bone-marrow transplantation**

Under Investigation #2
- **New chemotherapy drugs, immunologic agents, and cancer vaccines**
- ◆ Ask your doctor about any clinical trials that might benefit you.

STAGE III MULTIPLE MYELOMA

A relatively large number of cancer cells has spread throughout the body, and there may be one or more of the following: a decrease in the number of red blood cells, causing anemia; abnormally high levels of calcium in the blood; more than three bone tumors; high levels of M proteins in the blood or urine.

- Chemotherapy, frequently consisting of melphalan and prednisone, or one of several other drug combinations • *and*
- External-beam irradiation, to relieve symptoms

Under Investigation

- High-dose chemotherapy, frequently consisting of melphalan, cyclophosphamide, or busulfan, alone or in combination • *with or without*
- Total-body irradiation • *followed by*

- Autologous peripheral-blood stem-cell transplantation *or* bone-marrow transplantation • *followed by*
- Immunotherapy, frequently consisting of alpha-interferon • *or*

- Allogeneic bone-marrow transplantation
- ◆ Ask your doctor about any clinical trials that might benefit you.

PRIMARY REFRACTORY MULTIPLE MYELOMA (UNRESPONSIVE)

Your treatment will depend on which therapy you received initially.

If you do not have symptoms:
- Observation

If you have symptoms:
- Chemotherapy, consisting of a different combination of drugs • *or*
- High-dose hormonal therapy, frequently consisting of dexamethasone

Under Investigation

- New chemotherapy drugs, immunologic agents, and cancer vaccines
- ◆ Ask your doctor about any clinical trials that might benefit you.

SECONDARY REFRACTORY MULTIPLE MYELOMA (RELAPSING)

- Observation

Or:
- Chemotherapy, consisting of either the same drugs used successfully before or a new drug combination

Or:
- High-dose hormonal therapy, frequently consisting of dexamethasone

Or:
- High-dose chemotherapy • *with or without*
- Total-body irradiation • *followed by*

- Autologous peripheral-blood stem-cell transplantation • *followed by*
- Immunotherapy, consisting of alpha-interferon

Or:
- **High-dose chemotherapy** · *followed by*
- **Growth factors such as erythropoietin and filgrastim, to stimulate the production of blood cells**

Or:
- **External-beam radiation therapy, to relieve symptoms**

Under Investigation
- **New chemotherapy drugs, immunologic agents, and cancer vaccines**
- ◆ **Ask your doctor about any clinical trials that might benefit you.**

See treatment options for bone metastases.

I disease: Their bone marrow contains an excess of myeloma cells, and blood or urine specimens reveal elevated levels of M proteins, the antibodies produced by the abnormal plasma cells. Yet they may go for years without any symptoms. Because starting chemotherapy early has not been found to bring about longer remissions or survival, treatment is delayed until signs of progression emerge, such as low blood counts, impaired kidney function, or bone destruction. Your medical oncologist will probably want to see you for quarterly checkups.

Chemotherapy

Multiple myeloma is incurable, but patients can live with the disease for many years. Since around 1970, the standard induction chemotherapy regimen has consisted of melphalan (brand name: Alkeran), an *alkylating agent,* and the *steroid* prednisone (Deltasone), given for a minimum of one year.

Several equally effective drug combinations have come along since. Oncologists generally start patients on melphalan-prednisone, then switch them to another protocol should the cancer fail to respond.

One drawback to melphalan is that it can permanently injure the normal stem cells found in the bone marrow. These are the precursor cells that mature into red blood cells, white blood cells, and blood platelets. Why is this important? The most significant advance in the treatment of multiple myeloma has been high-dose chemotherapy with autologous stem-cell "rescue." Patients receive megadoses powerful enough to wipe out more cancer cells than conventional drug treatment. In the process, though, the alkylating agents also destroy the marrow, the production site for all blood cells. To replenish the marrow, stem cells can be harvested from the patient's marrow and/or skimmed from the bloodstream prior to the high-dose chemotherapy (and possibly total-body irradiation), then reinfused afterward.

Having too few stem cells due to the toxic effects of melphalan puts autologous transplantation out of reach. Dr. Jill Lacy, a medical oncologist at the Yale Cancer Center, has witnessed this dilemma many times. "We get patients referred to us for high-dose chemotherapy and stem-cell support when they are fairly far along in their disease," she says. "But they've been so heavily treated with drugs that deplete their stem-cell population, it's no longer an option for them."

High-dose chemotherapy isn't appropriate for all patients with multiple myeloma. The disease mainly afflicts men and women between the ages of fifty and seventy. Although the cutoff age for autoBMT varies from one institution to the next, most doctors would draw the line at around age seventy. But a person at the younger end of the age spectrum who is in reasonably good overall health might be a candidate for the rigorous procedure.

What can you do to ensure that doors to future treatment aren't closed inadvertently? The first step, says Dr. Lacy, is to find an expert in multiple myeloma, "someone who is up-to-date on recent developments and aware of potential therapies that could perhaps be pursued down the road." This needs to be mapped out at the time of diagnosis,

---

MULTIPLE MYELOMA/ Drug Therapy

First-line therapy frequently consists of one of the following regimens:
- **MP: melphalan + prednisone (H)**
- **VAD: vincristine + doxorubicin + dexamethasone (H)**
- **CP: cyclophosphamide + prednisone (H)**

Other drugs that may be used include:
- **VBMCP: vincristine + carmustine + melphalan + cyclophosphamide + prednisone (H)**
- **VMCP/VBAP: vincristine + melphalan + cyclophosphamide + prednisone (H)** *alternating with* **vincristine + carmustine + doxorubicin + prednisone (H)**
- **dexamethasone (H)**
- **busulfan**
- **alpha-interferon (I)**
- **pamidronate (B)**

(B) = bone-resorption inhibitor
(H) = hormonal agent
(I) = immunologic agent

---

she stresses, "because you don't want a doctor embarking on an induction therapy that could possibly compromise the marrow.

"Newer regimens have been developed that aren't as toxic." One alternative is to substitute cyclophosphamide (Cytoxan) for melphalan. While also an alkylating agent with antimyeloma activity, it inflicts less damage on stem cells. (The drug may also be the better choice for patients with moderate kidney failure or a low blood-platelet count.) Another is the widely used protocol VAD, comprised of three non-alkylating agents: vincristine (Oncovin), doxorubicin (Adriamycin), and dexamethasone (Decadron).

Bone-Marrow Transplantation

Administering heavy doses of chemotherapy, then infusing patients with identically matching marrow stem cells from a sibling may offer the hope of a cure. In one British study of 162 allogeneic BMT recipients, nearly one in three were alive seven years later. The procedure is seldom performed, though, on account of its high risk; patients face up to a 30 percent chance of dying from complications. BMT using an identical twin's stem cells, while far safer, is rarer still, as are syngeneic transplants in general.

The incidence of mortality from high-dose chemotherapy followed by autologous marrow or peripheral-blood stem-cell rescue is less than 5 percent. It is not a cure, emphasizes Dr. Lacy. "The treatment 'resets the clock,' returning the disease to an earlier stage and, hopefully, extending people's lives." Half of all patients to receive high-dose chemo go into complete remission and see their symptoms vanish.

A French clinical trial of two hundred patients compared conventional chemotherapy to high-dose chemotherapy and autoBMT. The estimated five-year survival rate for the more intensive protocol was over four times higher (52 percent versus 12 percent), yet with a similarly low number of treatment-related deaths. "The sense is that the outcome is probably better for patients with early-stage disease," says Dr. Lacy, "although we have yet to answer that definitively. But certainly patients with stage II and stage III disease can be eligible for this therapy."

Immunotherapy

It is now common practice to follow high-dose chemotherapy and stem-cell rescue with alpha-interferon (Intron-A and Roferon-A). Patients self-inject the drug three times a week. Another British study tracked two groups of people with multiple myeloma for nearly four and a half years. Those patients put on maintenance immunotherapy experienced far longer remissions than the participants who received no posttransplant therapy.

Interferon's effect after standard induction chemotherapy isn't nearly as dramatic. According to the National Cancer Institute, it has not been shown to prolong patients' lives. "Because alpha-interferon has side effects and is very expensive," says Dr. Lacy, "there is a great deal of variability in how frequently it's used." Other substances that stimulate the immune system are being evaluated.

Radiation Therapy and Drug Therapy (Palliative Treatments)

Controlling Bone Pain—"Far and away, the complication of multiple myeloma that has the most impact on the quality of life is bone pain," says Dr. Lacy. The myeloma cells cause bone to resorb itself faster than it can grow new bone, until holes form. "The bones become so fragile that fractures develop. It can become a major problem: Their weakened bones are breaking, and they're in constant pain.

"Bone pain can occur in any bone that has a hole in it," she continues, "but back pain is extremely common." The bones that make up the spine are especially susceptible to fracture, as is the femur bone in the upper leg. Surgery to stabilize the bone with a pin may be necessary.

Chemotherapy goes after myeloma cells throughout the body. One to two weeks of external-beam radiation may be given to problem spots that are causing pain. Radiotherapy impairs bone-marrow stem cells in the treatment field, however, and therefore should be limited to small areas.

Many patients now receive monthly intravenous infusions of the *bone-resorption inhibitor* pamidronate (Aredia). Not an anticancer agent, pamidronate belongs to the class of agents known as *bisphosphonates.* It binds to the surface of damaged bones and slows excessive resorption, thus giving the bones a chance to heal and regain their density and strength. In a large national study published shortly before pamidronate won FDA approval in 1996, the drug was found to reduce bone fractures, spinal-cord compression, or the need for surgery or radiation by nearly half.

See "Pain Management" in Chapter Eight, "Take Control: Managing Symptoms, Side Effects, and Complications."

Controlling Hypercalcemia—Pamidronate is also effective for preventing and treating hypercalcemia, a frequent complication of this and other cancers. The destruction of bone seen in myeloma releases calcium into the circulation. Too much of this mineral can cause a range of problems, beginning with listlessness and muscle weakness. The calcium may also collect in the kidneys, possibly leading to impaired renal function. Drinking plenty of water is one way to help the organs clear out the excess calcium in the blood. Should hypercalcemia develop, your physician will almost certainly order IV fluids.

See "Hypercalcemia" in Chapter Eight, "Take Control: Managing Symptoms, Side Effects, and Complications."

TREATMENTS FOR REFRACTORY MULTIPLE MYELOMA

Thirty to 50 percent of people with multiple myeloma will not respond to first-line chemotherapy. Even when a patient appears to be in complete remission—no evidence of myeloma cells or M proteins—minute levels of malignant cells are still present. For this reason, all patients are said to have refractory disease. *Primary refractory* means the myeloma resisted treatment and continued to progress. The terms *secondary refractory* and *relapsing refractory* refer to plasma-cell cancers that regress but eventually relapse.

Primary Refractory Multiple Myeloma

Observation

One in ten myeloma patients will have what is referred to as *stable disease.* Although largely immune to chemotherapy, the cancer cells are so inactive that no treatment is necessary until the disease advances. And that can be a long time, says Dr. Lacy. "We have patients who have been followed for years without any substantial progression of their myeloma."

Hormonal Therapy

High doses of dexamethasone can induce partial remissions in patients who did not respond to their initial round of chemotherapy. (In multiple myeloma, partial remission is defined as a reduction of 50 percent or more in the level of M proteins.) The drug is a steroid, like prednisone, only more potent. High-dose chemotherapy with anticancer agents, however, is not recommended.

Secondary Refractory Multiple Myeloma (Relapsed)

Chemotherapy

Patients whose cancer stayed in remission at least six months before relapsing are re-treated with the same regimen of chemotherapy. More than half will go into remission a second time, although the symptom-free intervals become progressively shorter. The myeloma cells may still be chemosensitive, but upon relapse they proliferate too rapidly for the drugs to destroy them all. High-dose dexamethasone or prednisone may be prescribed at this point.

The VAD combination (vincristine, doxorubicin, dexamethasone) has been highly effective when relapse occurs within six months of the initial chemotherapy. The three drugs will induce a partial remission in about three in four patients. What's more, VAD can be administered again at the time of a second relapse.

High-dose chemotherapy with stem-cell support or growth-factor support *may* be an option, even if you've undergone the procedure previously. *Growth factors* are substances that stimulate the production of blood cells. You may also want to consider investigating clinical trials.

OTHER THERAPIES THAT MAY BE USED IN THE TREATMENT OF MULTIPLE MYELOMA

Kidney Dialysis—"Multiple myeloma can affect the kidneys in many different ways," says Dr. Lacy. Renal function rarely dwindles to the point where the organs can no longer skim waste and excess fluid from the blood adequately, but if it should, a patient must go on artificial dialysis throughout treatment. Kidney function usually rebounds once the myeloma is brought under control.

There are two types of dialysis. In *hemodialysis,* administered three times a week in a hospital or dialysis clinic, the blood is run through a machine that purifies it like a healthy kidney. This takes about three to five hours. Another method, *peritoneal dialysis,* performs the same task, but inside the person's body. Instead of traveling to a dialysis facility, patients *dialyze* themselves at home, at work—anywhere there's a clean rest room—by infusing a cleansing solution into their abdomen through a surgically implanted catheter tube. While they go about their daily activities, the impurities and fluid pass through the *peritoneal membrane* lining the abdomen and into the solution, which is then drained back into its plastic bag. Patients repeat the process several times a day.

Plasmapheresis—If the kidneys aren't working properly, too many M proteins may build up in the blood. To quickly reverse this potentially dangerous condition, patients are connected to a machine that is not unlike a hemodialyzer. By filtering out the excess myeloma antibodies, plasmapheresis thins the blood and eases the workload on the kidneys and heart.

◆ *Ask your doctor about any investigational therapies that might benefit you.*

Cancer of the Cervix

Overview

TREATMENTS FOR CERVICAL CANCER THAT
HAS NOT METASTASIZED

Cervical Carcinoma in Situ (High-Grade SIL/Moderate or Severe Dysplasia)

Surgery

Physicians vary in their approaches to mild dysplasia, the precancerous condition also known as low-grade squamous intraepithelial lesion (SIL). "Many doctors will treat it," says Dr. Mitchell Morris of M. D. Anderson Cancer Center. "But some of us will simply keep a watchful eye on the patient, because frequently the dysplasia disappears on its own." High-grade SIL, or cervical carcinoma in situ (CIS), is one step closer to invasive disease and "should certainly be treated."

The most widely practiced methods for removing a precursor lesion are loop electrosurgical excision procedure (LEEP), cryosurgery, and surgical conization. Laser surgery is fading from use.

LEEP and cryosurgery, both office procedures, require no general anesthesia. "LEEP is increasingly becoming the procedure of choice," says Dr. Morris, "though cryosurgery is a reasonable alternative." Patients must be put to sleep for "cold knife" (scalpel) conization, which takes place in an operating room but is almost always an outpatient procedure. The cone biopsy often doubles as a diagnostic and therapeutic measure. If the margins of the cone-shaped specimen of cervical tissue are negative, no further treatment should be necessary.

Most women diagnosed with CIS of the cervix are between the ages of thirty and forty. One point of contention in gynecologic oncol-

---

CERVICAL CANCER/ Surgical Procedures

Loop electrosurgical excision procedure (LEEP): an office procedure that uses an electrically charged wire loop to slice off the outermost layer of the cervix. Average hospital stay: outpatient procedure

Cryosurgery: applies extreme cold to cancer cells, destroying them. Average hospital stay: outpatient procedure

Surgical conization: surgery to remove a cone-shaped section of tissue from the cervix and cervical canal, with either a scalpel ("cold knife" conization) or a laser. Average hospital stay: outpatient procedure; in the rare event of complications, 1–2 days

Total hysterectomy: surgery to remove the cervix and uterus; also referred to as a *simple* hysterectomy.

continued on page 528

CERVICAL CANCER/Treatment Options

CERVICAL CARCINOMA IN SITU

The cancer is found only in the cervical lining's first layer of cells.

- Loop electrosurgical excision procedure (LEEP), to remove the lesion using an electrified wire loop • *or*
- Laser therapy, to destroy the cancer cells using a narrow beam of light • *or*
- Conization, to surgically remove a cone-shaped piece of tissue where the lesion was found • *or*
- Cryosurgery, to destroy the cancer cells by freezing them • *or*
- Total hysterectomy, to surgically remove the cervix and the uterus

If the cancer is inoperable:
- Internal radiation therapy

STAGE IA CERVICAL CANCER

The cancer involves the deeper tissues of the cervix but is visible only under a microscope.

- Conization • *or*
- Total hysterectomy, *with or without* bilateral salpingo-oophorectomy, to surgically remove the ovaries and fallopian tubes • *or*
- Radical hysterectomy, to surgically remove the cervix, uterus, and part of the vagina, *with* pelvic lymph-node dissection

If the cancer is inoperable:
- Internal radiation therapy

STAGE IB CERVICAL CANCER

A larger amount of cancer is found in the cervical tissue.

- External-beam radiation therapy • *and*
- Internal radiation

Or:
- Radical hysterectomy, *with* bilateral pelvic lymph-node dissection • *with or without*
- External-beam radiation therapy

STAGE IIA CERVICAL CANCER

The cancer has spread to the upper two-thirds of the vagina.

- External-beam radiation therapy • *and*
- Internal radiation

Or:
- Radical hysterectomy, *with* bilateral pelvic lymph-node dissection • *with or without*
- External-beam radiation therapy

STAGE IIB CERVICAL CANCER

The cancer has spread to the tissue around the cervix.

- **Chemotherapy, frequently consisting of cisplatin and fluorouracil · *given concurrently with***
- **External-beam radiation therapy · *with or without***
- **Internal radiation**

Under Investigation
- **New methods of delivering radiation therapy**
- ◆ **Ask your doctor about any clinical trials that might benefit you.**

STAGE III CERVICAL CANCER

The cancer has spread to the lower third of the vagina.

The cancer has spread to the pelvic wall or has caused kidney distension or kidney failure.

- **Chemotherapy, frequently consisting of cisplatin and fluorouracil · *given concurrently with***
- **External-beam radiation therapy · *with or without***
- **Internal radiation**

Under Investigation
- **New methods of delivering radiation therapy**
- ◆ **Ask your doctor about any clinical trials that might benefit you.**

STAGE IVA CERVICAL CANCER

The cancer has invaded the bladder or rectum.

- **Chemotherapy, frequently consisting of cisplatin and fluorouracil · *given concurrently with***
- **External-beam radiation therapy · *with or without***
- **Internal radiation**

Under Investigation
- **New methods of delivering radiation therapy**
- ◆ **Ask your doctor about any clinical trials that might benefit you.**

STAGE IVB CERVICAL CANCER

The cancer has spread to distant organs.

- **External-beam radiation therapy, to relieve symptoms · *or***
- **Chemotherapy, frequently consisting of cisplatin, ifosfamide, or other agents**

See treatment options for metastases of the bone, liver, and lung.

RECURRENT CERVICAL CANCER

Your therapy will depend on how you were treated initially.

If the cancer recurs in the pelvis:
- **Chemoradiation**

Or:
- **Chemotherapy, frequently consisting of cisplatin, ifosfamide, or other agents, to relieve symptoms**

If the cancer recurs in the central pelvis:
- **Pelvic exenteration surgery, to surgically remove the cervix, uterus, ovaries, fallopian tubes, vagina, bladder, lower ureter tubes, rectum, anus, pelvic floor, and usually the pelvic lymph nodes. Occasionally, a less radical procedure may be performed.**

---

ogy is whether or not a patient beyond child-bearing age should undergo one of the minimally invasive procedures described above or have her cervix and uterus removed in a total hysterectomy. Through the late 1980s and early 1990s, hysterectomy was the most common treatment for women who fit that profile.

But a cone biopsy for cervical CIS has a 97 percent cure rate. "If you're a compliant patient who's going to come in every few months for a Pap smear," says Dr. Morris, "it's far less risky to do a conization. Even though hysterectomy is a very common and safe operation, complications such as bleeding and infection can occur."

Some women who are told they have a precancerous condition choose hysterectomy for the psychological relief of not having to worry about a recurrence in the cervix. Another advantage is that they return to the doctor's office only for an annual gynecologic exam.

In a total hysterectomy for cancer of the uterus, the surgeon also removes both ovaries and fallopian tubes. *Bilateral salpingo-oophorectomy,* as this is called, is considered optional for cervical cancer. "Nowadays," says Dr. Morris, "hysterectomy is also being done laparoscopically. Much of the surgery is performed through a laparoscope, then the uterus

---

The operation can be performed one of three ways: (1) through an incision in the abdomen, (2) laparoscopically, also through the abdomen, or (3) vaginally, for which no incision is required.
Average hospital stay:

- **Abdominal hysterectomy: 3–7 days**

- **Vaginal hysterectomy: 1–2 days**

- **Laparoscopic hysterectomy: 1–2 days**

Radical hysterectomy: surgery to remove the cervix, uterus, and part of the vagina, along with the pelvic lymph nodes.
Average hospital stay: 4–5 days

Pelvic exenteration: surgery to remove the cervix, uterus, ovaries, fallopian tubes, vagina, bladder, lower ureter tubes, rectum, anus, pelvic floor, and usually the pelvic lymph nodes. Occasionally a less radical procedure may be performed. Because the bladder and rectum are taken out, artificial openings are made to relieve urine and to permit stool to pass. A new vagina can be fashioned by plastic surgery.
Average hospital stay: 14–21 days

is removed through the vagina." Instead of one long incision in the abdomen, the physician makes three or four quarter-inch slits. The hospitalization from laparoscopic hysterectomy is significantly shorter than from traditional surgery. So is the recovery time: one to two days versus six to eight weeks.

Invasive Cervical Cancer

In cervical cancer, only stages IA, IB, and IIA are operable. Stage IA is referred to as *microinvasive* disease; that is, the tumor has burrowed into healthy tissue, but so minimally that it can be seen only under a microscope. If a cone biopsy reveals that the depth of the lesion is less than 3 millimeters, no further treatment is necessary. As with cervical carcinoma in situ, women for whom preserving fertility is not an issue may opt for a total hysterectomy. In either case, says Dr. Morris, "the cure rate is 99 percent plus."

Deeper stage IA tumors (3 to 5 millimeters) call for a radical hysterectomy, which removes part of the vagina in addition to the cervix and uterus. The operation, also performed for stages IB and IIA, includes a *pelvic lymphadenectomy,* because the risk of spread to the pelvic lymph nodes is roughly one in five.

Why See a Gynecologic Oncologist?

A gynecologic oncologist is an obstetrician-gynecologist who has studied an additional three years in cancer care. These doctors are unique among cancer specialists in that they are trained in the three major treatments for gynecologic tumors: surgery, radiotherapy, and chemotherapy.

The obvious benefit of seeing a gynecologic oncologist is continuity of care. "When a woman comes to us," says Dr. Morris, "we take care of her for the entire disease. It's not like being treated by a general surgeon, who then hands you off to a radiation oncologist, who then hands you off to a medical oncologist."

Call the Gynecologic Cancer Foundation Information Hotline at 800-444-4441 for a free list of gynecologic oncologists who practice in your area, or conduct your own search on the GCF's Women's Cancer Network Web site: *http:www.wcn.org/ referral.*

"Radical hysterectomy can be carried out only by a gynecologic oncologist," notes Dr. Morris. "Most of us perform the surgery through an abdominal incision. It can be done vaginally, although not enough women have undergone the procedure that way for us to say what the cure rate is or if it truly benefits patients in terms of shorter hospitalizations and lower cost." Other gynecologic oncologists are incorporating the laparoscopic technique into radical hysterectomy.

Radiation Therapy for Operable Cervical Cancer—Patients with stage IB or stage IIA cervical cancer have two options: radiotherapy or a radical hysterectomy. Both boast high cure rates: for stage IB disease, 85 to 90 percent; for stage IIA, 75 to 80 percent. Since that's the case, why would any woman choose major surgery over radiation?

"One of the benefits of radical hysterectomy," explains Dr. Morris, "is that the ovaries are left intact. That is very important to a woman who might be twenty-five, thirty, thirty-five years old, because, on average, menopause doesn't begin until around fifty-one." *Menopause* is the phase of life when the ovaries gradually secrete less and less of the female sex hormone estrogen and menstruation ceases. A woman in the age range cited by Dr. Morris might have another fifteen to twenty-five years of normal ovarian function.

Radiation therapy will destroy the ovaries, inducing immediate menopause. Natural menopause typically unfolds over the course of several years. When estrogen production is halted abruptly, common menopausal symptoms (hot flashes, night sweats, vaginal dryness, irritability) tend to be more severe.

Yet another consideration when deciding between radical hysterectomy and radiation: If you are relatively young and receive radiotherapy, you will have to take *hormone replacement therapy* (HRT) indefinitely. The purpose of restoring your estrogen is not only to reverse the unwelcome effects of menopause but to provide protection against the crippling bone disease *osteoporosis*, which escalates in the absence of estrogen. HRT is not without side effects, including breast tenderness, bloating, headaches, mood swings, and depression.

According to Dr. Morris, radiation is often the preferable course for "elderly patients, or women who are extremely obese or have other medical problems that would make surgery more risky, or women who have large tumors." Although tumor size isn't included in the staging for cervical cancer, it is a major factor in influencing the choice of surgery versus radiotherapy. Large malignancies or those that do not respond completely to radiotherapy may be treated with external/intracavitary radiation *and* radical hysterectomy, in either order. Some studies have found that the combined-modality treatment reduces the chance of a relapse. Nevertheless, this more aggressive approach remains controversial.

Extended-Field Radiation—When an invasive cervical tumor measures 4 centimeters (1½ inches) or more, the radiation field may be extended to encompass the *para-aortic lymph nodes* in the upper abdomen, even if there is no evidence of nodal involvement. One large study showed a significantly higher ten-year survival rate for women with stage IB, IIA, or IIB cervical carcinoma who received *prophylactic* (preventive) para-aortic irradiation and pelvic irradiation as compared to pelvic irradiation alone.

Inoperable Cervical Cancer

Chemoradiation

Once cervical cancer has spread to the surrounding tissues (stages IIB to IVA), simultaneous chemotherapy and radiation therapy replace surgery as the principal form of treatment. For nearly fifty years, going back to the 1950s, external-beam radiation had been the sole treatment for "locally advanced" tumors. Later, *intracavity radiation therapy* was added. The five-year survival rate hovered around 50 percent.

In 1999, the National Cancer Institute took the unusual step of mailing letters to thousands of oncologists, urging them to administer chemotherapy at the same time as radiotherapy. The basis for this rare "clinical alert" was the results of five patient trials that had pitted external and internal pelvic radiation and chemotherapy against radiation alone. In all five studies, made public the same day, the dual-therapy approach outperformed the single-therapy method. When the drug cisplatin (brand name: Platinol) was used, deaths from cervical cancer were reduced by a remarkable 30 to 50 percent.

It's not fully understood why combined chemoradiation should be so much more effective than radiotherapy, although researchers theorize that the anticancer agents somehow sensitize the tumor to the high-energy rays and impede the damaged malignant cells from repairing themselves. What is clear, says Dr. Morris, one of the principal investigators, is that "this is the way to go."

The chemotherapy is given during the four to five weeks of external-beam radiation. About a week after the last treatment, patients check into the hospital for the first of two intracavitary implants. A capsule containing a radioactive substance is inserted directly into the cervix and left in place for one to three days. The treatment is typically repeated the following week.

At M. D. Anderson and other major cancer centers, doctors are experimenting with *high-dose-rate brachytherapy,* which is an outpatient procedure. Over a two-week period, expect to receive from two to five treatments, each lasting no more than a few minutes. Internal radiation alone would be offered to a woman with microinvasive disease (stage IA) who is ineligible for surgery.

TREATMENTS FOR ADVANCED CERVICAL CANCER

Radiation Therapy and Chemotherapy (Palliative Treatments)

At stage IVA, the cancer has extended to either the bladder or the rectum. Treatment consists of some form of radiation; most frequently a combination of internal and external-beam radiotherapy.

**CERVICAL CANCER/
Drug Therapy**

Drugs that may be used include:

- cisplatin
- fluorouracil
- carboplatin
- paclitaxel
- vinorelbine
- ifosfamide
- irinotecan

Stage IVB cervical cancer has metastasized, usually to the bone, lung, or liver. "The main thrust of treatment is to relieve symptoms," explains Dr. Morris, using either radiation or chemotherapy to shrink the primary tumor. Drug therapy, he says, hasn't been very effective at controlling metastatic lesions in other organs. Of the agents tried, cisplatin has evoked the best response. Sometimes it is used in conjunction with fluorouracil (5-FU). But few patients achieve a complete remission, much less a sustained one. Dr. Morris uses cisplatin's chemical cousin carboplatin (Paraplatin), "because there are fewer side effects with it."

TREATMENTS FOR RECURRENT CERVICAL CANCER

Surgery

Cervical cancer recurs most often in the cervix, if it hasn't been resected previously, or in the upper vagina, bladder, rectum, or the pelvic wall. Up to 50 percent of patients whose tumor comes back in the center of the pelvis can be *cured* with a radical surgery called pelvic exenteration. The surgeon takes out all of the pelvic reproductive organs, along with parts of the urinary and intestinal tracts. Extensive reconstructive surgery becomes necessary, in order to fashion a new vagina and create openings for both a *urostomy* and a *colostomy.*

"We've also managed to cure people through early detection of a recurrence in the lung," says Dr. Morris. Most of the time, secondary pulmonary cancer is terminal. "But there is a group of patients where you find just a single lesion in the lung, and removing it surgically can cure it."

Chemotherapy/Chemoradiation

In women who were treated initially with hysterectomy, other cures may be possible through combining chemotherapy and radiotherapy. Again, the recurrence must be confined to the central pelvis. More commonly, chemotherapy is administered palliatively. "I tell patients, 'This is not going to cure you,' " says Dr. Morris, " 'but it can slow down the cancer, shrink it, and perhaps prolong your life.' "

♦ *Ask your doctor about any investigational therapies that might benefit you.*

Cancer of the Esophagus

Overview

TREATMENTS FOR ESOPHAGEAL CANCER
THAT HAS NOT METASTASIZED

Surgery

The mainstay of treatment for invasive esophageal cancer, carcinoma in situ, and precancerous dysplasia is surgery to excise the lesion along with part of the gullet. The surgeon then pulls up the stomach into the chest cavity and joins it to what remains of the esophagus.

At first you'll want to eat smaller meals several times a day. Most patients are already familiar with this way of eating, having lived with an obstruction of the esophagus for months prior to being diagnosed. After the esophagectomy, "the movement of food through the esophagus improves," says Dr. Charles Fuchs of the Dana-Farber Cancer Institute in Boston, and patients usually return to a relatively normal meal schedule.

Sometimes, he notes, more extensive surgery is necessary. When much of the esophagus and part of the stomach must come out, the surgeon fashions a new passageway from the throat to the stomach using a segment of colon or small bowel. "It's a difficult operation, with a greater chance of complications. You want to go to a surgeon who performs this surgery regularly," Dr. Fuchs emphasizes, "because in experienced hands, the rates of complications and mortality are reasonably low." But when performed by surgeons who treat esophageal cancer only

---

**ESOPHAGEAL CANCER/
Surgical Procedures**

Esophagectomy: surgery to remove the cancerous portion of the esophagus. Depending on how much of the gullet must come out, the surgeon either pulls up the stomach and reconnects it to the remnant of the esophagus *(gastric pull-up)* or uses a segment of intestine to create a new gullet *(colon/bowel interposition)*.

Average hospital stay: 7–10 days

ESOPHAGEAL CANCER/Treatment Options

ESOPHAGEAL CARCINOMA IN SITU

Cancer cells are found solely in the first layer of cells that make up the lining of the esophagus.

- Esophagectomy, to surgically remove the cancerous portion of the esophagus

STAGE I ESOPHAGEAL CANCER

The cancer is confined to a small portion of the esophagus.

- Esophagectomy

Or:
- Chemoradiation, frequently consisting of fluorouracil and cisplatin • *with or without*
- Esophagectomy

STAGE II ESOPHAGEAL CANCER

The cancer covers much of the esophagus and may have spread to nearby lymph nodes, but it has not infiltrated other tissues.

- Esophagectomy

Or:
- Chemoradiation, frequently consisting of fluorouracil and cisplatin • *with or without*
- Esophagectomy

STAGE III ESOPHAGEAL CANCER

The cancer has spread to neighboring tissues or lymph nodes.

- Esophagectomy, to relieve symptoms

Or:
- Chemoradiation, frequently consisting of fluorouracil and cisplatin • *with or without*
- Esophagectomy

STAGE IV ESOPHAGEAL CANCER

The cancer has metastasized to other parts of the body.

- Esophagectomy *or* laser surgery *or* electrosurgery, to relieve symptoms • *or*
- External-beam or internal radiation therapy, to relieve symptoms • *or*
- Photodynamic therapy, to relieve symptoms

Or:

Under Investigation

- **Chemotherapy, frequently consisting of fluorouracil and cisplatin**

◆ **Ask your doctor about any clinical trials that might benefit you.**

See treatment options for metastases of the bone, liver, and lung.

RECURRENT ESOPHAGEAL CANCER

Your therapy will depend on how you were treated initially.

- **Esophagectomy, to relieve symptoms**

If the cancer comes back locally and you were previously treated surgically:

- **External-beam radiation therapy, to relieve symptoms**

If the cancer has spread to a distant site:

- **Chemotherapy, frequently consisting of fluorouracil and cisplatin, or other agents, to relieve symptoms**

---

on occasion, esophagectomy has the highest operative mortality rate of any elective surgery.

As with a gastric pull-up, anticipate eating smaller meals for a while. Before long, says Dr. Fuchs, the transplanted intestinal tissue "develops the type of inner lining necessary to function like an esophagus in terms of peristalsis," the wavelike motion that propels food down to the stomach. Still, "most patients find that eating is never altogether the same as before. If they eat too much at one sitting, they may experience indigestion." Other occasional problems are heartburn and regurgitation from stomach acid that backs up into the esophagus.

Radiation Therapy and Chemoradiation

Two nonsurgical treatments are radiation and chemoradiation. An oncologist might recommend either approach to a patient who is ineligible for surgery, perhaps due to a coexisting disease or because the cancer is inoperable.

Giving chemotherapy and radiation together is superior to radiation alone. In a federally funded clinical trial, 123 men and women with esophageal cancer received external-beam radiation. Sixty-one were additionally administered cisplatin (brand name: Platinol) and fluorouracil (5-FU). Those in the chemoradiation group lived for fourteen months on average, compared to nine months for the radiation-only group.

Esophagectomy has traditionally been preferred over radiotherapy. "That may be because surgery is better, but it also probably reflects the fact that we tend to send the sickest patients to the radiation oncolo-

---

**ESOPHAGEAL CANCER/
Drug Therapy**

*First-line therapy frequently
consists of:*
- fluorouracil
- cisplatin

*Other drugs that may be used
include:*
- mitomycin
- paclitaxel
- docetaxel
- irinotecan
- porfimer (PS)

(PS) = photosensitizer

---

gist," says Dr. Fuchs. He notes the intriguing results of a European study that compared surgery to radiotherapy. All of the participants, including those slated for radiation, had resectable tumors and were deemed healthy enough to withstand the operation. In contrast to earlier research, radiotherapy was found to be as effective.

"Increasingly," says Dr. Fuchs, "we're looking at administering patients radiation and chemotherapy before definitive surgery." The neoadjuvant strategy is investigational, he stresses, "because only one study has shown a benefit." There is no evidence that *post*operative chemotherapy and/or radiation confers any advantage.

Most clinical studies testing chemotherapy and/or radiation have focused on squamous-cell esophageal carcinoma. Adenocarcinoma, which makes up half of all cases, may not be as sensitive to cisplatin and 5-FU or to radiotherapy. Surgery is the standard treatment for these malignancies, which develop in the lower third of the gullet.

TREATMENTS FOR ADVANCED ESOPHAGEAL CANCER

By the time of diagnosis, one in four esophageal cancers have spread to distant organs. Therapy, which is no longer curative, centers on preserving quality of life. The main concern is to keep the primary tumor from obstructing the esophagus and interfering with swallowing *(dysphagia)*. Esophagectomy may be an option, though most physicians would probably lean away from major surgery for someone with stage IV disease. "The two most common approaches," says Dr. Fuchs, "are to give chemotherapy—in the hopes of treating both the distant metastasis and the local cancer—or to add radiation in order to open up that part of the esophagus."

See "Esophageal Dilation/Stent Placement," page 537.

TREATMENTS FOR RECURRENT ESOPHAGEAL CANCER

Recurrences in the same area typically call for radiotherapy or esophagectomy, depending on how you were treated initially. Radiation is the more frequent method, says Dr. Fuchs, "because locally recurrent esophageal cancer often cannot be removed successfully by surgery."

For disease that comes back elsewhere in the body, chemotherapy is usually prescribed. If the cisplatin-fluorouracil regimen was used previously, your oncologist will probably choose any of several newcomers that have demonstrated activity against esophageal cancer, including paclitaxel (Taxol), docetaxel (Taxotere), and irinotecan (Camptosar).

OTHER THERAPIES THAT MAY BE USED IN THE TREATMENT OF ESOPHAGEAL CANCER

Photodynamic Therapy/Laser Therapy (palliative treatment)— Porfimer (Photofrin), the first photosensitizing drug to win commercial approval for treating cancer, is used in combination with laser light to shrink cancers that are blocking the esophagus. PDT is also an experimental treatment for eradicating carcinoma in situ from the inner lining. The laser may be employed without the light-activated agent.

See "Photodynamic Therapy" in Chapter Four, "How Cancer Is Treated."

Esophageal Dilation/Stent Placement (palliative treatment)—Each of these endoscopic outpatient procedures enables patients to eat normally. In dilation the doctor attempts to widen the esophagus by passing a series of progressively larger rubber tubes down the throat and past the narrowed part of the gullet one at a time.

Should dilation cease to be effective, a cylindrical metallic prosthesis called a *stent* may be placed to open up the obstruction. "Stents are by no means a panacea," says Dr. Fuchs. The small tubes, he explains, cannot move food along like the esophagus can, and so solid food sometimes gets stuck. "Patients are often restricted to a soft or liquid diet." Stent placement, he adds, is typically reserved for those who have exhausted other means of relieving an obstruction.

Gastrostomy/Jejunostomy—Malnourishment is a frequent complication of esophageal cancer. If you're scheduled to receive six weeks of preoperative radiation, along with two courses of chemotherapy, it is essential that you maintain adequate nutrition. According to Dr. Fuchs, studies suggest that progressive weight loss in the weeks leading up to surgery increases the risk of not surviving the operation.

"We want patients to be in the best physical condition they can be," he says. "Often, in preparation for the chemoradiation, we'll put in a temporary feeding tube and instruct them on using liquid nutritional supplements." A catheter implanted in the stomach is called a gastrostomy, or *G tube*. A *J tube* (short for jejunostomy) goes in the jejunum, the middle part of the small intestine. Nowadays both procedures can usually be conducted through an endoscope. An intravenous catheter, for injecting or infusing the anticancer drug(s), may be inserted in a blood vessel at the same time.

> *See "Tube Feedings" under "Appetite Loss (Anorexia)" in Chapter Eight, "Take Control: Managing Symptoms, Side Effects, and Complications."*

◆ *Ask your doctor about any investigational therapies that might benefit you.*

Cancer of the Larynx

Overview

TREATMENTS FOR LARYNGEAL CANCER IN SITU

No additional treatment beyond the initial biopsy may be necessary for carcinoma in situ of the larynx. But if the superficial lesion is extensive, the physician might want to schedule a second procedure to cut out the affected area of the organ's lining or eradicate it using a laser. External-beam radiation therapy is an option for patients whose health dictates nonsurgical measures or who simply would prefer radiotherapy over an operation.

TREATMENTS FOR LARYNGEAL CANCER THAT HAS NOT METASTASIZED

A diagnosis of laryngeal cancer is no longer synonymous with total laryngectomy, the operation performed to remove the voice box. "There are many options available to patients today that didn't exist even just a few years ago," says Dr. William Richtsmeier of Duke Comprehensive Cancer Center. Early-stage tumors can often be treated with radiation alone or with surgical procedures that remove part of the larynx, preserving the voice. At Duke and other state-of-the-art cancer centers, an experimental organ-sparing approach combining hyperfractionated radiotherapy and chemotherapy is commonplace even for stage III and stage IV disease.

Radiation Therapy

External-beam radiotherapy is generally the preferred treatment for stage I and stage II laryngeal cancers. Later-stage tumors that require surgery may be irradiated postoperatively.

Chemoradiation

According to Dr. Richtsmeier, treating stage III or IV laryngeal cancer with chemotherapy and radiation is "at least as effective as laryngectomy and radiation. The key, though, is that they be given together."

You may have to search for a hospital that offers this alternative to surgery, because the investigational therapy is intensive and requires vigilant monitoring for side effects. In the event that the anticancer drugs do not reduce the tumor by at least half or the tumor persists following irradiation, laryngectomy can still be carried out with the intent of achieving a cure.

Certain situations may rule out chemoradiation, says Dr. Richtsmeier. "For instance, a person would not be a candidate if the tumor was so large that it had virtually destroyed the larynx. Or if a patient presented with a large lesion that was obstructing the airway, we would go right to surgery." The concern is that if the cancer did not respond to chemo and radiation, it could shut off the airway entirely, whereas surgery relieves that problem immediately.

LARYNGEAL CANCER/ Drug Therapy

First-line therapy frequently consists of:
- **cisplatin + fluorouracil**

Others drugs that may be used include:
- **hydroxyurea**
- **bleomycin**
- **carboplatin**
- **doxorubicin**
- **mitomycin**

Surgery

Total laryngectomy is rarely necessary when a laryngeal tumor remains limited to the region where it originated (stage I)—the supraglottis, glottis, or subglottis—or has progressed throughout the voice box (stage II). The other three operations for early-stage laryngeal carcinoma remove only part of the two-inch-long tube. Cordectomy, the least invasive, "leaves patients with a soft, hoarse quality of speech," says Dr. Richtsmeier. Partial laryngectomy and vertical hemilaryngectomy also preserve the voice, though it may sound slightly different than before.

LARYNGEAL CANCER/Treatment Options

LARYNGEAL CARCINOMA IN SITU

The cancer is present but has not invaded laryngeal tissue.

- **Endoscopic excisional biopsy, to surgically remove the cancerous area** · *followed by*
- **Observation** · *or*
- **Endoscopic reexcision, if necessary**

Or:
- **External-beam radiation therapy**

If the cancer in situ is extensive:
- **Laser surgery**

STAGE I LARYNGEAL CANCER

Supraglottic cancer: **The cancer is confined to one area of the supraglottis, and the vocal cords can move normally.**
Glottic cancer: **The cancer is confined to the vocal cords, which can move normally.**
Subglottic cancer: **The cancer is confined to the subglottis.**

Supraglottic Cancer

- **External-beam radiation therapy** · *or*
- **Supraglottic laryngectomy, to surgically remove the upper portion of the larynx**

Glottic Cancer

- **External-beam radiation therapy** · *or*
- **Cordectomy, to surgically remove one vocal cord** · *or*
- **Partial laryngectomy or hemilaryngectomy, to surgically remove part of the larynx** · *or*
- **Total laryngectomy, to surgically remove the entire larynx** · *or*
- **Laser surgery**

Subglottic Cancer

- **External-beam radiation therapy** · *or*
- **Hemilaryngectomy**

STAGE II LARYNGEAL CANCER

Supraglottic cancer: **The cancer is in more than one area of the supraglottis, but the vocal cords can move normally.**
Glottic cancer: **The cancer has spread to the supraglottis, the subglottis, or both. The vocal cords may or may not be able to move normally.**
Subglottic cancer: **The cancer has infiltrated the vocal cords, which may or may not be able to move normally.**

Supraglottic Cancer

- **External-beam radiation therapy**

Or:
- **Supraglottic laryngectomy** · *or*
- **Total laryngectomy**

If the surgical margins are too narrow or are found to contain cancer:
- **Postoperative external-beam radiation therapy**

Glottic Cancer

- **External-beam radiation therapy** · *or*
- **Partial laryngectomy** · *or*
- **Hemilaryngectomy** · *or*
- **Total laryngectomy**

Subglottic Cancer

- **External-beam radiation therapy** · *or*
- **Hemilaryngectomy** · *or*
- **Total laryngectomy**

Under Investigation (for all stage II laryngeal cancers)
- **Hyperfractionated external-beam radiation therapy**
- ◆ **Ask your doctor about any clinical trials that might benefit you.**

STAGE III LARYNGEAL CANCER

(1) The cancer has not spread outside the larynx but impairs movement of the vocal cords; or (2) the cancer has spread to neighboring tissues; or (3) the cancer has spread to one lymph node measuring no more than 3 centimeters (1¼ inches) on the same side of the neck as the cancer.

Supraglottic Cancer

{
- **Supraglottic laryngectomy** · *or*
- **Total laryngectomy** · *with or without*
- **External-beam radiation therapy**

Or:
- **External-beam radiation therapy alone**

If the radiation fails to shrink the tumor:
- **Total laryngectomy**

Under Investigation #1
- **Chemotherapy, frequently consisting of cisplatin and fluorouracil** · *and*
- **External-beam radiation therapy,** *administered at the same time or sequentially*

If the combined treatment fails to shrink the tumor:
- **Total laryngectomy**

Under Investigation #2

- Hyperfractionated external-beam radiation therapy and other new methods of delivering radiotherapy

◆ Ask your doctor about any clinical trials that might benefit you.

Glottic Cancer

- Surgery to remove the cancer • *with or without*
- External-beam radiation therapy

Or:
- External-beam radiation therapy

If the radiation fails to shrink the tumor:
- Total laryngectomy

Under Investigation #1

- Chemotherapy, frequently consisting of cisplatin and fluorouracil • *and*
- External-beam radiation therapy, *administered at the same time or sequentially*

If the combined treatment fails to shrink the tumor:
- Total laryngectomy

Under Investigation #2

- Hyperfractionated external-beam radiation therapy and other new methods of delivering radiotherapy

◆ Ask your doctor about any clinical trials that might benefit you.

Subglottic Cancer

- Total laryngectomy, *with* lymph-node dissection • *plus*
- Total thyroidectomy, to surgically remove the thyroid gland • *followed by*
- External-beam radiation therapy

Or:
- External-beam radiation therapy

STAGE IV LARYNGEAL CANCER

(1) The cancer has spread to nearby tissues, such as the throat and possibly area lymph nodes; or (2) the cancer has spread to more than one lymph node on the same side of the neck as the cancer, or to lymph nodes on one or both sides of the neck, or to any lymph node that measures more than 6 centimeters (about 2¼ inches); or (3) the cancer has spread to other parts of the body.

Supraglottic Cancer

- Total laryngectomy • *followed by*
- External-beam radiation therapy

Under Investigation #1

- Chemotherapy, frequently consisting of cisplatin and fluorouracil • *and*

- External-beam radiation therapy, *administered at the same time or sequentially*

If the combined treatment fails to shrink the tumor:
- Total laryngectomy

Under Investigation #2
- Hyperfractionated external-beam radiation therapy and other new methods of delivering radiotherapy

◆ Ask your doctor about any clinical trials that might benefit you.

Glottic Cancer

- Total laryngectomy • *followed by*
- External-beam radiation therapy

Under Investigation #1
- Chemotherapy, frequently consisting of cisplatin and fluorouracil • *and*
- External-beam radiation therapy, *administered at the same time or sequentially*

If the combined treatment fails to shrink the tumor:
- Total laryngectomy

Under Investigation #2
- Hyperfractionated external-beam radiation therapy and other new methods of delivering radiotherapy

◆ Ask your doctor about any clinical trials that might benefit you.

Subglottic Cancer

- Total laryngectomy, *with* lymph-node dissection • *plus*
- Total thyroidectomy • *followed by*
- External-beam radiation therapy

Or:
- External-beam radiation therapy

Under Investigation #1
- Hyperfractionated external-beam radiation • *with or without*
- Chemotherapy

Under Investigation #2
- Other new methods of delivering radiotherapy

◆ Ask your doctor about any clinical trials that might benefit you.

See treatment options for metastases of the lung, bone, and liver.

RECURRENT LARYNGEAL CANCER

Your therapy will depend on how you were treated initially.

If you were treated initially with surgery:
- A second surgery to remove the cancer • *and/or*
- External-beam radiation therapy

> *If you were treated initially with radiotherapy:*
> - **Partial laryngectomy** • *or*
> - **Total laryngectomy** • *or*
> - **External-beam radiation therapy**
>
> *If you were treated initially with chemoradiation:*
> - **Laryngectomy**
>
> *If both surgery and external-beam radiation therapy were used initially:*
> - **Chemotherapy, to relieve symptoms**

Patients who undergo a partial laryngectomy will have to relearn how to swallow through rehabilitation therapy with a *speech-language pathologist.* "As a group, they experience more difficulty swallowing after surgery than patients who've had a total laryngectomy," explains Dr. Richtsmeier. The procedure (also called a supraglottic laryngectomy) removes the upper part of the larynx, including the epiglottis—the flap of cartilage that normally moves down over the voice box when we swallow, to prevent food and liquid from slipping down the windpipe and into the lungs. The speech-language pathologist teaches patients to compensate by using their tongue and a pair of small cartilage that also make up the skeletal structure of the larynx.

Total Laryngectomy and Tracheostomy—During any open surgery on the larynx, the surgeon creates an opening in the *trachea,* or windpipe, at the front of the neck and inserts a curved plastic tube. You can expect your throat to swell following the operation, impeding your ability to swallow for a short time. The *tracheostomy* will help you to breathe. To prevent mucus and saliva from accumulating in the airway, a nurse will periodically apply gentle suction to the hole (called a *stoma*) with a small aspirating device. "The vast majority of patients who un-

LARYNGEAL CANCER/
Surgical Procedures

Endoscopic re-excision: a second endoscopic surgical procedure to remove a wider area of laryngeal tissue found to contain carcinoma in situ. Often performed using a laser.
Average hospital stay: outpatient procedure

Cordectomy: surgical removal of one of the two vocal cords; can be performed endoscopically or through an incision in the neck.
Average hospital stay: outpatient procedure

Partial/supraglottic laryngectomy: surgical removal of part of the larynx. In a standard partial laryngectomy, the upper portion of the voice box is taken out—but not the vocal cords. A vertical hemilaryngectomy removes the left or right side of the larynx.
Average hospital stay: 3–7 days

Total laryngectomy: surgical removal of the entire voice box. In addition, the surgeon creates a permanent opening in the neck and

(cont.)

dergo a partial laryngectomy can have the tracheostomy removed in about a week to ten days," says Dr. Richtsmeier. By then they should be talking again.

If a total laryngectomy had to be performed, the stoma is permanent, because in taking out the voice box, he explains, "the windpipe is cut off at the top and sewn to the skin," thus closing off the air passage. From now on, breathing takes place through the stoma. One of your nurses will teach you how to clean the stoma and the surrounding skin, change the trach (pronounced *trake*) tube, suction secretions, and other routine care. It may be difficult to believe right now, but in time this does become routine. You'll also be instructed on precautions to take, such as preventing water from getting into the tube. Although you may not shower or swim, you can bathe as often as you wish.

See "Tracheostomy," page 494.

Learning New Ways to Speak After a Total Laryngectomy— People without a voice box must learn to talk in a new way. Anyone scheduled for a total laryngectomy should request a consultation with a speech-language pathologist beforehand to get an idea of the communication options that are available:

Electrolarynx—The electrolarynx is a handheld battery-powered device that emits high-frequency vibrations. The technique is easy to learn. To speak, you hold it against your neck and use your mouth and tongue to form words as you would normally. If you've ever heard someone use the electrolarynx, you're familiar with its monotonic sound.

Dr. Cathy Lazarus, associate director of the voice, speech, and language service and swallowing center at Northwestern University Medical School in Chicago, begins speech therapy before patients are discharged. "For the first day or two, they have to communicate by writing, since the throat

---

inserts a tube in the windpipe. Patients with advanced subglottic laryngeal cancer also have their thyroid gland taken out *(thyroidectomy)*. The thyroid, located just below the voice box, secretes two essential hormones that influence a number of vital functions. Following thyroid removal, patients must take oral thyroid hormone for the rest of their lives.

Average hospital stay: 7–10 days *See treatment options for thyroid cancer, page 489.*

For free referrals to a certified speech-language pathologist in your area, contact:

American Speech-Language-Hearing Association Action Center 10801 Rockville Pike Rockville, MD 20852-3279 800-638-8255 *http://www.asha.org*

is too swollen for them to use an electrolarynx," she explains. "Then we'll give them one to try out. Even if they can't place it against their neck because they still have their surgical staples in, holding it to the cheek and articulating works fairly well."

Some mechanical larynxes come equipped with a flexible pipe-shaped adapter on top, which you insert in the corner of your mouth when talking. The drawback to this *intraoral electrolarynx* is that the mouthpiece tends to get in the way of the tongue, making speech harder to decipher.

Another, similar device fits over the roof of the mouth like a denture, freeing both hands. The user flicks the switch on and off with his tongue. Dr. Lazarus recommends against this type. "When a person places an electrolarynx against his neck," she says, "other people can see that he's going to sound different." With the unseen retainer-type prosthesis, however, listeners may be disconcerted by the robotic voice that comes out.

Esophageal Speech—Dr. Richtsmeier describes esophageal speech as a sort of "controlled burp." Patients are taught to forcefully gulp air down into their esophagus. Then they deliberately release it and use the sound generated by the rumbling in the throat for speech. In his experience, "not all patients can learn esophageal speech. And of those that do, not all attain a quality of speech that allows them to be understood and to speak in fairly long sentences." The sound tends to be deep-pitched and husky. One practical advantage is that esophageal speech enables you to speak without using your hands.

Tracheoesophageal Puncture (TEP Voice)—In many respects, this may be the most satisfactory choice for restoring speech. During the laryngectomy, or shortly thereafter in a separate procedure, an opening is made from the windpipe into the adjacent esophagus, and a small plastic silicone valve is inserted.

In order to talk, you take a deep breath, then cover the stoma in the front of your neck with a finger. This diverts air from the trachea through the prosthesis, into the esophagus and out the mouth. "The quality of the voice is similar to esophageal speech," says Dr. Lazarus, "but it's a much more efficient method."

To free your hands, a mechanical one-way valve can be added to the stoma. Normally, it stays in an open position, to allow air into the windpipe. When you speak, the pressure forces the device shut, shunting the air through the tracheoesophageal opening. According to Dr. Lazarus, relatively few of her patients have had long-term success with the one-way valve, because the seal loosens. Most who tried it, she says, eventually went back to using their thumb.

TREATMENTS FOR ADVANCED LARYNGEAL CANCER

With most forms of cancer, stage IV usually denotes that the disease has metastasized to a distant organ. Laryngeal carcinoma differs in that a person can have no secondary lesion or malignant lymph nodes yet still be classified as stage IV: The tumor, a *T4*, has either penetrated the surrounding thyroid cartilage or encroached upon the throat or the soft tissue of the neck.

Therapy for advanced cancer of the upper and middle parts of the larynx typically consists of (1) total laryngectomy followed by irradiation or (2) a clinical trial of

> **Tips for Making Yourself Better Understood**
>
> 1. **Eliminate background noise when speaking. Turn off the TV, radio, and so on.**
>
> 2. **Stand or sit no more than three feet away from the person you're speaking to, and look directly at him.**
>
> 3. **Encourage listeners to carefully watch your lips and tongue.**
>
> 4. **Speak slowly and overarticulate. "I always tell patients to pretend their speaker is ten feet away," says Dr. Lazarus. "Just slowing down their rate of speech can make a huge difference."**

chemoradiation. Subglottic laryngeal carcinoma, which accounts for only about one in twenty cases, frequently necessitates extensive surgery. In addition to total laryngectomy, the neighboring thyroid gland is taken out, as are lymph nodes on both sides of the neck.

It is believed that the larger the tumor, the higher the risk of its metastasizing to the regional lymph nodes in the neck. The cancer status of the nodes, says Dr. Richtsmeier, "is the strongest predictor of the probable outcome." Unless the cancer is treated successfully, it generally progresses to other nodes in the neck and then to other parts of the body.

Of the three types of laryngeal carcinoma, supraglottic cancer is by far the most likely to affect the nodes; one-quarter to one-half of patients are diagnosed with node-positive disease. During the surgery to remove the voice box, the surgeon would dissect all of the lymph nodes in the neck. A *radical neck dissection* also takes out three important structures that run through the neck: a major blood vessel called the *internal jugular vein;* the *spinal accessory nerve,* which governs movement of one of the shoulder muscles; and the *sternocleidomastoid muscle.* If one of these structures can be preserved, the operation is referred to as a *modified radical neck dissection.*

Glottic cancer rarely spreads to the lymph nodes. When it does, the involved nodes are taken out along with the larynx, and the area irradiated. Because the chance of nodal metastasis is so remote, most oncologists would order elective neck irradiation—a preventive measure—only if the tumor was large.

TREATMENTS FOR RECURRENT LARYNGEAL CANCER

If the cancer returns following primary radiation or chemoradiation, total or partial laryngectomy would probably be recommended. Normally, the same area of the body cannot be reirradiated, but the larynx is often able to withstand a second treatment. Patients treated surgically would undergo a second operation, radiotherapy, or both.

Second Primary Cancers of the Larynx—People with laryngeal cancer face a substantial risk of developing a second cancer of the head and neck or esophagus, particularly if they continue to smoke tobacco and use alcohol. This is a new tumor, mind you, *not* a recurrence of the original lesion.

Traditionally, if radiotherapy had been employed to manage the first cancer, a subsequent tumor would be treated surgically, in the belief that the voice box could not tolerate further irradiation. Now it appears that the larynx is more resilient than previously thought.

TABLE 6.3	Potential Side Effects of Neck Dissection Surgery
General effects of neck dissection	▪ In many patients, temporary or permanent numbness in the skin of the neck and the ear
If one jugular vein is removed . . .	▪ Few side effects, other than temporary swelling
If both jugular veins are removed . . .	▪ More severe swelling
If the spinal accessory nerve is removed . . .	▪ Limited shoulder movement ▪ Some difficulty raising the arm over the head ▪ Mild pain due to inflammation at the shoulder joint ◆ *Physical therapy is essential for maintaining good shoulder function. Ask the surgeon for a referral.*
If one sternocleidomastoid muscle is removed . . .	▪ No side effects, although the neck may take on a slightly sunken appearance
If both muscles are removed . . .	▪ Reduced strength in flexing your head forward

A small study evaluated twenty patients whose laryngeal cancer had been treated with radiation. Then history repeated itself. The participants, most of whom had stage I or stage II disease, were administered high-dose radiation in lieu of laryngectomy. Five years later, more than 90 percent were still alive.

◆ *Ask your doctor about any investigational therapies that might benefit you.*

Cancer of the Throat (Pharyngeal Cancer)

Overview

TREATMENTS FOR THROAT CANCER THAT
HAS NOT METASTASIZED

Surgery and Radiation Therapy

Though the throat measures just five inches from top to bottom, a tumor's location in this hollow tube greatly determines the treatment that will be used.

Nasopharyngeal Cancer—The upper segment, the nasopharynx, is located behind the nasal cavity. It is an area inaccessible through surgery. Consequently, "radiation is the standard therapy for nearly all stages of nasopharyngeal cancer," says Dr. Randal Weber of the University of Pennsylvania Cancer Center. As many as nine in ten patients with small lesions can be cured this way. If surgery is used at all, it may be to remove large lymph nodes in the neck that have withstood radiation treatment.

Oropharyngeal Cancer—Radiation vies with surgery as the primary treatment for early-stage cancer of the middle part of the throat. The oropharynx includes several structures at the back of the oral cavity: the base of the tongue *(posterior tongue);* the arch-shaped *soft palate* in the rear roof of the mouth and its fleshy U-shaped protuberance, the *uvula;* and the *tonsils.* Tumors of the soft palate and the tonsils generally have a brighter prognosis than those in the tongue or the oropharyngeal wall itself.

The decision whether to irradiate or to operate varies from one center to another. The University of Pennsylvania Cancer Center leans toward radiation, says Dr. Weber, "and our experience has been that it's

**THROAT CANCER/
Surgical Procedures**

Pharyngectomy: surgical removal of part of the throat. Lymph nodes in the neck may be taken out as well *(neck dissection)*.
Average hospital stay: 5–7 days

Laryngopharyngectomy: surgical removal of the larynx and all or part of the throat. Neck dissection is almost always performed. When the entire pharynx is removed, a new throat is reconstructed using tissue transferred from another part of the body. Sometimes part of the voice box can be preserved, in what is called a *partial laryngopharyngectomy*. If the whole larynx has to be taken out, the surgeon creates an opening through the neck and into the windpipe. Patients now breathe through this *tracheostomy* and must learn a new technique for speaking.
Average hospital stay: 7–10 days

quite effective." Tumor site may also dictate the modality used. For an early-stage lesion on the base of the tongue (measuring up to 4 centimeters, or 1½ inches), most oncologists would recommend combination external-beam radiation followed by interstitial radioactive implants, to preserve speech and swallowing. External and internal radiotherapies are significantly more effective than external-beam radiation alone and equally effective as surgery plus radiation, the standard approach to stage III cancer of the posterior tongue. When pharyngectomy is necessary for tumors of the oropharynx, only part of the throat is typically cut out.

Hypopharyngeal Cancer—Radiation may still be an option for stage I disease, when the cancer is limited to one of three parts of the hypopharynx: (1) the *pyriform sinus,* site of two in three hypopharyngeal cancers; (2) the *pharyngoesophageal junction,* where the throat meets the esophagus; and (3) the rear wall of the lower throat.

At stage II, the malignancy has invaded a second part of the hypopharynx or involved neighboring tissue. Cancers of the pharyngoesophageal junction or the rear hypopharyngeal wall respond equally well to surgery or radiation. Pyriform-sinus tumors, though, usually require surgery followed by radiation.

Hypopharyngeal carcinoma is one of the so-called silent cancers, typically discovered in an advanced state. Therefore, most men and women are treated surgically, then given external-beam radiation. Because the bottom of the throat wraps around the larynx, Dr. Weber explains, "it's very infrequent that we can remove just the cancer without taking out all or part of the voice box." This operation, a laryngopharyngectomy, usually resects the diseased part of the throat and the whole larynx. Total laryngectomy entails a permanent tracheostomy: an opening made through the neck and into the airway, to facilitate breathing.

See "Total Laryngectomy and Tracheostomy," page 544.

THROAT CANCER/Treatment Options

Nasopharyngeal Cancer

STAGE I NASOPHARYNGEAL CANCER

The cancer is found in only one part of the nasopharynx.

- External-beam radiation therapy

STAGE II NASOPHARYNGEAL CANCER

The cancer is found in more than one part of the nasopharynx.

- External-beam radiation therapy

STAGE III NASOPHARYNGEAL CANCER

The cancer has spread into the nose or to the oropharynx; or the cancer is in the nasopharynx or has spread to the nose or the oropharynx; and it involves only one lymph node, measuring 3 centimeters (1 1/4 inches) or less, on the same side of the neck as the tumor.

{
- External-beam radiation therapy • *or*
- Hyperfractionated external-beam radiation therapy • *with or without*
- Lymph-node dissection

Under Investigation #1

{
- Chemotherapy, frequently consisting of cisplatin and fluorouracil • *followed by*
- External-beam radiation therapy • *or*
- Pharyngectomy, to remove the cancerous portion of the neck

Under Investigation #2

- Chemotherapy, frequently consisting of cisplatin and fluorouracil • *given before, during, or after*
- External-beam radiation therapy
- ◆ Ask your doctor about any clinical trials that might benefit you.

STAGE IV NASOPHARYNGEAL CANCER

The cancer has spread to the bones or nerves in the head, with or without area lymph-node involvement; or the cancer is in the nasopharynx or has spread to the nose, another part of the nasopharynx, or the bones or nerves in the head; and it involves more than one lymph node on the same side of the neck as the tumor, or lymph nodes on one or both sides of the neck, or any lymph node that measures more than 6 centimeters (2 1/4 inches); or the cancer has spread to other parts of the body.

- External-beam radiation therapy *or* hyperfractionated external-beam radiation therapy to the primary tumor and cancerous lymph nodes on both sides of the neck • *with or without*
- Lymph-node dissection

Under Investigation #1

{
- Chemotherapy, frequently consisting of cisplatin and fluorouracil • *followed by*
- External-beam radiation therapy • *or*
- Pharyngectomy
}

Under Investigation #2

- Chemotherapy, frequently consisting of cisplatin and fluorouracil • *given before, during, or after*
- External-beam radiation therapy
- ◆ Ask your doctor about any clinical trials that might benefit you.

Oropharyngeal Cancer

STAGE I OROPHARYNGEAL CANCER

The cancer measures no more than 2 centimeters (³/₄ inch).

- Pharyngectomy • *or*
- External-beam radiation therapy

Under Investigation #1

- Hyperfractionated external-beam radiation therapy

Under Investigation #2

- Internal radiation therapy

Under Investigation #3

- Mohs' micrographic surgery • *followed by*
- External-beam radiation therapy
- ◆ Ask your doctor about any clinical trials that might benefit you.

STAGE II OROPHARYNGEAL CANCER

The cancer measures more than 2 centimeters but less than 4 centimeters (1¹/₂ inches).

- Pharyngectomy • *or*
- External-beam radiation therapy

Under Investigation #1

- Hyperfractionated external-beam radiation therapy

Under Investigation #2

- Internal radiation therapy
- ◆ Ask your doctor about any clinical trials that might benefit you.

STAGE III OROPHARYNGEAL CANCER

The cancer measures more than 4 centimeters; or the cancer is any size but has spread to only one lymph node on the same side of the neck, and the cancerous lymph node measures no more than 3 centimeters (1¹/₄ inches).

- Pharyngectomy, *with or without* lymph-node dissection · *followed by*
- External-beam radiation therapy

Under Investigation #1

- Chemotherapy, frequently consisting of cisplatin, alone or in combination with fluorouracil · *followed by*

{
- External-beam radiation therapy · *or*
- Pharyngectomy

Under Investigation #2

- Internal radiation therapy

Under Investigation #3

- Hyperfractionated external-beam radiation therapy

Under Investigation #4

- Chemoradiation, frequently consisting of cisplatin, alone or in combination with fluorouracil

◆ Ask your doctor about any clinical trials that might benefit you.

STAGE IV OROPHARYNGEAL CANCER

(1) The cancer has spread to surrounding tissues and possibly to area lymph nodes; or (2) the cancer is any size and has spread to more than one lymph node on the same side of the neck, or to lymph nodes on one or both sides of the neck, or to any lymph node measuring more than 6 centimeters (about 2¼ inches); or (3) the cancer has spread to other parts of the body.

If the cancer is operable:

{
- Pharyngectomy · *or*
- Laryngopharyngectomy, to surgically remove the larynx and part or all of the throat · *with*

- Lymph-node dissection · *followed by*
- External-beam radiation therapy

Under Investigation #1

- Chemotherapy, frequently consisting of cisplatin and fluorouracil · *followed by*

{
- Pharyngectomy · *or*
- External-beam radiation therapy

Under Investigation #2

- Hyperfractionated external-beam radiation therapy · *with or without*
- Chemotherapy

Under Investigation #3

- Internal radiation therapy

◆ Ask your doctor about any clinical trials that might benefit you.

If the cancer is inoperable:

- External-beam radiation therapy

Under Investigation #1

- Chemotherapy, frequently consisting of cisplatin, alone or in combination with fluorouracil • *followed by*

{
- External-beam radiation therapy • *or*
- Pharyngectomy

Under Investigation #2

- Chemoradiation, frequently consisting of cisplatin, alone or in combination with fluorouracil

Under Investigation #3

- Hyperfractionated external-beam radiation therapy

Under Investigation #4

- Internal radiation therapy

◆ Ask your doctor about any clinical trials that might benefit you.

Hypopharyngeal Cancer

STAGE I HYPOPHARYNGEAL CANCER

The cancer is found in only one part of the hypopharynx.

{
- Partial laryngopharyngectomy, to surgically remove part of the larynx and part or all of the throat • *or*
- Laryngopharyngectomy • *with*
- Lymph-node dissection • *followed by*
- External-beam radiation therapy

Or:
- External-beam radiation therapy alone, to the tumor and to both sides of the neck

STAGE II HYPOPHARYNGEAL CANCER

The cancer is found in more than one part of the hypopharynx.

- Laryngopharyngectomy, *with* lymph-node dissection • *followed by*
- External-beam radiation therapy

Under Investigation

- Chemotherapy, frequently consisting of cisplatin and fluorouracil • *followed by*

{
- External-beam radiation therapy • *or*
- Laryngopharyngectomy

◆ Ask your doctor about any clinical trials that might benefit you.

STAGE III HYPOPHARYNGEAL CANCER

The cancer is in more than one part of the hypopharynx or has spread to adjacent tissue and has invaded the larynx; or the cancer is in the hypopharynx or has spread to adjacent tissue, has spread to only one lymph node on the same side of the neck, and the cancerous lymph node measures no more than 3 centimeters (1¼ inches).

- Laryngopharyngectomy, *with* lymph-node dissection · *followed by*
- External-beam radiation therapy

Under Investigation #1
- Chemotherapy, frequently consisting of cisplatin and fluorouracil · *followed by*

{
- External-beam radiation therapy · *or*
- Laryngopharyngectomy

Under Investigation #2
- Chemoradiation, frequently consisting of cisplatin, alone or in combination with fluorouracil

◆ Ask your doctor about any clinical trials that might benefit you.

STAGE IV HYPOPHARYNGEAL CANCER

(1) The cancer has spread to the connecting tissue or soft tissues of the neck and may or may not have affected area lymph nodes; or (2) the cancer is in the hypopharynx or has spread to adjacent tissues and has spread to more than one lymph node on the same side of the neck, or to lymph nodes on one or both sides of the neck, or to any lymph node measuring more than 6 centimeters (about 2¼ inches); or (3) the cancer has spread to other parts of the body.

If the cancer is operable:

- Laryngopharyngectomy, *with* lymph-node dissection · *followed by*
- External-beam radiation therapy

Under Investigation
- Chemotherapy, frequently consisting of cisplatin and fluorouracil · *followed by*

{
- External-beam radiation therapy · *or*
- Laryngopharyngectomy

◆ Ask your doctor about any clinical trials that might benefit you.

If the cancer is inoperable:

- External-beam radiation therapy

Under Investigation
- External-beam radiation therapy *or* hyperfractionated external-beam radiation therapy · *with or without*
- Chemotherapy, frequently consisting of cisplatin, alone or in combination with fluorouracil

◆ Ask your doctor about any clinical trials that might benefit you.

See treatment options for metastases of the lung and liver.

RECURRENT THROAT CANCER
Your therapy will depend on how you were treated initially.

Nasopharyngeal Cancer

- **External-beam radiation therapy** · *and*
- **Internal radiation therapy**

Or:
- **Pharyngectomy**

If the cancer has recurred in a distant part of the body, or if it has recurred locally but cannot be treated by surgery or radiation:

- **Chemotherapy, frequently consisting of cisplatin and fluorouracil**

Under Investigation
- **New chemotherapy drugs and immunologic agents**
- ◆ **Ask your doctor about any clinical trials that might benefit you.**

Oropharyngeal Cancer

If the cancer was treated previously with radiation therapy:
- **Pharyngectomy**

If the cancer was treated previously with surgery:
- **External-beam radiation therapy** · *or*
- **A second surgery, to remove the cancer**

Under Investigation
If the cancer was treated previously with surgery and radiation therapy:
- **Chemotherapy, frequently consisting of cisplatin and fluorouracil**

If the cancer has recurred in a distant part of the body:
- **Chemotherapy, frequently consisting of cisplatin and fluorouracil**
- ◆ **Ask your doctor about any clinical trials that might benefit you.**

Hypopharyngeal Cancer

If the cancer was treated previously with radiation therapy:
- **Pharyngectomy**

If the cancer was treated previously with surgery:
- **External-beam radiation therapy** · *or*
- **A second surgery, to remove the cancer**

Under Investigation
If the cancer was treated previously with surgery and radiation therapy:
- **Chemotherapy, frequently consisting of cisplatin and fluorouracil**

If the cancer has recurred in a distant part of the body:
- **Chemotherapy, frequently consisting of cisplatin and fluorouracil**
- ◆ **Ask your doctor about any clinical trials that might benefit you.**

Lymph-Node Dissection—Cancers of the throat frequently metastasize to lymph nodes in the neck by the time of diagnosis. In nasopharyngeal carcinoma, diseased nodes are irradiated at the same time as the primary tumor. Most patients with tumors lower down in the pharynx have their malignant nodes removed as part of pharyngectomy or laryngopharyngectomy.

A *radical neck dissection* excises all two hundred nodes in the neck, along with a major muscle, nerve, and vein; a *modified radical neck dissection* preserves one of these three vital structures. More commonly, the surgeon performs a less extensive *functional neck dissection,* taking out only the nodes in an area of the neck.

Throat-Reconstruction Surgery—Most of the time, surgery for throat cancer resects a portion of the tube. If a total or near-total pharyngectomy is necessary, the operation includes throat reconstruction using tissue from the small intestine or the forearm. "Both of these are *microvascular* procedures," says Dr. Weber. "We disconnect the blood supply to where the tissue is located, then reimplant it in the neck and hook it up to the blood vessels there." Recovery from microvascular surgery is usually quick enough that patients can begin radiotherapy within four weeks, the recommended period of time. Postoperative radiation is more effective when it is initiated promptly.

The transplanted tissue doesn't contract like the muscles of the throat to propel food down toward the esophagus. To what degree swallowing is affected depends on the extent of the surgery and the site of the cancer. A tumor on either side of the pharyngeal wall will impact less on a person's swallowing ability than a cancer in the back of the throat—particularly one that lies immediately behind the base of the tongue. If food can't clear that area, it may lodge in the throat.

A less popular approach to reestablishing the upper digestive tract is *gastric transposition,* also known as a *gastric pull-up.* "That's to replace the throat and the entire esophagus," explains Dr. Weber. The upper part of the J-shaped stomach is brought up and surgically attached to the remaining pharynx.

If your treatment plan calls for throat reconstruction, ask the surgeon for a referral to a *speech-language pathologist,* who can teach you techniques for swallowing more efficiently.

Glossectomy (Tongue-Removal Surgery)—Surgery to treat cancer in the posterior tongue impairs speech and swallowing less than resecting a tumor in the front two-thirds of the muscular organ. (Carcinoma of the *anterior* tongue is classified as a cancer of the oral cavity.) Frequently, the physician can perform a *hemiglossectomy*, which cuts out one side at the back of the tongue yet leaves the tongue intact. Many patients who lose their tongue entirely *(total glossectomy)* can speak surprisingly clearly. However, most have to give up solid foods for an all-liquid diet.

See "Will Treatment Affect Your Speech, Voice, or Swallowing?," page 485.

Side Effects of Radiation to the Throat—Irradiation can inflame the throat, making it difficult to swallow. The high-energy rays also damage the glands that produce saliva. Because saliva helps to prevent tooth decay, a reduction in the flow of saliva *(xerostomia)* can open the door to cavities. Therefore, conscientious oral hygiene is a must.

See "Dry Mouth (Xerostomia)" under "Oral Complications" in Chapter Eight, "Take Control: Managing Symptoms, Side Effects, and Complications."

Chemotherapy

Larger or more extensive tumors may warrant chemotherapy, administered in conjunction with either radiation or surgery. The two drugs typically relied upon are cisplatin (brand name: Platinol) and fluorouracil (5-FU).

Though drug treatment is still considered investigational in pharyngeal cancer, says Dr. Weber, "there have been some studies published showing that the addition of chemotherapy significantly improves survival for patients with stage III and stage IV cancer of the nasopharynx."

The evidence is less compelling for tumors elsewhere in the throat. Still, in hypopharyngeal carcinoma, chemo may be considered as early as stage II. One French study compared the conventional treatment of surgery plus radiotherapy to cisplatin-fluorouracil plus radiotherapy. The five-year survival rates were the same, but 35 percent of the patients in the second group did well enough that they never had to lose their voice box and retained the ability to speak normally.

TREATMENTS FOR ADVANCED THROAT CANCER

Radiation, alone or preceded by chemotherapy, remains the principal strategy for metastatic nasopharyngeal cancer, while stage IV oropharyngeal and hypopharyngeal carcinomas usually call for surgery and radiation. Larynx removal, associated mainly with hypopharyngeal tumors, may be necessary for oropharyngeal cancer if the lesion has grown deep into the muscle of the tongue base (the reason is to prevent patients from accidentally ingesting food or liquid into the lungs, which can bring about *aspiration pneumonia*) or if it has spread to the voice box.

**THROAT CANCER/
Drug Therapy**

First-line therapy frequently consists of:
- cisplatin + fluorouracil

Other drugs used may include:
- bleomycin
- hydroxyurea
- carboplatin
- doxorubicin
- mitomycin

TREATMENTS FOR RECURRENT THROAT CANCER

Generally, oropharyngeal and hypopharyngeal cancers that were treated surgically receive radiation, and vice versa. A second operation to take out the cancer may be possible. Prior surgery *and* radiation rules out either modality, says Dr. Weber, "in which case chemotherapy is given as a palliative measure."

Since nasopharyngeal tumors are rarely resectable, pharyngectomy is attempted only on occasion. Patients who were previously irradiated may be re-treated with a combination of external-beam and internal radiotherapy. If the recurrent cancer is not amenable to surgery or radiation, many oncologists would recommend chemotherapy.

OTHER THERAPIES THAT MAY BE USED IN THE TREATMENT OF THROAT CANCER

Hyperfractionated External-Beam Radiation Therapy—Delivering smaller doses of radiation two or more times per day is now a standard treatment for advanced nasopharyngeal and oropharyngeal cancers, and experimental for early-stage tumors of the middle throat. Clinical trials have also evaluated the potential benefits of giving chemotherapy at the same time for locally advanced oropharyngeal and hypopharyngeal carcinomas. In one study, at Duke University Medical Center, the addition of chemotherapy was clearly superior: After three years, more than half the patients in the combined-therapy group were alive, compared to one in three of those who received hyperfractionated radiation alone.

Mohs' Micrographic Surgery (investigational)—Some cancer centers have evaluated this operative technique for early-stage oropharyngeal cancer. The objective of micrographic surgery is to remove the cancer and as little normal tissue as possible. After taking out the tumor, the surgeon inspects the surrounding area through a microscope to ensure that the margins are free of disease.

◆ *Ask your doctor about this and any other investigational therapies that might benefit you.*

Soft-Tissue Sarcomas

Overview

TREATMENTS FOR SOFT-TISSUE SARCOMAS THAT
HAVE NOT METASTASIZED

Surgery

Localized soft-tissue sarcomas are staged according to how well differentiated their cells appear under the microscope (expressed as grade I, II, or III, or low, intermediate, or high grade) and by their size (A or B). The classification IB, for example, tells the doctor that the cancer is larger than 5 centimeters in diameter and that its cells look very much like normal cells.

Equally important as grade and size is the tumor's location. Forty percent of soft-tissue malignancies originate in the legs; another 15 percent in the arms. Compared to sarcomas of the head and neck, upper trunk, and abdomen, "tumors in the extremities can be removed more readily, without having to sacrifice vital anatomic parts," explains Dr. Kenneth Yaw, chief of the division of musculoskeletal oncology at the University of Pittsburgh Cancer Institute. "Also, a tumor in the upper torso or abdomen can grow to a much larger size before it becomes detectable than, say, a tumor in the wrist can."

During the operation, the surgeon attempts to excise the cancer plus a cuff of disease-free tissue. Ideally, the margin should be wide enough to ensure that no tumor cells remain in the area around the lesion. Of equal concern, though, is minimizing the surgery's effect on function and appearance. The procedure of choice, called a wide surgical excision, removes 2 to 3 centimeters of normal tissue *in all directions.*

Radiation Therapy

Stage I sarcomas of the extremities can frequently be managed with surgery alone. But because of the cancer's close proximity to vital nerves, vessels, and bone, achieving a wide margin in the trunk or the head and

SOFT-TISSUE SARCOMAS/Treatment Options

Stages I through III of soft-tissue sarcomas are divided into A and B, with A denoting that the tumor measures 5 centimeters (2 inches) or less; B sarcomas are larger than 5 centimeters.

STAGE I SOFT-TISSUE SARCOMA

The cancer cells appear well differentiated, or similar to normal cells.

Sarcoma of the Extremities

- Wide surgical excision, to remove the cancer and a margin of normal tissue extending 2 to 3 centimeters (³/₄ inch to 1¹/₄ inches) in all directions from the tumor site

Or:
- Conservative surgical excision, to remove the cancer and a margin of normal tissue less than 2 centimeters · *followed by*
- External-beam radiation therapy

If the cancer is inoperable:
- High-dose external-beam radiation therapy · *followed by*
- Surgical excision, to remove the cancer and a margin of normal tissue · *followed by*
- External-beam radiation therapy (high-dose if the sarcoma is still unresectable)

Sarcoma of the Trunk, Abdomen, or Head and Neck

- Surgical excision

If the margins are positive for cancer:
- Surgical excision · *preceded or followed by*
- External-beam radiation therapy

STAGE II SOFT-TISSUE SARCOMA

The cancer cells appear moderately well differentiated.

Sarcoma of the Extremities

- Wide surgical excision · *with or without*
- External-beam radiation therapy

Or:
- Amputation, to remove the cancerous part of the body

Or:
- Conservative surgical excision · *preceded and/or followed by*
- External-beam radiation therapy

If the cancer is inoperable:
- High-dose external-beam radiation therapy

Under Investigation #1
- Preoperative regional or systemic chemotherapy, frequently consisting of doxorubicin

Under Investigation #2
- Excisional surgery · *with or without*
- External-beam radiation therapy · *followed by*
- Chemotherapy, frequently consisting of doxorubicin

Under Investigation #3
- New forms of external-beam radiation therapy
◆ Ask your doctor about any clinical trials that might benefit you.

Sarcoma of the Trunk, Abdomen, or Head and Neck

- Wide surgical excision · *with or without*
- High-dose external-beam radiation therapy

Or:
- External-beam radiation therapy · *followed by*
- Conservative surgical excision · *followed by*
- External-beam radiation therapy

If the cancer cannot be completely removed surgically:
- High-dose external-beam radiation therapy *and* chemotherapy, to relieve symptoms

Under Investigation #1
- Intraoperative external-beam radiation therapy, administered during surgery

Under Investigation #2
- Chemotherapy · *alone or following*
- Surgical excision
◆ Ask your doctor about any clinical trials that might benefit you.

STAGE III SOFT-TISSUE SARCOMA
The cancer cells appear poorly differentiated or undifferentiated.

Sarcoma of the Extremities

- Wide surgical excision · *with or without*
- External-beam radiation therapy

Or:
- Amputation

Or:
- Conservative surgical excision · *preceded and/or followed by*
- External-beam radiation therapy

If the cancer is inoperable:
- High-dose external-beam radiation therapy

Under Investigation #1

{
- Excisional surgery • *with or without*
- External-beam radiation therapy • *followed by*
- Chemotherapy, frequently consisting of doxorubicin in combination with one or more other drugs

Under Investigation #2

- Preoperative regional chemotherapy, frequently consisting of doxorubicin

Under Investigation #3

- New forms of external-beam radiation therapy

Under Investigation #4

- External-beam radiation therapy before and after surgery
- ◆ Ask your doctor about any clinical trials that might benefit you.

Sarcoma of the Trunk, Abdomen, or Head and Neck

- Wide surgical excision • *with or without*
- High-dose external-beam radiation therapy

Or:

- External-beam radiation therapy • *followed by*
- Conservative surgical excision • *followed by*
- External-beam radiation therapy

If the cancer cannot be completely removed surgically:

- High-dose external-beam radiation therapy *and* chemotherapy, to relieve symptoms

Under Investigation #1

- Intraoperative external-beam radiation therapy, administered during surgery

Under Investigation #2

- Chemotherapy • *alone or following*
- Surgical excision
- ◆ Ask your doctor about any clinical trials that might benefit you.

STAGE IVA SOFT-TISSUE SARCOMA

The cancer has spread to regional lymph nodes.

- Surgical excision *or* amputation, *with* lymph-node dissection • *with or without*
- External-beam radiation therapy

Or:

- External-beam radiation therapy • *followed by*
- Amputation • *followed by*
- External-beam radiation therapy

STAGE IVB SOFT-TISSUE SARCOMA

The cancer has metastasized to other parts of the body.

- **Wide surgical excision of the primary cancer**

Or:
- **Conservative surgical excision of the primary cancer ·** *followed by*
- **External-beam radiation therapy**

Or:
- **External-beam radiation therapy ·** *followed by*
- **Amputation ·** *followed by*
- **External-beam radiation therapy**

If the cancer is inoperable:
- **High-dose external-beam radiation therapy ·** *or*
- **Chemotherapy—frequently consisting of doxorubicin, alone or in combination with dacarbazine; or ifosfamide, alone or in combination with other agents—to relieve symptoms**

If the cancer has spread only to the lung or lungs:
- **Surgical excision of the primary cancer ·** *followed by*
- **High-dose external-beam radiation therapy ·** *or*
- **Chemotherapy, possibly consisting of doxorubicin alone or in combination with ifosfamide, or as part of a regimen known as CYVADIC (see "Drug Therapy" box) ·** *plus*
- **Surgical excision of cancerous lesions in the lung(s)**

Under Investigation #1
- **Surgical excision ·** *followed by*
- **Chemotherapy**

Under Investigation #2
- **New chemotherapy drugs and immunologic agents**
- ◆ Ask your doctor about any clinical trials that might benefit you.

See treatment options for metastases of the brain and lung.

RECURRENT SOFT-TISSUE SARCOMA

Your therapy will depend on how you were treated initially.

If the cancer has recurred locally:
- **Surgical excision ·** *followed by*
- **External-beam radiation therapy**

Or:
- **Amputation**

Or, in selected patients:
- **External-beam radiation therapy ·** *followed by*
- **Wide surgical excision**

{
If the cancer recurs in the lung or lungs:
- **Surgical excision of the primary cancer** • *followed by*
- **High-dose external-beam radiation therapy** • *or*
- **Chemotherapy, possibly consisting of doxorubicin alone or in combination with ifosfamide, or as part of a regimen known as CYVADIC** • *plus*
- **Surgical excision of secondary lesions in the lung(s)**

Under Investigation
- **New chemotherapy drugs and immunologic agents**

♦ **Ask your doctor about any clinical trials that might benefit you.**

neck is seldom possible. Wherever the tumor develops, when the rim of noncancerous tissue is too narrow for comfort, low-grade soft-tissue cancers generally call for radiotherapy. "With high-grade sarcomas," says Dr. Yaw, "more often than not patients receive radiation regardless of the margin. The controversy in the field is over whether we need to give radiation following a radical excision." This more extensive operation, once the preferred treatment for high-grade sarcomas, is rarely required nowadays.

For stage II or stage III disease, external-beam radiotherapy may be supplemented by interstitial radiation. The surgeon, having removed the tumor and finding cancer in the margin, implants a catheter. Then a radioactive substance is loaded in the tube a few days later.

Limb-Sparing Surgery Versus Amputation—"Radiation has made a huge difference in our ability to remove tumors in the extremities without having to amputate," says Dr. Yaw. Administering high-dose radiation as the first step of treatment may shrink an otherwise inoperable soft-tissue sarcoma to a resectable size. Additional irradiation is given postoperatively.

Before proceeding with this approach, the doctor must be satisfied that it will control the cancer at least as well as an amputation and that the preserved limb will be functional. Once again, the site of the cancer is a key determinant.

SOFT-TISSUE SARCOMAS/ Surgical Procedures

Surgical excision: surgical removal of the cancer with or without a margin of normal tissue. Average hospital stay: 5–7 days

Wide excision takes out the cancer and 2 to 3 centimeters of negative tissue on all sides. A margin less than 2 centimeters is referred to as a *conservative* excision.

Radical excision takes out the entire "compartment" containing cancer, with margins extending approximately 5 centimeters on all sides.

Marginal excision cuts through the tumor's surrounding *pseudo capsule*, or *reactive zone*. This narrow belt, filled with fluid, tissue, and various cells, including cancer cells, separates the tumor from normal tissue. Marginal excision leaves behind microscopic malignant cells; the National Cancer Institute strongly discourages its use.

"For distal tumors of the leg, amputations are very real considerations," says Dr. Yaw. "In the foot, for example, amputating below the knee is preferable to attempting to save the foot and winding up with a less-than-adequate margin *and* a mutilated foot.

Medical Terms You're Likely to Hear

Distal: situated away from the point where a limb or bone is attached.

Proximal: situated toward the point of attachment.

"The hand can tolerate more extensive surgery than the foot," he continues, "because its main functions are sensation and fine-motor, as opposed to durability and bearing the weight of the body. So whereas I might do a partial hand amputation for a distal sarcoma of the hand, an equivalent sarcoma in the foot might require an amputation below the knee.

"With more proximal tumors," meaning those closer to the hip or shoulder, "we can often surgically excise a tumor that is pressing against major nerves and blood vessels. But if they are actually encased by the cancer, we would probably opt for amputation, no matter how high up the tumor is."

Physical Therapy—Imagine losing a two-inch block of tissue from your upper arm—one possible outcome of a wide surgical excision of a small sarcoma. "The operation usually takes away a significant amount of muscle," explains Dr. Yaw, "which may impair function. It may also involve resecting important nerves that can affect function and leave areas of numbness."

For the names of licensed physical therapists in your area, contact:

American Physical Therapy Association
1111 North Fairfax Street
Alexandria, VA 22314
703-684-2782
http://www.apta.org

For the names of certified occupational therapists in your area, contact:

American Occupational Therapy Association
4720 Montgomery Lane
Bethesda, MD 20824-1220
301-652-2682 (ask for Direct Mail Service)
http://www.aota.org

Virtually all men and women with soft-tissue sarcomas receive physical therapy and occupational therapy following surgery. Rehabilitation may commence in the hospital, but the ongoing program takes place mainly at a facility near your home.

According to Leslie Freeman, clinical manager of physical medicine at Georgetown University Medical Center, "physical therapy focuses on strengthening muscles and improving mobility." Patients who lost part or all of an arm or a leg to amputation are taught to walk using artificial limbs *(prostheses)* or adaptive equipment.

"Occupational therapy works on compensatory strategies for self-care and general independence: dressing, bathing, eating, child care, driving a car, getting back to work." Depending on the goals set by the patient and the therapist, she says, rehab can last anywhere from two weeks to six months.

Chemotherapy

Clinical trials are evaluating the effectiveness of incorporating chemotherapy into the treatment of intermediate- and high-grade soft-tissue sarcomas as well as large tumors at any stage. "This is a highly controversial area," says Dr. Yaw. "On the one hand, we know that chemotherapy makes a profound difference in improving survival from rhabdomyosarcoma," a group of malignant soft-tissue cancers that is extremely sensitive to anticancer drugs.

"With the rest of the adult soft-tissue sarcomas, though, we have to tell patients honestly that we're not sure whether it will really make a difference. Also, the regimens used tend to be very aggressive." Of the many combinations that have been tried, none has proved superior to doxorubicin (brand name: Adriamycin) alone.

Dr. Yaw's criteria for recommending chemotherapy to patients include the person's age and the severity of the cancer. "Because a high-grade sarcoma has a relatively poor prognosis, patients who could reasonably be expected to tolerate the drugs—that would be aged fifty or younger—should be offered them. The other role for chemotherapy is in metastatic disease, either at the time of diagnosis or later."

TREATMENTS FOR ADVANCED OR RECURRENT
SOFT-TISSUE SARCOMAS

Stage IVA indicates that the cancer has spread to regional lymph nodes, a rare occurrence most often seen in synovial-cell sarcomas, epithelioid sarcomas, and rhabdomyosarcomas. "The other soft-tissue sarcomas almost never metastasize to the lymph nodes," says Dr. Yaw.

"It's also rare for these cancers to spread to other organs besides the lung." If the number of secondary tumors is limited, treatment consists of lung-resection surgery, possibly supplemented by radiation or chemotherapy. "Generally speaking, there is little hope for a cure by surgically removing the metastases—with one exception. When a patient develops one or two metastatic lesions in the lung a year or so after treatment of the primary sarcoma, there is reasonable potential for him to be rendered disease free." The cure rate for this scenario ranges from 20 to 40 percent. High-

---

**SOFT-TISSUE SARCOMAS/
Drug Therapy**

*First-line therapy frequently
consists of:*
- doxorubicin
- ifosfamide

*Other drugs or drug regimens
that may be used include:*
- cyclophosphamide
- dacarbazine
- cisplatin
- carboplatin
- doxorubicin + dacarbazine
- doxorubicin + ifosfamide
- CYVADIC: cyclophosphamide + vincristine + doxorubicin + dacarbazine
- MAID: mesna + doxorubicin + ifosfamide + dacarbazine
- MAP: mitomycin + doxorubicin + cisplatin
- alpha-interferon (for AIDS-related Kaposi's sarcoma) (I)

(I) = Immunologic Agent

---

grade sarcomas that recur usually turn up in the lung; low-grade soft-tissue cancers rarely come back at all.

OTHER THERAPIES THAT MAY BE USED IN THE TREATMENT OF SOFT-TISSUE SARCOMAS

Mohs' Micrographic Surgery—In cases where conserving the maximum amount of tissue possible is a priority, Mohs' surgery may be used to remove small, low-grade sarcomas. Doctors receive special training in the technique, which essentially requires them to assume a pathologist's role.

First the physician removes all the tumor she can see with the naked eye, plus a thin circumference of normal tissue. Then she slices the specimen and analyzes it under a microscope. If cancer remains, more tissue is cut out of that specific area. The process continues until the margin is cancer free.

Arterial Perfusion (investigational)—Some centers have utilized arterial-perfusion chemotherapy prior to surgery for intermediate-grade and high-grade sarcomas of the extremities, though Dr. Yaw characterizes the treatment as uncommon. "It has met with mixed reviews," he says.

In arterial perfusion, blood from the arm or leg is routed through a special bypass machine, which adds chemotherapy (typically doxorubicin) "at a far higher level than we could ever give systemically. Theoretically, the idea is to sterilize any microscopic disease that might be left after we've resected the tumor."

◆ *Ask your doctor about these and any other investigational therapies that might benefit you.*

Cancer of the Testicle

Overview

TREATMENTS FOR TESTICULAR CANCER THAT
HAS NOT METASTASIZED

Surgery

All men suspected of having nonmetastatic testicular cancer undergo a radical inguinal orchiectomy to remove the testicle through an incision in the groin. Many cancer centers now perform the procedure as same-day surgery.

Usually, the cancer diagnosis has been tentatively established prior to the operation, based on an ultrasound scan coupled with positive alpha-fetoprotein (AFP) and beta human chorionic gonadotropin (HCG) tumor-marker blood tests. The crucial piece of information yielded by the orchiectomy is the malignancy's cell type, which will dictate the next step of treatment.

Under standard protocols, seminoma testicular tumors call for radiation to the retroperitoneal lymph nodes located in the rear of the abdomen, near the spine. For nonseminoma cancers, the doctor will schedule a second operation, called a retroperitoneal lymph-node dissection. Generally, the nodes are treated whether or not a CT scan turns up evidence that the cancer has spread there.

Surgery, Radiation Therapy, and Observation

Nonseminoma: Lymph-Node Dissection Versus Observation—
Even with a negative CT scan and negative tumor-marker blood tests following surgery, approximately one in three men will be found to harbor microscopic nodal disease. "The CT scan is only so accurate," explains Dr. Bruce Redman of the University of Michigan Comprehensive Cancer Center. The flip side is that two in three patients are subjected to unnecessary surgery, because testicular carcinoma can usually be cured with chemotherapy should it come back, even as metastatic disease to the lung, liver, or bone.

This led oncologists to consider forgoing node dissection for some patients with stage I

**TESTICULAR CANCER/
Surgical Procedures**

Radical inguinal orchiectomy: surgical removal of a cancerous testicle through an incision in the groin. It is both diagnostic and therapeutic.
Average hospital stay: outpatient procedure

Retroperitoneal lymph-node dissection: surgical removal of the retroperitoneal lymph nodes.
Average hospital stay: 5–7 days

TESTICULAR CANCER/Treatment Options

STAGE I TESTICULAR CANCER

The cancer is confined to the testicle.

Seminoma

- **Radical inguinal orchiectomy, to surgically remove the testicle containing the mass · *followed by***
- **External-beam radiation therapy**

Under Investigation
- **Radical inguinal orchiectomy · *followed by***
- **Observation**
- ◆ **Ask your doctor about any clinical trials that might benefit you.**

Nonseminoma

- **Radical inguinal orchiectomy · *followed by***
- **Lymph-node dissection**

Under Investigation #1
- **Radical inguinal orchiectomy · *followed by***
- **Observation**

Under Investigation #2
- **Radical inguinal orchiectomy · *followed by***
- **Chemotherapy, consisting of cisplatin in combination with one or more other drugs**
- ◆ **Ask your doctor about any clinical trials that might benefit you.**

STAGE II TESTICULAR CANCER

The cancer has spread to the retroperitoneal lymph nodes in the back of the abdomen or the para-aortic lymph nodes in the upper abdomen. Patients who have cancerous retroperitoneal nodes larger than 5 centimeters (2 inches) are said to have bulky disease.

Nonbulky-Tumor Seminoma

- **Radical inguinal orchiectomy · *followed by***
- **External-beam radiation therapy**

Bulky-Tumor Seminoma

- **Radical inguinal orchiectomy · *followed by***
- **Chemotherapy, consisting of cisplatin in combination with one or more other drugs · *or***
- **External-beam radiation therapy**

Nonseminoma

- **Radical inguinal orchiectomy · *followed by***
- **Lymph-node dissection · *followed by***
- **Observation · *or***
- **Chemotherapy, consisting of cisplatin in combination with one or more other drugs**

If the cancer is too large to resect completely:
- **Radical inguinal orchiectomy · *followed by***
- **Chemotherapy, consisting of cisplatin in combination with one or more other drugs · *followed by***
- **Additional surgery, to remove the remainder of the cancer**

Under Investigation
- **Chemotherapy alone, consisting of cisplatin in combination with one or more other drugs**
- ◆ **Ask your doctor about any clinical trials that might benefit you.**

STAGE III TESTICULAR CANCER

In nonbulky stage III, the cancer has spread to lymph nodes beyond the abdomen and to the lung, but no mass measures larger than 2 centimeters ($^3/_4$ inch). Bulky stage III testicular cancer is characterized by extensive involvement of the retroperitoneal lymph nodes plus metastasis to the lung and sometimes to the liver or the brain.

Seminoma

- **Radical inguinal orchiectomy · *followed by***
- **Chemotherapy, consisting of cisplatin in combination with one or more other drugs**

Nonseminoma

- **Chemotherapy, consisting of cisplatin in combination with one or more other drugs**

Or:
- **Chemotherapy, consisting of cisplatin in combination with one or more other drugs · *followed by***
- **Surgery, to remove any remaining cancer · *with or without***
- **Additional chemotherapy**

Or:
- **Chemotherapy, consisting of cisplatin in combination with one or more other drugs · *followed by***
- **Radical inguinal orchiectomy**

If the cancer has metastasized to the brain:
- **Chemotherapy, consisting of cisplatin in combination with one or more other drugs · *with***
- **Whole-brain irradiation**

Under Investigation #1
- **High-dose chemotherapy • *followed by***
- **Autologous bone-marrow transplantation**

Under Investigation #2
- **New chemotherapy drugs**
- ◆ **Ask your doctor about any clinical trials that might benefit you.**

See treatment options for metastases of the liver, lung, and brain.

RECURRENT TESTICULAR CANCER

Your therapy will depend on how you were treated initially.
- **Chemotherapy, frequently consisting of ifosfamide, cisplatin, and either etoposide or vinblastine**

If the cancer is limited to one site and is unresponsive to chemotherapy:
- **Surgery, to remove the cancer**

Under Investigation #1
- **High-dose chemotherapy • *followed by***
- **Autologous bone-marrow transplantation**

Under Investigation #2
- **New chemotherapy drugs**
- ◆ **Ask your doctor about any clinical trials that might benefit you.**

---

nonseminoma. (At stage II, the cancer has spread to the nodes.) In a study at Indiana University, doctors divided participants into two groups. One underwent retroperitoneal lymph-node dissection. The men in the other group were followed; if they relapsed, they were treated with chemotherapy. Nearly ten years later, the cure rate is exactly the same. According to Dr. Redman, only about one in four men who elect observation over dissection experience a recurrence. "So the potential is there to avoid a retroperitoneal lymph-node dissection in a large percentage of patients.

"Why is this important? I don't want to imply that chemotherapy is easy," says Dr. Redman, a medical oncologist, "but there are more competent medical oncologists to give chemotherapy for testicular cancer than there are surgical oncologists competent at performing retroperitoneal lymph-node dissection, which is a very doctor-dependent procedure." In experienced hands—"someone who does ten to fifteen a year"—the operation is extremely safe, with minimal complications. "The problem," he says, "is that most community-hospital surgeons do maybe one a year."

The major potential side effect is *retrograde ejaculation*. Instead of semen being discharged through the urethra and out the penis, it goes in the opposite direction, landing in the bladder. Retrograde ejaculation is a common complication of a surgical technique called TURP, used to treat prostate cancer. But most of those patients are of an age where having children is no longer a priority. Testicular cancer primarily afflicts men thirty-four and younger. For them this is often a serious concern.

A negative CT scan and negative tumor markers put a patient at clinical stage I. If this describes you, you would almost certainly qualify for a *modified* retroperitoneal node dissection. The less extensive surgery rarely causes retrograde ejaculation, thereby preserving fertility. It may also be an option for men whose CT scan shows minimal nodal involvement (designated $N1$), meaning the cancer has metastasized to a single regional lymph measuring no larger than 2 centimeters. "In that situation," says Dr. Redman, "we might have to clear out a greater area of nodes," but without affecting normal ejaculation.

See *"Sperm Banking: Why Every Patient Should Make a Deposit," page 575.*

The majority of nonseminomas are made up of two or more cell types. In order to determine whether or not a patient with clinical stage I disease can avoid a second operation, the doctor needs to know the relative proportions of each type.

Example: "People whose tumor contains 50 percent or more of embryonal carcinoma are much more likely to have involvement of the retroperitoneal lymph nodes and therefore should undergo the dissection surgery," says Dr. Redman, "whereas patients whose tumor includes a good percentage of teratoma or yolk-sac tumor and a low percentage of embryonal carcinoma are perfect candidates for observation. Don't have surgery, don't have chemo, we're going to keep an eye on you."

Dr. Redman treats a number of patients referred from other hospitals. "Many times," he says, "their pathology reports will say simply 'nonseminoma embryonal tumor.' That means nothing to us. We need to know the percentages of the subtypes, so we send the slides down to our pathologist, who is an expert in genitourinary pathology. He then determines those percentages.

"Most cancer centers," he adds, "enjoy the luxury of having a pathologist dedicated to reading only genitourinary cancers." You're less likely to find this attention to crucial histologic detail at a smaller, nonacademic medical facility, for the simple fact that with fewer than eight thousand testicular cancers diagnosed annually, a general pathologist may go for months, maybe years, without encountering a single case. Request that your testicular biopsy be interpreted by a genitourinary pathologist.

"The other criterion we use when considering someone for observation is, How compliant will he be?" The recommended surveillance consists of monthly doctor's visits for two years and periodic checkups after that. At each appointment, the physician conducts a physical exam; X rays are taken of the chest; and blood is drawn to assess the levels of AFP, HCG, and a third serum marker, *lactate dehydrogenase* (LDH). CT scans of the abdomen are performed every three months for the first year, every six months for the second year, and annually thereafter.

"You would think that if you told a young man with cancer that he needed to come in for follow-up checkups, of course he would," observes Dr. Redman. In his experience, "the vast majority of them do, until they get out to about six, seven months. Then they start forgetting their appointments," he says, "because they feel so healthy."

Seminoma: Radiation Therapy Versus Observation—In seminoma, too, oncologists are looking at the possibility of sparing clinical stage I patients from additional treatment—in this case, radiotherapy to the retroperitoneal lymph nodes. In one study comparing postorchiectomy radiation to surveillance, after five years the group of men who were observed had four times the relapse rate as those treated with radiation: approximately 20 percent to 5 percent. But because even recurrent testicular cancer is so treatable, the overall cure rate for stage I seminoma approaches 100 percent.

Since radiotherapy is mild compared to node dissection, there isn't the same urgency to answer the question of whether or not early-stage seminoma patients can go without it. Irradiating the retroperitoneal lymph nodes has no effect on ejaculation and, according to Dr. Redman, "hardly causes any side effects whatsoever." The dose given—over the course of three weeks—is significantly lower than that administered for most cancers.

Chemotherapy

Drug treatment for testicular cancer centers around cisplatin (brand name: Platinol). Several regimens have been used, but the current standard is BEP, an abbreviation for bleomycin (Blenoxane), etoposide (VePesid, VP-16), and cisplatin.

Generally, adjuvant chemotherapy is not indicated for stage I disease. Anticancer drugs would be added to treatment for stage II seminoma if the tumor measured more than 5 centimeters on the CT scan; and possibly for stage II nonseminoma after retroperitoneal node dissection. Occasionally, when a CT scan reveals limited retroperitoneal involvement, the oncologist may tap chemotherapy as the primary treatment, in an effort to avoid lymph-node surgery.

Sperm Banking: Why Every Patient Should Make a Deposit— When a man must lose a testicle due to some form of trauma, most of the time he retains his fertility; the other testicle compensates by stepping up its production of sperm. "But for some reason," says Dr. Redman, "about two-thirds of young men who undergo orchiectomy on account of testicular cancer will have an abnormally low sperm count or sperm motility afterward." *Motility* refers to the sperm cells' ability to move forward, which of course they must do in order to travel from the vagina to the fallopian tube, where fertilization takes place.

A normal sperm count is approximately 60 million sperm per milliliter of semen. "Below that," says Dr. Redman, "the ability to conceive becomes progressively poorer." Prospects for fathering a child also fall if less than 60 percent of the sperm are motile.

Chemotherapy, should it be necessary, renders patients sterile for one and a half to two years afterward. Once drug treatment ends, more than half of those who had adequate sperm counts before will return to normal. (Of the three major modalities, radiation is the least likely to cause permanent infertility.) Dr. Redman recommends sperm banking to *all* of his patients.

Testicular Cancer and Sexuality— When Dr. Redman sat in on some initial meetings of a newly formed support group for testicular-cancer survivors, he admits to having been unprepared for the anguish that filled the room. Many of his patients lamented that the disease had somehow stripped them of their masculinity.

TESTICULAR CANCER/ Drug Therapy

First-line therapy frequently consists of:
- **BEP: bleomycin + etoposide + cisplatin**

Other drugs or drug combinations used may include:
- **EP: etoposide + cisplatin**
- **PVB: cisplatin + vinblastine + bleomycin**
- **VAB VI: vinblastine + dactinomycin + bleomycin + cyclophosphamide + cisplatin**
- **VPV: vinblastine + cisplatin + etoposide**
- **carboplatin + etoposide + bleomycin**
- **POMB/ACE: cisplatin or carboplatin + vincristine + methotrexate + bleomycin + dactinomycin + cyclophosphamide + etoposide**
- **high-dose carboplatin**
- **ifosfamide + cisplatin + etoposide or vinblastine**
- **plicamycin**
- **doxorubicin**

This, despite the fact that they were all but assured a full, healthy life and had retained normal sexual function and testosterone levels. "It was an eye-opener," the doctor recalls. "The disease exerts a greater impact on men's perceptions about their sexuality than physicians realize." If you find yourself feeling this way, don't suffer in silence. Given the low incidence of testicular cancer, few patient support groups exist, but your oncologist or the hospital's department of psycho-oncology may be able to refer you to a psychiatrist, psychologist, or psychotherapist who specializes in treating sexual problems related to serious illness.

See "Sexual Problems" in Chapter Eight, "Take Control: Managing Symptoms, Side Effects, and Complications."

TREATMENTS FOR ADVANCED TESTICULAR CANCER

Metastatic seminomas are treated with orchiectomy, then chemotherapy. For nonseminomas, the sequence is reversed: chemotherapy, alone or followed by surgery to take out any remaining masses. Only about one in five of those metastatic lesions will prove to be cancerous, says Dr. Redman, "but there's no way to tell without our removing them."

Testicular cancer is rarely diagnosed in an advanced stage. When it is, chemotherapy may be initiated prior to orchiectomy. "The testicle frequently acts as a sanctuary from the effects of the drugs," Dr. Redman explains. "Many times, what we find is that the testicle still contains residual cancer, even though it's been eradicated everywhere else."

OTHER THERAPIES THAT MAY BE USED IN THE TREATMENT OF TESTICULAR CANCER

High-Dose Chemotherapy/Autologous Bone-Marrow Transplantation (investigational)—Two groups of patients may be eligible for high-dose chemotherapy followed by an autologous BMT to replenish the damaged marrow: those whose cancer failed to respond to cisplatin-based chemotherapy and those who achieved remission with standard-dose cisplatin-based chemo but relapsed.

The principal agent used is carboplatin (Paraplatin), often in combination with other drugs. Studies conducted at Memorial Sloan-Kettering Cancer Center in New York have been encouraging. As many as two in five patients saw their cancer go into remission, in many cases for a number of years. Initiating the experimental therapy sooner rather than later seems to be beneficial, resulting in fewer blood-cell-related complications. Researchers are also considering high-dose chemotherapy with autologous rescue as a first-line treatment for men who have one of the high-risk forms of testicular cancer.

◆ *Ask your doctor about this and any other investigational therapies that might benefit you.*

Cancer of the Small Intestine

Overview

TREATMENTS FOR SMALL-INTESTINE CANCER THAT
HAS NOT METASTASIZED

Observation

Small-intestine lymphoma takes hold in the organ's lymph tissue. If the tumor is slow-growing and has yet to produce symptoms, the doctor might choose to defer any treatment until the cancer progresses. Carcinoid tumors of the small intestine also follow an indolent course. Odd as it may seem, an oncologist may recommend "watchful waiting" even after the disease has spread to the lymph nodes or to the liver.

Surgery

Surgical resection is the cornerstone of treatment for small-bowel cancer. "The operative approach may differ slightly from one section of the small intestine to another," explains Dr. Fred Richards of the Comprehensive Cancer Center of Wake Forest University, "but generally the surgeon cuts out the tumor plus 5 centimeters [2 inches] of bowel on either side." Then the two segments are sutured together. The coiled small intestine, twenty feet in length, usually withstands the loss of tissue without adversely affecting eating and bowel habits.

"Very few patients will require a permanent ileostomy," says Dr. Richards. Like a colostomy, an *ileostomy* is a surgically constructed opening, or *stoma,* for evacuating stool into a detachable soft-plastic pouch. The surgeon brings the small bowel up to the surface of the abdomen and sews it into position.

A *conservative local excision* is often sufficient for carcinoid tumors measuring less than 1 centimeter across (just under ½ inch). In this operation, the doctor cuts out the tumor through a flexible endoscope.

See "Ostomies" in Appendix A for the names of organizations that offer information and support to people with ileostomies.

SMALL-INTESTINE CANCER/Treatment Options

Small-Intestine Adenocarcinoma

ALL STAGES

If the cancer is resectable:
- Bowel resection, to remove the tumor

If the cancer is unresectable:
- Bypass surgery, to allow food to travel around the tumor • *or*
- External-beam radiation therapy, to relieve symptoms • *or*
- Chemotherapy, frequently consisting of fluorouracil and leucovorin

Under Investigation
If the primary cancer is inoperable:
- External-beam radiation therapy incorporating radiosensitizing drugs • *with or without*
- Chemotherapy, frequently consisting of fluorouracil and leucovorin

If the secondary cancer is inoperable:
- New chemotherapy drugs and immunologic agents

◆ Ask your doctor about any clinical trials that might benefit you.

Small-Intestine Lymphoma

LOCALIZED SMALL-INTESTINE LYMPHOMA

The cancer is confined to the wall of the small bowel.

- Observation

Or:
- Bowel resection, *with* lymph-node dissection • *with or without*
- External-beam radiation therapy • *or*
- Chemotherapy, frequently consisting of cyclophosphamide for low-grade lymphoma; cyclophosphamide, doxorubicin, vincristine, and prednisone for intermediate-grade or high-grade lymphoma

REGIONAL SMALL-INTESTINE LYMPHOMA

The cancer has invaded the regional lymph nodes.

- Bowel resection, *with* lymph-node dissection • *followed by*
- Chemotherapy, frequently consisting of cyclophosphamide, doxorubicin, vincristine, and prednisone

METASTATIC SMALL-INTESTINE LYMPHOMA

The cancer has spread to other parts of the body.

- Chemotherapy, frequently consisting of cyclophosphamide, doxorubicin, vincristine, and prednisone • *with or without*
- External-beam radiation therapy

Small-Intestine Leiomyosarcoma

LOCALIZED, REGIONAL, OR METASTATIC

If the cancer is resectable:
- Bowel resection

If the primary cancer is inoperable:
- Bypass surgery · *followed by*
- External-beam radiation therapy

If the secondary cancer is inoperable:
- Surgery, to relieve symptoms · *or*
- External-beam radiation therapy, to relieve symptoms · *or*
- Chemotherapy, frequently consisting of cyclophosphamide, doxorubicin, and dacarbazine, to relieve symptoms

Under Investigation
- New chemotherapy drugs and immunologic agents
- ◆ Ask your doctor about any clinical trials that might benefit you.

Small-Intestine Carcinoid Tumor

LOCALIZED SMALL-INTESTINE CARCINOID TUMOR

The cancer is confined to the small intestine.

- Observation · *or*
- Local excision, to remove the cancer through an endoscope · *or*
- Bowel resection, *with or without* lymph-node dissection

If the cancer is unresectable:
- External-beam radiation therapy

REGIONAL SMALL-INTESTINE CARCINOID TUMOR

The cancer has spread to nearby lymph nodes.

- Observation · *or*
- Bowel resection

If the cancer is inoperable:
- Surgery, to resect or bypass a tumor obstructing the small bowel

METASTATIC SMALL-INTESTINE CARCINOID TUMOR

The cancer has spread to other parts of the body.

- Observation · *or*
- Surgery, to resect or bypass a tumor obstructing the small bowel · *or*
- Systemic chemotherapy, frequently consisting of fluorouracil in combination with other agents, to relieve symptoms

If the cancer has spread to the liver:
- Hepatic-artery embolization, frequently consisting of fluorouracil or doxorubicin, which is infused into the artery serving the liver

If you have the array of symptoms that makes up carcinoid syndrome, with metastasis to the liver:
- Observation

Or:
- Hepatic resection, to remove one or more secondary tumors in the liver · *or*
- Cryosurgery, to destroy the cancer with extreme cold · *or*
- Hepatic-artery ligation, to surgically cut and tie the main artery that serves the liver

Or:
- Hepatic-artery embolization, frequently consisting of fluorouracil or doxorubicin · *with or without*
- Systemic chemotherapy

Or:
- Regional (intra-arterial) chemotherapy, to deliver a high dose of anticancer drugs into the main artery serving the liver

Or:
- Alcohol ablation therapy, to destroy the cancer by injecting it with pure alcohol

Under Investigation
- Immunotherapy consisting of alpha-interferon given alone or in conjunction with chemotherapy, frequently consisting of fluorouracil
- ◆ Ask your doctor about any clinical trials that might benefit you.

See treatment options for metastases of the liver and lung.

RECURRENT SMALL-INTESTINE CANCER

Your therapy will depend on how you were treated initially.

If the cancer recurs in the small intestine:
- Bowel resection · *or*
- External-beam radiation therapy, to relieve symptoms · *or*
- Chemotherapy, to relieve symptoms

If the cancer recurs elsewhere in the body:
- Hepatic resection
- ◆ There is no standard effective chemotherapy for recurrent metastatic adenocarcinoma or leiomyosarcoma of the small bowel.

Under Investigation
- New chemotherapy drugs and immunologic agents
- ◆ Ask your doctor about any clinical trials that might benefit you.

Chemotherapy

Chemotherapy enters the treatment plan when the tumor cannot be completely removed surgically or when it has spread to the regional lymph nodes or to distant sites. Doctors draw on different agents to treat each of the four types of small-bowel cancer, which begin in different parts of the organ.

Adenocarcinoma is treated much like large-bowel cancer, also a malignancy of the intestinal lining. The drugs of choice are fluorouracil (5-FU) and leucovorin (brand name: Wellcovorin).

Men and women with small-intestine lymphoma normally receive the same four-drug regimen often prescribed for non-Hodgkin's lymphomas: cyclophosphamide (Cytoxan), doxorubicin (Adriamycin), vincristine (Oncovin), and prednisone (Deltasone). CHOP, as it is acronymed, "is an aggressive regimen," says Dr. Richards. "Cyclophosphamide alone may be more appropriate for patients who are not experiencing many symptoms, especially if they're elderly."

Half of all leiomyosarcomas of the small intestine are curable. The cancer, which develops in the bowel's smooth muscle, responds best to cyclophosphamide, doxorubicin, and dacarbazine (DTIC-Dome) delivered by way of a portable *continuous-infusion pump*.

Carcinoid tumors, found in certain hormone-producing cells of the small intestine, generally call for chemotherapy only if the symptoms can be attributed to the cancer's size.

Radiation Therapy

External-beam irradiation is employed mainly for inoperable cancers of the small in-

---

SMALL-INTESTINE CANCER/ Surgical Procedures

Local excision: surgical removal of the cancer through an endoscope inserted down the throat.
Average hospital stay: 7–10 days

Small-bowel resection: surgical removal of the cancerous part of the small intestine. A *duodenectomy* resects part or all of the duodenum, the upper portion; a *jejunectomy*, part or all of the jejunum, the middle section; and an *ileectomy*, part or all of the ileum, the portion that leads to the colon. Regional lymph nodes are usually dissected as well.
Average hospital stay: 7–10 days

SMALL-INTESTINE CANCER/ Drug Therapy

First-line therapy frequently consists of:

Adenocarcinoma
- fluorouracil + leucovorin

Lymphoma
- cyclophosphamide
- CHOP: cyclophosphamide + doxorubicin + vincristine + prednisone (H)

Leiomyosarcoma
- cyclophosphamide + doxorubicin + dacarbazine

Carcinoid Tumor
- fluorouracil + streptozocin
- fluorouracil + streptozocin + cyclophosphamide
- fluorouracil + doxorubicin + dacarbazine
- octreotide (H)

(H) = hormonal agent

testine, although it may be given postsurgically when a lymphoma is localized and able to be resected.

TREATMENTS FOR ADVANCED SMALL-INTESTINE CANCER

Surgery

"When small-intestine cancer spreads," says Dr. Richards, "it often involves other abdominal organs, such as the liver. Many times it travels to the lungs." If the primary lesion is obstructing the intestinal tract, the patient may undergo *tumor-debulking surgery* to cut away as much tumor as possible, or *bypass surgery* to route semidigested food around the blockage. The operation is succeeded by radiation.

Chemotherapy

Combination chemotherapy is the treatment of choice for advanced lymphoma. However, it is a palliative measure for unresectable metastatic leiomyosarcoma and is still considered experimental for adenocarcinoma. Drug therapy for metastatic carcinoid tumors consists of 5-FU in combination with one or more of the following anticancer agents: doxorubicin, dacarbazine, cyclophosphamide, and streptozocin (Zanosar). Because chemotherapy hasn't been shown to prolong the lives of people with carcinoid tumors, the National Cancer Institute recommends its use only to relieve symptoms, and preferably as part of a clinical trial.

Malignant Carcinoid Syndrome

Surgery, Cryosurgery, and Hepatic-Artery Ligation

As long as secondary malignancies in the liver are surgically accessible, they can sometimes be resected—through either a conventional operation or *cryosurgery*—even when they arise in multiple areas of the organ. The same is true of recurrent metastatic carcinoid tumor.

The principle behind *hepatic-artery ligation* "is to destroy the cancer by cutting off its blood supply," explains Dr. Richards. "Carcinoid tumors happen to be extremely vascular." In this surgical procedure, the physician severs and ties off the *hepatic artery*, the main blood vessel that delivers blood to the liver.

Hepatic-Artery Chemoembolization and Percutaneous Alcohol Ablation Therapy

Hepatic-artery chemoembolization achieves the same result as ligation, only nonsurgically. Fluorouracil or doxorubicin is injected directly into the hepatic artery, along with a substance that blocks the vessel and starves the tumor of blood. Although as many as three in five patients will see their liver metastases shrink by at least half, the major drawback to embolization is its harsh potential side effects, which include abdominal pain, nausea, and fever. Not only that, the symptoms of carcinoid syndrome can worsen temporarily. On the positive side, the treatments often induce long-lasting remissions and can be repeated from time to time.

Percutaneous *alcohol ablation therapy* entails injecting pure alcohol through the skin and directly into the tumor, killing the cells.

Hormonal Therapy (Palliative Treatment)

People with carcinoid syndrome frequently experience attacks of severely flushed skin, swelling, diarrhea, difficulty in catching their breath, and abrupt drops in blood pressure because the cancer secretes excessive amounts of certain hormones. The hormonal agent octreotide (Sandostatin) "is extremely effective for preventing the symptoms of carcinoid syndrome," says Dr. Richards. "Patients are taught to give themselves the injections under the surface of the skin, one to three times a day."

OTHER THERAPIES THAT MAY BE USED IN THE TREATMENT OF SMALL-INTESTINE CANCER

Immunologic Therapy (investigational)—Alpha-interferon (Roferon-A, Intron-A), given alone or with chemotherapy, has been tested in patients with carcinoid syndrome. Its impact on arresting cancer growth has been minimal. However, interferon may be useful as a palliative agent, particularly for men and women who do not respond to octreotide.

◆ *Ask your doctor about this and any other investigational therapies that might benefit you.*

Metastatic Cancers

A secondary tumor forms when malignant cells separate from a primary cancer and colonize another part of the body, having traveled through the bloodstream or the lymphatic system. The cells often take refuge in the nearest cluster of blood vessels; for instance, the portal vein frequently whisks colon-cancer cells to the liver. The liver is one of the most common sites of metastasis, along with the lungs, brain, bones, and lymph nodes. A secondary lesion may subsequently give rise to another metastasis, which in turn may spawn a tumor elsewhere in the body, and so on.

The inherited cancer contains the same abnormal cells as those in the original tumor. Metastatic breast cancer of the lung is made up of breast-cancer cells, *not* lung-cancer cells. This is a crucial distinction, because breast-cancer cells respond to different regimens of chemotherapeutic agents than do the two main types of lung-cancer cells: small-cell and non-small-cell. (As a matter of fact, early-stage non-small-cell lung carcinoma doesn't warrant drug treatment at all.) Furthermore, some women with secondary breast cancer of the lung might receive hormonal therapy, a strategy that has no place in primary lung cancer.

How late-stage disease is treated depends on several factors, beginning with the type of cancer. Ordinarily, the focus of therapy shifts from effecting a cure to prolonging life and relieving symptoms. That isn't true of all cancers. For example, secondary testicular cancer is curable more than 70 percent of the time, while nearly half of all men and women with stage IV thyroid cancer will be alive five years after diagnosis, and presumably cured. The five-year survival rates for advanced carcinomas of the larynx, prostate, breast, and endometrium range from 20 to 40 percent—encouraging enough to perhaps warrant aggressive treatment.

When the prognosis is less optimistic, as with stage IV cancer of the esophagus, conservative measures may be in order. Given that only one in fifty patients live five years, on average, few oncologists would recommend a major operation like esophagectomy, which removes part of the esophagus. More likely, the recommendation would be to use chemotherapy to control both the local and the distant tumors, adding local irradiation should the primary lesion in the gullet interfere with swallowing.

Two other major factors in determining treatment are the site and extent of the metastasis. Secondary cancers that blanket vital organs are usually considered inoperable. But if the spread is limited, not only may surgery still be feasible but a cure may still be within reach.

A fourth consideration: Has the cancer been treated before, or was the disease diagnosed in an advanced state? Among the cancers that most often evade detection until they have disseminated to other organs are ovarian, pancreatic, lung, stomach, esophageal, kidney, liver, and several types of soft-tissue sarcomas.

If no therapy has been given previously, treatment may take any of a number of directions. For metastatic cancers that are operable: perhaps surgery to remove or debulk the primary tumor, the secondary tumor, or both lesions. Radiation or chemotherapy may be administered preoperatively, postoperatively, or on both sides of surgery.

The purpose of surgical resection may be to cure the cancer. Or it may be to relieve symptoms or to enhance the effectiveness of chemotherapy by reducing the volume of the local mass. Should a cancer be obstructing a crucial passageway, inhibiting swallowing, urination, or another bodily function, the surgeon may attempt to cut away the tissue or to construct a *bypass* around the blockage.

For inoperable metastatic disease, treatment is typically systemic, consisting of chemotherapy, hormonal therapy, and/or immunologic therapy, with or without irradiation.

Fewer options may be available when patients have undergone prior treatment. Either the tumor has come back following a period of remission, or it has continued to progress, impervious to therapy. Whether advanced disease is recurrent, resistant (refractory), or newly diagnosed, now may be an appropriate time to weigh the benefits and risks of an experimental protocol.

Metastatic Cancer of the Bone

CANCERS THAT FREQUENTLY SPREAD TO THE BONE
- Breast ▪ Prostate ▪ Lung ▪ Kidney ▪ Pancreatic ▪ Lymphomas ▪ Multiple myeloma

WARNING SIGNS/SYMPTOMS
- Bone pain ▪ Swelling of a bone or area of bone

You may undergo any number of these diagnostic procedures:
- Physical exam

Laboratory Tests
- Blood tests, to detect elevated level of calcium and/or the enzyme alkaline phosphatase

Imaging Studies
- X rays ▪ Bone scan

Biopsy
- Bone biopsy

Primary sarcomas of the bone are rare, striking some 2,400 men and women each year. Metastatic bone cancer, however, eventually touches roughly half of all cancer patients. "We see more of it nowadays," says Dr. Franklin Sim of the Mayo Clinic Cancer Center in Rochester, Minnesota, "because medical treatment of primary cancers is more effective, and patients are living longer." Carcinomas of the breast, prostate, and lung account for four in five secondary lesions of the bone. The most vulnerable sites, in descending order, are the spinal column, the pelvis, the long bones of the arms or legs, and the base of the skull.

Metastatic bone disease can seriously undermine a patient's quality of life. Pain, the most common symptom, typically comes on over a period of weeks or months. Unless controlled, it becomes progressively more debilitating. Large cancers can weaken a bone until it snaps; the *femur* in the upper leg is particularly prone to *spontaneous fracture*. Being immobilized, even for a short time, places a person at risk for a number of complications, including chronic constipation, bedsores, and indigestion. Should a cancer spread to the vertebrae of the spine, it may compress the spinal cord housed within, inflicting severe neurologic damage.

Another frequent consequence of bone metastasis is *hypercalcemia,* in which excessive amounts of calcium build up in the blood. This can produce a variety of problems, including dehydration, appetite loss, confusion, and an irregular heartbeat. Though potentially fatal, hypercalcemia is quickly reversible using any of several types of medications.

Treatment of secondary bone tumors consists of a two-prong attack: systemic therapy to control the underlying malignant disease; and surgery, irradiation, and/or drug therapy to manage symptoms caused by the bone lesion itself. "We're very aggressive in treating skeletal lesions," says Dr. Sim, an orthopedic oncologist, "because we now have methods for relieving pain and improving function that we didn't have before. And if we're able to enhance a patient's quality of life, the oncologists can be more aggressive in treating the primary tumors."

Surgery (Palliative Treatment)

Internal Bone Fixation—"In the past," notes Dr. Sim, "there used to be a sense of hopelessness when a person with end-stage cancer experienced a pathological fracture of a bone. But today most doctors realize that a lot can be done to restore a bone's structure and keep patients active." Metal rods, plates, wires, and other materials can be used to mechanically put the bone back together. As for joints damaged by the tumor, they can be replaced with artificial, or *prosthetic,* implants. "Internal fixation and joint reconstruction have been very effective," says Dr. Sim, adding that most patients who fracture a bone are able to resume their former level of activity. The operation is usually succeeded by external-beam radiation.

Internal fixation may be performed as a preventive measure, particularly when a patient has a secondary lesion in a weight-bearing area such as the leg. "Fixing the bone before it breaks is a lot less traumatic for the patient," says Dr. Sim. "This way they retain their function and have a shorter hospitalization."

When is it advisable to intervene with prophylactic surgery? One major consideration is the location of the cancer. "If a person has a tumor in an area of high stress, like the upper femur, normally we would want to fix it." Size is the other significant factor. The standard guideline calls for operating on a metastatic lesion that arises in a bone other than the spine if it is larger than 2.5 centimeters (about 1 inch) in diameter. Amputation is almost never necessary for bone metastases of the extremities.

Laminectomy—"Metastasis to the spine can be a devastating problem," says Dr. Sim, "so there we're more aggressive as well. New techniques in spinal surgery enable us to prevent many of the catastrophic complications." A *laminectomy* removes much of the tumor and any surrounding bone that might be impinging on the spinal cord, to decompress the central nervous system. Rods may be inserted on either side of the vertebrae, for support.

Radiation Therapy (Palliative Treatment)

"If a patient has a painful lesion of the bone and none of the high-risk factors for fracture, radiation is the treatment of choice," says Dr. Sim. Even at low doses, "it usually provides very good pain relief for up to a year."

Bone metastases typically arise in more than one site, however.

Bone Biopsy

After administering intravenous sedation and an injection of local anesthetic, the physician pushes a hollow needle into the bone, using a twisting motion. You may feel some pain as it penetrates the *periosteum,* the bone's outer lining. The instrument's ratchetlike cutting device cuts out a tiny piece of bone measuring about $1/6$ inch across. Then the needle is twisted out and the site bandaged.

Patients who undergo a bone biopsy of the spine may be asked to remain in the hospital for twenty-four hours. Otherwise, they can usually go home after about one hour. The area where the needle was inserted may be sore for several days. Baths are off-limits for forty-eight hours, but you are allowed to shower, so long as you keep the biopsy site covered.

Typical setting:	outpatient
Anesthesia:	local, occasionally general
Sedation:	yes

**BONE METASTASES/
Surgical Procedures**

Internal fixation: the surgical
insertion of metal rods, screws,
plates, wires, pins, or a combination
into bone fragments in order to
stabilize the bone.
Average hospital stay: 2–5 days

Laminectomy: surgical removal of
as much tumor as possible from the
spine, to relieve pressure on the
spinal cord or a nerve emanating
from the spinal cord.
Average hospital stay: 5–7 days

This often rules out external-beam radiotherapy, because irradiating multiple tumors spread out over a wide area of bone would damage too much marrow and suppress blood-cell production. Instead, diffuse bone disease may be treated systemically with an injectable *radiopharmaceutical* or a type of drug known as a *bone-resorption inhibitor*.

Systemic Radionuclide Therapy and Drug Therapy (Palliative Treatments)

When primary cancer of the prostate, breast, or lymphatic system spreads to the bone, the new tumor is said to be *osteoblastic,* whereas a secondary bone tumor that has traveled from the lung, kidney, or plasma cells (multiple myeloma) is *osteolytic.*

Osteoblastic lesions are characterized by the growth of new bone. "Bone reacts to the presence of the cancer cells and forms bone and mineral around them," Dr. Sim explains. Nascent bone happens to absorb the radioactive isotopes strontium 89 and samarium 153. Both have been developed into intravenous radiopharmaceuticals named Metastron and Quadramet, respectively. The agents deliver their cancer-killing doses of radiation by insinuating themselves directly into the tumor. A single injection has been shown to relieve bone pain for months at a time and can be repeated if necessary.

**BONE METASTASES/
Drug Therapy**

• **pamidronate (B)**

• **samarium 153 (R)**

• **strontium 89 (R)**

B = bone-resorption inhibitor
R = radiopharmaceutical

Osteolytic tumors cause bone to be resorbed, or literally eaten up. This leaves gaping holes known as *lytic lesions.* The drug pamidronate (brand name: Aredia), a *bisphosphonate,* inhibits the bone-resorption process. Not only does it provide effective pain control, it slows the progression of bone metastases. In a study of women with stage IV breast cancer that had spread to the bone, Aredia delayed the onset of bone-related symptoms by six months.

Pamidronate also counteracts hypercalcemia. Another drug used for this purpose is calcitonin (Miacalcin, Calcimar). It, too, decreases the rate of bone resorption and curbs pain.

Certain hormonal therapies used to treat advanced breast cancer, such as *estrogens* and *antiestrogens,* may trigger hypercalcemia. Should hypercalcemia develop, your doctor will temporarily discontinue the drug until your calcium level returns to normal.

> *See "Hypercalcemia" in Chapter Eight, "Take Control: Managing Symptoms, Side Effects, and Complications."*

OTHER THERAPIES THAT MAY BE USED IN THE TREATMENT OF BONE METASTASES

Pain Medications/Nerve Blocks—Bone pain can also be controlled systemically with pain-relieving drugs *(analgesics)* or *corticosteroid* medications. When pain is unremitting, it may be necessary to inject an agent directly into or around a nerve, to block the sensation.

> *See "Pain Management" in Chapter Eight, "Take Control: Managing Symptoms, Side Effects, and Complications."*

◆ *Ask your doctor about any investigational therapies that might benefit you.*

Metastatic Cancer of the Brain

CANCERS THAT FREQUENTLY SPREAD TO THE BRAIN OR THE LEPTOMENINGES

- Lung ▪ Breast ▪ Melanoma ▪ Soft-tissue sarcomas ▪ Kidney ▪ Colon ▪ Acute lymphocytic leukemia ▪ Non-Hodgkin's lymphomas

At approximately 100,000 newly diagnosed cases per year, secondary brain cancers outnumber primary brain cancers by more than five to one. No matter where they originate, 25 percent of all malignant cells shed into the circulation are destined to migrate to the brain, where they form metastatic lesions. Primary tumors of the lung, colon, and kidney spawn 80 percent of secondary brain cancers in men, while primary melanoma and carcinomas of the lung, colon, and breast are responsible for the same percentage of cerebral metastases in women.

Often, brain metastases are detected at the same time as the original cancer, after neurologic symptoms bring a patient to her doctor. Even when no primary tumor can be found, as occurs 15 percent of the time,

**Medical Terms You're
Likely to Hear**

Leptomeninges: the *pia mater* and
the *arachnoid*, the thin set of
membranes that covers the brain and
spinal cord. *Cerebrospinal fluid* flows
between them, in what's called the
subarachnoid space.

secondary brain lesions are readily distinguished from primary brain lesions. One telltale characteristic: The vast majority grow in the junction dividing the cerebrum's gray and white matter, an area rich in blood vessels.

The leptomeningeal membrane that surrounds the brain and spinal cord is also a destination for stray tumor cells from other parts of the body, although far less frequently than the brain. Breast cancer, small-cell lung cancer, and melanoma may involve either site. Acute lymphocytic leukemia and non-Hodgkin's lymphomas typically spread to the leptomeninges only, whereas non-small-cell carcinoma of the lung manifests mainly in the brain. However, because the latter is one of the most common types of cancer, "we see quite a lot of leptomeningeal metastases from non-small-cell lung cancer," says Dr. Paul Moots of the Vanderbilt Cancer Center in Nashville. Certain primary brain tumors, most of them relatively rare, can seed cancer cells in the leptomeninges as well.

Brain Metastases

Surgery

Innovative surgical techniques have made it possible to resect metastatic brain lesions that previously would have been declared inoperable and treated with radiation to the entire brain. According to Dr. Steven Rosen, director of Chicago's Lurie Comprehensive Cancer Center, "Now surgery may be the first consideration for metastatic brain cancer. There is good evidence that an aggressive strategy benefits a patient's quality of life more than a mere palliative approach." About one in four people with secondary brain deposits undergo resection followed by whole-brain radiotherapy. The operation is safe, with a mortality rate of less than 3 percent.

When weighing whether to proceed with surgery or with whole-brain radiation therapy, a neurologic oncologist takes the following factors into account:

**BRAIN METASTASES/
Surgical Procedures**

For a description of *craniotomy*
to remove a tumor from the
brain, see "Brain Cancers/Sur-
gical Procedures," page 499.

Has the primary tumor spread to areas other than the brain? "If someone had widely metastatic cancer," explains Dr. Rosen, "we might not be as aggressive with treatment as we would if they had metastasis to the brain only."

How much time has elapsed since the primary cancer was diagnosed and the secondary disease in the brain detected? In a study of cancer patients over a six-year period, those who didn't develop cerebral metastases for at least a year after the initial diagnosis lived significantly longer than patients whose cancer disseminated to the central nervous system within one year. The interval between diagnosis and CNS metastasis tends to be longest for melanoma and carcinomas of the breast and colon.

How is the patient's overall health? And how severe are the patient's neurological symptoms? One criterion in selecting candidates for brain surgery is the person's estimated life span. For instance, at Houston's M. D. Anderson Cancer Center, patients must be expected to live for at least four months after the operation in order to be considered.

A patient's level of neurological function suggests how well or how poorly he may fare postsurgically. In general, people who have minimal neurological symptoms (meaning they can essentially care for themselves, perhaps with occasional assistance) live longer. Yet the presence of neurological deficits doesn't necessarily eliminate brain surgery as an option, because the procedure frequently restores many lost abilities. To help gauge a person's prospective recovery, some centers administer *corticosteroid* drugs beforehand. A marked improvement in neurological function is taken as a favorable sign and may tip the balance in favor of surgery.

Does the patient have one or more secondary brain lesions? Roughly half of all tumors that spread to the brain form a single malignant mass—carcinomas of the kidney, colon, and lung (nonsmall-cell) in particular. According to Dr. Michael Gruber of New York University Medical Center, as long as a patient is in good health and the primary cancer is contained, "physicians should be very aggressive in trying to remove a solitary metastasis."

Primary melanoma and cancers of the breast and lung (small-cell) tend to produce multiple cerebral metastases. As a general rule, surgery may still be attempted for up to four secondary tumors. To remove only some of the deposits has no effect on prolonging life. However, if all of the lesions are successfully resected, the survival benefit is virtually equivalent to that for surgery to excise an isolated cancer.

How responsive is the primary cancer to nonsurgical therapies? Brain metastases that originated in the testicle, lung (small-cell), or lymphatic system are highly sensitive to radiotherapy and chemotherapy; therefore, one or both modalities are often used in lieu of surgery. The opposite is true of secondary cerebral tumors from the kidney, soft tissue, or melanoma, all of which are resistant to radiation. Breast and non-small-cell lung carcinomas typically call for a combination of surgery and radiation.

Is the lesion(s) surgically accessible? As with primary brain tumors, says Dr. Rosen, "there are certain areas that are not safe for operating. A surgical procedure could rob the patient of brain function." The *brain stem,* the *thalamus* (a relay terminal for body sensations, located at the base of the cerebrum), and the *basal ganglia* (areas of gray matter, made up of nerve cells) are usually considered off-limits to surgery. Other metastases may be situated too deep within the brain or too close to parts of the brain that regulate vital functions, such as speech or movement, to chance an operation.

Radiation Therapy

The high rate of complications from irradiating the entire brain has led radiation oncologists to reconsider the long-standing practice of administering whole-brain radiation therapy after surgery. "Among the patients we would consider not giving whole-brain irradiation are those with metastatic renal-cell carcinoma or melanoma, which are relatively resistant to radiation," says neurosurgeon Frederick Lang of the M. D. Anderson Cancer Center in Houston. Some cancer centers now limit its routine use to people with multiple secondary brain lesions. In that situation, the likelihood of a recurrence in the brain is great enough to justify risking radiation-induced brain impairment. In spite of its potential hazards, whole-brain irradiation is still the primary therapy for three in four people with cerebral metastases. "If you're not getting whole-brain irradiation after surgery," says Dr. Lang, "that is a deviation from the standard of treatment, and you should ask the doctor to explain why it's not being given."

In a study conducted at the University of Kentucky Medical Center in Lexington, ninety-five patients underwent surgery to remove a single metastatic cancer from the brain. Forty-nine received radiation immediately; the other forty-six had no further therapy. The group that was administered postoperative radiation exhibited far lower rates of the cancer's recurring either in the original site (just 10 percent, as compared to 46 percent among the surgery-only group) or in another part of the brain (18 percent versus 70 percent). Forty-four percent of the participants in the observation group eventually succumbed to complications brought on by the secondary brain cancer, whereas only 14 percent in the radiation group died of neurologic causes. They also lived a good deal longer. However, the men and women treated with surgery and radiation were nearly twice as likely to die of their primary cancer, so that overall the benefit from postoperative irradiation amounted to an additional five weeks of life.

Stereotactic Radiosurgery—Stereotactic radiosurgery, described in more detail on page 508, attacks tumors from many angles with pencil-thin shafts of radiation. Minimally invasive, it can eradicate metastases in the most remote regions of the brain while sparing vital structures, all in a single treatment.

Nevertheless, conventional surgery remains the accepted technique for removing solitary secondary lesions. For one thing, stereotactic radiosurgery is effective only against small cancers. There are other drawbacks as well: Unlike surgery, its effects are not immediate. Nor does it provide pathologists with a tissue specimen for confirming the diagnosis. (As many as one in ten people with advanced cancer have a brain mass that upon being biopsied is found to be either a primary tumor or an abscess.) Currently, stereotactic radiosurgery is reserved for metastases that are inaccessible to the surgeon's scalpel or for patients whose health precludes craniotomy.

Chemotherapy

Chemotherapy has a limited role in treating cerebral metastases, for the same reasons that hamper its effectiveness against primary brain cancer. "Most types of tumors that spread to the brain are not very responsive to chemotherapy," explains Dr. Rosen. There are several exceptions. When set against chemosensitive primary cancers (breast, small-cell lung carcinoma, testicular, lymphomas), anticancer drugs can induce complete remissions.

As in primary brain cancer, oncologists face the dilemma of how to traverse the *blood-brain barrier*, the network of cells and blood vessels that prevents most substances in the circulation from reaching the brain. The approximately half dozen institutions to offer *blood-brain-barrier-disruption therapy* for certain primary brain cancers also do so for secondary cerebral tumors, "particularly when there's a tumor in the brain but no disease elsewhere in the body," says Dr. Edward Neuwelt of Oregon Health Sciences University Hospital in Portland. Dr. Neuwelt, a neurosurgeon, developed this technique for overcoming the

---

**BRAIN METASTASES/
Drug Therapy**

- cyclophosphamide
- fluorouracil
- methotrexate
- tamoxifen (H)

(H) = hormonal therapy

---

protective barrier. With the patient having been put to sleep, a sugar called mannitol is injected into one of the blood vessels that feed the brain. The medical team then has a thirty-minute window in which to deliver the anticancer drug before gaps in the barricade close off.

Leptomeningeal Metastases

Symptoms of leptomeningeal metastases include pain, headache, difficulty in walking, loss of bladder and bowel control, confusion, seizures, memory loss, and mood changes. "With such a tremendous spectrum of symptoms," says Dr. Paul Moots, "it frequently goes unidentified for quite a while. Usually, the diagnosis is made by performing a spinal tap or a cisternal puncture and detecting tumor cells in the cerebrospinal fluid."

Involvement of the leptomeninges often occurs in conjunction with widespread metastasis to other organs. In view of the fact that therapy is rarely if ever curative, says Dr. Moots, a neurologic oncologist, "sometimes it is appropriate *not* to treat these patients other than palliatively."

Radiation Therapy and Intrathecal Chemotherapy

Surgery does not figure in the treatment of leptomeningeal metastases, which are diffuse by nature. A single lesion, says Dr. Moots, "is really quite the oddity. Normally, the spectrum runs from patients with two, three, or four pea-sized nodules scattered throughout the membranes, to those who have too many to count. Then there are people whose entire leptomeninges are coated with a frosting of tumor cells, from the head to the bottom of the spine."

Symptomatic disease is typically treated with external-beam radiation followed by chemotherapy, irrespective of the type of primary cancer. "The radiation can be given either to the whole brain or to the area that's producing the symptoms," explains Dr. Moots. "In some instances, we irradiate the brain and the entire spine, because that happens to be the distribution of the tumor cells."

Chemotherapy may sometimes be administered systemically, but most of the time it is injected directly into the cerebrospinal fluid. This can be done through one of two routes. The needle is inserted either between the vertebrae of the lower spine and into the subarachnoid space *(intrathecally)* or into a small reservoir that has been surgically implanted below the scalp *(intraventricularly)*. A thin tube conveys the drug to one of the fluid-filled ventricles in the brain.

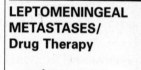

LEPTOMENINGEAL METASTASES/ Drug Therapy

- methotrexate
- cytarabine
- thiotepa
- mercaptopurine

Most cancer-killing agents are too toxic to be given safely via the cerebrospinal fluid. Oncologists rely mainly on methotrexate and cytarabine (also known as ara-C; brand name: Cytosar-U). As with metastatic tumors of the brain, secondary cancers from the breast, lung (small-cell), and lymphatic system are sensitive to these and the few other medicines available for intrathecal or intraventricular injection. Leukemia, too, responds to chemotherapy.

CNS Prophylaxis—"With several hematologic malignancies," says Dr. Moots, "involvement of the leptomeninges is so common that we treat the brain and spinal-cord meninges prophylactically," meaning before symptoms emerge. Lymphoblastic lymphoma, Burkitt's lymphoma, and acute lymphocytic leukemia (ALL) fall into this category. According to the National Cancer Institute, preventive therapy takes one of several forms: for metastatic acute leukemia, intrathecal methotrexate and cranial irradiation, *or* intrathecal or intraventricular methotrexate alone, *or* high-dose systemic methotrexate alone; for metastatic lymphomas, intrathecal chemotherapy and high-dose systemic methotrexate.

The same protocols are used to treat confirmed CNS metastases from ALL and acute myeloid leukemia (AML). When lymphomas infiltrate the membranes, standard therapy consists of cranial irradiation and intrathecal methotrexate. Once the cerebrospinal fluid tests negative for cancer cells, patients receive monthly injections of methotrexate, or methotrexate alternating with cytarabine, for one year.

OTHER THERAPIES THAT MAY BE USED IN THE TREATMENT OF BRAIN AND LEPTOMENINGEAL METASTASES

Steroid Therapy/Shunt Surgery (palliative treatment)—A buildup of water in the brain, or *hydrocephalus,* is a common complication of CNS metastases. The cancer may block the channels that carry the cerebrospinal fluid. Or it may damage the protective linings of cerebral blood vessels, permitting substances that would normally be filtered out to enter the brain. In response, the brain produces more fluid to dilute these substances. Either way, brain tissue expands dangerously against the unyielding skull.

Corticosteroid drugs such as dexamethasone (Decadron) and prednisone (Deltasone) usually bring down the swelling within twenty-four hours. Another way to relieve *cerebral edema* is to surgically implant a tube called a *shunt* "to release the pressure and drain off the extra fluid," says Dr. Moots. The procedure is performed under general anesthesia and requires a hospital stay of three to five days.

Interstitial Radiation Therapy—Surgically placing a radioactive material directly into a tumor may be an option for patients with a single metastatic cranial lesion, particularly if it is one of the cancers known not to respond to radiotherapy. Interstitial radiation can be given to men and women who have undergone external-beam irradiation to the brain.

Hyperfractionated Radiation Therapy (investigational)—Radiation oncologists are experimenting with delivering external-beam radiation two or three times a day instead of the conventional once-a-day treatments.

◆ *Ask your doctor about these and any other investigational therapies that might benefit you.*

Metastatic Cancer of the Liver

CANCERS THAT FREQUENTLY SPREAD TO THE LIVER
  ▪ Colon and rectal ▪ Lung ▪ Breast ▪ Stomach ▪
  Lymphomas ▪ Pancreatic ▪ Small intestine

The liver is a common site for metastases—especially from the large organs of the abdomen, whose blood passes through it on the return trip to the heart. When metastasis from the gastrointestinal tract is confined to the liver, as often happens, "it is worthwhile to treat aggressively, if possible, with surgery," says Dr. John Butler, chief of surgical oncology at the Chao Family Comprehensive Cancer Center at Irvine in Orange, California. "There are cases where secondary liver cancer has been controlled for long periods of time by chemotherapy, but by and large, if you look at who has survived metastatic disease in the liver for more than five years, the overwhelming majority have done so due to liver-resection surgery."

Surgery

"If patients are carefully selected for the operation," continues Dr. Butler, "we can achieve five-year survival rates on the order of 30 to 50 percent. By 'carefully selected,' I mean that the primary tumor is controlled; the liver is the sole site of metastatic disease; and the patient is a reasonable candidate for surgery."

Although this criterion applies to all types of cancers, most operations to remove liver metastases are performed for stage IV (Dukes D) colorectal cancer. Cells that shed to the liver usually form multiple tumors. As a rule, hepatic resection can be performed so long as the organ bears no more than three metastatic lesions. Approximately one in five of these patients will be cured, even if they have relapsed. Postoperative intra-arterial chemotherapy, explained below, may help lower the odds of a recurrence.

> **LIVER METASTASES/ Surgical Procedures**
>
> For a description of hepatic resection, or *partial hepatectomy*, to remove the cancerous portion of the liver, see "Liver Cancer/Surgical Procedures," page 475.

Cryosurgery—Men and women with unresectable colorectal metastases limited to the liver may qualify for cryosurgery. In one study of 136 volunteers, patients lived for an average of two and a half years following the procedure, and five-year survival rates as high as 20 percent have been reported. Cryosurgery, carried out using a liquid-nitrogen probe instead of a knife, has about the same complication rate as liver-resection surgery.

Chemotherapy

Combination chemotherapy can produce cures in advanced lymphomas and testicular cancer of the liver (the latter of which is seldom seen). Anticancer drugs have also demonstrated activity against lesions that originated in the breast and the lung (small-cell). Although the agents usually shrink the tumors, rarely do they induce complete remissions.

Inoperable liver metastases from the colon or rectum may be treated with systemic fluorouracil (5-FU) given alone or in conjunction with *intra-arterial chemotherapy,* a method of targeting drugs to the cancer. Liver tumors derive most of their blood supply from the *hepatic artery.* By slowly infusing one or more agents directly into this large vessel, oncologists are able to deliver a high dose of cancer-killing medicine to the lesion. Relatively little makes its way to healthy liver tissue, which receives its blood from the portal vein, not the hepatic artery.

**LIVER METASTASES/
Drug Therapy**

- cisplatin
- doxorubicin
- floxuridine
- fluorouracil

A variety of agents may be used for intra-arterial chemotherapy (also referred to as *regional chemotherapy* or *hepatic-artery infusion),* including cisplatin (brand name: Platinol), doxorubicin (Adriamycin), and floxuridine (FUDR). "FUDR has an advantage in that the vast majority of it is taken up on its first pass through the liver," says Dr. Butler, "so patients get little systemic toxicity." In other words, milder side effects. The tumor response rates from hepatic infusion are far higher than those achieved with systemic therapy, although this has yet to translate into improved longevity.

OTHER THERAPIES THAT MAY BE USED IN THE TREATMENT
OF LIVER METASTASES

Arterial Embolization (investigational)—Embolization similarly attempts to minimize the system-wide side effects of anticancer drugs. In addition, it deprives the metastatic tumor of blood. Doxorubicin, fluorouracil, or another agent is infused into the hepatic artery along with a material that obstructs, or *occludes,* the vessel. Blood can't enter; the chemotherapy saturates the tumors. The infusions are repeated once a month until the liver enzymes normalize, which can take up to eighteen months.

Chemoembolization has been used experimentally as a treatment for several secondary cancers of the liver. In a study at the University of Pennsylvania Cancer Center, the procedure doubled the life expectancy of patients with colon cancer that had metastasized to the liver, from one year to two years.

Other techniques intended to close off the hepatic artery—*hepatic-artery ligation* and percutaneous *alcohol ablation therapy*—are among the options that may be offered to patients diagnosed with the relatively rare *malignant carcinoid syndrome,* which almost always includes liver metastases.

See "Malignant Carcinoid Syndrome," page 582.

◆ *Ask your doctor about this and any other investigational therapies that might benefit you.*

Metastatic Cancer of the Lung

CANCERS THAT FREQUENTLY SPREAD TO THE LUNG

- Breast - Colon and rectal - Stomach - Pancreatic - Kidney - Melanoma - Testicular - Soft-tissue sarcomas - Lymphomas - Leukemia

As many as two in five patients believed to have secondary tumors in one lung *(unilateral metastases)* are found to have lesions in both lungs *(bilateral metastases)*. Often the new growths broke away from a tumor in the opposite lung. The saclike organs are frequent harbors for metastases borne by the circulation because all blood flows through the lungs to receive a fresh supply of oxygen.

Chemotherapy and Hormonal Therapy

Since metastases of the lung behave similarly to the original tumor, "ordinarily we treat them the same way we would treat any stage IV cancer from that particular primary site," explains Dr. Paul A. Bunn, Jr., a lung-cancer specialist, and director of the University of Colorado Cancer Center in Denver. "For example, if breast cancer went to the lung, and the patient was a postmenopausal woman whose tumor tested positive for hormone receptors, we'd consider hormone therapy." Colon cancer, another carcinoma that commonly spreads to the lung, does not respond to hormonal agents. "In that situation," he continues, "we'd typically rely on the same chemotherapy that's used to treat primary colon cancer."

Surgery

"The most complicated issue in metastatic lung cancer," says Dr. Bunn, "is determining when metastases should be removed surgically." Involvement of both lungs doesn't necessarily rule out *pulmonary metastasectomy*, although bilateral disease is considered a less favorable indicator of how well a patient can be expected to fare. Besides the person's general health, other pressing questions need to be answered before a doctor would recommend the operation:

How many metastases are in the lung?

LUNG METASTASES/ Surgical Procedures

Thoracotomy: surgical removal of metastases from one lung (unilateral) or both lungs (bilateral).
Average hospital stay:

- **Unilateral thoracotomy: 4–7 days**
- **Bilateral thoracotomy: 5–10 days**

Three or fewer tumors is preferable to four or more. "But it's possible to remove many pulmonary metastases," says Dr. Bunn. "One of my patients had fifty-eight taken out at once."

Has the cancer spread anywhere else in the body? Soft-tissue sarcomas metastasize almost exclusively to the lung and can sometimes be cured by treating the primary tumor and resecting the pulmonary metastases.

Is the tumor slow-growing or fast-growing? The longer the interval between the time the primary cancer was treated and the lung metastases detected, the better the chances that surgery will lead to long-term survival. Another prognostic indicator is the time it takes secondary lesions in the lung to double in size. In a study of patients with metastatic soft-tissue sarcoma of the lung, those whose cancers took forty days or more to double in size lived more than twice as long as those whose cancer doubled in under forty days. Kidney cancers and other primary tumors sometimes spawn slow-developing lung metastases. Pulmonary metastasectomy may not be curative, but it can extend patients' lives.

Can the metastases be removed completely? In order for the surgery to be beneficial, there must be reasonable confidence that all disease in the lung can be successfully resected.

If you're a candidate for surgery, consider finding a surgeon experienced in a relatively new technique to operate on both lungs, nicknamed the *"clamshell" incision.* "It used to be that when a patient had bilateral lung metastases, we'd do what's called a *median sternotomy* and cut the sternum [breastbone] in half," says Dr. Bunn. In the clamshell operation, "we make a clamshell-shaped incision just below both breasts." This affords the surgeon better access to any disease that might be present in the lower sections, or *lobes.* (The medical term for this procedure, just so you know, is *bilateral anterior thoracotomies with transverse sternotomy.*)

Sometimes bilateral metastases are removed in two separate surgeries. First one lung is operated on. Then following approximately two weeks of recuperation, the patient checks back into the hospital for a unilateral thoracotomy of the other lung.

◆ *Ask your doctor about any investigational therapies that might benefit you.*

Chapter Seven

What You Can Expect
During Treatment

Circumstances prevented me from learning about my cancer treatment ahead of time. When I checked into the hospital for what was presumed to be an emergency appendectomy, I fully expected to be home within a matter of days. Two or three weeks of recuperation, I thought, and I could put this relatively minor incident behind me. Was *I* in for a surprise.

I wish I'd had the opportunity to prepare for the ordeal, mentally and otherwise. Most patients who have faced a major medical treatment would probably agree that having a sense of what to expect eased their fears and anxiety. If you're the type of person who finds it comforting to visualize potentially stressful situations beforehand, ask the doctor or nurse to describe in detail the procedure to you so that you can rehearse the scene in your mind.

Knowing in advance what the coming weeks or months may bring also enables you *and your family* to get a head start on rearranging your lives to accommodate this unwelcome intruder. That might mean recruiting neighbors and friends to drive the kids here and there during the month that you'll be recovering from abdominal surgery. Or what if you have an important project due at work around the time that you'll be undergoing six weeks of radiotherapy? It's helpful to be aware that the fatigue that frequently accompanies radiation often comes on toward the end of treatment and may linger for weeks afterward. Knowing this, you'll be better able to pace yourself.

In this chapter, we walk you through the most common forms of cancer therapy—surgery, radiation, chemotherapy, and bone-marrow transplantation—and acquaint you with the potential side effects of each. We've also suggested questions you can ask your doctor or nurse prior to the procedure. Chapter Eight describes the steps you and your medical team may take to prevent or arrest the symptoms and complications of cancer treatment and the disease itself.

Surgery: What You Can Expect

Questions to Ask . . . Before Surgery

- Please describe the operation to me in detail. Is there a diagram or an illustration that you could show me to help me understand what will happen during the surgery?

- Do you recommend that I bank blood beforehand?

- What form of anesthesia will I receive? Local? Regional? General?

- Where will I most likely wake up from the operation? In my hospital room? The recovery room? The intensive-care unit?

- How should I expect to feel afterward? If I have pain, what can you do to relieve it?

- Would you suggest that I order a private-duty nurse for the first twenty-four hours after surgery? If so, who at the hospital can help me make these arrangements?

- How should I expect to look after the operation? Will I have tubes or drains in me?

- Will I have a scar? If so, where? What will it look like?

- Will a skin graft or reconstructive surgery be necessary? Will this be done at the same time as the operation to remove the cancer or at a later date?

- How long do you anticipate that I will be hospitalized?

- What potential complications should I be aware of once I return home? What symptoms should I report to you?

- Do you anticipate my needing on a temporary basis either skilled home-nursing care or a home health aide? Will you prescribe these services for me, so that my health-insurance plan pays for them?

- When will I be able to resume my normal activities?

- Will I have to undergo any rehabilitation, such as occupational therapy, physical therapy, speech-language therapy, and/or pulmonary-rehabilitation therapy? If so, can you refer me to an experienced therapist or rehabilitation facility?

See "Occupational Therapists/Physical Therapists," "Pulmonary-Rehabilitation Therapists," and "Speech-Language Pathologists" in Appendix B.

- When do I need to schedule a follow-up appointment?

- What can I do to help ensure a safe recovery?

- Are there any exercises that you recommend I do?

Blood Donations

Unless your case is considered an emergency, definitive cancer surgery is typically scheduled within several weeks of a diagnosis. Prior to the operation, ask your surgeon if he recommends that you have some of your blood stored, in the event that you need a transfusion during surgery.

Not all cancer operations warrant autologous blood donation. Three frequently performed procedures—mastectomy, total hysterectomy, and transurethral resection of the prostate—all carry a low risk of significant blood loss. Liver resection, radical hysterectomy, and radical prostatectomy to remove the prostate, on the other hand, are among the surgeries associated with a higher-than-average loss of blood. *Intraoperative blood collection,* a technique for continuously recycling blood shed during the procedure, has eliminated the need for transfusions in many operations.

Age has no bearing on who can or can't bank their own blood. However, fragile health or an infection may rule out a person as a candidate. The time element, too, may render autologous donations unfeasible. The window of opportunity opens six weeks before surgery—because blood can be stored in its liquid form for up to forty-two days—and closes three days before the operation, to give the body sufficient time to recover. Normally, one *unit* of blood is drawn per week. However, if time is running out before surgery, this can be done every seventy-two hours, provided your doctor approves. During the period that you are giving blood, you may be prescribed an iron supplement to help restore depleted red blood cells.

Being reinfused with your own blood as opposed to blood from a donor safeguards you from exposure to blood-borne diseases such as the human immunodeficiency virus (HIV, the precursor to AIDS) and viral hepatitis. But given the tight screening process for donor blood in the United States, the odds of contracting an illness from a single unit of transfused allogeneic blood are negligible:

HIV: 1 in 1 million
Hepatitis C: less than 1 in 100,000
Hepatitis B: 1 in 66,000

Some patients, unable to stockpile blood before an operation and hoping to minimize their chances of incurring disease, ask relatives and friends with compatible blood types to donate expressly for them. You may be surprised to learn that such *directed donations* "may be less safe than anonymous donations," says Dr. Visalem Chandrasekarian, chief for the division of blood banking at Long Island Jewish Medical Center in Lake Success, New York.

The reason, she explains, is that "most volunteer donors are repeat donors; their blood has been tested multiple times before. Most designated donors, though, are giving blood for the first time, so there is a higher incidence of screening picking up an infectious marker." The lesson, in this era of AIDS and other sexually transmitted diseases, is that you never truly know another person's sexual history.

Your surgeon's office can help arrange autologous or directed blood donations. Or you can call the hospital *blood bank* yourself.

Preoperative Testing

Assuming that you've completed all of your tests to clinically stage the extent of the cancer, only routine exams should be necessary. Typically, presurgical testing consists of a thorough medical history, blood and laboratory tests, and, for patients over age forty, a chest X ray and an electrocardiogram (EKG) to evaluate the heart.

If your doctor admits you to the hospital the day before surgery, these procedures are usually performed after you've checked in. One growing trend in medicine is for patients to report to the hospital mere hours before being wheeled off to the operating room. In that situation, the tests are conducted on an outpatient basis in the days leading up to the operation. Men and women scheduled for *ambulatory surgery*—going home the same day—generally complete their testing the morning of the procedure.

A Visit from the Anesthesiologist

The *anesthesiologist* relies on information from the preoperative tests when calculating how much anesthetic to administer during the operation. You can expect to meet this specialist the day of your pre-op testing, although sometimes the interview takes place over the phone.

Besides seeing to it that you feel no pain during surgery, the anesthesiologist is responsible for monitoring your vital functions and correcting any problems that might arise. In order for him to accurately tailor the anesthesia to you, be prepared to answer the following questions.

- Do you have any allergies?
- Have you ever suffered an allergic reaction to anesthesia before?
- Do you have any medical conditions in addition to cancer, such as heart disease, diabetes, hypertension, and so on?
- Do you smoke tobacco, drink alcohol, or use any illicit drugs?
- Are you currently on any medications? If so, at what dosage? If you're not sure what you're taking or how much, bring all your medicine bottles with you. That includes over-the-counter drugs as well as prescription medications.

The table below summarizes the four major types of anesthesia. For some surgeries, you may be offered a choice of techniques. At the Lombardi Cancer Center, for instance, selected women undergoing lumpectomy or mastectomy can opt for intravenous sedation and a regional nerve block in lieu of general anesthesia.

TABLE 7.1 Methods of Anesthesia

Local anesthesia—A small area of tissue is numbed, as when excising a small melanoma of the skin. The injected anesthetic prevents the nerves from transmitting the pain impulse to the brain. Only local anesthesia may be given without a member of the anesthesiology team present.

Monitored anesthesia care—local anesthesia supplemented by systemic pain relievers and sedation.

Regional anesthesia—blocks pain throughout a larger region of the body. A local anesthetic is injected near a major nerve serving the area to be operated on; for example, in the arm, leg, hand, or foot. Or a tube, placed into the back, delivers small, precise doses of a local painkiller near the spinal cord, in what is referred to as *epidural block* or a *spinal block.* Although you are conscious, most likely you'll be given a sedative to make you comfortably drowsy and cloud your memory. You should have little or no recollection of the procedure afterward.

General anesthesia—Most cancer operations call for general anesthesia, which renders patients unconscious and unaware of pain or other sensations. It also induces a temporary state of amnesia.

The anesthetic may be injected intravenously or inhaled as a vapor through a mask. If you're slated for same-day surgery, you'll be administered one of the newer shorter-acting anesthetics that wear off more quickly and are less likely to cause nausea and prolonged drowsiness. Once you are asleep, a flexible *endotracheal tube* is fed down your throat and into your windpipe to maintain an airway.

The anesthesiologist juggles a variety of agents during the operation. In addition, he may administer drugs that regulate your heart rate and rhythm, blood pressure, breathing, kidney function, and brain activity to keep all systems functioning normally.

Once the surgery is completed, anesthesia is discontinued. You may receive still other medications intended to reverse the effects of the anesthesia and return you to consciousness.

Medical Terms You're Likely to Hear

NPO: a doctor's order denoting no food or liquid. The initials are an abbreviation for the Latin words *nil per os,* meaning "nothing by mouth."

Preoperative Precautions

Wherever you spend the night prior to surgery, your doctor will probably give you the following instructions:

1. Do not eat *or drink* after midnight. Most operations require that the stomach be empty so that food or liquid isn't accidentally regurgitated into the lungs.
2. Do not smoke after midnight. Nicotine interferes with the blood's ability to clot.
3. Do not chew gum after midnight.
4. Take only those medications that have been approved by your physician or the anesthesiologist.
5. You may be required to take a laxative and/or an enema in order to thoroughly cleanse the bowel.
6. Bathe or shower the night before your operation.
7. If you shave, do so the night before surgery; you may not get another opportunity for several days.

The Day of Surgery

Patients admitted the day of their operation are usually sent to a presurgical area where nurses and other medical personnel finalize any details. Otherwise, if you spent the night in the hospital, there is little else to do but wait to be wheeled into surgery. Family members will probably be invited to sit in a special waiting room. Once the surgical team has outfitted you with assorted monitoring devices and inserted an intravenous (IV) line in your arm, anesthesia is administered and the procedure begins.

Afterward, you are transferred to either the *intensive-care unit* (ICU) or the *recovery room.* A nurse will check on you regularly and monitor your vital signs. Most cancer patients will have received intravenous sedation or general anesthesia. As you gradually regain consciousness, you're liable to feel groggy. If you are in any pain at all, let the staff know, so they can dispense *analgesic* medication as necessary.

The endotracheal tube often irritates the throat. Sucking on throat lozenges should ease the soreness within a day or two. A dry mouth is another common aftereffect of general anesthesia.

Depending on the nature of the surgery, you may wake up to find tubes emanating from your body: the IV, which is keeping you hydrated, and perhaps drainage tubes for suctioning off blood and fluids from the surgical site. Patients who've had throat surgery experience swelling that prevents them from eating for a few days, so they typically have a soft *nasogastric tube* (NG tube, for short) inserted through a nostril and into the stomach for feeding purposes. Following prostate-removal surgery, men can expect to temporarily have an indwelling *urinary catheter* drain their urine into a plastic bag. The thin, flexible tube is introduced into the penis's urethral opening and advanced until it reaches the bladder. Then a small bulb is inflated in the bladder to hold the instrument in place. Any operation expected to last several hours generally requires the placement of a urinary catheter.

If you are to go home the same day, typically one to four hours postsurgery, you *must* have someone accompany you to the hospital. A patient's not having an appointed driver is grounds for canceling the operation. The lone exception would be if you had local anesthesia only. Furthermore, it is recommended that a family member or friend stay with you until the next day.

During the first twenty-four hours after regional or general anesthesia, do not operate a motor vehicle or dangerous machinery. Because it's impossible to predict how clearheaded you'll be, "don't do anything that requires a great deal of thought," advises Dr. Margaret Pratila, an anesthesiologist at New York's Memorial Sloan-Kettering Cancer Center. "This is not the time to sign a will or give away property!"

What if you don't have anyone at home to assist you? Some medical institutions provide postoperative recovery facilities or home nurses. To find out if a hospital offers these services, call its department of social work or ask a member of your surgeon's office staff.

Your Recovery

Between the physical trauma of surgery and the effects of lying on the operating table and in bed, a major operation can impair virtually every system. During abdominal surgery, for instance, manipulation of the intestines brings peristalsis to a halt for a few days. *Peristalsis* is the rhythmic muscular contractions that propel food through the digestive tract. Narcotic pain medications also make the bowel sluggish. Patients are temporarily restricted to a *clear-liquid diet* consisting of water, juices, tea, coffee, gelatin, ginger ale, seltzer, and fat-free broth. It isn't until the bowels "wake up" and patients pass gas or stool that they can move on to heartier liquids and then to soft, easily digested foods before finally resuming their normal diet.

Two potentially serious postsurgical complications involve the respiratory tract. Inactivity and the pain from the incision can make it painful to breathe deeply. "When a patient doesn't fully expand his lungs," explains Dr. Marie Pennanen, a breast surgeon at the Lombardi Cancer Center, "the tiny air sacs in the lungs can collapse upon themselves. This is called *atelectasis.* Secretions then accumulate there, and that can set the stage for pneumonia."

> **Potential Side Effects of Surgery**
>
> - **Pain at the incision site**
> - **Shallow breathing**
> - **Constipation and gas pain**
> - **Appetite loss**
> - **Indigestion**
> - **Venous thrombosis**
> - **Infection**
> - **Bleeding or discharge from the surgical wound**

Major surgery and immobilization also predispose you to the formation of a blood clot in the leg, or *venous thrombosis.* "The danger there," says Dr. Pennanen, "is that the clot will dislodge and ultimately plug up one of the vessels that supply the lungs." The hallmarks of a *pulmonary embolism* are chest pain and labored breathing. If clot-dissolving intravenous drugs aren't administered promptly (typically the *blood thinner* heparin, or, for patients in severe respiratory distress, a more potent *thrombolytic* agent such as streptokinase), an embolism in the lungs can be fatal.

> **Medical Terms You're Likely to Hear**
>
> **Ambulatory: able to walk; not confined to bed.**

Exercise and gravity are two of your staunchest allies in helping to reduce the likelihood of atelectasis and venous thrombosis, not to mention indigestion, constipation, and urinary-tract infections. The day after surgery—possibly the same day—the nurses will help you out of bed and assist you as you pad around the hospital corridors. If you're not ambulatory just yet, a nurse or physical therapist will demonstrate exercises you can perform in bed or she'll manipulate your limbs for you. The goal is to improve circulation, which promotes quicker healing, and to keep muscles and joints from atrophying. Whenever resting in bed or in a chair, elevate your legs; this prevents blood from pooling in the lower extremities.

You'll also be encouraged to cough, to rid the respiratory tract of mucus, and to practice inhaling and exhaling deeply. "Most of our surgical patients," says Dr. Pennanen, "are given a small plastic device called an *incentive spirometer,* which measures how deep a breath they are taking."

When You're Discharged from the Hospital

Your doctor will send you home with various instructions: how to relieve pain, which medications to avoid, and when you can resume vigorous exercise, driving, and other daily activities. You'll also be instructed to notify your physician immediately of any evidence that the surgical wound has become infected:

- Pain, swelling, redness, or warmth around the incision
- Bleeding or drainage from the surgical site
- Other signs of infection, such as a temperature exceeding 101 degrees, headache, aching muscles, dizziness, nausea, vomiting, and chills

Radiation Therapy: What You Can Expect

Questions to Ask . . . Before Radiation Therapy

- How will the radiation be administered? External beam? A radioactive implant?
- For how many weeks will I receive radiation? How many treatments per week?
- How can I expect to feel during treatment and in the weeks afterward?
- Will I be able to continue my normal activities?
- What side effects may occur from the radiation and how are they managed?
- What can I do to take care of myself?
- If you are having radiation to the head and neck: Do you recommend that I have a dental checkup before radiation begins?
- If you are having radiation to the pelvis or to the reproductive or-

gans: Will the treatment affect my sex life or my ability to bear or father children?

External-Beam Radiation

Simulation

Before your first treatment, you visit the department of radiation oncology for a planning session. This is known as a *simulation*. You lie on a table, just as you will during the actual procedure, while the radiation therapist uses a special X-ray machine to outline the treatment field, or *port*. From this information, one or more lead shields, called *blocks,* are custom-molded. During each treatment, the blocks slide into the head of the radiation machine and contour the beam to the precise dimensions of the area to be irradiated, thus protecting as much healthy tissue as possible. Other molds may be fashioned from plastic or plaster, to help you to remain in the same position day after day.

To further ensure that the radiation is targeted accurately, the therapist will mark the skin around the treatment site with a felt pen. Corresponding marks are made on any molds that will be used. It's important that you not wash off the temporary "bull's-eye," says Dr. Christine Berg, director of the breast radiation-therapy program at the Lombardi Cancer Center. "Patients can bathe and shower while they're undergoing radiation; we just ask them not to soap or scrub the area." Should the mark begin to fade, don't attempt to do any "touch-up work" yourself; let one of the nurses or technicians reapply it. The marks can rub off on clothing, incidentally, so you might want to consider wearing older, discardable garments until you're through with treatment.

Many centers, including Lombardi, also permanently tattoo tiny dots around the field in India ink. "I had one done on my wrist to show to patients," says Dr. Berg, "because some get frightened when they hear the word 'tattoo.' We try to make them as unobtrusive as possible." The reason for the tattoo is this: In most cases, though not all, radiation cannot be given to the same area twice. If you were ever to develop a second cancer that required radiotherapy, Dr. Berg explains, "we would know from the tattoo where the previous radiation stopped, so that we didn't overlap the two fields."

In all, expect this initial session to last anywhere from half an hour to two hours.

A Typical Radiotherapy Treatment

Adapting your daily routine to accommodate outpatient radiation therapy is surprisingly easy. Each patient is assigned a set time, Monday through Friday. Barring an equipment malfunction or an emergency, appointments usually run according to schedule.

Eating prior to treatment poses no problem, except for patients receiving radiation to the abdomen. "Many of them feel nauseous afterward if they have food in their stomach," says Merilyn Francis, a radiation-therapy nurse at Lombardi. Should you experience queasiness, try fasting for several hours before and after each treatment. If the nausea is still a problem, ask your radiation oncologist to prescribe an antinausea medication, which you take about half an hour before your appointment.

Most days, you breeze in and out of the radiation facility in under an hour. You change into a hospital gown, if necessary, and are brought into the treatment room and assisted onto the mechanical table or into a special chair. From time to time, blood may be drawn first. This is to check your levels of white cells and platelets, which may be abnormally low during treatment.

Patients are also weighed once a week to see if they're maintaining their normal weight and getting adequate nutrition. Although some people put on pounds during therapy, it's more common to lose weight. Treatment to the chest and the head and neck may make swallowing painful, while the indigestion, nausea, and diarrhea associated with radiation to the abdomen and the pelvis can dull one's enthusiasm for eating.

It should take the radiation therapist no more than fifteen minutes to position you beneath the radiation unit, which revolves 360 degrees in order to treat from any angle. Depending on where the cancer is located, you may be lying on your side, on your back, or on your stomach. "Sometimes we take films just before we treat," says Merilyn Francis, "to make sure that the field is aligned properly." Then he closes the door behind him and heads to the brightly lit control booth. Although you are alone during the procedure, a two-way intercom allows you to communicate back and forth with the therapist, who is observing you on a closed-circuit television monitor or through the control-room window.

After all the preparation, the treatment itself can seem almost anticlimactic, lasting one to five minutes. Unlike during a diagnostic X ray, you don't have to hold your breath; just breathe naturally. The large, imposing apparatus grunts and whirs as it moves into position, but you will not hear or see the radiation beam.

"Some patients worry that they're going to get zapped by the radiation and that it's going to hurt," says nurse Francis. In fact, the delivery of the dose is completely painless. Should you feel ill or uncomfortable, though, alert the therapist. The machine can be shut off at any point.

Potential Side Effects of Radiation Therapy

One common misconception that patients have about radiotherapy, says Dr. Berg, is that its effects are systemic, like chemotherapy. Therefore, a woman about to begin radiation following a lumpectomy might fear that the treatment is going to leave her bald, all because a cousin's hair had fallen out after cranial irradiation to treat a brain tumor. Irradiating the breast does not cause hair loss. In Dr. Berg's initial consultation with patients, "I stress that many issues come up only with radiation therapy to certain sites."

General Effects

Two complications that can occur, regardless of location, are fatigue and skin irritation.

Fatigue—Beginning midway through treatment, you may find yourself feeling weary. This is an accumulative effect of the extra energy your body has been expending in order to absorb the ionizing rays and to repair damaged normal cells. The fatigue typically persists for four to six weeks following the last dose of radiation.

How You Can Help Yourself: Rest. Be sure to get plenty of sleep at night, stay active during the day, but nap whenever you feel tired. Just how much rest you'll need depends partly on the area being irradiated. According to Dr. Berg, "Radiation to the head is the most fatiguing."

See "Fatigue" in Chapter Eight, "Take Control: Managing Symptoms, Side Effects, and Complications."

Skin Irritation—About two to three weeks into radiation, the skin in the treatment area often becomes red and dry, but no more severe than a mild sunburn. The days when patients developed ulcerative "radiation burns" ended with the widespread use of the high-energy linear accelerator, introduced in the 1960s. "These machines are more deeply penetrating than the older ones," explains Dr. Berg. "They can get to the tumor and spare more of the overlying tissue."

Nurse Merilyn Francis suggests checking your skin every day. Alert the radiation-oncology department right away if the skin appears bright red or purple or if you notice any blistering, scaling or peeling, or "weeping" (that's when the skin turns moist and sore, particularly in between folds in fleshy areas). Most radiation "tans" fade away a few weeks after radiotherapy ends, even for patients who've experienced a dramatic change in their skin color.

How It Is Treated: Some hospitals treat routine skin reactions with an ointment called Aquaphor. The Lombardi Cancer Center takes a preventive approach. "Beginning with the first treatment, we have our patients apply an aloe-vera gel to the radiation site," says Francis. "It soothes the skin, and for some people it seems to cut down on the amount of irritation they have."

Should the skin show signs of breaking down, your doctor may suspend treatment for a few days to allow it to recover. "Depending on the severity, we might simply aim a fan at the area, to blow cool air on it. Or, if there's a lot of blistering, we might put on a gel-type dressing, which helps the skin to heal."

How You Can Help Yourself: Be extra kind to your skin during treatment by following these skin-care do's and don'ts:

- Wear loose-fitting, soft clothing over the area being irradiated; avoid tight garments such as girdles or shirts with snug collars. Women receiving radiotherapy to the breast might want to consider wearing a sports bra or forgoing a bra altogether.
- Don't starch your clothes or wear garments made of abrasive materials.
- Switch to a hypoallergenic perfume- and dye-free laundry deter-

gent. Don't add fabric softener to your wash or put fabric-softener sheets in your dryer.

- Choose fabrics that breathe, such as cotton. Orlon, rayon, and many other synthetics retain body heat.

- Always use lukewarm water when washing, bathing, and showering. Hot water can damage the tissue.

- Avoid extremes of temperature: no ice packs or heating pads.

- Never rub or scrub the treated skin. Wash gently, then pat it dry.

- If bandaging is necessary, substitute paper tape for adhesive tape. Apply it outside the irradiated area.

- If your head is being treated, wash your hair gently and use only baby shampoo.

- Don't shave the area without your doctor's consent. Use an electric razor only and avoid shaving lotions and hair-removal products.

- Before you venture out in the sun for more than a few minutes at a time, make sure that the treated skin is covered by lightweight clothing. Your physician may recommend smoothing on either a sunscreen containing PABA (para-aminobenzoic acid) or a sunblock with a sun-protection factor (SPF) of at least 15. An over-the-counter product, Alra, is specially formulated for people undergoing radiation therapy. Continue to protect your skin from the sun's rays for at least one year posttreatment. *Some doctors may advise avoiding sun exposure altogether during radiation treatment.*

- If you are receiving radiation to the head and neck, wear a wide-brimmed hat and a cotton shirt with a collar whenever you are out in the sun.

- Check with your doctor before using any soaps, lotions, deodorants, perfumes, powders, depilatories, petroleum jelly, or medications. Not only can these products irritate the skin and delay healing, some actually interfere with the radiation's cancer-destroying effects. *For the first two weeks following treatment, keep using a mild, hypoallergenic, perfume-free soap.*

- Instead of deodorant or powder, try cornstarch, which also helps to reduce itching. Just remember to wash off the old cornstarch before putting on the new. *Don't use any skin product the morning of a radiation treatment.*

Local Effects

Irradiation can injure any organ that happens to be in the line of fire. Damage to tissue provokes an *inflammatory response,* characterized by redness, warmth, swelling, and pain at the site of injury. The reaction can progress to *ulceration,* in which the dead tissue sloughs off, creating shallow sores.

Because inflammation also temporarily interferes with organ function, patients experience other symptoms unique to the affected part of the body. For instance, inflammation of the bowels gives rise to nausea, diarrhea, and other gastrointestinal problems, while inflammation of the lung causes coughing and difficulty in breathing.

Most inflammatory conditions brought on by radiation generally arise during weeks two or three and subside several weeks after treatment ends. In the meantime, the medical focus is on managing the symptoms. Some disorders, though, develop into chronic problems and can be potentially serious.

Radiation Mucositis—inflammation of the membranous lining *(mucosa)* of the mouth or throat, caused by radiation to the oral cavity or to the head and neck. *Mucositis* describes a virulent inflammatory reaction that can ravage the entire digestive tract, from mouth to anus. But in everyday usage, the term often refers strictly to inflammation of the mouth or throat. Your oncologist may call mouth sores by another name: *stomatitis.*

> To learn how these and other radiation-related complications are controlled, see Chapter Eight, "Take Control: Managing Symptoms, Side Effects, and Complications."

Symptoms: a red, swollen, sore mouth or throat; difficulty in swallowing and speaking; dry mouth, due to lack of saliva; altered taste, from lack of saliva and/or damaged taste buds; infections.

How It Is Treated: There is no treatment for mucositis as such; care consists of oral hygiene and relieving symptoms. Most cases resolve two to three weeks following the completion of therapy, although severe symptoms can take up to six weeks to heal.

Radiation Pneumonitis—inflammation of the lung, caused by radiation to the chest. Features usually appear two to six months after treatment.

Symptoms: fever, coughing, difficulty in breathing.

How It Is Treated: The condition may resolve on its own or progress to respiratory failure. Corticosteroid drugs can be effective, but only if they are initiated early on.

Radiation Fibrosis—permanent scarlike changes in lung tissue, caused by radiation to the chest. Fibrosis, which frequently takes one to two years to develop, can interfere with the lung's ability to furnish the body with oxygen.

Symptoms: shortness of breath upon exertion.

How It Is Treated: No treatment has proved successful. Fortunately, radiation fibrosis is usually mild, although in some patients it can culminate in chronic respiratory failure.

Radiation Enteritis—inflammation of the large and small intestines, caused by radiation to the abdomen, pelvis, or rectum. Virtually all men and women receiving radiotherapy to these areas will exhibit signs of acute enteritis during treatment or up to eight weeks later, although sometimes years pass before symptoms occur. The disorder becomes chronic in about 10 percent of patients.

Acute Symptoms: nausea and vomiting, abdominal cramping, painful bowel movements, diarrhea.

Chronic Symptoms: attacks of abdominal pain, bloody diarrhea, painful bowel movements, nausea and vomiting, weight loss.

How It Is Treated: A combination of medications, changes in diet, and rest can usually solve acute enteritis. Should the effects worsen, radiation may have to be suspended temporarily. Chronic enteritis can cause such severe intestinal damage that an operation to bypass or resect the diseased portion of the bowel may be necessary. Fortunately, in more than 98 percent of cases, the symptoms can be controlled without surgical intervention.

Radiation Proctitis—inflammation of the rectum or anus, caused by radiation to the abdomen, pelvis, or rectum. A history of hemorrhoids predisposes you to rectal irritation.

Symptoms: rectal pain, a mucuslike discharge, rectal bleeding.

How It Is Treated: Radiation proctitis often produces mild symptoms and heals on its own. If it persists, however, it can cause potentially serious bleeding. Although chronic proctitis responds poorly to local drug treatment, surgery is regarded as a last resort, due to its high rate of postoperative complications. Endoscopic laser surgery has been used successfully to stem mild to moderate bleeding.

If you have hemorrhoids, don't use ointments such as Preparation H and Anusol *before* radiation treatments.

Radiation Cystitis—inflammation of the lining of the bladder, caused by radiation to the pelvis.

Symptoms: painful or difficult urination, frequent urination, blood in the urine.

How It Is Treated: Bladder irritation due to radiation is rarely a serious problem. Should it occur, your doctor will recommend that you drink eight to ten glasses of fluid a day, particularly water and juice. Sometimes patients are prescribed *blood-pressure medications* such as terazosin (brand name: Hytrin) and doxazosin (Cardura). Both drugs relax the smooth muscle in the neck of the bladder, improving urine flow and relieving symptoms.

Effects on Fertility

Since radiation may be harmful to a fetus, women of childbearing age are advised to avoid conceiving while treatment is under way. Abstaining from sex during the five and a half weeks of therapy is one option. The other is to use birth control; discuss with your doctor which form may be preferable.

Men receiving pelvic radiation can continue to have sexual intercourse, but they or their partners should use contraception to prevent a pregnancy during this time. When the treatment field includes the testicles, the output and the effectiveness of the sperm cells *may* temporarily drop below the level at which fertilization can take place. Most of the time, sperm production rebounds within several months of treatment. If you're hoping to father a child, you might consider banking your sperm prior to the first session.

TABLE 7.2   **Potential Side Effects from Radiation Therapy**

Short-term effects typically arise during or shortly after treatment and subside within three months. They tend to be mild. *Long-term* effects, though rare, can spring up anywhere from six months to three years following radiation therapy.

Cancer of the Prostate

Short-Term	Long-Term
■ Fatigue	■ Impotence
■ Frequent, urgent urination	■ Incontinence
■ Discomfort or pain while urinating	■ Rectal bleeding
■ Bloody urine	
■ Bloody bowel movements	
■ More frequent bowel movements	
■ Diarrhea	
■ Burning and itching during bowel movements	

Cancer of the Breast

Short-Term	Long-Term
■ Fatigue	■ Breast discomfort or pain
■ Mild to moderate skin irritation	■ Swelling (may subside gradually)
■ Severe blistering (rare)	■ Decreased breast size
■ Breast swelling, discomfort, or pain	■ Increased risk of arm swelling or nerve injury due to lymph-node radiation
■ Dry cough within three months of treatment	

Cancer of the Lung

Short-Term	Long-Term
▪ Fatigue	▪ Lung scarring, causing shortness of breath (rarely may require treatment with steroids)
▪ Dry, sore throat	
▪ Difficulty swallowing, painful swallowing	
▪ Coughing with or without shortness of breath	
▪ Skin irritation	

Cancer of the Colon or Rectum

Short-Term	Long-Term
▪ Fatigue	▪ Rectal bleeding
▪ Diarrhea	▪ Fecal incontinence
▪ Abdominal pain and cramping	▪ Mucus discharge from the rectum
▪ Straining while urinating or defecating	
▪ Rectal pain	
▪ Rectal bleeding	
▪ Mucus discharge from the rectum	

Hodgkin's Disease and Non-Hodgkin's Lymphomas

Short-Term	Long-Term
Treatment to the Neck and Chest	Treatment to the Neck and Chest
▪ Fatigue	▪ Coughing
▪ Dry, sore mouth and/or throat	▪ Shortness of breath (rarely may require treatment with steroids)
▪ Difficulty swallowing	▪ Temporary tingling in arms, legs, and lower back when flexing head
▪ Dry cough	
▪ Nausea	
▪ Skin irritation	
▪ Hair loss at the nape of the neck	

Hodgkin's Disease and Non-Hodgkin's Lymphomas

Short-Term	Long-Term
Treatment to the Neck and Chest	**Treatment to the Neck and Chest**
▪ Swollen saliva glands after the first few days of treatment; subsides after several days	

Short-Term	Long-Term
Treatment to the Abdomen	**Treatment to the Abdomen**
▪ Nausea, vomiting	▪ Radiation of spleen may increase the risk of infection
▪ Diarrhea	
▪ Abdominal cramping	▪ Bowel obstruction if surgery is performed

Cancer of the Bladder

Short-Term	Long-Term
▪ Frequent urination	▪ Decreased bladder capacity causing frequent urination
▪ Difficulty starting urination	
▪ Painful urination	
▪ Diarrhea	
▪ Abdominal pain	
▪ Straining while urinating or defecating	

Melanoma

Radiation is used only for metastatic melanoma to other organs or to distant lymph nodes. Therefore, potential side effects depend on where the cancer has spread. Melanoma most often metastasizes to the brain, lung, and bone.

Cancer of the Endometrium

Short-Term	Long-Term
▪ Diarrhea	▪ Bowel obstruction
▪ Discomfort while urinating	▪ Painful sexual intercourse due to narrowing of the vagina
▪ Vaginal dryness, itching, burning	▪ Rectal bleeding
	▪ Mucus discharge from the rectum

Leukemia

Potential side effects depend on the site treated. Radiation, rare in leukemia, is most often given to the brain, spleen, and sometimes bone.

Cancer of the Kidney

Short-Term	Long-Term
▪ Nausea, vomiting	
▪ Diarrhea	
▪ Abdominal pain	
▪ Straining while urinating or defecating	

Cancer of the Pancreas

Short-Term	Long-Term
▪ Fatigue	▪ Bowel obstruction if surgery is performed
▪ Nausea, vomiting	
▪ Diarrhea	
▪ Abdominal pain	
▪ Appetite loss	

Cancer of the Ovary

Short-Term	Long-Term
▪ Diarrhea	▪ Bowel obstruction if surgery is performed
▪ Cramping, abdominal pain	▪ Possible infertility

Cancer of the Stomach

Short-Term	Long-Term
■ Fatigue	■ Feeling of fullness after eating small amount
■ Appetite loss	
■ Nausea, vomiting	■ Bowel obstruction
■ Diarrhea, possibly with cramping	

Cancer of the Liver

Short-Term	Long-Term
■ Nausea, vomiting	
■ Diarrhea	

Cancer of the Oral Cavity

Short-Term	Long-Term
■ Fatigue	■ Dry mouth
■ Sensation of lump in throat	■ Reduction in saliva flow, possibly leading to tooth decay
■ Painful swallowing, difficulty eating and drinking	
■ Mouth sores	■ Altered taste
■ Skin irritation	■ Change in contour of the gums, causing dentures to no longer fit properly
■ Hoarseness	
■ Altered taste, bitter taste, loss of taste	■ Damage to tooth socket, with subsequent tooth extraction
■ Increased sensitivity of the tongue	■ If the temporomandibular joint (TMJ) is in the radiation field, may have pain or difficulty opening jaw
■ Swollen saliva glands after the first few days of treatment; subsides after several days	
■ Swelling near surgical site	

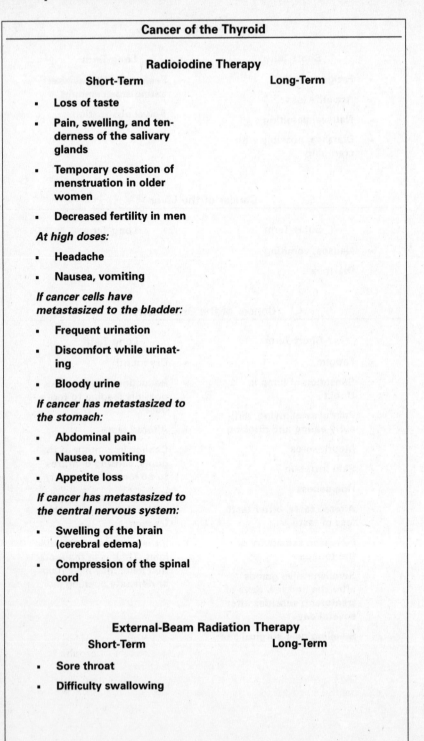

Cancer of the Thyroid

Radioiodine Therapy

Short-Term	Long-Term

- Loss of taste
- Pain, swelling, and tenderness of the salivary glands
- Temporary cessation of menstruation in older women
- Decreased fertility in men

At high doses:

- Headache
- Nausea, vomiting

If cancer cells have metastasized to the bladder:

- Frequent urination
- Discomfort while urinating
- Bloody urine

If cancer has metastasized to the stomach:

- Abdominal pain
- Nausea, vomiting
- Appetite loss

If cancer has metastasized to the central nervous system:

- Swelling of the brain (cerebral edema)
- Compression of the spinal cord

External-Beam Radiation Therapy

Short-Term	Long-Term

- Sore throat
- Difficulty swallowing

Cancers of the Brain

Short-Term	Long-Term
▪ Fatigue	▪ Small risk of impaired intellectual functioning, particularly when radiation is combined with chemotherapy
▪ Headaches	
▪ Skin irritation	
▪ Hair loss	
▪ Difficulty hearing due to middle-ear congestion	

Multiple Myeloma

Potential side effects depend on the site treated. When radiation is used in multiple myeloma, it is often to relieve pain in the lower back, thus exposing the lower digestive tract to radiation.

Short-Term	Long-Term
▪ Nausea, vomiting	▪ Diminished blood counts
▪ Diarrhea	
▪ Abdominal pain	

Cancer of the Cervix

Short-Term	Long-Term
▪ Frequent or painful urination	▪ Bowel obstruction (from internal radiation)
▪ Diarrhea	▪ Painful sexual intercourse due to narrowing of the vagina
▪ Abdominal cramping	
▪ Vaginal itching, burning, dryness	▪ Infertility

Cancer of the Esophagus

Short-Term	Long-Term
▪ Dry, sore throat	▪ Difficulty swallowing due to stricture of esophagus; requires dilation
▪ Dry cough	
▪ Difficulty swallowing, painful swallowing	▪ Shortness of breath

Cancer of the Larynx

Short-Term	Long-Term
▪ Hoarseness	▪ Dry mouth
▪ Sensation of a lump in throat	▪ Reduction in saliva flow, possibly leading to tooth decay
▪ Sore throat	

Cancer of the Throat (Pharynx)

Short-Term	Long-Term
▪ Fatigue	▪ Dry mouth
▪ Sensation of lump in throat	▪ Reduction in saliva flow, possibly leading to tooth decay
▪ Painful swallowing, difficulty eating and drinking	▪ Altered taste
▪ Mouth sores	▪ Change in contour of the gums, causing dentures to no longer fit properly
▪ Skin irritation	▪ Damage to tooth socket, with subsequent tooth extraction
▪ Hoarseness	
▪ Altered taste, bitter taste, loss of taste	▪ If the temporomandibular joint (TMJ) is in the radiation field, may have pain or difficulty opening jaw
▪ Increased sensitivity of the tongue	
▪ Swollen saliva glands after the first few days of treatment; subsides after several days	
▪ Swelling near surgical site	

Soft-Tissue Sarcoma

Potential side effects depend on the area treated. Radiation to the limbs may irritate the skin temporarily and (rarely) produce leg swelling. Radiation to the chest, abdomen, and pelvis, or to the head and neck cause side effects similar to those listed for other diseases at those sites.

Cancer of the Testicle

Short-Term	Long-Term
▪ Nausea, vomiting	▪ Reduced fertility
▪ Diarrhea	

Cancer of the Small Intestine	
Short-Term	**Long-Term**
▪ **Nausea, vomiting**	
▪ **Diarrhea**	
▪ **Abdominal pain**	
▪ **Straining while urinating or defecating**	

Low-Dose Internal Radiation

One fringe benefit of internal radiation, apart from reduced side effects, is a private hospital room. That is where *loading* takes place: The radioactive material is set into the container that was surgically implanted in your body earlier in the day. You are awake while this is done. The lead-alloy shields placed at the sides of the bed and under the bed, explains Dr. Berg, "are to protect the medical personnel from radiation."

For the next few days, your body is emitting radioactivity. Nurses and other health-care professionals will take care of all your needs, but will do so quickly. And although family and friends may visit you, they must sit a safe distance away—typically six feet or more. At the Lombardi Cancer Center, says Dr. Berg, "we put tape on the floor and ask visitors to stay behind it." Children under eighteen and pregnant women will not be permitted in your room.

Effects from internal radiation are usually mild. You might experience some discomfort, however, if you have a special applicator holding the radioactive substance inside a body cavity. You may also be asked to lie reasonably still in bed to prevent the implant from shifting. Ask your doctor in advance to order you pain medication and antianxiety medication in the event you need either one.

If you notice any unusual side effects, such as sweating or a burning sensation, alert the nurse.

Temporary implants are removed at the bedside, typically without anesthesia. You are now free of radiation, but you may have to spend another day or two in the hospital. People with permanent implants are discharged even though the radionuclide inside them is still active. The energy gradually dissipates until it becomes inert.

Most patients can return immediately to their normal daily activities, although for the first few days you may find that you need some extra sleep. One lingering reminder of internal radiation is sensitivity or soreness in the area of the implant.

Chemotherapy: What You Can Expect

Questions to Ask . . . Before Chemotherapy

- What drug or drugs will I be given to treat my cancer?

- How long can I expect to be on chemotherapy?

- How frequently is the chemotherapy given?

- How is it delivered? Orally? By way of injection? Infusion?

- Will the chemotherapy be injected directly into a vein, or will I have a temporary or permanent catheter?

- What side effects or complications might occur?

- Are these side effects usually temporary, or can they become chronic?

- How are the side effects managed?

- Are there medications you can give me prior to each treatment to prevent certain side effects?

- Will the treatment affect other medical conditions I have or other medications I am currently taking? *Inform your oncologist about all other medicines you use, including over-the-counter brands. Certain drugs can interfere with the cancer-killing agents. While you're on chemotherapy, never take any medication without your doctor's knowledge.*

- What side effects should I report to you during and after treatment?

- Will I be able to continue my normal activities?

- Will the treatment affect my sex life or my ability to bear or father children?

- Can the chemotherapy affect my mood or personality?

- What can I do to take care of myself while I am on chemotherapy?

- Do you recommend that I have a dental checkup before chemo begins?

- Are there any potential long-term effects from this chemotherapy?
- When will we be able to tell if the treatment is effective?

A Typical Chemotherapy Treatment

Maureen Sawchuk, an oncology nurse since the early 1980s, remembers when cancer patients receiving chemotherapy frequently had to be hospitalized for each cycle. "They would vomit for days and days on end," she says. What's more, the medications that were administered to try to relieve the vomiting and keep the patients hydrated produced side effects of their own.

In the early 1990s, a new class of *antiemetic* drugs called *serotonin-receptor antagonists* came along. Ondansetron (Zofran), the first, and granisetron (Kytril) work by blocking a brain chemical from triggering the vomiting mechanism. I took a Zofran tablet before each treatment, and in six months of chemotherapy, I never threw up or even felt nauseous.

Recent years have produced medications that help control chemotherapy's other complications, including agents that stimulate damaged bone marrow to step up its production of blood cells. These advances in supportive care now make it possible for more than 90 percent of people with cancer to receive chemotherapy as outpatients.

Typically, your oncologist sees you the first day of each cycle. In addition to performing a full physical exam, he'll want to know in detail how you tolerated the previous round. You may have been asked to keep a log of your diet and your bowel habits between treatments.

The doctor walks you through the symptoms: "How did you feel? Were you tired all the time? Any trouble eating? Concentrating? Sleeping?" Your feedback helps the doctor decide whether to (1) proceed with treatment at the full dose, (2) reduce the dose to make it more bearable, or (3) withhold treatment until you recover from the effects. Another option would be to change any medications being given to manage side effects. "In extreme instances," says nurse Sawchuk, "a regimen might be so toxic for a person that we have to switch him to a different chemotherapy.

"It's extremely important for patients to be honest with their physician about the symptoms they're having and how the treatment is impacting on their lives," she continues. "Many people so desperately want to stay on schedule that they tend to downplay the true extent of their symptoms." Either that, or they feel they are somehow "letting the doctor down" by reporting news that's less than positive.

> *See "How to Describe Symptoms to the Doctor" in Chapter Eight, "Take Control: Managing Symptoms, Side Effects, and Complications."*

A Word to Family and Friends: When a loved one with cancer is naturally on the stoic side, prompt him during doctor's visits not to minimize side effects: "Come on, Dad, you're not really telling Dr. Hackett how bad you've been feeling." Or take the physician aside and describe the symptoms yourself. If you can't accompany the patient, phone the doctor with any concerns you have about how he seems to be withstanding therapy.

How Chemotherapy Is Administered

My chemotherapy treatments were shorter than most. An injection of fluorouracil, one minute to infuse the leucovorin, and I was on my way to work or back home, depending on how I was feeling. The average infusion, though, takes six hours, so you may want to bring reading material, a battery-powered portable CD player or audiocassette player (with headphones), and other items for passing the time as you lie in a comfortable reclining chair. Many outpatient clinics reserve a few private rooms for patients with long treatments. The rooms often have televisions in them.

Some patients experience what is called *anticipatory nausea:* The sights, sounds, and smells associated with treatment trigger memories of how they felt after previous appointments, and they become sick to their stomach before chemo has been given—or even before they arrive at the medical facility. Doctors and nurses have their own name for this phenomenon: "parking-lot syndrome." Since you never know how you'll feel, coming or going, stock your car with a small plastic bucket, bottled water, mouthwash, spray disinfectant, and a change of clothing.

The antiemetic medications administered prophylactically take the edge off anxiety as well as reduce nausea. One widely used drug, lorazepam (Ativan), is first and foremost a sedative, but it suppresses nausea and induces temporary amnesia. According to nurse Sawchuk, "Patients will sleep through therapy, then wake up and ask, 'My chemo is all done?' "

Methods of Delivery: Venipunctures

Inserting a needle into a vein in the lower arm or the hand—hopefully on the first try—requires considerable skill, particularly once a patient is well into treatment. The intravenous cancer-destroying agents are highly caustic and can cause blood vessels to collapse. In addition, a poorly executed *needle stick* can "blow" a vein.

"Even when the drugs are given properly," Maureen Sawchuk points out, "the veins may become thick and hardened and difficult to access." The medical term for this is *sclerosed*. After just two cycles, the veins in my arm turned so leathery that the nurses had one heck of a time trying to draw blood and start IVs.

Six, twelve, eighteen, or more months of venipunctures eventually deplete the supply of healthy blood vessels in the area. Normally, the next site would be the other arm or hand, but before the end of treatment, veins elsewhere in the body may have to be utilized. "We have patients who receive chemo in their thumbs and fingers," says Sawchuk. Some people have poor veins to begin with. In elderly or overweight men and women, the vessels tend to "roll," so that attempting to inject medication into the circulation becomes the equivalent of hitting a moving target.

Protect Your Veins

Blood tests become part of your weekly schedule when you're receiving anticancer drugs. Be sure that the *phlebotomist* who draws your blood is aware that you're on chemotherapy so that she'll take extra care not to further damage your veins.

Fortunately for me, my regular oncology nurse, Kathryn Unruh, was exceptionally talented at needle sticks. In fact, the only painful treatment I experienced during the entire time occurred at the hands of another nurse, who missed the vein and began injecting the 5-FU into the surrounding tissue. She quickly corrected her mistake, but the chemical burned my hand, leaving it discolored for more than a week.

At a teaching hospital, venipunctures may be entrusted to resident doctors and interns. In general, they are not as proficient as oncology nurses, members of chemotherapy teams or IV teams, or anesthesiologists. You have a right to request that someone more experienced place the needle, especially when it's for delivering chemo.

Not long after I finished treatment, I returned to Georgetown for a colonoscopy. A nurse I didn't recognize attempted to start an IV for fluids and sedation. She was nervous and kept jabbing me like I was an orange.

After her third painful try, I insisted that she stop and asked an older nurse to please take over. She deftly eased the needle into a vein in a matter of seconds. Nurse Sawchuk recommends that patients allow for two unsuccessful sticks, perhaps three, "then ask for a more skilled practitioner."

Tips for Making Needle Sticks Less Painful

- Unless the doctor advises otherwise, eat well and drink plenty of water the morning of each treatment. Good nourishment and hydration cause the veins to dilate, or "open," and improve blood flow.

- Go scouting the halls while waiting for a chemo treatment or a blood drawing. Mild exercise enhances circulation and makes the veins protrude, so that they're easier for the nurse to find.

- Exercise your hands and arms. At home, lift small weights and squeeze rubber balls. This too will enlarge the blood vessels.

- Before inserting the needle, the health-care professional should "open" the vein by lightly tapping the area or wrapping a warm, wet cloth or compress around it.

- Moisturize your arms, hands, and fingertips daily. Venipunctures won't hurt as much if the needle doesn't have to pierce dry, hard skin.

- Don't look at the needle while it is being placed.

- Practice techniques to help you relax, such as rhythmic breathing or progressive muscle relaxation.

See "Noninvasive Mind-Body-Control Interventions" in Chapter Eight, "Take Control: Managing Symptoms, Side Effects, and Complications."

The needle is attached to one or more flexible plastic tubes. For IV infusion therapy, the drugs flow from a hanging plastic bag through the catheter and needle and into the circulation. In an IV push, a syringe is used to squirt the medication through the tubing.

Leakage from a Vein: What to Do

If the anticancer agent should seep out of the blood vessel and into the surrounding tissue during infusion, you may feel a sensation of cold or warmth in the area—more often the latter. Or you may notice only that something doesn't "feel right." In either case, tell a nurse.

Chemotherapy can leak from a vein after patients have gone

home, explains Maureen Sawchuk, "even when there was no indication of any difficulty while the drug was being administered." With some medications, at most you might temporarily experience moderate pain at the injection site. Other agents used in cancer treatment, though, are *vesicants,* capable of producing blisters.

"If one of these drugs leaks out," says Sawchuk, "it can cause tremendous damage to the tissue, to the point of requiring plastic surgery. There are antidotes, but we need to respond immediately in order for them to be effective." When seepage of a vesicant is suspected, patients are advised to come in for observation. If they report blistering, "we refer them to a plastic surgeon right away."

Notify your oncologist or oncology nurse of any pain, discomfort, burning, blistering, or changes in the skin at the injection site.

Methods of Delivery: Venous-Access Devices

Surgically implanting a *venous-access catheter* or *port* into a large vein, usually in the upper chest, eliminates most of the complications that can arise from venipunctures.

The catheter, a flexible tube, protrudes from the skin and is capped with a special port for administering injections and connecting intravenous lines. Chemotherapy, *transfusions,* and *IV hydration* and *antibiotics* can all be given, and blood sampled, without having to pierce the skin with the needle.

Implantable ports, made from metal, plastic, or other materials, are inserted beneath the skin. The small, round device is attached to a catheter that feeds into the large vein known as the *superior vena cava,* which returns blood to the heart. When delivering IV therapy or drawing blood, the nurse or physician inserts the needle through the surface of the skin and into the port.

Certain circumstances all but dictate the need for a vascular-access device. For instance, says nurse Sawchuk, "the treatment protocols for some cancers can go on for years. The best veins in the world are not going to last that long. We would advise those patients to get catheters right from the start." Highly toxic regimens and having difficult-to-access veins also usually warrant one. And if a person is just plain squeamish

> **Medical Terms You're Likely to Hear**
>
> Broviac
> Groshong
> Hickman
> Mediport
> Port-a-Cath
>
> . . . all brand names of venous-access devices

about needles, "we'll go straight to a catheter." A central line is always put in for continuous-infusion chemotherapy using a portable pump.

No one likes being poked with needles, so why don't all chemotherapy patients automatically receive a vascular-access device? One reason is the expense. The procedure, performed in an operating room, using local anesthesia, costs roughly $1,500 to $2,000. With external catheters, there is also the cosmetic consideration of having a tube extruding from the chest, which some patients find unappealing.

Both devices require varying amounts of home care. To prevent clotting, the ports are flushed with an *anticoagulant* called heparin between uses and at least once a month. Maintaining a catheter is more involved. The Hickman and Broviac models call for daily heparin flushes, while the Groshong must be irrigated weekly with saline solution. You'll also be shown how to change the cap and the sterile dressing covering the site where the tube enters the body. This is done approximately three times a week. Always remember to wash your hands with soap and running water before touching the dressing or the catheter so that you don't introduce germs into the bloodstream.

Each type of device has its advantages over the other: The port is superior in terms of appearance and ease of care. There are no restrictions on swimming, as there are with a catheter (although you can shower). A catheter spares you the nuisance of even a single needle stick. It can be easily removed without surgery, whereas taking out the port entails a minor operative procedure.

If the medical oncologist has prescribed combination chemotherapy, she'll almost certainly recommend the catheter rather than the internal port. The tube's exposed end can have up to three branches, or *lumens,* which makes it possible for multiple IVs to be given at the same time. "Patients who are considering a bone-marrow transplant would want to go with the catheter," says Sawchuk, "because they're going to need lumens for chemotherapy, probably transfusions of blood products, and possibly intravenous nutrition."

Ports and catheters can remain in the body for years. A temporary vascular-access device called a *peripherally inserted central catheter* (PICC, for short) can be placed in a vein in the crook of the arm, without surgery. A PICC functions much like a Hickman or Groshong catheter, except that it must be rinsed and dressed every day. After several weeks, or at most a few months, the tube is removed.

When considering a central line, ask your doctor to show you pictures of what the devices look like after they're implanted. It's always valuable to solicit opinions from people who have a catheter or port. Perhaps the oncologist can put you in touch with some patients who are willing to share their experiences. Or ask around at patient support-group meetings, post questions on Internet bulletin boards, and so on.

Methods of Delivery: Continuous Infusion/Home Infusion

The advent of the portable continuous-infusion pump has given new meaning to the term "outpatient treatment." In the past, patients requiring continuous infusions had to check into the hospital for the duration of therapy, which can last several hours, several days, or several weeks. The computerized pump, small enough to wear on a belt or slip into a pocket, is preprogrammed to dispense a steady dose of chemotherapy.

"It gives patients tremendous freedom," says Maureen Sawchuk. "They can go to work, work in their garden—do just about anything you can imagine." The method is particularly convenient for those who are too ill to travel back and forth for treatment or who don't drive and have no one to take them.

On day one, you report to the hospital to have a venous-access device threaded into a vein. The pump is then connected to the catheter. Before you go home, your doctor and an oncology nurse will review the device's operation with you and any family members. They will instruct you about how to change the cassettes containing the drug and what to do should an alarm beep to warn you that the battery is low or the tubing leading to the access device has become closed off, or *occluded.* This can happen if there's a kink in the line, a clamp on the tubing, or a problem with the access device itself.

Like anyone dependent upon a mechanical medical device, you may feel apprehensive at first. What if something goes wrong? A medical oncologist is on call after hours to handle any emergencies. Moreover, you return to the hospital for periodic checkups, at which time a nurse will make sure that the pump is functioning properly and delivering the precise dose of medicine.

Not all chemotherapy can be administered this way. "Certain drugs have a high risk of causing an allergic reaction," Sawchuk explains. "With any of those agents, patients need to be in a setting where there is emergency medical personnel nearby." Another obstacle to receiving continuous infusion—and to home chemotherapy infusions in general—is insurance. Although many private health plans cover home infusions, Medicare and Medicaid do not.

Between Cycles

Among its other potential effects, chemotherapy can suppress the bone marrow's production of blood components. This commonly results in abnormally low amounts of red cells (anemia), white cells (leukopenia, also called neutropenia), and platelet cells (thrombocytopenia). Depending upon the drug(s) used, blood-cell production reaches its *nadir,* or lowest level, seven to fourteen days after treatment. Then, typically, the blood counts begin to return to a normal range.

If one or more counts rebound too slowly, the next cycle may have to be postponed. This step is always taken reluctantly, says nurse Sawchuk, "because it's believed that the more you can stay on schedule, the better the chances of killing cancer cells." In addition, patients have often rearranged their lives in anticipation of receiving therapy. Perhaps they've enlisted a friend to drive them to and from the outpatient clinic, taken time off from work, or arranged for day care. You should be prepared for this possibility, although "most patients stay right on time," she emphasizes.

Between cycles your blood is tested regularly. The usual timetable is once a week; several times a week if you're receiving one of the more toxic drugs. "When a person's blood counts reach their nadir, we might consider doing her blood work every day for a couple of days," says Sawchuk. A blood test may be conducted the first day of each cycle.

Since Georgetown University Medical Center was just twenty minutes from my office, I went there for my blood tests. I'd come in at eight in the morning and be at work with time to spare. You don't have to go to the facility where you receive treatment, though. Phlebotomies can be carried out at nearby community hospitals or medical laboratories, or even at home, provided your health insurer approves.

What Circumstances Might Delay Chemotherapy?

Other side effects can force treatment to be postponed, but chemo-related blood disorders are most often to blame, particularly deficiencies of white cells and platelets.

"If a person has only a low red-cell count, we try not to delay giving chemotherapy," says nurse Sawchuk. "With most solid tumors, we support patients with a transfusion because they usually won't need many blood transfusions over the course of their treatment." A lesser-used alternative is to inject anemic patients with epoetin alfa (Epogen, Procrit), which spurs red-cell production. It belongs to the group of biologic agents known as *hematopoietic growth factors,* also known as *colony-stimulating factors.*

A shortage of white cells depletes your defenses against infections that would normally pose little threat. White cells are the lone solid particle in the blood that cannot be replenished through a transfusion. Another intravenous growth factor, filgrastim (Neupogen) is frequently used to boost patients' white-cell production.

Following my second cycle of chemotherapy, my white count plummeted and was taking its time returning to normal. I suggested to one of the nurses, "Why don't you give me some Neupogen?"

"That's a very good idea," she replied, and went off to ask one of my doctors. I knew of the drug, which had just recently been approved by the FDA, because its manufacturer, Amgen, Inc., happened to be a client of my public-relations firm. Two years later, I joined the company as vice-president for government public relations.

I was feeling pretty proud of myself for being an informed patient when the nurse came back in the room. "Mr. Teeley, I can't give you any Neupogen," she said apologetically. It turned out that the experimental protocol I was on did not allow the use of growth factors as part of supportive care. We had to wait until the count came back up naturally.

Thrombocytopenia is also cause for withholding chemotherapy. When your platelet count is down, you're predisposed to hemorrhaging and bruising because the blood doesn't clot adequately. Three things can be done to reverse this situation: transfuse platelets, hold off until the marrow begins pumping them out again in sufficient numbers, or administer platelet growth factor. The first to win FDA approval for commercial use was oprelvekin (Neumega); others are expected to follow.

See "Blood Disorders" in Chapter Eight, "Take Control: Managing Symptoms, Side Effects, and Complications."

Potential Side Effects of Chemotherapy

Blood cells forming in the marrow aren't the only normal fast-growing cells to attract the attention of chemotherapy as it ferrets out cancer cells. The cells that make up hair follicles and the lining of the entire digestive system also replicate at an accelerated pace. Consequently, hair loss, sores in the mouth or throat, nausea and vomiting, abdominal cramping, and diarrhea join blood disorders as some of the more common side effects associated with drug treatment.

Table 7.3 shows the possible side effects for each chemotherapeutic, hormonal, and immunologic agent used to attack cancer. Bear in mind that these are *potential* unwanted consequences. No one can predict which ones, if any, will affect you and to what extent. Everybody and *every body* are different. It's important to be aware of the possibilities, though, so that you can notify your doctor at the first hint of a symptom and initiate treatment.

"The first cycle or two can be very unpredictable," observes Maureen Sawchuk. "You may do beautifully; you may become sick and have to be admitted to the hospital." Both scenarios describe me.

I underwent my first treatment in early November, still weakened from the two abdominal surgeries and the near-fatal bout of aspiration pneumonia. The first three days went by without incident. *Hey,* I thought, *maybe I'll sail through this.* Thursday's dose brought fierce side effects, which continued for about ten days. The drugs inflamed the lining of the intestinal tract, causing relentless diarrhea and cramps that at times doubled me over. By Thanksgiving, though, I was feeling reasonably well.

Cycle number two followed the same pattern: Monday, Tuesday, Wednesday, no adverse effects to speak of; Thursday and Friday, *whoa* . . . I went to work the following week, but I wasn't bouncing back. In fact, the symptoms grew progressively worse. I couldn't keep anything down, and between that and the diarrhea, I became severely dehydrated. In the course of a month and a half, my weight plunged from about 180 to 145 pounds. That's on a six-foot frame.

Plus, my blood counts were down. I was so exhausted that I bowed out of the Bushes' annual Christmas party, a small get-together they threw for friends. The president and the first lady thoughtfully called later that night to see how I was feeling, and we talked for a long time.

That weekend, I was reading when I heard Valerie's voice from the other room. ". . . I'm not sure I can get him in there . . . No, I think you ought to send an ambulance."

I looked up. "Ambulance? What are you talking about?"

She had called one of my oncology nurses, concerned about how I wasn't getting better. Frankly, *I* didn't think I was all that sick, which in itself should have been an indication of how sick I was! Barbara Lewis urged Valerie to get me to the hospital so they could rehydrate me with intravenous fluids. To be honest, I felt relieved to get back to Georgetown.

I didn't go home for eight days. My doctors weren't sure if I was merely suffering the toxic effects of the 5-FU and leucovorin, or whether I'd developed an infection of the GI tract. On top of this, while I was hospitalized, my intestine twisted again. Dr. Woolley remarked that I might have to undergo yet another operation.

"Forget it," I snapped. "I'm not having any more surgery."

He thought for a moment. "Well," he said, "there is one other thing we can do." He suggested inserting a tube down my mouth and into my stomach to drain the fluids. It was miserable as hell, but after three days, the bowel untangled itself, and I was discharged just in time for Christmas.

When I returned to Lombardi to begin my third cycle during the first week of the new year, my physical was performed by one of the fellows, an Indian woman named Dr. Chitra Rajagopal. I was crazy about Dr. Raj, as everyone called her. She was upbeat and full of life.

The first thing she said to me was, "We're going to cut back your chemotherapy by 25 percent." I wasn't sure how to feel. On the one hand, I was thrilled that the side effects would almost certainly not be as debilitating; on the other hand, I wanted to have as potent a dose as possible to wipe out any cancer cells that might still be inside me. In response to my concern, she said, "Mr. Teeley, we want to kill the cancer, not the patient."

Just then Dr. Woolley walked into the examining room. "I've told Mr. Teeley that we're going to cut back his dosage by 25 percent," Dr. Raj said.

"I don't think so," he replied. Looking me in the eye, Dr. Woolley said, "I think he can take the full dose."

At that point, I was politely asked to step outside and sit in the waiting room. Normally, the cancer center at Georgetown was a model of efficiency. But one hour went by, then another, as my medical team discussed whether or not to lower the dosage.

"The concern on my part," Dr. Raj recalls, "was that Pete had lost a significant amount of weight and was fairly neutropenic. I was worried that it might be unnecessary exposure. To reduce the dose by 25 percent is standard practice. Dr. Woolley wanted to see if there was some way Pete could ride out the entire six months of treatment."

According to Dr. Woolley, "If a patient isn't tolerating a drug, we cut the dose, but we don't like to unless absolutely necessary. It's a judgment call that we make each time." Eventually, Dr. Woolley was satisfied that reducing the dosage wouldn't compromise treatment. After he and Dr. Raj had recalculated the dosage and remixed it, I began my third cycle.

Thereafter I still experienced side effects, but not nearly as severe, and for only a few days. Instead of missing a full week of work, I might stay home sick the Thursday and Friday of treatment. Throughout the remaining months of chemotherapy, I grew continually stronger and it became easier and easier for me to pick up the pace. Psychologically, it gave me a tremendous lift to feel that I would be able to complete treatment. Following the brutal second cycle, I wasn't so sure.

During my hospital stay, I was worried that I'd never get to pull my daughters on their sled again. At the time, we used to spend virtually every weekend on a farm that we'd bought near Charlottesville, Virginia. One hundred thirty-five acres of lush greenery on a gently sloping pasture.

I loved to walk up this one small hill about seventy-five yards from the house. If you looked west, you were treated to one of the most spectacular views you've ever seen. I set myself two goals: One, I wanted to have the energy to make it up that hill again. The second was to give the girls a sled ride.

A few weeks after my third cycle, in February, we had a snowfall and I felt strong enough to pull Randall and Adrienne up and down the street. Valerie took pictures and put them in the family album. She captioned them: "So that the kids would remember."

TABLE 7.3   Potential Drug Side Effects

Key

HOW COMMON IS THE SIDE EFFECT?

RC (or rc) = Relatively common
LC (or lc) = Less common
R (or r) = Rare
LC/R (or lc/r) = Less common or rare

HOW SERIOUS IS THE SIDE EFFECT?

boldface = Contact your doctor or nurse at once   nonboldface = Contact your doctor or nurse as soon as possible lowercase = Side effect usually requiring no medical attention unless persistent or bothersome

♦ *The following drugs were approved too late to be included in the 1999 USP DI, Vol. 2, Advice for the Patient, from which this material has been adapted: denileukin, diftitox, epirubicin, methoxsalen, temozolomide, uracil/tegafur, valrubicin, yttrium-90 radiolabeled carcinoembryonic-antigen antibody. Their most common potential side effects are listed in table 7.4.*

♦ *An empty box next to a given side effect doesn't rule out the possibility that it might occur. If you're unsure whether a new side effect is serious or not, always err on the side of caution and contact your doctor's office.*

Notify your doctor about any of the following side effects

- A fever of 101 degrees or higher
- Nosebleeds
- Black-and-blue marks
- Tiny red dots under your skin
- Fatigue
- Sores in your mouth or throat
- A persistent cough
- A tingling in your fingers or toes
- A ringing in your ears
- Nausea or vomiting
- Diarrhea
- Constipation
- Rapid weight gain or weight loss of ten or more pounds
- Losing your hair

Chemotherapy Drugs

(For epirubicin, temozolomide, uracil/tegafur, and valrubicin, see table 7.4)

Symptoms	Altretamine	Asparaginase	Bleomycin	Busulfan	Capecitabine	Carboplatin	Carmustine (BCNU)	Chlorambucil	Cisplatin	Cladribine	
Aches and Pains											
Back pain											
Bone pain											
Breast tenderness and/or enlargement											
Chest pain			R		LC/R						
Generalized pain											

Symptoms	Chemotherapeutic Agents Alphabetically by Generic Name										
	Altretamine	Asparaginase	Bleomycin	Busulfan	Capecitabine	Carboplatin	Carmustine (BCNU)	Chlorambucil	Cisplatin	Cladribine	
Headache		rc			lc/r					rc	
Headache, severe		R									
Jaw pain											
Joint or muscle pain or stiffness		RC		LC	lc/r			LC	RC	lc	
Pain at the injection site						RC	RC		LC	LC	
Pain in the lower back or the side		LC								LC	
Pain in the lower legs		R									
Testicular pain											
Blood-Related											
Bloody urine or stool	LC/R			RC	LC/R	LC	LC	LC	LC	RC	
Red spots on the skin	LC/R			RC	LC/R	LC	LC	LC	LC	RC	
Unusual bleeding or bruising	LC/R	R		RC	LC/R	LC	LC	LC	LC	RC	
Cardiac-Related											
Decreased blood pressure					LC/R						
Elevated blood pressure					LC/R						
Irregular heartbeat					LC/R						
Rapid heartbeat					LC/R				LC	LC	
Digestion-Related											
Appetite loss	lc	rc	rc	lc	rc	lc	lc		lc	rc	
Black, tarry stools	LC/R			RC	LC/R	LC	LC	LC	LC	RC	
Bloating, gas											
Bloody vomit					LC/R						
Constipation					LC/R	lc				rc	
Diarrhea	lc			lc	RC	lc	lc			rc	
Difficulty in swallowing					LC/R		lc				
Heartburn/indigestion					lc/r						
Intense hunger											
Nausea and/or vomiting	rc	rc	rc	lc	rc	rc	rc	lc	rc	rc	
Severe stomach pain accompanied by nausea or vomiting		RC			LC/R						

Symptoms	Chemotherapeutic Agents Alphabetically by Generic Name										
	Altretamine	Asparaginase	Bleomycin	Busulfan	Capecitabine	Carboplatin	Carmustine (BCNU)	Chlorambucil	Cisplatin	Cladribine	
Stomach pain or cramps	lc	rc			**RC**					LC	
Weight gain											
Weight loss		rc	lc	lc							
Genitourinary-Related											
Bladder inflammation and bleeding											
Discolored or cloudy urine					LC/R						
Decreased urination							**R**				
Frequent urination		**LC**									
Painful or difficult urination											
Gynecologic											
Missing or irregular menstruation			rc					lc			
Vaginal bleeding											
Vaginal burning, dryness, or itching											
Mouth-Related											
Dry mouth											
Lip or mouth sores		LC	RC	LC	RC	R	LC	**LC**	R		
Red, sore, swollen tongue											
Swollen lips					RC						
Neurologic											
Clumsiness, difficulty walking	R				LC/R		ic	R	LC		
Convulsions	RC	R		r				R	LC		
Forgetfulness											
Hallucinations		LC						R			
Numbness in the arms or legs	R										
Numbness in the face											

Symptoms	Chemotherapeutic Agents Alphabetically by Generic Name									
	Altretamine	Asparaginase	Bleomycin	Busulfan	Capecitabine	Carboplatin	Carmustine (BCNU)	Chlorambucil	Cisplatin	Cladribine
Numbness or tingling in the hands/fingers or feet/toes					RC	LC			LC	
Tremors or twitching								R		
Weakness or paralysis	RC	R	R	lc		rc	LC	R	RC	lc
Other Symptoms										
Changes in fingernails or toenails			lc		lc/r					
Confusion		LC	LC	lc				R	R	
Dizziness	RC			lc	lc/r		lc		LC	lc
Drowsiness		LC								
Extreme thirst		LC								
Fatigue	LC/R	LC		lc	LC/R		LC		LC	rc
Feeling faint			LC						LC	
Fever or chills accompanied by coughing or hoarseness	LC/R		LC		LC/R	LC	LC	LC	LC	RC
Fever or chills accompanied by pain in the lower back or side	LC/R		LC		LC/R	LC	LC	LC	LC	RC
Fever or chills accompanied by painful or difficult urination	LC/R		LC		LC/R	LC	LC	LC	LC	RC
Flushed face							LC			
Freckles										
General feeling of discomfort or illness									lc	
Hair loss			lc			lc	lc			
Hot flashes										
Nightmares										
Profuse sweating									lc	
Puffy face		RC			LC/R				LC	
Sleep disturbance					lc/r				lc	
Sore throat					LC/R					

Symptoms	Chemotherapeutic Agents Alphabetically by Generic Name										
	Altretamine	Asparaginase	Bleomycin	Busulfan	Capecitabine	Carboplatin	Carmustine (BCNU)	Chlorambucil	Cisplatin	Cladribine	
Swollen feet, ankles, or calves		LC		LC	LC/R		R	LC	RC	LC	
Swollen fingers			rc		LC/R						
Swollen or tender neck											
Water retention											
Psychological											
Agitation		LC						R	R		
Anxiety	RC										
Behavioral changes											
Depression	RC	LC									
Mood swings											
Respiratory-Related											
Coughing or hoarseness			RC								
Noisy, rattling breathing											
Shortness of breath		RC	RC	LC	LC/R		RC	R		LC	
Stuffy or runny nose					LC/R						
Thick phlegm											
Tightness in the throat or chest					LC/R						
Wheezing			LC			R			LC		
Sensory Disturbances											
Blurry vision				R		R			R		
Color blindness									R		
Difficulty in hearing									RC		
Discoloration of the whites of the eyes											
Drooping eyelids											
Earache											
Loss of taste									LC		
Metallic taste											
Red, sore eyes					lc/r						
Ringing in the ears						R			RC		
Slurred speech											
Sudden vision changes											

Symptoms	Chemotherapeutic Agents Alphabetically by Generic Name										
	Altretamine	Asparaginase	Bleomycin	Busulfan	Capecitabine	Carboplatin	Carmustine (BCNU)	Chlorambucil	Cisplatin	Cladribine	
Sexually-Related											
Decreased sexual desire									rc		
Skin-Related											
Acne											
Blistered, peeling, or scaling skin					RC			R			
Boils											
Burning, crawling, or tingling sensation											
Darkened or thickened skin and/or fingernails			rc	rc							
Discolored skin along vein of injection							lc				
Dry skin											
Increased sensitivity of the eyes to light											
Increased sensitivity of the skin to sunlight					1/cr						
Itching (Pruritus)										lc	
Red, tender skin			rc		lc/r						
Skin rash and itching (mild)	R	RC	rc		LC/R	LC	lc	LC		RC	
Skin rash and itching (severe)								R			
Yellow eyes or skin					LC/R			R			

Symptoms	Chemotherapeutic Agents Alphabetically by Generic Name										
	Cyclophosphamide	Cytarabine	Dacarbazine	Dactinomycin	Daunorubicin	Docetaxel	Doxorubicin	Estramustine	Etoposide	Floxuridine	Fludarabine
Aches and Pains											
Back pain									R		
Bone pain		R									
Breast tenderness and/or enlargement								rc			
Chest pain		R				R		R			
Generalized pain											RC
Headache	lc	lc/r				R					lc
Headache, severe							R				
Jaw pain											
Joint or muscle pain or stiffness	RC	LC	lc	R	LC	lc	LC				lc
Pain at the injection site	R	R	RC	R	LC	lc	LC		R		
Pain in the lower back or the side	RC	LC			LC	LC	LC		R	R	RC
Pain in the lower legs								R			
Testicular pain											
Blood-Related											
Bloody urine or stool	R	LC	LC	LC	R	LC	R	R	LC	R	LC
Red spots on the skin	R	LC	LC	LC	R	LC	R	R	LC	R	LC
Unusual bleeding or bruising	R	LC	LC	LC	R	LC	R	R	LC	R	LC
Cardiac-Related											
Decreased blood pressure						R					
Elevated blood pressure						R					
Irregular heartbeat		R			LC	R	LC				
Rapid heartbeat	RC					R	LC		RC		
Digestion-Related											
Appetite loss	rc	rc	rc						rc	lc/r	lc
Black, tarry stools	R	LC	LC	LC	R	LC	R	R	LC	LC	LC
Bloating, gas						RC					
Bloody vomit											
Constipation											
Diarrhea	lc/r	lc/r		RC	lc	rc	lc	rc	lc	RC	rc

Symptoms	Chemotherapeutic Agents Alphabetically by Generic Name										
	Cyclophosphamide	Cytarabine	Dacarbazine	Dactinomycin	Daunorubicin	Docetaxel	Doxorubicin	Estramustine	Etoposide	Floxuridine	Fludarabine
Difficulty in swallowing		R		RC					R	LC	
Heartburn/indigestion		R		RC						LC	
Intense hunger											
Nausea and/or vomiting	rc	rc	rc	rc	rc	rc	rc	rc	rc	LC	rc
Severe stomach pain accompanied by nausea or vomiting											
Stomach pain or cramps	lc		R	RC			LC			RC	
Weight gain						RC					
Weight loss											
Genitourinary-Related											
Bladder inflammation and bleeding											
Discolored or cloudy urine					rc		lc				
Decreased urination											
Frequent urination	R	R									
Painful or difficult urination		LC		LC	LC	LC		R		R	RC
Gynecologic											
Missing or irregular menstruation	RC										
Vaginal bleeding											
Vaginal burning, dryness, or itching											
Mouth-Related											
Dry mouth											
Lip or mouth sores	R	RC	R	RC	RC	rc			LC	RC	LC
Red, sore, swollen tongue										LC	
Swollen lips	lc										
Neurologic											
Clumsiness, difficulty walking								R	R	R	
Convulsions											

Symptoms	Chemotherapeutic Agents Alphabetically by Generic Name										
	Cyclophosphamide	Cytarabine	Dacarbazine	Dactinomycin	Daunorubicin	Docetaxel	Doxorubicin	Estramustine	Etoposide	Floxuridine	Fludarabine
Forgetfulness											
Hallucinations											
Numbness in the arms or legs						rc		R			
Numbness in the face			lc								LC
Numbness or tingling in the hands/fingers or feet/toes		LC				rc			R		LC
Tremors or twitching											
Weakness or paralysis	RC	R				rc		R	R		LC
Other Symptoms											
Changes in fingernails or toenails						lc					
Confusion	RC										LC
Dizziness	RC	lc/r				R					
Drowsiness		LC									
Extreme thirst	R										
Fatigue	RC	LC		rc		RC		R	lc		LC
Feeling faint		R				R			R		
Fever or chills accompanied by coughing or hoarseness	LC		LC				LC		LC		LC
Fever or chills accompanied by pain in the lower back or side	LC		LC				LC		LC		LC
Fever or chills accompanied by painful or difficult urination	LC		LC				LC		LC		
Flushed face	lc		lc								
Freckles		r									
General feeling of discomfort or illness		R									lc
Hair loss	lc	lc	lc	rc	rc	rc	lc		rc	lc	r
Hot flashes											
Nightmares											
Profuse sweating	lc										
Puffy face			R			RC			R		

Symptoms	Chemotherapeutic Agents Alphabetically by Generic Name										
	Cyclophosphamide	Cytarabine	Dacarbazine	Dactinomycin	Daunorubicin	Docetaxel	Doxorubicin	Estramustine	Etoposide	Floxuridine	Fludarabine
Sleep disturbance								Ic	R		
Sore throat											
Swollen feet, ankles, or calves	RC			R	LC	RC	LC	RC			LC
Swollen fingers						RC					
Swollen or tender neck											
Water retention											
Psychological											
Agitation	RC										LC
Anxiety		Ic									
Depression											
Mood swings											
Respiratory-Related											
Coughing or hoarseness	RC	LC		LC	LC	LC		R		R	RC
Noisy, rattling breathing						LC					
Shortness of breath	RC	R	R		LC	R	LC	R	R		RC
Stuffy or runny nose											
Thick phlegm											
Tightness in the throat or chest									R		
Wheezing				R			LC		R		
Sensory Disturbances											
Blurry vision											LC
Color blindness											
Difficulty in hearing											LC
Discoloration of the whites of the eyes		R									
Drooping eyelids											LC
Earache											
Loss of taste											
Metallic taste											
Red, sore eyes		R									
Ringing in the ears											
Slurred speech								R			

Symptoms	Chemotherapeutic Agents Alphabetically by Generic Name										
	Cyclophosphamide	Cytarabine	Dacarbazine	Dactinomycin	Daunorubicin	Docetaxel	Doxorubicin	Estramustine	Etoposide	Floxuridine	Fludarabine
Sudden vision changes								R			
Sexually-Related											
Decreased sexual desire								rc			
Skin-Related											
Acne											
Blistered, peeling, or scaling skin						LC					
Boils											
Burning, crawling, or tingling sensation											
Darkened or thickened skin and/or fingernails	rc				rc	lc/r	lc				
Discolored skin along vein of injection							LC				
Dry skin											
Increased sensitivity of the eyes to light											
Increased sensitivity of the skin to sunlight											
Itching (Pruritus)		lc/r									
Red, tender skin					rc	lc				**LC**	
Skin rash and itching (mild)	lc	R			rc	R	rc	R	R	lc/r	rc
Skin rash and itching (severe)											
Yellow eyes or skin	R	R	**R**	R						R	

Symptoms	Chemotherapeutic Agents Alphabetically by Generic Name										
	Fluorouracil	Gemcitabine	Hydroxyurea	Idarubicin	Ifosfamide	Irinotecan	Leucovorin	Lomustine (CCNU)	Mechlorethamine	Melphalan	Mercaptopurine
Aches and Pains											
Back pain											
Bone pain											
Breast tenderness and/or enlargement											
Chest pain	R	LC									
Generalized pain						LC					
Headache		LC		rc		Ic			Ic		Ic
Headache, severe		LC	R								
Jaw pain											
Joint or muscle pain or stiffness		rc	R	LC					LC	LC/R	LC
Pain at the injection site		Ic		LC	LC				LC		
Pain in the lower back or the side			LC	RC				LC	LC	LC	LC
Pain in the lower legs											
Testicular pain											
Blood-Related											
Bloody urine or stool	R	RC	R	RC	RC	R		LC	LC	LC	LC
Red spots on the skin	R	RC	R	RC	R	R		LC	LC	LC	LC
Unusual bleeding or bruising	R	RC	R	RC	R	R		LC	LC	LC	LC
Cardiac-Related											
Decreased blood pressure											
Elevated blood pressure		LC									
Irregular heartbeat		LC		LC							
Rapid heartbeat		LC		LC							
Digestion-Related											
Appetite loss	rc	rc	rc		LC	rc		rc	Ic		LC
Black, tarry stools	LC	RC	R	RC	R	R		LC	LC	LC	LC
Bloating, gas						LC					
Bloody vomit											
Constipation		rc	Ic			rc					
Diarrhea	RC	rc	rc	rc		RC		Ic	Ic		Ic

Symptoms	Chemotherapeutic Agents Alphabetically by Generic Name										
	Fluorouracil	Gemcitabine	Hydroxyurea	Idarubicin	Ifosfamide	Irinotecan	Leucovorin	Lomustine (CCNU)	Mechlorethamine	Melphalan	Mercaptopurine
Difficulty in swallowing											
Heartburn/indigestion	RC					Ic					
Intense hunger											
Nausea and/or vomiting	Ic	rc	rc	rc	rc	rc		rc	rc	Ic	LC
Severe stomach pain accompanied by nausea or vomiting											
Stomach pain or cramps	LC			R		rc					
Weight gain											
Weight loss						rc					
Genitourinary-Related											
Bladder inflammation and bleeding											
Discolored or cloudy urine		RC			rc						
Decreased urination		R				LC		LC			
Frequent urination		R			RC						
Painful or difficult urination				LC	RC	RC		LC	LC	LC	LC
Gynecologic											
Missing or irregular menstruation									RC		
Vaginal bleeding											
Vaginal burning, dryness, or itching											
Mouth-Related											
Dry mouth						Ic					
Lip or mouth sores	RC	Ic	LC	RC	R	Ic		LC	R	LC/R	R
Red, sore, swollen tongue											
Swollen lips											
Neurologic											
Clumsiness, difficulty walking	R							LC			
Convulsions			R		R		R				

Symptoms	Chemotherapeutic Agents Alphabetically by Generic Name										
	Fluorouracil	Gemcitabine	Hydroxyurea	Idarubicin	Ifosfamide	Irinotecan	Leucovorin	Lomustine (CCNU)	Mechlorethamine	Melphalan	Mercaptopurine
Forgetfulness											
Hallucinations			R		RC						
Numbness in the arms or legs											
Numbness in the face									R		
Numbness or tingling in the hands/fingers or feet/toes	R	lc			lc				R		
Tremors or twitching											
Weakness or paralysis	rc	**LC**			LC	RC		LC	lc		RC
Other Symptoms											
Changes in fingernails or toenails											
Confusion			R		RC			LC	lc		
Dizziness			R		LC	LC			LC		
Drowsiness		lc	rc						lc		
Extreme thirst						LC					
Fatigue		**RC**			RC	**RC**		LC			RC
Feeling faint						LC					
Fever or chills accompanied by coughing or hoarseness	LC	LC			LC	LC					
Fever or chills accompanied by pain in the lower back or side	LC	LC			LC	LC					
Fever or chills accompanied by painful or difficult urination	LC	LC				LC					
Flushed face						lc					
Freckles											
General feeling of discomfort or illness		rc									
Hair loss	rc	lc		rc	rc	lc		lc	lc		
Hot flashes											
Nightmares											
Profuse sweating		rc				lc					
Puffy face											

Symptoms	Chemotherapeutic Agents Alphabetically by Generic Name										
	Fluorouracil	Gemcitabine	Hydroxyurea	Idarubicin	Ifosfamide	Irinotecan	Leucovorin	Lomustine (CCNU)	Mechlorethamine	Melphalan	Mercaptopurine
Sleep disturbance		rc				LC					
Sore throat						LC					
Swollen feet, ankles, or calves	R	RC	R	LC		LC		LC	LC	LC/R	LC
Swollen fingers		RC									
Swollen or tender neck											
Water retention						LC					
Psychological											
Agitation					RC						
Anxiety											
Depression											
Mood swings											
Respiratory-Related											
Coughing or hoarseness	R	R	LC	RC	R		R	LC	LC	LC	LC
Noisy, rattling breathing		R									
Shortness of breath	R	RC		LC	R	RC		R	R		
Stuffy or runny nose		rc				LC					
Thick phlegm											
Tightness in the throat or chest		LC									
Wheezing		LC					R		R		
Sensory Disturbances											
Blurry vision											
Color blindness											
Difficulty in hearing									LC		
Discoloration of the whites of the eyes											
Drooping eyelids											
Earache											
Loss of taste											
Metallic taste									lc		
Red, sore eyes											
Ringing in the ears									LC		
Slurred speech		LC						LC			
Sudden vision changes											

Symptoms	Chemotherapeutic Agents Alphabetically by Generic Name										
	Fluorouracil	Gemcitabine	Hydroxyurea	Idarubicin	Ifosfamide	Irinotecan	Leucovorin	Lomustine (CCNU)	Mechlorethamine	Melphalan	Mercaptopurine
Sexually-Related											
Decreased sexual desire											
Skin-Related											
Acne											
Blistered, peeling, or scaling skin											
Boils											
Burning, crawling, or tingling sensation											
Darkened or thickened skin and/or fingernails				Ic				Ic			Ic
Discolored skin along vein of injection											
Dry skin	Ic					LC					
Increased sensitivity of the eyes to light											
Increased sensitivity of the skin to sunlight											
Itching (Pruritus)											
Red, tender skin			Ic								
Skin rash and itching (mild)	rc	RC	Ic	R		Ic	**R**	Ic	RC		Ic
Skin rash and itching (severe)									RC	**LC**	**LC**
Yellow eyes or skin		R							R		RC

Symptoms	Chemotherapeutic Agents Alphabetically by Generic Name										
	Mesna	Methotrexate	Mitomycin	Mitotane	Mitoxantrone	Paclitaxel	Pamidronate	Pegasparagase	Pentostatin	Plicamycin	Procarbazine
Aches and Pains											
Back pain		LC							Ic		
Bone pain											
Breast tenderness and/or enlargement											
Chest pain									LC		R
Generalized pain									RC		
Headache		LC			rc			Ic	rc	Ic	Ic
Headache, severe											R
Jaw pain											
Joint or muscle pain or stiffness		RC		Ic		rc	Ic	Ic	rc	LC	rc
Pain at the injection site			R		R	R	rc	Ic		Ic	
Pain in the lower back or the side			LC		LC			R	RC		LC
Pain in the lower legs									LC		
Testicular pain											
Blood-Related											
Bloody urine or stool		RC	LC	LC	LC	LC		R	LC		LC
Red spots on the skin		LC	LC		LC	LC		R	LC		LC
Unusual bleeding or bruising		LC	LC		LC	LC		R	LC		LC
Cardiac-Related											
Decreased blood pressure											
Elevated blood pressure											
Irregular heartbeat					LC						
Rapid heartbeat					LC			Ic			R
Digestion-Related											
Appetite loss		rc	rc	RC				Ic	rc	rc	Ic
Black, tarry stools		RC	LC		RC	LC		R	LC		LC
Bloating, gas									Ic		
Bloody vomit		RC	R								LC
Constipation								RC	Ic		Ic
Diarrhea	Ic	RC			rc	rc			rc	rc	LC

Symptoms	Chemotherapeutic Agents Alphabetically by Generic Name										
	Mesna	Methotrexate	Mitomycin	Mitotane	Mitoxantrone	Paclitaxel	Pamidronate	Pegasparagase	Pentostatin	Plicamycin	Procarbazine
Difficulty in swallowing								LC			lc
Heartburn/indigestion											
Intense hunger								LC			
Nausea and/or vomiting	lc	rc	rc	RC	rc	rc	rc	RC	rc	rc	rc
Severe stomach pain accompanied by nausea or vomiting											
Stomach pain or cramps		RC			RC		RC	RC	LC	LC	
Weight gain											
Weight loss								RC	lc		
Genitourinary-Related											
Bladder inflammation and bleeding											
Discolored or cloudy urine		LC			lc						
Decreased urination			LC		LC						
Frequent urination								RC			
Painful or difficult urination			LC		LC			R	RC		LC
Gynecologic											
Missing or irregular menstruation											RC
Vaginal bleeding											
Vaginal burning, dryness, or itching											
Mouth-Related											
Dry mouth											lc
Lip or mouth sores		RC	LC		RC	R			LC	rc	LC
Red, sore, swollen tongue											
Swollen lips											
Neurologic											
Clumsiness, difficulty walking											LC
Convulsions		LC			LC			lc			RC

Symptoms	Chemotherapeutic Agents Alphabetically by Generic Name										
	Mesna	Methotrexate	Mitomycin	Mitotane	Mitoxantrone	Paclitaxel	Pamidronate	Pegasparagase	Pentostatin	Plicamycin	Procarbazine
Forgetfulness											
Hallucinations								LC			RC
Numbness in the arms or legs											
Numbness in the face											
Numbness or tingling in the hands/fingers or feet/toes			lc			rc		LC	LC		LC
Tremors or twitching				lc			RC				rc
Weakness or paralysis	LC	lc						**LC**	lc	lc	RC
Other Symptoms											
Changes in fingernails or toenails											
Confusion		**LC**					RC	lc	LC		RC
Dizziness		LC	RC								lc
Drowsiness		LC	RC					lc	LC	lc	rc
Extreme thirst											
Fatigue		LC	lc	RC				RC	RC	lc	RC
Feeling faint								RC			R
Fever or chills accompanied by coughing or hoarseness		LC				RC					
Fever or chills accompanied by pain in the lower back or side		LC				RC					
Fever or chills accompanied by painful or difficult urination		LC				RC					
Flushed face						RC					
Freckles											
General feeling of discomfort or illness								rc	lc		
Hair loss		lc	lc		rc	rc					lc
Hot flashes											lc
Nightmares								lc			rc
Profuse sweating											R
Puffy face								LC	RC		

Symptoms	Chemotherapeutic Agents Alphabetically by Generic Name										
	Mesna	Methotrexate	Mitomycin	Mitotane	Mitoxantrone	Paclitaxel	Pamidronate	Pegasparagase	Pentostatin	Plicamycin	Procarbazine
Sleep disturbance								Ic	LC		rc
Sore throat							RC				
Swollen feet, ankles, or calves		RC	LC		LC				LC		
Swollen fingers											
Swollen or tender neck											R
Water retention											
Psychological											
Agitation											rc
Anxiety								Ic	LC		
Depression				RC					LC	Ic	
Mood swings											
Respiratory-Related											
Coughing or hoarseness		LC	LC		RC			R	RC		LC
Noisy, rattling breathing											
Shortness of breath		LC	LC	R	RC	R		LC	RC		RC
Stuffy or runny nose											
Thick phlegm											RC
Tightness in the throat or chest											
Wheezing				R							R
Sensory Disturbances											
Blurry vision		LC		LC				RC			
Color blindness											
Difficulty in hearing											
Discoloration of the whites of the eyes					Ic						
Drooping eyelids											
Earache											
Loss of taste											
Metallic taste	Ic										
Red, sore eyes				LC					LC		
Ringing in the ears											
Slurred speech								Ic			
Sudden vision changes									LC		

Symptoms	Chemotherapeutic Agents Alphabetically by Generic Name										
	Mesna	Methotrexate	Mitomycin	Mitotane	Mitoxantrone	Paclitaxel	Pamidronate	Pegasparagase	Pentostatin	Plicamycin	Procarbazine
Sexually-Related											
Decreased sexual desire											
Skin-Related											
Acne		Ic									
Blistered, peeling, or scaling skin											
Boils		Ic									
Burning, crawling, or tingling sensation											
Darkened or thickened skin and/or fingernails			Ic	RC	R						
Discolored skin along vein of injection											
Dry skin								RC	Ic		
Increased sensitivity of the eyes to light											
Increased sensitivity of the skin to sunlight											
Itching (Pruritus)											
Red, tender skin		**RC**		Ic				LC			
Skin rash and itching (mild)	R	Ic	Ic	RC	R	RC		RC	RC		R
Skin rash and itching (severe)							**R**				
Yellow eyes or skin		LC			LC						LC

Symptoms	Chemotherapeutic Agents Alphabetically by Generic Name										
	Streptozocin	Teniposide	Testolactone	Thioguanine	Thiotepa	Topotecan	Tretinoin	Uracil Mustard	Vinblastine	Vincristine	Vinorelbine
Aches and Pains											
Back pain											
Bone pain							RC		lc		
Breast tenderness and/or enlargement											
Chest pain							RC				LC
Generalized pain							LC				
Headache	LC					rc	rc		R	RC	
Headache, severe							LC				
Jaw pain									R	RC	lc
Joint or muscle pain or stiffness				LC	LC		rc	LC	LC	RC	lc
Pain at the injection site	LC				LC				LC	LC	RC
Pain in the lower back or the side	R	R		LC	LC		LC	LC	RC	RC	LC
Pain in the lower legs											
Testicular pain									R	RC	
Blood-Related											
Bloody urine or stool	R	RC		LC	LC	RC		LC	R	R	R
Red spots on the skin	R	RC		LC	LC	RC		LC	R	R	R
Unusual bleeding or bruising	R	RC		LC	LC	RC		LC	R	R	R
Cardiac-Related											
Decreased blood pressure							RC				
Elevated blood pressure							RC				
Irregular heartbeat							RC				
Rapid heartbeat	LC	RC									
Digestion-Related											
Appetite loss			lc	lc	lc	rc	rc			LC	
Black, tarry stools	R	RC		LC	LC	RC		LC	R	R	R
Bloating, gas							RC			lc	
Bloody vomit				LC							
Constipation						rc	rc			RC	rc
Diarrhea	lc	rc	lc	lc		rc	rc	rc		lc	lc

Symptoms	Chemotherapeutic Agents Alphabetically by Generic Name										
	Streptozocin	Teniposide	Testolactone	Thioguanine	Thiotepa	Topotecan	Tretinoin	Uracil Mustard	Vinblastine	Vincristine	Vinorelbine
Difficulty in swallowing											
Heartburn/indigestion							LC				
Intense hunger	LC										
Nausea and/or vomiting	rc	rc	lc	lc	lc	rc	LC	rc	lc	lc	rc
Severe stomach pain accompanied by nausea or vomiting											
Stomach pain or cramps						rc	LC			RC	
Weight gain							**RC**				
Weight loss							rc			lc	
Genitourinary-Related											
Bladder inflammation and bleeding											R
Discolored or cloudy urine											
Decreased urination	RC	R					RC			LC	
Frequent urination							lc			LC	
Painful or difficult urination	**R**	**RC**		LC	LC		LC	**LC**		LC	
Gynecologic											
Missing or irregular menstruation						lc					
Vaginal bleeding											
Vaginal burning, dryness, or itching											
Mouth-Related											
Dry mouth							rc				
Lip or mouth sores		RC		R	R	rc	RC	R	LC	R	LC
Red, sore, swollen tongue			lc								
Swollen lips											
Neurologic											
Clumsiness, difficulty walking				LC			lc	RC	R		
Convulsions							**LC**			LC	

Symptoms	Chemotherapeutic Agents Alphabetically by Generic Name										
	Streptozocin	Teniposide	Testolactone	Thioguanine	Thiotepa	Topotecan	Tretinoin	Uracil Mustard	Vinblastine	Vincristine	Vinorelbine
Forgetfulness							lc				
Hallucinations							LC				
Numbness in the arms or legs											
Numbness in the face			LC								
Numbness or tingling in the hands/fingers or feet/toes			LC			rc	rc		R	RC	LC
Tremors or twitching							lc				
Weakness or paralysis	LC					rc	LC		R	RC	RC
Other Symptoms											
Changes in fingernails or toenails											
Confusion							rc			LC	
Dizziness					lc		rc		R	LC	
Drowsiness	LC						LC				
Extreme thirst											
Fatigue	LC	RC				rc					RC
Feeling faint										LC	
Fevor or chills accompanied by coughing or hoarseness						RC			RC		
Fever or chills accompanied by pain in the lower back or side						RC					
Fever or chills accompanied by painful or difficult urination						RC			RC		
Flushed face		RC				R	rc				
Freckles											
General feeling of discomfort or illness							rc				
Hair loss		rc			lc	lc	rc	lc	rc	rc	
Hot flashes											
Nightmares											
Profuse sweating											
Puffy face		R				R	RC				

Symptoms	Chemotherapeutic Agents Alphabetically by Generic Name										
	Streptozocin	Teniposide	Testolactone	Thioguanine	Thiotepa	Topotecan	Tretinoin	Uracil Mustard	Vinblastine	Vincristine	Vinorelbine
Sleep disturbance							rc			LC	
Sore throat							RC				RC
Swollen feet, ankles, or calves	RC	R	Ic	LC	LC		RC	LC	LC	RC	
Swollen fingers		R					RC				
Swollen or tender neck											
Water retention											
Psychological											
Agitation	LC						Ic	Ic		LC	LC
Anxiety	LC						rc	Ic			
Depression							RC	Ic	R	LC	LC
Mood swings							LC				
Respiratory-Related											
Coughing or hoarseness	R	RC			LC	LC	RC	LC		R	
Noisy, rattling breathing											
Shortness of breath		RC				RC	RC				LC
Stuffy or runny nose							RC				
Thick phlegm											
Tightness in the throat or chest		RC			R	R	RC				
Wheezing		RC			R	R	RC				
Sensory Disturbances											
Blurry vision									R	RC	
Color blindness											
Difficulty in hearing							LC		R		
Discoloration of the whites of the eyes											
Drooping eyelids									R	RC	
Earache							RC				
Loss of taste											
Metallic taste											
Red, sore eyes											
Ringing in the ears											
Slurred speech							LC				
Sudden vision changes							RC				

Symptoms	Chemotherapeutic Agents Alphabetically by Generic Name										
	Streptozocin	Teniposide	Testolactone	Thioguanine	Thiotepa	Topotecan	Tretinoin	Uracil Mustard	Vinblastine	Vincristine	Vinorelbine
Sexually-Related											
Decreased sexual desire											
Skin-Related											
Acne											
Blistered, peeling, or scaling skin											
Boils											
Burning, crawling, or tingling sensation							rc				
Darkened or thickened skin and/or fingernails								lc			
Discolored skin along vein of injection											
Dry skin							rc				
Increased sensitivity of the eyes to light											
Increased sensitivity of the skin to sunlight											
Itching (Pruritus)							rc				
Red, tender skin											
Skin rash and itching (mild)		LC		lc	R	R	RC	lc		lc	R
Skin rash and itching (severe)		RC			lc	R					
Yellow eyes or skin	R	R		R			LC	R			

Hormonal Drugs

Symptoms	Hormonal Agents Alphabetically by Generic Name								
♂ = In men ♀ = In women	Aminoglutethimide	Anastrozole	Androgens	Bicalutamide	Corticosteroids	Estrogens	Flutamide	Goserelin	Ketoconazole
Aches and Pains									
Back pain									
Bone pain		rc						R	
Breast tenderness and/or enlargement		lc	RC♂	rc		RC	rc	lc	
Chest pain		RC		LC				LC	R♂
Generalized pain		LC			R				
Groin pain									R♂
Headache	lc/r	rc		rc	lc/r	lc	rc	lc	
Headache, severe			LC			lc	R		
Joint or muscle pain or stiffness	lc/r	lc		lc	lc/r			R	
Pain at the injection site			lc		R			lc	
Pain in the lower back or the side		LC						LC	
Pain in the lower legs								R♂	
Pelvic pain								lc♀	
Pressure in the skull							R		
Testicular pain			LC						
Blood-Related									
Bloody urine or stool	R			LC	R			LC	
Red spots on the skin	R		R	R				R	
Unusual bleeding or bruising	R		LC	R	R			R	
Wounds that won't heal					R				
Cardiac-Related									
Decreased blood pressure								R	
Elevated blood pressure		LC							
Irregular heartbeat					R				LC
Rapid heartbeat	LC							R	LC
Digestion-Related									
Appetite loss	rc		R	rc		rc	rc	lc	
Black, tarry stools	R		R	LC	R			LC	
Bloating, gas				lc		rc	lc		

Symptoms	Hormonal Agents Alphabetically by Generic Name								
	Aminoglutethimide	Anastrozole	Androgens	Bicalutamide	Corticosteroids	Estrogens	Flutamide	Goserelin	Ketoconazole
Bloody vomit			R						
Constipation			LC†	rc				rc	lc†
Diarrhea		rc	lc	rc		lc	rc		
Difficulty in swallowing									
Heartburn/indigestion				lc	rc		lc		
Intense hunger					rc				
Light-colored stools			R						
Nausea and/or vomiting	rc	rc	LC	rc	R	rc	rc	lc	
Stomach pain or cramps		rc	lc	R	R		R		
Weight gain		lc	LC		R	RC		lc	
Weight loss									
Endocrine-Related									
Hyperglycemia, or abnormally elevated blood sugar: dry mouth, flushed, dry skin, increased urination, appetite loss, stomach ache, nausea or vomiting, hyperventilation, extreme thirst, unusual fatigue, rapid weight loss									
Hypoglycemia, or abnormally low blood sugar: anxiety, chills, cool, pale skin, poor concentration, headache, hunger, nausea, nervousness, shakiness, sweating, unusual fatigue, weakness									
Genitourinary-Related									
Discolored or cloudy urine			R	R			R		

Symptoms	Hormonal Agents Alphabetically by Generic Name								
	Aminoglutethimide	Anastrozole	Androgens	Bicalutamide	Corticosteroids	Estrogens	Flutamide	Goserelin	Ketoconazole
Frequent urination			RC♀/LC♀		LC				
Painful or difficult urination		LC	LC♀						
Gynecologic									
Change in vaginal discharge									
Enlarged clitoris			RC						
Missing or irregular menstruation	lc/r		RC		RC/L	LC		rc	
Vaginal bleeding		LC			RC/L				
Vaginal burning, dryness, or itching		lc						lc	
Mouth-Related									
Dry mouth		rc							
Lip or mouth sores									
Swollen tongue									
Neurologic									
Clumsiness, difficulty walking	LC								
Hallucinations					R				
Numbness or tingling in the hands/fingers or feet/toes		lc			LC		LC	R	
Tremors or twitching									
Weakness or paralysis	LC	LC			LC	R	LC		
Other Symptoms									
Chronic bad breath			R						
Confusion			LC♀	lc	R		lc		
Decreased breast size			RC♀						
Deepened voice	lc/r♀		RC♀					R♀	
Dizziness	LC	rc	LC	R	lc/r	lc	R	lc	
Drowsiness	RC				lc		lc		
Extreme thirst		rc	LC♀		LC				

Symptoms	Hormonal Agents Alphabetically by Generic Name								
	Aminoglutethimide	Anastrozole	Androgens	Bicalutamide	Corticosteroids	Estrogens	Flutamide	Goserelin	Ketoconazole
Fatigue	LC	LC	LC	LC	R		LC	lc	
Feeling faint							R	R	
Fever or chills accompanied by coughing or hoarseness	R	LC							
Fever or chills accompanied by pain in the lower back or side	R								
Fever or chills accompanied by painful or difficult urination	R								
Flulike symptoms (such as headache, muscle or joint pain, and fatigue, occurring together)					lc		lc		
Flushed face		rc			lc/r			R	
General feeling of discomfort or illness			R						
Hair loss		lc	RC♦						
Hot flashes		rc			rc		rc	rc	
Increased hair growth	lc/r♦		lc		lc/r			R♦	
Increased sensitivity to heat									
Lumpy breasts and/or nipple discharge						LC/R			
Profuse sweating		rc			lc/r				
Puffy face				LC	R		LC	R	
Sleep disturbance			lc	lc	rc		lc	lc	
Sore throat		LC	R	RC			RC		
Swollen feet, ankles, or calves		RC	LC	LC	R	RC	LC	lc	
Swollen or tender neck	R								
Unexpected or increased flow of breast milk									
Psychological									
Agitation				lc	R		lc	R♦	
Anxiety	LC			lc	R		LC	R♦	
Depression	LC		LC♦	LC	R		LC	R♦	

Symptoms	Hormonal Agents Alphabetically by Generic Name								
	Aminoglutethimide	Anastrozole	Androgens	Bicalutamide	Corticosteroids	Estrogens	Flutamide	Goserelin	Ketoconazole
False sense of well-being					R				
Mood swings					R			R♀	
Paranoia or delusion of grandeur					R				
Respiratory-Related									
Coughing or hoarseness		LC		RC			RC		
Shortness of breath	R	RC		LC		R♀	LC	R	
Stuffy, runny nose		lc		RC			RC		
Tightness in the chest				RC			RC	R	
Wheezing				RC			RC	R	
Sensory Disturbances									
Blurry vision					LC			lc	
Difficulty in wearing contact lenses						lc			
Red, sore eyes									
Slurred speech	LC					R♀			
Sudden vision changes					LC				
Uncontrolled eye movements	LC								
Sexually-Related									
Decreased sexual desire			lc	rc		lc♀	rc	lc	
Decreased testicle size			lc					lc	
Frequent or continuing erections			RC						
Heightened sexual drive			lc			lc♀			
Impotence				rc			rc	lc	
Skin-Related									
Acne			lc		R				
Blue-tinged lips, finger-nails, palms								R	
Brown spots on exposed skin, possibly long-lasting									

Symptoms	Hormonal Agents Alphabetically by Generic Name								
	Aminoglutethimide	Anastrozole	Androgens	Bicalutamide	Corticosteroids	Estrogens	Flutamide	Goserelin	Ketoconazole
Darkened, lightened, or thickened skin and/or fingernails	LC		LC†		lc/r		R		
Dry skin									
Infection, itching, redness, or other skin irritation of the scrotum			LC						
Itching (Pruritus)		Ic	LC	RC			RC		
Pitting, scarring, or depression of the skin at the injection site					R				
Red, tender skin			LC			rc			
Reddish-purple lines on the arms, face, legs, trunk, or groin					R				
Skin rash and itching (mild)		rc	LC	LC			LC		RC
Skin rash and itching (severe)	RC		R					R	
Thin, shiny skin					R				
Yellow eyes or skin	R	R	LC	R		LC/R	R		

Symptoms	Hormonal Agents Alphabetically by Generic Name							
	Letrozole	Leuprolide	Levothyroxine	Nilutamide	Octreotide	Progestins	Tamoxifen	Toremifene
Aches and Pains								
Back pain						R		
Bone pain		R					lc	lc
Breast tenderness and/or enlargement		lc		rc		lc		
Chest pain	LC	RC†	R	LC				R
Groin pain		R†						
Headache	lc	lc	LC	rc	lc	rc	lc	
Headache, severe								
Joint or muscle pain or stiffness	lc	R						
Pain at the injection site		lc			rc	rc		
Pain in the lower back or the side								
Pain in the lower legs		R†	LC				LC/R	R
Pelvic pain		lc†					LC/R†	LC
Pressure in the skull								
Testicular pain								
Blood-Related								
Bloody urine or stool				LC				
Red spots on the skin				R				
Unusual bleeding or bruising				R				
Wounds that won't heal								
Cardiac-Related								
Decreased blood pressure		R						
Elevated blood pressure						rc		
Irregular heartbeat		LC	R					
Rapid heartbeat		LC	R					
Digestion-Related								
Appetite loss	lc		LC	rc		RC		LC
Black, tarry stools				LC				
Bloating, gas				lc				

Symptoms	Hormonal Agents Alphabetically by Generic Name							
	Letrozole	Leuprolide	Levothyroxine	Nilutamide	Octreotide	Progestins	Tamoxifen	Toremifene
Bloody vomit								
Constipation	lc	lc†		rc				
Diarrhea	lc		LC	rc	rc			
Difficulty in swallowing								
Heartburn/indigestion				lc				
Intense hunger								
Light-colored stools								
Nausea and/or vomiting	rc	lc	LC	rc	rc	R	rc	rc
Stomach pain or cramps	lc			R	rc	rc		
Weight gain	lc	lc				rc	rc†	
Weight loss			LC					
Endocrine-Related								
Hyperglycemia, or abnormally elevated blood sugar: dry mouth, flushed dry skin, increased urination, appetite loss, stomachache, nausea or vomiting, hyperventilation, extreme thirst, unusual fatigue, rapid weight loss					RC	RC		
Hypoglycemia, or abnormally low blood sugar: anxiety, chills, cool pale skin, poor concentration, headache, hunger, nausea, nervous-ness, shakiness, sweating, unusual fatigue, weakness					RC			
Genitourinary-Related								
Discolored or cloudy urine				R				

Symptoms	Hormonal Agents Alphabetically by Generic Name							
	Letrozole	Leuprolide	Levothyroxine	Nilutamide	Octreotide	Progestins	Tamoxifen	Toremifene
Frequent urination								LC
Painful or difficult urination								
Gynecologic								
Change in vaginal discharge								
Enlarged clitoris								
Missing or irregular menstruation		rc	LC			RC	lc	
Vaginal bleeding	R						LC/R	LC
Vaginal burning, dryness, or itching		lc					lc	
Mouth-Related								
Dry mouth								
Lip or mouth sores								
Swollen tongue								
Neurologic								
Clumsiness, difficulty walking								
Hallucinations								
Numbness or tingling in the hands/fingers or feet/toes		R		LC				
Tremors or twitching			LC					
Weakness or paralysis	lc			LC	lc	R	LC/R	
Other Symptoms								
Chronic bad breath								
Confusion				lc			LC/R	LC
Decreased breast size								
Deepened voice		R♀						
Dizziness	lc	lc		R	lc	rc		lc
Drowsiness	lc			lc		rc	LC/R	
Extreme thirst								

Symptoms	Hormonal Agents Alphabetically by Generic Name							
	Letrozole	Leuprolide	Levothyroxine	Nilutamide	Octreotide	Progestins	Tamoxifen	Toremifene
Fatigue	Ic	Ic		LC	Ic	R		LC
Feeling faint		R						
Fever or chills accompanied by coughing or hoarseness								
Fever or chills accompanied by pain in the lower back or side								
Fever or chills accompanied by painful or difficult urination								
Flulike symptoms (such as headache, muscle or joint pain, and fatigue, occurring together)				Ic				
Flushed face		R			Ic			
General feeling of discomfort or illness								
Hair loss	Ic					Ic		
Hot flashes	Ic	rc		rc		Ic	rc♀	rc
Increased hair growth		R♀				Ic		
Increased sensitivity to heat			LC					
Lumpy breasts and/or nipple discharge								
Profuse sweating	Ic		LC					rc
Puffy face		R		LC		R		
Sleep disturbance		Ic	LC	Ic		Ic		
Sore throat				RC				
Swollen feet, ankles, or calves	LC	Ic		LC	Ic	rc		
Swollen or tender neck								
Unexpected or increased flow of breast milk						LC		
Psychological								
Agitation		R♀	LC	Ic		R		
Anxiety	Ic	R♀	LC	Ic		rc		
Depression	LC	R♀		LC		LC		

Symptoms	Hormonal Agents Alphabetically by Generic Name							
	Letrozole	Leuprolide	Levothyroxine	Nilutamide	Octreotide	Progestins	Tamoxifen	Toremifene
False sense of well-being								
Mood swings		R♀				rc		
Paranoia or delusion of grandeur								
Respiratory-Related								
Coughing or hoarseness	lc			RC				
Shortness of breath	LC	**R**	R	**LC**		**R**	LC/R	R
Stuffy, runny nose				RC				
Tightness in the chest		**R**		RC				
Wheezing		**R**		RC				
Sensory Disturbances								
Blurry vision		lc					LC/R	LC
Difficulty in wearing contact lenses								
Red, sore eyes								lc
Slurred speech						**R**		
Sudden vision changes				lc		**R**		LC
Uncontrolled eye movements								
Sexually-Related								
Decreased sexual desire		lc		rc		lc	lc	
Decreased testicle size		lc						
Frequent or continuing erections								
Heightened sexual drive								
Impotence		lc		rc		**R**	lc	
Skin-Related								
Acne						lc		
Blue-tinged lips, finger-nails, palms								
Brown spots on exposed skin, possibly long-lasting						lc		

Symptoms	Hormonal Agents Alphabetically by Generic Name							
	Letrozole	Leuprolide	Levothyroxine	Nilutamide	Octreotide	Progestins	Tamoxifen	Toremifene
Darkened, lightened, or thickened skin and/or fingernails								
Dry skin							Ic	
Infection, itching, redness, or other skin irritation of the scrotum								
Itching (Pruritus)				RC				
Pitting, scarring, or depression of the skin at the injection site								
Red, tender skin								
Reddish-purple lines on the arms, face, legs, trunk, or groin								
Skin rash and itching (mild)	Ic		R	LC		LC	Ic	
Skin rash and itching (severe)		R	R					
Thin, shiny skin								
Yellow eyes or skin				R			LC/R	

Immunologic Drugs

(For denileukin diftitox and yttrium-90 radiolabeled carcinoembryonic-antigen antibody, see table 7.4)

Symptoms	Immunologic Agents Alphabetically by Generic Name					
	Alpha-Interferons	Bacillus Calmette-Guérin	Interleukin-2	Levamisole	Rituximab	Trastuzumab
Aches and Pains						
Back pain	lc/r				lc	
Chest pain	R		LC		R	
Headache	rc		lc	lc	RC	RC
Jaw pain						
Joint or muscle pain or stiffness	lc/r	RC	lc	lc	lc	
Leg cramps	lc/r					
Pain at the injection site			R		LC	
Pain in the lower back or the side			LC	R	LC	
Blood-Related						
Bloody urine or stool	R	RC	LC	R	LC	
Red spots on the skin	R		LC	R	LC	
Unusual bleeding or bruising	R		LC	R	LC	
Cardiac-Related						
Irregular heartbeat	R		LC		R	LC
Rapid heartbeat			LC			LC
Digestion-Related						
Appetite loss	rc		rc		lc	lc
Black, tarry stools	R		LC	R	LC	
Bloating, gas			LC		lc	
Bloody vomit			LC			
Constipation			lc			
Diarrhea	lc/r		RC	rc	lc	rc
Heartburn/indigestion					lc	
Nausea and/or vomiting	rc	RC	RC	rc		RC
Stomach pain or cramps			LC		lc	
Weight gain			RC			
Weight loss	lc/r					

Symptoms	Immunologic Agents Alphabetically by Generic Name					
	Alpha-Interferons	Bacillus Calmette-Guérin	Interleukin-2	Levamisole	Rituximab	Trastuzumab
Genitourinary-Related						
Decreased urination			RC			
Frequent urination		RC				R
Painful or difficult urination		RC	**LC**	**R**	LC	
Gynecologic						
Missing or irregular menstruation			R			
Mouth-Related						
Dry mouth	lc/r					
Lip or mouth sores	lc/r		RC	LC		
Red, sore, swollen tongue			LC		RC	
Neurologic						
Clumsiness, difficulty walking			R	R		
Convulsions			R	R		
Involuntary movements of arms and legs				R		
Numbness or tingling in the hands/fingers or feet/toes	LC		RC	R	lc	lc
Poor concentration or thinking	LC					
Puffing or smacking of the lips			R			
Puffing of the cheeks				R		
Rapid or wormlike tongue movements				R		
Tremors or twitching				R		
Weakness or paralysis			R		LC	**RC**
Other Symptoms						
Cold sensation			R			
Confusion	LC		RC	R		
Dizziness	lc/r		RC	lc	RC	**RC**
Drowsiness			RC	lc		
Fatigue	rc		RC	lc	RC	R
Feeling faint			LC			

Symptoms	Immunologic Agents Alphabetically by Generic Name					
	Alpha-interferons	Bacillus Calmette-Guérin	Interleukin-2	Levamisole	Rituximab	Trastuzumab
Fever or chills accompanied by coughing or hoarseness	R					R
Fever or chills accompanied by pain in the lower back or side	R					R
Fever or chills accompanied by painful or difficult urination	R					R
Flushed face					RC	
General feeling of discomfort or illness	rc		rc	**LC**	lc	
Hair loss	lc			lc		
Nightmares				lc		
Profuse sweating	lc/r					
Sleep disturbance	LC			lc	lc	lc
Sore throat					lc	
Swollen feet, ankles, or calves			R		LC	LC
Swollen or tender neck			R			
Psychological						
Agitation	LC		RC		lc	
Anxiety	LC			lc	lc	
Depression	LC		RC	lc		
Paranoia				R		
Respiratory-Related						
Coughing or hoarseness		R	**LC**	**R**	LC	rc
Rapid breathing			**LC**			
Shortness of breath			**RC**		RC	**RC**
Tightness in the chest					RC	**lc**
Sensory Disturbances						
Blurry vision	lc/r		LC	R		
Loss of taste			LC			
Metallic taste	rc			rc	lc	

Symptoms	Immunologic Agents Alphabetically by Generic Name					
	Alpha-Interferons	Bacillus Calmette-Guérin	Interleukin-2	Levamisole	Rituximab	Trastuzumab
Red, sore eyes					LC	
Slurred speech			LC			
Skin-Related						
Blistered, peeling, or scaling skin			**LC**			
Dry skin	lc/r		rc			
Itching (Pruritus)	lc/r					R
Skin rash and itching (mild)	rc	R	rc	lc	RC	**RC**
Yellow eyes or skin			LC			

Other Drugs
(For methoxsalen, see table 7.4.)

Symptoms	Photosensitizing Agent		Radiopharmaceutical Agents Alphabetically by Generic Name			
	Porfimer		Chromic Phosphate P-32	Samarium 153	Sodium Iodide -131	Strontium 89
Aches and Pains						
Bone pain				lc		rc
Chest pain	LC		LC/R			
Pain in the lower back or the side				RC	R	R
Blood-Related						
Bloody urine or stool	RC			RC	R	R
Red spots on the skin				RC	R	R
Unusual bleeding or bruising			LC/R	RC	R	R
Cardiac-Related						
Irregular heartbeat	RC			LC		
Rapid heartbeat	RC					
Digestion-Related						
Appetite loss			rc			
Black, tarry stools				RC	R	R
Constipation	rc					
Diarrhea	rc		rc			
Difficulty in swallowing	RC					
Nausea and/or vomiting	rc		rc	lc	lc	
Severe stomach pain accompanied by nausea or vomiting	LC		LC/R			
Stomach pain or cramps	RC		rc			
Weight gain	RC					
Genitourinary-Related						
Discolored or cloudy urine	RC					

Symptoms	Photosensitizing Agent		Radiopharmaceutical Agents Alphabetically by Generic Name			
	Porfimer		Chromic Phosphate P-32	Samarium 153	Sodium Iodide-131	Strontium 89
Frequent urination	RC					
Painful or difficult urination	RC			**RC**	R	R
Mouth-Related						
Lip or mouth sores	RC					
Neurologic						
Weakness or paralysis	RC		rc			
Other Symptoms						
Dizziness	RC					
Fatigue	RC		LC/R			
Feeling faint	RC					
Fever or chills	RC		LC/R		R	R
Flushed face	RC					rc
General feeling of discomfort or illness			rc			
Puffy face	RC					
Sleep disturbance	rc					
Sore throat			LC/R			
Swollen feet, ankles, or calves	RC					
Swollen or tender neck	LC					
Respiratory-Related						
Coughing or hoarseness	RC		LC/R	RC	R	R
Shortness of breath	**RC**		LC/R			
Tightness in the throat or chest	RC					
Wheezing	RC					
Sensory Disturbance						
Blurry vision	lc					
Heightened sensitivity to light	lc					
Loss of taste					lc	

Symptoms	Photosensitizing Agent		Radiopharmaceutical Agents Alphabetically by Generic Name			
	Porfimer		Chromic Phosphate P-32	Samarium 153	Sodium Iodide -131	Strontium 89
Skin-Related						
Blistered, peeling, or scaling skin	rc					
Yellow eyes or skin	LC					

Adapted from the *USP DI, Vol. 2, Advice for the Patient, Drug Information in Lay Language,* 19th ed. Copyright © 1999, the USP Convention, Inc. Permission granted.

TABLE 7.4   More Drugs and Their Potential Side Effects

These drugs were approved after mid-1998, too late for inclusion in the 1999 USP DI, Vol. 2, Advice for the Patient, from which the material in table 7.3 was adapted. Below are the most common side effects for each.

Chemotherapeutic Agents

Epirucibin: Hair loss, nausea, vomiting, mouth sores, low white-blood-cell count

Temozolomoide: Nausea, vomiting, headache, fatigue, constipation

Uracil/Tegafur: Diarrhea, nausea, vomiting, abdominal cramping, fatigue

Valrubicin: Painful straining during bowel movements, itching, loss of taste, skin irritation, poor urine flow, bladder inflammation

Immunologic Agents

Denileukin diftitox: Fever and chills, nausea, vomiting, diarrhea

Yttrium-90 radiolabeled carcinoembryonic-antigen antibody: No major side effects.

Photosensitizing Agent

Methoxsalen: No major side effects.

Know the Signs of a Drug-Induced Allergic Reaction

Any medication, not just chemotherapy, has the potential to provoke the immune system into overreacting. Among the drugs most often associated with severe reactions *(anaphylaxis)* are antibiotics, local anesthetics, enzymes, and codeine.

The effects are typically mild at first. Recognizing the early symptoms can save your life, because anaphylactic reactions, though rare, can quickly escalate into a serious medical crisis. A person's airway may close up, leading to respiratory failure. The other major cause of death is *anaphylactic shock,* in which fluid escapes from the blood vessels into the spaces between body tissues until the circulatory system collapses.

Mild Symptoms	Severe Symptoms
• Flushed face	• Puffy face, particularly around the eyes
• Skin rash (hives), accompanied by intense itching and swelling	• Difficulty in breathing and asthmalike wheezing
• Nausea or vomiting	• Rapid heartbeat
• Severe headache	• Chills and tremors
	• Clammy skin
	• Blurry vision
	• Low blood pressure *(hypotension)*
	• Progressive loss of consciousness

A liquid *antihistamine* can bring mild anaphylaxis under control. Considering that everything from food to insect stings to pollen can trigger an allergic reaction, every household should have some Benadryl or another brand on hand at all times. After ingesting the antihistamine, call your doctor for further instructions. If the symptoms don't subside within about fifteen minutes, dial 911, then take a second dose while you wait for the emergency medical service to arrive. A delay of just a few minutes sometimes spells the difference between life and death. Severe anaphylactic reactions are treated with injections of the hormone epinephrine, which reverses the airway and blood-vessel constriction.

◆ Summon an ambulance immediately if you experience dizziness, heart palpitations, or difficulty catching your breath.

Bone-Marrow Transplantation: What You Can Expect

Questions to Ask . . . Before Bone-Marrow Transplantation

- Since I will be hospitalized for a while, can I bring my own pillows and items for decorating the room?

- What clothes should I bring?

- Can my family bring me food from home?

- What personal-hygiene supplies should I bring?

- Can you describe the room I will be in?

- Can I leave my room or the transplant unit once I'm admitted?

- Can you please explain the procedure for infusing marrow stem cells?

- Can my spouse or another family member stay overnight in my room?

- What are the visiting hours? Can children visit me?

- What can I expect in the weeks after the transplant?

- When will I be able to go home?

- I have children at home. Does this pose a problem?

- What about pets?

- What precautions do I need to take to avoid infection, and for how long?

- Can I eat normally once I'm home?

- When can I return to my regular activities?

- How frequently do I need to return to the transplant center for follow-up visits?

- How long will the BMT team follow me?

- When can I go back to the physician who referred me?

- Once I am home, what medical symptoms should I report to the transplant center?

Preparation

The Lombardi Cancer Center's Bone Marrow Transplantation Program, one of approximately two hundred in the United States, has an eighteen-bed unit. Within days of beginning high-dose chemotherapy, alone or followed by total-body irradiation, patients have little or no defense against infectious agents. Even once the donor or autologous marrow begins manufacturing blood cells, transplant recipients will be *immunocompromised* for months to come. Therefore, from the time you are admitted until some immunity is restored, you are quarantined in a private room equipped with high-efficiency particulate air (HEPA) filters.

The hallways, too, are HEPA-filtered. Your level of neutrophils, a type of white blood cell, will be monitored regularly. Autologous-BMT patients can roam the unit at any time but must wear a special type of surgical mask. Until their *absolute neutrophil count* (ANC) exceeds 500 for three days in a row, they cannot leave the unit, except for tests. Allogeneic-BMT patients must have an ANC higher than 500 for three days in order to leave their room.

Lombardi and other major cancer centers reserve several *laminar airflow (LAF) rooms* for patients who will be receiving marrow from a matched unrelated donor. These rooms have special one-way airflow systems that rid the air of germs, greatly reducing the risk of severe infection. However, tests notwithstanding, you must remain in the room at all times.

During the weeks that your immunity is impaired, you can have visitors, including children. Before entering the unit, though, they must thoroughly wash their hands and put on a mask, surgical gloves, a cover gown, and possibly shoe covers too. Lombardi allows the patient's spouse or another family member or close friend to spend the night "throughout the transplant," says Dr. Kenneth Meehan, acting director of the BMT program. Before children under twelve are allowed onto the unit, their parents must fill out a health questionnaire detailing their history of immunizations.

As much as you may crave company, your health takes precedence. "Until a patient's blood counts come back up, only immediate family should visit," says Dr. Meehan. "And children's visits should be kept to a minimum." Remind prospective visitors that in your immunocompromised state, exposure to any sort of infection could be fatal. According to Dr. Meehan, "If they even *think* they might have a cold or were around someone with a cold, they shouldn't visit."

You might want to think twice about allowing younger children into the room. Besides the fact that you may not feel well, the environment could be upsetting to a youngster. Because patients often have to travel some distance from home for a bone-marrow transplant, many BMT units have video phones in the rooms.

High-Dose Chemotherapy and Total-Body Irradiation (TBI)

The conditioning regimen, intended to suppress or eradicate the recipient's bone marrow, usually commences five to ten days before transplantation, depending on the type of cancer. Marrow infusion is referred to as "day 0," with the preceding days designated "day −10," "day −9," and so on, like a countdown.

Total-body irradiation is generally administered two or three times a day for three to five days. Multiple doses of approximately 125 *grays* per treatment instead of 400 grays in a single daily session significantly reduce acute side effects and diminish the danger of serious long-term complications.

> **Free Housing/Lodging During BMT**
>
> When marrow transplants are performed at a facility away from home, family members may be able to find free accommodations through the American Cancer Society or the National Association of Hospital Hospitality Houses.
>
> *See "Housing/Lodging Assistance" in Appendix B.*

When preparative therapy calls for both high-dose chemotherapy and TBI—as in leukemia and lymphoma—drug treatment comes first. With the average regimen lasting four days, you might undergo chemo on days −8, −7, −6, and −5, and radiotherapy on days −4, −3, and −2.

Patients usually get to rest on day −1. "The induction regimens are basically the same for autologous and allogeneic transplantations," explains Dr. Meehan, "except that in the allogeneic setting we give a number of medications to suppress the immune system the day before transplantation." This step is to help prevent graft-versus-host disease, in which white blood cells from the donor marrow perceive their new surroundings as foreign and attack the body.

Posttransplantation

Now begins the most treacherous phase of the procedure. Following an autoBMT, it will be a week to a week and a half before healthy marrow begins to generate new blood cells; following an alloBMT, two to four weeks. This presumes that the graft "takes" properly.

The specially trained nursing staff will monitor you around the clock. Their main concern during this time is to fend off infection. To that end, patients are kept in isolation and receive prophylactic infusions of antiviral medications, antifungals, and antibiotics. "Despite this," says Dr. Meehan, "99 percent of patients develop a fever," the first sign of infection. These are usually *opportunistic* infections already present in the body. Ordinarily, microorganisms such as herpes simplex, herpes zoster, and cytomegalovirus do not cause disease. But in a person with weakened immunity, they can be life-threatening. "When an infection develops," says Dr. Meehan, "we put patients on even more infection-fighting medications."

You will have a central catheter with multiple tubes so that your blood counts can be measured frequently. The first indication that the transplanted marrow has engrafted is the emergence of new white cells in the bloodstream. (Interestingly, if you've had an allogeneic transplant, your blood type should now be the same as the donor's.) As part of an investigational study, at the Lombardi Center recipients are given the immunologic agent interleukin-2, in an attempt to speed renewal of the immune system. According to Dr. Meehan, "All transplant patients will be asked to participate in a variety of clinical trials, regardless of the institution." Other experimental approaches include injecting patients with growth factors that accelerate production of each type of blood cell.

Levels of red cells and platelets take longer than white cells to rebound. To prevent anemia and bleeding complications, patients regularly receive transfusions of both blood products. "The problem," explains Dr. Meehan, "is that transplant patients get so many products, their bodies start developing antibodies against them. If we kept giving them random donor platelets, after two or three days they would become resistant to the new platelets. A person admitted to the hospital after an accident might receive platelets from six to eight different donors, but with transplant patients we keep it to a single donor."

While whole blood can be donated only once every six to eight weeks, platelets can be given twice a week up to twenty-four times a year. Ask a family member or friend to line up several volunteers to donate platelets for you. *Plateletpheresis* is similar to a conventional blood donation, except that two needles are placed: one in each arm. While the donor lies in a reclining chair, his blood is routed through a special machine that skims off platelets, then returns the blood to the other arm. The process takes about two hours. Platelets can be typed, just like bone marrow. A volunteer whose platelets match yours will be asked to make repeat donations as necessary.

"I advise all patients to arrange for getting donor-directed platelets or even red cells," says Dr. Meehan. You should know in advance that many insurance companies will not pay for designated donations of whole blood or blood products.

The toxic effects of the conditioning regimen usually don't come crashing down until shortly after the transplant. Mouth sores, digestive problems, or diarrhea may interfere with your desire to eat, in which event you will be fed intravenously. This is called *total parenteral nutrition* (TPN) or *hyperalimentation*. Whatever food you are able to eat will have been carefully prepared in order to reduce the chances of your contracting a bacterial or fungal infection. Raw fruits and vegetables are eliminated from your diet for a while, although you can eat cooked veggies and canned fruits.

Home from the Transplant Center

Different centers have their own discharge criteria, but in general you will not be allowed to go home until your absolute neutrophil count has topped 500 for at least three days in a row. At Lombardi, BMT patients must also meet these requirements in order to leave:

- They must need no more than three or four platelet transfusions per week.
- They must be able to consume one thousand calories per day.
- They must have less than a quart or so of diarrhea per day.
- They must have gone forty-eight hours without a fever.
- They must be off all IV medications, although exceptions may be made if they're medically stable and able to arrange for home health care.

- Any nausea and vomiting must be controllable with oral medications.

The hospitalization for a bone-marrow transplant varies in length but can range from two weeks to two months. Even though by this time your marrow is pumping out blood cells, you may still be somewhat anemic and thrombocytopenic.

Full immunity doesn't return for a year or more. Once you're released from the hospital, you will have to take a number of precautions to avoid incurring an infection, especially if you're on cyclosporine (Sandimmune) or other immunosuppressive drugs to prevent or treat graft-versus-host disease. "An allogeneic patient on immunosuppressants is basically like a newborn baby or a person with HIV," explains Dr. Meehan. "They have virtually no immune system. So a virus that might cause a mere upper respiratory infection for a healthy person can be lethal for them."

See "Steps for Preventing Infection Following Bone-Marrow Transplantation," in Chapter Eight, "Take Control: Managing Symptoms, Side Effects, and Complications."

When to Contact Your Doctor

Call the transplant unit if you experience any of the following:

- A temperature higher than 100.4 degrees Fahrenheit
- Coughing or shortness of breath that persists for more than a day
- Redness, pain, drainage, or swelling at the catheter site
- Changes in the color, consistency, amount, or frequency of bowel movements
- Discolored urine
- Skin rash
- Lack of appetite for more than two or three days
- Nausea and vomiting that resists medication
- Inability to take your prescribed medications
- Sudden new pain

- Bleeding gums or a nosebleed
- Mouth sores or cold sores
- Prolonged headache, abdominal discomfort, or muscle cramps
- Visual disturbances, dizziness, or weakness

Follow-up Outpatient Visits

Patients must return to the transplant center one to three times a week for the first several weeks after discharge. If you're from out of town, you'll have to make plans to remain nearby. The Lombardi Cancer Center asks that allogeneic-BMT patients stay in the Washington metropolitan area until day 100 posttransplant. At that time, you'll undergo a major workup to evaluate the effectiveness of the procedure. Barring any problems, your central catheter will be taken out. This and future follow-up testing can be conducted by your doctor at home. Tests are scheduled at six months, one year, and annually for the next four years.

Bone-Marrow Transplantation: A Long Ordeal

Depression, anxiety, and fears about the future are familiar to anyone being treated for a serious illness. But from an emotional and social standpoint, men and women who undergo bone-marrow transplantation face a unique set of issues.

BMT disrupts families' lives longer than other cancer therapies. Patients may have to spend months living out of suitcases in a strange city, and usually a full year passes before they can return to work or school full-time. They must cope with weeks of relative isolation in the hospital, then spend months trying to dodge infection while their immune system rebuilds. The enormous financial burden adds to the considerable stress. For people with leukemia, there is also the daunting prospect of possibly gambling away months or years by choosing bone-marrow transplantation, a procedure that could be fatal. Drug therapy, while not a cure, can prolong life, in some cases substantially.

In Dr. Meehan's experience, depression often sets in after patients leave the transplant center. "A lot of patients have been gearing up for months to have the procedure, so during transplant they can tolerate a lot, because they know they're going to go home in x number of days," he comments. "Plus, we keep them pretty busy, walking the halls and so on.

"Now they're home. They have to climb a flight of stairs for the first time in weeks, and that makes them tired. They're looking at their medication list; they're on ten different medications. How long is this going to go on? And suddenly it dawns on them: *Oh my God, I just had a bone-marrow transplant!*" BMT teams almost always include psychiatrists, psychologists, therapists, social workers, and chaplains to provide practical, emotional, and spiritual support to patients and their families. We urge you to make use of these services. Despite everything, observes Dr. Meehan, "I'm impressed by how well patients cope psychologically during transplant."

Chapter Eight

Take Control:

Managing Symptoms,

Side Effects, and Complications

The goal of aggressive symptom control isn't just to keep you comfortable, it's to keep you healthy enough to stay on schedule with your cancer therapy and to stay out of the hospital. Cost and inconvenience are two compelling reasons to avoid hospitalization, but the chief concern is the risk of infection. Each year as many as fifteen thousand people die from pneumonia and other infections acquired in the hospital.

Symptoms, side effects, and complications can develop as a result of the cancer itself or its treatment. Curative therapy to eradicate the underlying tumor may bring relief; at other times, treatment may be purely palliative.

When you have cancer, you want an oncologist who takes a proactive approach to symptom management: intervening promptly, before a bothersome effect snowballs into a major problem or sets off a chain reaction. For instance, feeling anxious intensifies a patient's perception of pain, which in turn can interfere with sleep, thereby exacerbating the pain and anxiety, in an interminable cycle. What's more, sleep deprivation weakens immunity, opening the door to infection.

You also want your doctor to spare you from symptoms whenever possible. My six months on chemotherapy were far more bearable because of the oral antiemetic medication I took before each treatment. As of this writing no effective measure exists to prevent chemo- and radiation-induced mucositis, which made me pretty sick for a while. But thank goodness I never had to deal with nausea on top of it. Pain, anxiety, and infection, too, may be minimized or avoided altogether through the prophylactic use of different agents and nonpharmacologic methods.

This chapter will familiarize you with treatments and techniques for controlling and preventing the effects most frequently associated with cancer, chemotherapy, radiation, and other therapies. You'll also learn simple, nonmedical steps you can take to help yourself feel better. As always, you want to be aware of your options so that you'll know what type of symptom relief to request in the event that one of your doctors doesn't volunteer information freely or is overly conservative when it comes to palliation.

Let's say that you've had violent diarrhea following each of your first two cycles of chemotherapy. Both times you had to call your oncologist, who prescribed an oral diarrhea medication. Your local druggist doesn't deliver. As sick and weak as you felt, you had to get dressed and drive to the pharmacy. When you see your doctor at the start of your next cycle, ask him to order the drug in advance. That way you can fill the prescription on your way home and have it on hand should you need it. Sometimes nausea, pain, and other symptoms are more tolerable if you know that relief is immediately available.

Or what if you've felt sick to your stomach, but no one has suggested taking an antinauseant shortly before the chemo is administered? Tell your oncologist or nurse, "I've read that many patients have success avoiding nausea and vomiting by taking Kytril or Zofran prophylactically. Is it possible to get a prescription for one of those or a similar medication?"

Few doctors will turn down a request for symptom control. But your physician may feel, based on experience and your particular circumstances, that an effect is so unlikely or so mild that only minimal medication or none at all is warranted. For instance, over-the-counter pain relievers like aspirin and ibuprofen often provide relief equal to prescription drugs such as Darvon and codeine, at significantly less cost and with far fewer potential side effects. Repeated battles with a doctor over adequate symptom management—a rare occurrence—are grounds for changing physicians. How much pain, nausea, depression, and so forth you can withstand is your call, no one else's.

How to Describe Symptoms to the Doctor

One of the keys to managing your symptoms effectively is to keep your doctor posted on *exactly* how you're feeling. Not everyone does. "Many people so desperately want to stay on schedule with treatment that they put on a brave face and downplay the true extent of their symptoms," observes Maureen Sawchuk, nursing coordinator at the Lombardi Cancer Center.

Or, she adds, "they don't want to seem like a complainer. Patients often view doctors as authority figures, and so they tend to want to please them by being the 'good' patient. But being a good patient doesn't mean that you have to put up with unbearable symptoms. The physician wants you to be truthful, because he wants you to be as comfortable as possible. We all do.

"If a patient on chemotherapy tells us that an antinausea regimen isn't working well, we'll bring in the pharmacy team to help us come up with the right combination." Inform your doctor or nurse about symptoms immediately. The sooner the medical team knows you have a problem, the easier it is to treat.

A Word to Family and Friends: When a loved one with cancer is naturally on the stoic side, encourage him at medical visits not to minimize his condition: "Come on, Dad, you're not really telling Dr. Hackett how sick you've been." Or take the physician aside and describe the symptoms yourself. If you can't accompany the patient, phone the doctor with any concerns you have about how he seems to be feeling.

What to Tell the Doctor

- Describe or point out where the symptom is occurring. Pain? Itching? Fluid retention? Where on the body?

- Describe the sensation and intensity in as much detail as you can. Would you

---

Descriptive Words for Characterizing Symptoms

- aching ▪ burning
- convulsive ▪ deep ▪ dull
- excruciating ▪ gnawing
- intense ▪ numbing
- palpitating ▪ periodic
- racking ▪ sharp ▪ sporadic
- stinging ▪ subtle
- throbbing ▪ tingling
- unbearable ▪ unrelenting

characterize the pain in your side as "dull"? Or "burning"? Is your stool "loose" or "watery"? The difference could provide your oncologist with an important clue.

- Use numbers to express the intensity at its worst and at its mildest. *"At its worst, my anxiety is about a seven on a scale of one to ten. Other times it's closer to a two."*

- How is the symptom affecting your life? Is it interfering with:
  General activity
  Sleep
  Eating
  Mood
  Your ability to walk or get around
  Your ability to work
  Your relations with other people

- What makes the symptom better or worse? *"If I hold a pillow to my stomach when I cough or take a deep breath, the pain from the incision doesn't hurt as much."*

- If you're presently on medication to relieve the symptom, tell the doctor what you're taking, how much, how often, and how it seems to be working. *"I'm currently taking a tablespoon of Metamucil one to three times a day. My constipation was a six on a scale of ten; by the third day it was about a three, but I'm still not regular."*

Keeping a chart in which you write down the frequency, duration, and intensity of any symptoms, may help your doctor discover a pattern to them. If you often feel queasy after eating, it could be diet-related. But your physician might attribute the nausea more to the narcotic analgesic you've been prescribed for pain. The solution could be to take an antinausea agent shortly before each dose.

Questions to Ask . . . Before Taking Any Medication

Be doubly safe: Ask your doctor or nurse *and* the pharmacist these questions:
- What is the medicine's generic name and brand name?
- What is this medication supposed to do?
- How frequently should I take it, and at what time(s) of day?

TABLE 8.1 Sample Symptoms Chart

Circle the day or days on which you underwent treatment.

Rate the severity of each symptom that occurs on a given day, using a scale of 1 to 5:

1 = discomfort

2 = mild

3 = distress

4 = severe

5 = the worst

Also note in the box how long the symptom lasted:

C = constant (present most of the time)

I = intermittent (comes and goes)

Week of _____

Cycle _____

Day of the Week	Mon.	Tues.	Wed.	Thurs.	Fri.	Sat.	Sun.
Date							
Aches and Pains							
Bone, muscle, or joint pain							
Breast tenderness and/or enlargement							
Chest pain or tightness							
Headache							
Pain at the injection site							
Testicular pain							
Blood-Related							
Bloody urine or stool, red spots on the skin, or unusual bleeding or bruising							
Cardiac-Related							
Irregular or rapid heartbeat							

Day of the Week	Mon.	Tues.	Wed.	Thurs.	Fri.	Sat.	Sun.
Date							
Digestion-Related							
Appetite loss							
Black, tarry stools or bloody vomit							
Bloating, gas							
Constipation							
Diarrhea							
Difficulty in swallowing							
Indigestion							
Nausea and/or vomiting							
Stomach pain or cramps							
Weight loss							
Endocrine-Related							
Hyperglycemia or hypoglycemia (abnormally elevated or abnormally low blood sugar)							
Genitourinary-Related							
Discolored urine, decreased or frequent urination, painful or difficult urination							
Gynecologic							
Enlarged clitoris							
Missing or irregular menstruation							
Vaginal bleeding, burning, dryness, or itching							
Mouth-Related							
Lip or mouth sores							
Neurologic							
Clumsiness, difficulty walking							
Convulsions							

Day of the Week	Mon.	Tues.	Wed.	Thurs.	Fri.	Sat.	Sun.
Date							
Hallucinations							
Numbness							
Tremors or twitching							
Weakness or paralysis							
Other Symptoms							
Changes in fingernails or toenails							
Confusion							
Decreased breast size							
Deepened voice							
Dizziness							
Drowsiness or fatigue							
Extreme thirst							
Faintness							
Fever or chills							
Hair loss							
Hot flashes							
Increased hair growth							
Lumpy breasts and/or nipple discharge							
Profuse sweating							
Sleep disturbance							
Swelling in the feet, ankles, fingers, or neck							
Unexpected or increased flow of breast milk							
Psychological							
Agitation, anxiety, depression, mood swings, paranoia, delusion of grandeur							
Respiratory-Related							
Coughing, hoarseness, or wheezing							
Shortness of breath							
Tightness in the throat							

Day of the Week	Mon.	Tues.	Wed.	Thurs.	Fri.	Sat.	Sun.
Date							
Sensory Disturbances							
Blurry or distorted vision							
Difficulty in hearing or ringing in the ears							
Metallic taste or loss of taste							
Slurred speech							
Sexually-Related							
Decreased or heightened libido							
Decreased testicle size							
Frequent or continuing erections							
Impotence							
Skin-Related							
Acne, boils, or skin rash							
Blistered, peeling, or scaling skin							
Darkened, thickened, or discolored skin and/or fingernails							
Itching							
Yellow eyes or skin							

- What dosage will I be taking?

- Is it necessary to ingest this medication with food or milk, or can I take it on an empty stomach?

  ♦ When taking oral medications with water, be sure to drink eight ounces. Too little water actually prevents some drugs from working properly.

- Are there any foods or beverages this medication cannot be taken with?

- Will this drug interfere with other medications I am taking, or vice versa?

♦ List for your doctor every medication you are currently on, including nonprescription drugs, nutritional supplements, and natural herbal remedies.

- What should I do if I miss a dose?

- While I'm on the medication, are there any restrictions on driving?

- How long should I take the medicine? Must I finish the entire prescription?

- Does the prescription include refills? If so, how many? What should I do if I need to refill the prescription?

- Can I expect the same results from the generic equivalent of this drug?

- Does the medication have any possible side effects? If I experience side effects, how will these be managed?

- Are there any side effects I should report to you?

- When will we be able to tell if the medication is effective?

- Do you have any print information on this medication that I can read?

- How much does this prescription cost? (Just to eliminate any surprises at the drugstore cash register.)

♦ If you have difficulty in swallowing pills, ask if the medication can be crushed, or if it comes in the form of a liquid, skin patch, rectal suppository, inhaler, or nose spray.

Common Symptoms, Side Effects, and Complications of Cancer and Cancer Treatment

Blood Disorders

One of the most common and serious effects of cancer is *cytopenia:* a reduction in the number of white blood cells, red blood cells, and platelets. Neutropenia, erythropenia, and thrombocytopenia can be dangerous in and of themselves. They pose an additional hazard to people receiving anticancer drugs because abnormally low blood counts may force treatment to be delayed or the dose reduced.

COMMON CAUSES

Chemotherapy and extensive radiotherapy often interfere with the formation and maturation of blood cells (hematopoiesis), mainly by inhibiting activity in the bone marrow *(myelosuppression)*. The disease itself can impair blood-cell production in several ways. Cancer cells may:

- Damage or destroy the marrow
- Displace or decimate the stem cells and immature blast cells from which all blood cells develop
- Curb production of growth factors, substances that stimulate hematopoiesis
- Induce production of substances that prevent stem cells and blast cells from dividing and developing

Certain secondary complications of cancer, too, can bring about cytopenia, such as:

- Severe malnutrition
- Blood loss
- Immune disorders that cause the body to destroy its own blood cells
- Hypersplenism, a condition in which the spleen enlarges as it accumulates blood cells. It is seen mainly in leukemia and lymphomas, but it can occur in any cancer that spreads to the spleen or the liver.

Leukopenia/Neutropenia

According to a Gallup poll of chemotherapy patients, nearly half had their treatment postponed at least once because their white counts were alarmingly low. White cells safeguard us against infection, particularly the neutrophils, which make up 60 percent of all white cells. Their job is to intercept and destroy bacteria.

A person is said to be mildly neutropenic when her absolute neutrophil count *(ANC)* is between 2,000 and 1,000. The ANC is determined by multiplying the percentage of neutrophils by the total white-blood-cell count. Oncologists will generally continue chemotherapy so long as the number stays in the 500-to-1,000 range, which is considered moderate neutropenia. "For some reason," says Dr. Chitra Rajagopal, one of my oncologists, "at 500 or greater the body's ability to fight bacterial infections remains almost normal." My neutrophil level had dipped to around 300—severe neutropenia—when it was decided to lower the dosage of 5-FU and leucovorin.

Normal Levels of White Blood Cells (Leukocytes)	
White Blood Cell Count (WBC) 4,100 to 10,600 in a single drop (microliter) of blood	
Type/Approximate Number	
Neutrophils	3,000 to 7,000
Lymphocytes	1,000 to 4,000
Monocytes	100 to 600
Eosinophils	50 to 400
Basophils	25 to 100

Of the three solid components in the blood, white cells are the least abundant. For every leukocyte, there are forty platelets and six hundred red cells. White cells are also the most sensitive to chemo and radiation, explains Dr. Rajagopal, "because they divide much more rapidly than the other cells."

Most chemo regimens suppress your immune system for perhaps a week to ten days, after which time the neutrophil count starts climbing back up. The other key players in fighting off disease are the lymphocytes, which track down viruses. "Although chemotherapy depletes the numbers of lymphocytes," says Dr. Rajagopal, "the ones that remain are functional."

During this period of impaired immunity, the major concern is to immediately treat any bacterial infections that develop. The GI tract, along with the skin and the respiratory tract, is a haven for bacteria. Normally, its lining prevents the microorganisms from migrating into your circulation. But when that fragile barrier sustains damage from chemotherapy, the bacteria easily find their way into the bloodstream. This can result in systemic *septicemia,* often referred to as blood poisoning. Or the germs may lodge in the lungs, the mouth, the urinary tract, or some other part of the body. "The type of bacteria is more important than the site of infection," says Dr. Rajagopal. "Most common bacteria are usually sensitive to antibiotic drugs. But then there are rarer organisms like the *Pseudomonas,* which can be deadly wherever they are."

Prolonged neutropenia lasting several weeks or more, as happens following a bone-marrow transplant, weakens the immune response against nonbacterial infections too. When several types of white cells are decimated, the medical term *leukopenia* may be used.

SYMPTOMS OF INFECTION

- Fever over 101°F ▪ Sweating ▪ Diarrhea ▪ Redness or swelling, particularly around a wound, sore, boil, or pimple
- Joint pain ▪ Flushed face ▪ Fatigue ▪ Chills ▪ Burning upon urination ▪ Severe cough or sore throat ▪ Unusual vaginal discharge or itching ▪ Headache ▪ Warm, dry skin
- Lack of appetite

At 104°F and above:
- Shortness of breath ▪ Rapid heartbeat ▪ Confusion, delirium, convulsions

If You Develop a Fever

Never ignore a fever or let it "run its course." Tell your oncologist. In cancer, an oral temperature over 101 degrees frequently heralds an infection. Contrary to popular belief, a fever does not "burn up" whatever's ailing you. If left untreated, the infection can become life-threatening, especially in people who are immunocompromised. A fever of 104 degrees or more can overstimulate the brain and overexert the heart.

♦ Family and friends should know that if you experience convulsions, delirium, or confusion, they should immediately take you to a hospital emergency room or call the local emergency medical service.

Other Causes of Fever

Some chemotherapy and immunotherapy agents can trigger flu-like symptoms that come on anywhere from a few hours to a few days after treatment. Taking diphenhydramine (brand name: Benadryl), an antihistamine, and the pain reliever acetaminophen before cancer therapy can help to prevent so-called drug fever. Discuss this with your oncologist.

A fever can also be a reaction to transfusions of donor blood products, particularly whole blood containing white cells. If this is a recurrent problem, ask your doctor about using Benadryl and acetaminophen prior to a transfusion. Another way to minimize *febrile* reactions is for all white cells to be extracted from the units of blood or for all blood products to be irradiated.

Several cancers may induce fevers, among them lymphomas, leukemia, and solid tumors that either metastasize to the liver or block vital passageways such as the digestive tract, the urinary tract, or the respiratory tract. Why this occurs is unclear, but the fevers typically subside once the underlying disease is brought under control.

HOW INFECTIONS ARE TREATED

Systemic Antimicrobial Therapy—Bacterial infections are treated with one or more systemic antibiotics, the largest group of antimicrobial drugs. If you are neutropenic, it is vital that intravenous antibiotics be administered promptly, even when the cause of the fever cannot be determined, as is often the case. "The antibiotics are started in the hospital," says Dr. Rajagopal, "because patients need to be evaluated. Then we try to get them home in twenty-four to thirty-six hours."

Typically, the drugs are discontinued after five to seven days, provided you're free of fever and infection, and your neutrophil count has risen to an acceptable range. If the neutropenia hasn't improved after a week and the fever persists or recurs, the doctor might add an *antifungal* medication and possibly an *antiviral*.

♦ When taking antibiotics, always finish the prescription, even once you're feeling better.

Managing the Fever

- Over-the-counter fever reducers such as acetaminophen (Tylenol), ibuprofen (Advil), naproxen (Aleve), and salicylic acid (aspirin) all bring down temperatures. But check with your doctor regarding which one to take.

- Drink more fluids than normal to cool down your system and keep you hydrated. The American College of Physicians recommends consuming four to six sixteen-ounce glasses of cool, noncaffeinated liquids every twelve hours, unless your doctor has instructed you otherwise.

See "Dehydration," page 729.

- Eat foods high in calories and carbohydrates. When you have a fever, you burn fuel faster than normal. Pasta, potatoes, bread, and fruit can help to restore your energy.

- Cover yourself with a single sheet, unless you're cold or experiencing chills, in which case add blankets as needed. Damp bedclothes and bed linens should be changed frequently. Not only will you feel more comfortable, you'll reduce your risk of developing a bedsore.

- A lukewarm bath or sponge bath can help to lower elevated temperatures, as can a cool compress placed on your forehead.

- If your temperature is 103 degrees or higher, place ice packs under your arms or in the groin area for approximately fifteen minutes at fifteen-minute intervals, or until the fever breaks.

  ◆ Don't use ice packs if you are receiving radiation therapy to any of these areas.

- Take your temperature every two to four hours and keep a log for the doctor. Record the time; your temperature; any related symptoms; and what steps were taken to lower the fever, such as a tepid bath or medication. If your fever went down, note by how many degrees.

HOW NEUTROPENIA/LEUKOPENIA IS TREATED

Granulocyte Growth Factor—White blood cells are the only component of the blood that is not transfused, except for infections that do not respond to antimicrobial drugs. A single platelet lives in the body for 10 days; a red cell, for 120 days. Leukocytes survive for only twenty-four to forty-eight hours, so the benefit from a transfusion is short-lived. In addition, recipients often experience severe reactions when their immune systems mobilize against the foreign cells.

An injectable immunologic agent, filgrastim (Neupogen), enables patients to continue with chemotherapy when they otherwise might not be able to. It is a synthetic version of a natural substance manufactured in the body, called colony-stimulating factor, which steps up production of neutrophils. The drug is usually administered shortly after your last treatment in a cycle and is continued for ten to fourteen days—before and during the time when blood-cell production sinks to its lowest point. Neupogen reduces both the duration and the severity of neutropenia. It is also given to patients following bone-marrow transplantation or peripheral-blood stem-cell transplantation to accelerate recovery.

HOW YOU CAN HELP YOURSELF

Steps for Preventing Infection During Chemotherapy

Being temporarily immunocompromised doesn't mean that you have to lock yourself in your bedroom and not venture out again until your white counts improve. "That's a real misconception among a lot of patients," observes Dr. John Marshall of the Lombardi Cancer Center. Naturally, you don't want to wipe a child's runny nose during this time, he says, "but more often than not, an infection is going to develop from *your own* bacteria, not because someone else sneezed."

General Precautions

- Stay away from anyone who has a communicable disease, such as a cold, the flu, measles, or chicken pox. Let people around you know that your resistance is low. Explain what could happen if you contracted an infection and ask them to keep their distance or alert you when they're sick. Avoiding crowds is a wise idea too.

- Wear protective gloves when you're gardening or cleaning up after pets.

- Try not to nick or cut yourself when handling knives, scissors, pins, or needles.

- Never share drinking glasses and other items that could contain another person's germs, including washcloths, towels, hairbrushes, combs, razors, and toothbrushes.

- Avoid sunburn by wearing sunscreen and staying out of the sun during the late-morning and early-afternoon hours. Peeling, blistered skin acts as a portal for infection.

Personal Hygiene

- Wash your hands. *A lot.* Washing away germs under running water is the single most effective way of protecting yourself. Lather well, using liquid soap from a pump bottle, then dry your hands with paper towels to cut down on the transmission of bacteria and other organisms. Be sure to clean under your nails and between the fingers, and wash any rings you may be wearing. Then liberally rub on lotion to keep your skin moist and free of cracks.

    ♦ Always wash your hands before and after handling food and after you use the bathroom.

- Take a warm bath, shower, or bed bath every day. Be sure to wash between folds of skin. Germs' favorite haunts include the groin, the area beneath a woman's breasts—anywhere that skin touches skin and is not exposed to air. Then pat your skin dry—don't rub.

- If you should cut or scrape yourself, clean the wound right away with soap and water, then apply antiseptic and cover it with a bandage.

- Clean your rectum gently but thoroughly after each bowel movement, wiping from front to back. The rectal area harbors bacteria that can live and grow without oxygen. According to Dr. Rajagopal, "They are much harder to treat than common bacteria." Alert your physician if you have hemorrhoids or if your anus becomes irritated, because any break in the barrier can allow several types of bacteria to infiltrate the body.

- Take your temperature orally, not rectally.

- Don't cut or tear your nail cuticles; use cuticle cream and remover instead.

- Use an electric shaver rather than a hand razor, so as not to cut yourself.

- Clean your teeth and gums with a soft-bristle toothbrush.

- Resist the urge to scratch or squeeze pimples.

- During menstrual periods, women should use sanitary napkins, not tampons, which are more likely to breed germs and possibly tear vaginal tissue.

Diet and Nutrition
- Defrost frozen foods in the refrigerator or microwave only and keep them covered. Never leave them out on the counter to thaw.

- Wash the lids of containers and the tops of cans before opening.

- When you're done preparing food—particularly meat, poultry, and eggs—disinfect countertops and cutting boards and anything else you may have touched, such as faucets, kitchen cabinets, stove and oven knobs, and the door handle to the refrigerator.

- Slice deli meats and cheeses yourself at home.

- Store food in sealable containers. The temperature in your refrigerator should be no higher than forty degrees, and the freezer, zero degrees.

- Cook food thoroughly. That means no runny eggs or pink meat or poultry.

- While you're on chemotherapy, do not eat raw oysters or alfalfa sprouts or drink unpasteurized juices, all of which have been cited by the Food and Drug Administration as sources of foodborne infections. Shellfish, though not on the FDA's list of foods carrying warnings for people with weakened immunity, should also be avoided during episodes of neutropenia, says Dr. Rajagopal, "because they contain many organisms that are difficult to kill through cooking. For a person with a normal immune system, it usually doesn't pose a problem, but in neutropenic patients, eating shellfish can cause profound diarrhea."

- Use a manual can opener, not an electric one, and clean it after each use.

- Fresh vegetables should be cooked, never eaten raw. You can eat any fruit that has a nonedible peel, such as bananas, melons, and oranges, but not apples, pears, and peaches. Wash all fruits and veggies first.

Vaccinations

- Ask your oncologist about whether or not you should be immunized against certain infectious diseases. For example, people with Hodgkin's disease receive vaccinations for pneumococcus, meningococcus, and *Hemophilus influenzae* type B (HIB), the bacteria responsible for such serious infections as meningitis, pneumonia, and septicemia. The shots are given before treatment begins, and booster shots are given two years or more after therapy has been completed. Patients who have undergone bone-marrow transplantation or splenectomy to remove the spleen are also at inordinate risk of bacterial infections and would be candidates for these and possibly other immunizations.

Steps for Preventing Infection Following Bone-Marrow Transplantation

Bone-marrow transplantation subjects patients to prolonged leukopenia. In addition to the preventive measures mentioned above, they should observe the following precautions.

General Precautions

- You must wear a mask *at all times* as long as you are on immuno-suppressants.

- Take your temperature in the morning, early afternoon, and later at night for the first month, and anytime you feel warm or have the chills.

- Spray doorknobs and faucets with disinfectant at least once a day and spray the toilet seat and the flushing lever after each use.

- Avoid crowds. If you need to do the grocery shopping, for instance, go early in the morning or at night, when the store is relatively empty. Restaurants, however, are off-limits for now.

- Avoid contact with anyone who has recently had a "live"-virus vaccination for polio, rubella, or another disease. This precaution remains in effect for up to one year; longer if you have chronic graft-versus-host disease.

- Stay away from construction sites, which may send bacteria and fungi from the soil into the air.

- Do not go camping.

- Avoid handling wood.

- If you underwent an allogeneic transplant or received interleukin-2, wear protective clothing and apply sunscreen with a sun-protec-tion factor (SPF) of at least 15 anytime you go outside. Exposure to the sun may spur or exacerbate graft-versus-host disease.

If You Have Children at Home

- Ask your child's teacher, baby-sitter, or day-care person to notify you immediately if any of the children your youngster has contact with develops any illness, including a cold.

- Instruct your children not to bring their friends home until you're fully recovered.

- Avoid any youngster who's been exposed to chicken pox, measles, strep, or other infections. "One of our autologous patients wanted to go home, but his child had developed strep throat," recalls Dr. Meehan. "So he went to live with his parents for a while."

  ◆ Alert your BMT physician if a child in your home (1) has been exposed to any of these diseases and (2) is due for any vaccination.

If You Have Pets at Home

- Prior to your discharge from the transplant center, arrange for a family member or friend to have pets tested for diseases that are contagious to humans. For instance, parrots and other pet birds can transmit a respiratory infection called *psittacosis.*

- You should not handle litter boxes, birdcage linings, fishbowls, and turtle bowls, and you should avoid contact with animal saliva, urine, and fecal matter. People who are immunocompromised can contract *toxoplasmosis,* a serious protozoal infection, from cat feces. Discourage pets from biting and scratching.

- Stay out of pet stores, animal shelters, and petting zoos.

Around the Home

- Before you come home, have someone change filters for air-conditioners, heaters, air purifiers, and so on. New filters should be installed regularly after that, but never while you're at home.

- Don't do housework for the first one hundred days after transplant.

- If you have plants, avoid contact with the soil or standing water. That includes emptying water from a flower vase.

- Refrain from gardening until your doctor advises you otherwise.

Diet and Nutrition

- Until day 50 following an autoBMT and day 100 following an alloBMT, do not eat raw vegetables; fresh shellfish; or raw fruit, except those that can be peeled, such as bananas, grapefruits, oranges, and melons. Wash peelable fruits before and after peeling.

- For the first few months, take a multivitamin supplement containing no iron.

Vaccinations and Transfusions

- Even if a marrow donor was inoculated against childhood diseases, the immunity is not transferred with the transplant. One year after alloBMT, patients should receive tetanus, diphtheria, and *inactivated* ("dead") polio vaccinations. Flu shots and the pneumococcal vaccine are also advised.

- Two years after transplant, your blood should be tested for *immunocompetence*—meaning that your immune system now produces adequate numbers of antibodies against various disease-causing organisms. Thereafter you will need inoculations for rubella, mumps, and measles three times every sixty to ninety days, the same schedule recommended for newborns.

- If you received donor marrow, you should wear a medical bracelet or carry a medical-alert wallet card at all times indicating that you had an allogeneic BMT and should be transfused *only* with blood products that have been irradiated.

Anemia (Erythropenia)

A complete blood count (CBC) expresses your level of red cells in three different ways. The *red-blood-cell count* tells your doctor the exact number of red cells in a drop of blood, while the *hematocrit* measures the percentage of red cells in the sample. The *hemoglobin* count tallies up the amount of hemoglobin in the blood. Hemoglobin, made of protein and iron, lends erythrocytes their red pigment and enables them to transport oxygen from the lungs to all the body's tissues. A substantial reduction in any of these numbers indicates anemia, the most common disorder of red blood cells. Patients tend to tire easily and may become short of breath because not enough red cells are making their rounds throughout the circulation.

> **Medic Alert**
>
> **The basic stainless-steel Medic Alert bracelet engraved with your personal medical information costs $35, plus a $15 annual renewal fee.**
> 800-432-5378
> *http://www.medicalert.org*

Anemia can also prevent the body from utilizing iron, which it needs to build new red blood cells as old ones die off. It is generally recommended that anemic patients load up on foods rich in this mineral, such as liver, lean red meat, kidney beans, whole-wheat bread, and green, leafy vegetables like kale and spinach. But not if you've had a bone-marrow transplant, cautions Dr. Rajagopal.

"Patients who go through transplantation receive an average of five to ten transfusions of red cells during the period where they have no bone marrow," she says. "When these cells are destroyed, the hemoglobin is excreted, but the iron gets deposited into the lining of the gastrointestinal tract." So although these men and women are still marginally anemic by the time they leave the hospital, "increased iron intake could trigger conditions of iron overload or destroy their liver." She instructs patients to avoid iron for one year. Gradually, as the cells in the GI mucosa are replaced by new ones, the level of iron in the body returns to normal.

> ### Normal Levels of Red Blood Cells (Erythrocytes)
>
> **Red-Blood-Cell Count (RBC)**
> * **Men: 4.6 to 6.2 million red blood cells in a single drop (microliter) of blood**
> * **Women: 4.2 to 5.4 million per microliter of blood**
>
> **Hematocrit (HCT)**
> * **Men: 45 to 57 percent**
> * **Women: 37 to 47 percent**
>
> **Hemoglobin (HGB)**
> * **Men: 14 to 18 grams per 100 milliliters of blood**
> * **Women: 12 to 16 grams per 100 milliliters of blood**

SYMPTOMS OF ANEMIA

- Fatigue ▪ Paleness of the palms of the hands, the fingernails, and the lining of the eyelids ▪ Dizziness, particularly upon standing up or sitting down ▪ Chills ▪ Shortness of breath ▪ Rapid pulse ▪ Chest pains

HOW ANEMIA IS TREATED

Erythrocyte Growth Factor—Epoetin alfa (Epogen, Procrit) does for red blood cells what granulocyte growth factor does for white blood cells. It is a synthetic form of *erythropoietin,* a colony-stimulating factor produced in the kidneys. Patients who become anemic during chemotherapy, radiation, or concurrent chemoradiation may be injected with epoetin alfa to increase their red cells and with it their hemoglobin.

Epogen and Procrit afford doctors the option of not having to order a transfusion of red cells. The fewer transfusions you need, the smaller your risk of acquiring a bloodborne infection, as remote as that may be. Should you require a bone-marrow transplant somewhere down the line, it's important to bear in mind that the possibility of graft failure rises slightly along with the number of transfusions a patient has undergone prior to transplant. Alfa epoetin takes several days to boost the hematocrit, so if the anemia is severe enough to defer cancer treatment, "most centers would intervene with a transfusion," says Dr. Rajagopal. The National Marrow Donor Program emphasizes that while it is reasonable to want to limit transfusions, they should always be administered when necessary.

Transfusions—Donor red cells can be refrigerated for up to forty-two days or frozen for a maximum of ten years.

HOW YOU CAN HELP YOURSELF

Anemia is just one of several causes of fatigue in people with cancer. For tips on how to conserve your energy, see "Fatigue," page 778.

Thrombocytopenia (Clotting Disorder)

At least one in four patients receiving chemotherapy develop thrombocytopenia, in which the bone marrow fails to turn out sufficient numbers of platelets, the tiny cells that promote clotting of the blood. Radiation can also lower the platelet count.

> **Normal Level of Platelets (Thrombocytes)**
>
> An average of 250,000 per cubic millimeter of blood

A person's platelet level can plummet from the normal range of 150,000 to 400,000 per cubic millimeter of blood to 20,000 before patients enter the danger zone. However, severe thrombocytopenia is serious enough to delay, reduce, or prematurely discontinue chemotherapy if the clotting problems can't be rectified. When blood doesn't clot properly, patients can bleed or hemorrhage spontaneously.

SYMPTOMS OF THROMBOCYTOPENIA

- Unexplained bruises ▪ Pinpoint red spots, called *petechiae,* under the skin or inside the mouth ▪ Reddish or pinkish urine
- Black or bloody stool ▪ Bleeding gums ▪ Nosebleeds

◆ Let your doctor know about any of these symptoms.

HOW THROMBOCYTOPENIA IS TREATED

Thrombocyte Growth Factor—Oprelvekin (Neumega), a synthetic version of the naturally occurring platelet growth factor human inter-leukin-11, acts in a manner similar to its counterparts for red and white cells. The agent, injected under the skin six to twenty-four hours after chemotherapy has been given, stimulates the bone marrow to increase its production of platelets. Other colony-stimulating factors for platelets are in development.

Transfusions—Oncologists try to avoid excessive transfusions of platelets, which are now transfused more than red cells. If your level fell to, say, 100,000 per cubic millimeter of blood, or perhaps even 50,000, your doctor would probably recommend utilizing thrombocyte growth factor. Below 20,000 "and certainly below 10,000," says Dr. Rajagopal, platelet transfusion becomes necessary, "because at those levels the risk for spontaneous bleeding is extremely high."

Platelets often have to be transfused on a daily basis. The drawback to repeated transfusions is that a patient's immune system reacts to the donor platelets, which can come from several different volunteers. According to Dr. Rajagopal, "Patients develop antibodies to the various proteins that sit on the surface of the transfused platelets." This happens, she points out, even in the absence of white cells. Before long, patients no longer respond to the transfusions.

To limit the number of antibodies your body forms, most centers try to obtain platelets from a specific donor. "This way," she explains, "the recipient will make antibodies only to that particular person's antigens." Siblings' platelets are frequently more compatible. "When a patient has significant antibody formation and doesn't respond to platelets no matter how many units he receives, we'll try to hunt down siblings and ask them to donate at their local Red Cross and have the platelets shipped to us."

HOW YOU CAN HELP YOURSELF

- When your platelet count is low, be extremely careful when handling sharp instruments or objects.

- If you must cook, wear heavily padded oven mitts. Similarly, put on thick gloves if you're working in the garden or around plants with thorns.

- Check with your doctor before drinking any alcoholic beverages, which can impair clotting.

- Also check with your physician before taking any medication. Aspirin, for instance, is an anticoagulant and should be avoided. Read the labels of all drugs. If you see *acetylsalicylic acid* listed among the ingredients, it means the product contains aspirin. Another pain reliever, ibuprofen, also interferes with clotting. Use acetaminophen instead.

- Use a soft-bristle toothbrush to gently clean your teeth after eating, then rinse. The idea is to rid the mouth of food particles, which can cause bleeding, sores, or abscesses of the gums. And no flossing!

- Blow your nose gently. The nose contains many tiny capillaries that can burst open if you blow too hard.

- Use petroleum jelly, K-Y jelly, or lip balm to moisten your lips and nasal passages.

> ### What to Do If You Have Bleeding
>
> **Press a clean cloth against the area for at least ten minutes. If the bleeding does not stop, have someone take you to a hospital emergency room or call your local emergency medical service.**

- Allow hot foods to cool down before eating, so as not to burn or tear the fragile lining of the mouth. If your mouth is sore, stay on a soft, bland diet for a while, which is less likely to cause a cut, scrape, or bleeding. Suggestions: soup, mashed potatoes, pudding, pureed meat, gelatin, custard.

- Do not take your temperature with a rectal thermometer. Rectal tissue is extremely delicate and prone to tearing. Enemas and suppositories should not be inserted in the rectum either.

- When shaving, use an electric razor only.

- Avoid activities that could cause a bump, bruise, burn, or fall, such as bicycling, ironing, and all contact sports. Ask family and friends to take over heavy lifting and strenuous activities.

- Don't eat coarse foods like popcorn and peanuts, which can irritate the gastrointestinal tract. Follow this chapter's steps for avoiding constipation too. Straining during bowel movements can rupture tiny vessels in the area.

See "Constipation," page 739.

- If you wear dentures, make sure they fit properly and don't irritate the gums. Whenever you remove them, rinse your mouth with an alcohol-free mouthwash.

- Women should not use vaginal douches when their platelet counts are low because the nozzle of the bag or bottle may scrape or scratch the vaginal tissue.

Digestive Disorders

Appetite Loss (Anorexia)

COMMON CAUSES

- Take your pick

Nausea, a metallic taste in the mouth, fatigue, difficulty in swallowing, depression—these are among the many reasons why a person with cancer may lose interest in food. However, sound nutrition must be viewed as an essential component of your recovery. Eating well doesn't kill cancer cells, but it helps you to better heal, combat infection, maintain your strength, and withstand the side effects of therapy. A healthful diet is beneficial from a psychological standpoint too, in that it is one of the few aspects of cancer care that patients can control.

Necessary Nutrients: Prioritizing Protein and Cramming Calories

Cancer and cancer therapy can compromise nutrition in one or more ways. Besides producing symptoms and side effects that make eating a chore, the disease can interfere with the body's ability to convert protein, carbohydrates, and fat in food into energy, or *calories*.

Tumor cells deprive normal cells of nutrients. Meanwhile the body is expending extra energy as it heals from the effects of cancer surgery, radiotherapy, or chemotherapy. In order to sustain vital functions, the

The Five Major Classes of Nutrients
Protein
Carbohydrates
Fats
Vitamins
Minerals

body retrieves nutrients stored in fatty tissue. Once all available fat has been broken down for fuel, it sets to work on muscle. Of all nutrients, protein is the one most essential for building muscle, bone, skin, and blood cells. If the body's cells consume more protein than you take in, muscle mass rapidly wastes away, causing the emaciated look often associated with cancer. About half of all cancer patients experience this condition, called *cachexia*. Because their body doesn't have the raw material from which to manufacture red and white blood cells, they frequently become anemic and immunocompromised as well.

A low-fat, high-fiber diet can reduce your risk of several cancers, including carcinomas of the breast, colon, and endometrium. But

TABLE 8.2	How Many Calories and How Much Protein Do I Need During Treatment?

Calories per Day	
Men and women who are underweight	Multiply your weight by 18
Men and women who are of normal weight	Multiply your weight by 16
Men and women who are overweight	Multiply your weight by 13

Grams of Protein per Day
Multiply your weight by 0.5

that's something to consider *after* you're fully on the mend from treatment. Your main concern right now is to load up on protein and calories. Before you begin therapy, a doctor, nurse, or dietician should review your eating habits with you and suggest ways for you to stay well nourished. A formula devised by the National Cancer Institute, shown in table 8.2, will give you an idea of how many calories and how much protein you'll need to maintain your weight.

Around Christmastime, when I weighed a skeletal 145 pounds, I required roughly 2,610 calories (145×18) and 72.5 grams of protein (145×0.5) per day. By the end of chemotherapy in late spring, I was back up around my ideal weight of 175 pounds. Yet I didn't need much more in the way of food: 2,800 calories (175×16) and 87.5 grams of protein (175×0.5) daily. A mere four-ounce serving of low-fat cottage cheese would supply the additional 15 grams of protein, along with 101 calories. A healthy adult man needs about 59 grams of protein per day; a healthy adult woman, about 49 grams.

On days when you don't have much of an appetite, aim for foods dense in high-quality protein. These come mainly from animal sources: meat, chicken, fish, eggs, and dairy products. Vegetables, grains, and other plant sources contain low-quality protein, with the exception of soybeans and soybean products such as tofu. Look at the difference between these *complete-protein* and *incomplete-protein* foods:

Complete Proteins			Incomplete Proteins		
Food	Serving Size	Grams of Protein	Food	Serving Size	Grams of Protein
Canned tuna in water	3 ounces	30	Cooked lima beans	¹/₂ cup	6
Skinless white-meat turkey	3 ounces	30	Baked potato	1	4.6
Smoked trout	3 ounces	29	Brown rice	²/₃ cup	3.3
Porterhouse steak	3 ounces	23.9	Orange	1	1.3
Roasted white-meat chicken	3 ounces	23	Cooked peas	¹/₂ cup	1
Protein-fortified milk	1 cup	9.7	Raw carrot	1	0.7

Recipes combining two or more plant proteins frequently add up to a complete protein. You can boost your protein and calorie counts by liberally adding sauces, gravies, and butter to cooked foods; breading meats and vegetables; and taking oral medications with milk shakes or nutritional supplements instead of water, unless a label specifies that you take the drug on an empty stomach. Tables 8.3 and 8.4 contain the National Cancer Institute's serving suggestions for increasing protein and calories.

Carbohydrates and Dietary Fat

Less attention is paid to the two other nutrients that contain calories. Cancer may cause you to temporarily rethink your attitudes toward dietary fat, which is normally considered a nemesis of good health. When you need to maximize your calorie intake but don't have much of an appetite, fat-laden foods get you to your goal more quickly. Each gram of fat delivers nine calories, as compared to four calories from a gram of protein or carbohydrates.

However, fatty foods should still be eaten in moderation. As clinical dietitian Susan Sloan of the Lombardi Cancer Center explains, "Even though cancer patients need calories, a high-fat diet sits in the digestive tract for so long that if they have a high-fat meal for lunch, they may not be hungry come dinnertime, which defeats the whole purpose."

TABLE 8.3 **Super Sources of Protein**

Food	Suggested Serving Ideas
Beans and bean curd (tofu)	• Add to soup, casseroles, pasta, rice dishes. • Mash with cheese and milk. • Whip into fruit-juice smoothies.
Cheeses, hard or semisoft	• Melt on sandwiches, bread, muffins, tortillas, hamburgers, hot dogs, other meat or fish, vegetables, eggs, stewed fruit, pies. • Grate and add to soup, sauces, casseroles, vegetable dishes, mashed potatoes, rice, noodles, meat loaf.
Cheeses, soft (cottage cheese, ricotta cheese)	• Add to fruit, vegetables, casseroles, pasta, egg dishes, crepes, gelatin, pudding, cheesecake, pancake batter.
Eggs	• Add chopped hard-boiled eggs to salads, dressing, vegetables, casseroles, creamed meats. • Add extra egg yolks to quiches, scrambled eggs, custard, pudding, pancake and French-toast batter, milk shakes. • Combine egg yolks, high-protein milk, and sugar to make a rich custard. • Add extra hard-boiled yolks to deviled-egg filling and sandwich spreads.
Ice cream, frozen yogurt, yogurt	• Stir into milk to make a milk shake or into carbonated beverages such as ginger ale to make an ice-cream soda. • Add to fruit, cereal, gelatin, pies. • Blend with fruit. • Make an ice-cream sandwich using cookies, graham crackers, or slices of firm cake.
Meat, poultry, fish	• Add chopped, cooked meat or fish to vegetables, salads, casseroles, soup, sauces, biscuit dough. • Use in omelets, soufflés, quiches, wraps, sandwiches, chicken and turkey stuffing. • Wrap in pie crust or a biscuit to make a turnover. • Add to stuffed baked potatoes. • Calves' or chicken livers or hearts are especially good sources of protein, vitamins, and minerals.
Milk, whole	• Add to beverages and cooking whenever possible, including hot cereal, soup, pudding, rice, cocoa. • Add cream sauces to vegetables and other dishes.
Milk, powdered	• Add a tablespoon of nonfat powdered dry milk to each cup of regular milk, milk shakes, pasteurized eggnog, cream soups, mashed potatoes.

	• Use in casseroles, meat loaf, bread, muffins, sauces, cream soups, pudding, custard, other milk-based desserts.
Nuts, seeds, wheat germ	• Add to casseroles and batters for bread, muffins, pancakes, cookies, waffles.
	• Sprinkle on fruit, cereal, ice cream, yogurt, vegetables, salads, toast; use in place of bread crumbs.
	• Blend with parsley or spinach, herbs, and cream for a sauce you can pour over pasta or vegetables.
Peanut butter and other nut butters	• Spread on sandwiches, toast, muffins, crackers, waffles, pancakes, fruit, raw vegetables. • Swirl through ice cream and yogurt.
	• Blend with milk drinks and other beverages.

TABLE 8.4 Super Sources of Calories

Food	Suggested Serving Ideas
Butter and margarine	• Add to soup, mashed and baked potatoes, hot cereal, grits, rice, pasta, and cooked vegetables.
Cream	• Use in cream soups, sauces, egg dishes, batters, pudding, custard, hamburgers, meat loaf, croquettes. • Pour on hot or cold cereal. • Mix with pasta, rice, mashed potatoes. • Pour on chicken and rice while baking. • Add to milk in recipes. • Make hot chocolate with cream and add marshmallows.
Cream cheese	• Spread on bread, muffins, fruit, crackers, raw vegetables. • Roll into bite-sized balls, then coat with chopped nuts, wheat germ, or granola.
Cream, whipped	• Use sweetened to top off hot chocolate, desserts, gelatin, pudding, fruit, pancakes, waffles. • Fold unsweetened into mashed potatoes or vegetable purees.
Cream, sour	• Add to cream soups, baked potatoes, macaroni and cheese, vegetables, sauces, salad dressings, stews, baked meat, fish. • Add a dollop to cake, fruit, gelatin, bread, muffins. • Use as a dip for fresh fruit and vegetables. • Spoon it on fresh fruit, sprinkle on some brown sugar, then let it sit in the refrigerator for a while.

Dried fruit	• Cook and serve for breakfast or as a dessert or snack.
	• Add to muffins, cookies, bread, cakes, rice and grain dishes, cereal, pudding, stuffing.
	• Bake in pies and turnovers.
	• Combine with cooked vegetables such as carrots, sweet potatoes, yams, squash.
	• Snack on dried fruit combined with nuts.
Granola	• Use in cookie, muffin, and bread batters.
	• Sprinkle on vegetables, yogurt, ice cream, pudding, custard, fresh or dried fruit.
	• Layer with fruit, then bake.
	• Use in place of bread or rice in pudding recipes.
Honey, jam, sugar	• Add to bread, cereal, milk drinks, fruit, and yogurt desserts.
	• Use as a glaze for chicken and other poultry.
Salad dressings and mayonnaise	• Spread on sandwiches and crackers.
	• Combine with meat, fish, egg, or vegetable salads.
	• Use in sauces, gelatin, croquettes.

◆ Frying and sautéing foods adds more calories than baking or broiling.

Your doctor, nurse, or dietitian will suggest general guidelines for how much fat and carbs to eat. Carbohydrates, found in starches and sugars, provide the body with its main fuel: the simple sugar *glucose*, also referred to as *blood sugar*. Starches consist of *complex carbohydrates*, which as a dividend provide many other nutrients and fiber. They are preferable to the "empty calories" of *simple carbohydrates* that make up sugar and sugary foods such as candy, cakes, and soft drinks.

A cancer patient's diet, says Susan Sloan, "should contain a reasonable amount of carbohydrates, but not a high percentage." As with fats, digestibility is an issue. "Fruits and vegetables are much easier to digest than pastas, potatoes, rice, and breads." Fresh vegetables are an especially good source of complex carbs because they're rich in fiber.

Cancer can slow down your body's ability to remove glucose from the blood, leading to an abnormally elevated blood-sugar level. In the event of *hyperglycemia,* your physician may advise you to cut down on carb consumption.

Vitamins and Minerals

Ideally, all of us should get our nutrients through our diet because vegetables and fruits contain many *phytochemicals* absent from vitamin and mineral supplements. Although much more needs to be learned about these plant substances, they are believed to lower the risk of cancer, heart disease, diabetes, high blood pressure, and other medical conditions through a variety of mechanisms.

For instance, the compound *genistein* appears to act as a natural antiangiogenesis agent by preventing tumors from forming the blood vessels they need to survive. It also inhibits rampant cell growth and may block the effects of estrogen on breast-cancer cells. Genistein is found primarily in soybean products and, in lower concentrations, in broccoli, cauliflower, kale, and other *cruciferous* vegetables. According to nutritionist Sloan, "Quite a bit of research has shown that phytochemicals help to protect normal cells and enhance the body's metabolism of food, even during chemotherapy."

Nevertheless, "if a patient is having difficulty consuming twelve hundred to fifteen hundred calories a day," she continues, "he isn't going to get enough vitamins and minerals. At that point it often becomes necessary to incorporate supplements into the diet." This may begin during treatment or afterward. "Breast-cancer patients frequently need calcium supplements posttreatment. Leukemics and people with cancer of the colon or lung usually require the *antioxidants*—vitamins A, C, and E—following therapy." All patients who've undergone extensive stomach surgery eventually become deficient in vitamin B_{12} and require monthly injections of this essential vitamin, which promotes red-blood-cell formation and a healthy central nervous system.

◆ Check with your doctor before taking any vitamins, because megadoses can interfere with radiotherapy and certain chemotherapy drugs.

HOW ANOREXIA IS MANAGED

Be conscientious about your diet, but don't allow eating to become a source of stress for you or a bone of contention between you and well-meaning loved ones (example: being nagged for not quite eating your fill of protein on a day when you're feeling queasy). Most people with cancer find that they're able to eat relatively normally throughout much of therapy. However, if an oncologist suspects that a patient is becoming undernourished, she will probably consult with a dietitian and order one of the following nutritional interventions.

Nutritional Supplements—A number of calorie-laden liquid supplements, available in most drugstores and supermarkets, provide a full spectrum of vital nutrients. Among the popular brands are Ensure, Isocal, Meritene, Resource, Sego, and Sustacal. An eight-ounce can of Ensure Plus packs 355 calories, 13 grams of protein, 47.3 grams of carbohydrates, and 12.6 grams of fat, as well as essential minerals.

The drinks come in assorted flavors and are usually lactose-free and low in cholesterol. They're best served cool or cold. Because they can be expensive, sample a few before you buy a case (or order it through the company's home-delivery service). "If you're on a limited budget," suggests Susan Sloan, "and you're able to digest milk, you can make a high-protein, high-calorie milk shake using Carnation Instant Breakfast or one of the other powdered products."

Appetite Stimulants—If you don't have much of an appetite, ask your oncologist about prescribing an appetite stimulant such as megestrol (Megace) or dronabinol (Marinol). Megace is a synthetic hormone; Marinol is the prescription form of delta-9-tetrahydrocannabinol (THC), the main *psychoactive* (mind-altering) ingredient in marijuana. Like natural marijuana, it relieves nausea as well. Although Marinol does not produce a euphoric "high," older men and women may be more sensitive to its psychoactive effects. The oral tablet, given in low doses, can also be habit-forming.

You may have heard about hydrazine sulfate, an inexpensive chemical that was once used as a fuel component for military rockets. In several small studies, it appeared to revive patients' appetites and increase their weight. The National Cancer Institute was sufficiently intrigued by the results to commission three clinical trials. Half of the more than six hundred volunteers received hydrazine sulfate; the other half, a placebo. None of the trials showed the agent to improve survival or prevent wasting. What's more, the participants assigned to the study group reported a lower quality of life than the men and women given the placebo. Consequently, hydrazine sulfate remains unapproved by the Food and Drug Administration as a supportive cancer therapy.

Tube Feedings—Tube feedings using specially formulated liquid nutritional supplements are usually a short-term measure for patients who can't swallow or metabolize food normally. For instance, many men and women recuperating from throat surgery must be fed through a nasogastric tube for several days until the swelling subsides. The flexible tube, inserted into a nostril, travels down the throat and esophagus and into the stomach. Typically, it is removed by the time a patient is ready to leave the hospital. Some people do go home with an NG tube, but rarely is it kept in for more than two weeks.

Gastrostomy, a surgical procedure, bypasses the upper digestive tract. It is indicated when a patient cannot take food by mouth for a long period of time and, in some cases, permanently. A tube is implanted directly into the stomach (a "G" tube) or lower down, in the jejunum portion of the small intestine (a "J" tube). Open gastrostomy requires that an incision be made in the abdominal wall. In percutaneous endoscopic gastrostomy, also known as a P.E.G. procedure, the surgeon places the tube with the aid of an endoscope that has been passed down the throat and into the stomach. Both operations call for local anesthesia and can usually be performed on an outpatient basis. However, the P.E.G. procedure is less time-consuming, less costly, and leaves a smaller scar.

Patients can also be fed *parenterally* through a central catheter inserted into a large vein. ("Parenteral" means "not through the alimentary canal"—the organs that constitute the digestive tract, from the mouth to the anus.) Oncologists generally try to avoid the intravenous route as long as the intestines are functioning. "There's less risk of infection with a gastrostomy," Susan Sloan explains, noting that many cancer patients who require alternative feeding techniques are immunosuppressed. IV nutrition is also more complicated to administer, although in her experience most patients and their loved ones adapt to either method of tube feeding. A nurse or dietitian will show you how. For instance, you must remember to sit upright throughout each feeding and for about half an hour afterward. It's helpful to have assistance, so request that all interested family members and caregivers receive training.

"The prospect of having to be fed through a tube is often scary to patients," says Dr. Jane Ingham, director of the palliative-care program at the Lombardi Cancer Center. "But I've had many of them say later on that it actually came as a relief. They no longer felt hungry, and eating ceased to be an extraordinarily time-consuming hassle."

HOW YOU CAN HELP YOURSELF

Tips for Reviving Your Appetite

How you eat is almost as important as what you eat. The major adjustment will be getting used to eating small meals or snacks every one to two hours, or whenever you're hungry, rather than the customary breakfast, lunch, and dinner. You'll probably find that your appetite peaks in the morning, then tapers off as the day goes on.

Because your desire to eat will wax and wane, nutritious snack foods become a dietary staple. To graze without guilt, stock up on the healthful items listed in table 8.5. A tablespoon of butter provides calories (one hundred) but little else: no protein, no carbohydrates, and a minimum of vitamins and minerals. Substitute the same amount of peanut butter, however, and you've just swallowed ninety-five calories, 4 grams of protein, and 3.5 grams of carbohydrates, plus iron, riboflavin, niacin, and vitamin E.

- Perk up your appetite by engaging in light exercise, like taking a short walk before meals.

- Certain beverages excite appetites. Drink a glass of orange juice, lemonade, wine, beer, or a cocktail prior to a meal.

  ◆ Be sure to ask your doctor first if alcohol is permissible. And never ingest alcohol before chemotherapy treatments because it can weaken or intensify the effect of the anticancer drugs.

- A little atmosphere, please. Make eating as enjoyable and aesthetically appealing as possible. Have a candlelight dinner with soft music playing in the background or create a festive table setting.

- Try not to let eating become routine. Your tastes may change from one day to the next, so vary your menu and experiment with new recipes, spices, and consistencies of food. Add parsley and other garnishes to the plate for an attractive presentation.

- Serve small portions on small plates. Big helpings on large dinner plates look overwhelming and impossible to finish.

- Whenever possible, eat with family members or friends. You're likely to eat more if you have conversation to distract your attention from the food on your plate. When eating alone, turn on the TV or radio.

- Have meals and snacks prepared in advance for times when you're too tired to cook. Make extra portions of your favorite foods and freeze them, remembering to mark the date on the storage bag or container. (Adding half a cup of liquid to casseroles before reheat-

TABLE 8.5 **Healthful Snacks to Have on Hand**	
• Applesauce	• Fruit (fresh or canned)
• Bread products, including crackers and muffins	• Gelatin
	• Granola
• Buttered popcorn	• Hard-boiled and deviled eggs
• Cakes and cookies made with whole grains, fruit, nuts, wheat germ, or granola	• Ice cream and frozen yogurt
	• Juices
• Cereal	• Nuts
• Cheese, cottage cheese, cream cheese	• Peanut butter
	• Pizza
• Cheesecake	• Pudding and custard
• Chocolate milk	• Sandwiches
• Cream soups	• Vegetables
• Dips made with cheese, beans, sour cream	• Whole-milk milk shakes and "instant breakfast" drinks
• Dried raisins, prunes, apricots, or other fruit	• Yogurt

ing will keep them from drying out.) Also fix yourself a milk shake and a small tray of cut-up fruit, cheese, vegetables, nuts, and crackers, and keep them in the refrigerator, so you can grab a ready-made snack anytime you're hungry.

- If relatives and friends offer to cook meals for you, let them! And don't be shy about specifying your likes and dislikes or what you can and can't eat.

◆ Ask your doctor when to call to report excessive weight loss or a lack of appetite.

Dehydration

COMMON CAUSES

▪ Vomiting ▪ Diarrhea ▪ Fever ▪ Frequent urination *(diuresis)*, a side effect of some medications ▪ Dry mouth or a disagreeable taste in the mouth ▪ Difficulty in swallowing ▪ Hypercalcemia, an abnormal buildup of calcium in the blood

---

Electrolytes

Sodium
Potassium
Calcium
Magnesium
Chloride
Bicarbonate
Phosphate

Keeping yourself sufficiently hydrated helps to prevent constipation, indigestion, urinary-tract infections, and electrolyte disturbances. Sixty percent of a healthy person's weight consists of water; two-thirds is distributed within the body's cells *(intracellular* fluid) and one-third outside the cells. The *extracellular* fluid comprises the liquid portion *(plasma)* of the blood and occupies the spaces between the blood vessels and the surrounding cells.

Electrolytes, electrically charged minerals found in all body fluids, regulate this delicate balance. Potassium controls the amount of intracellular fluid, while sodium and chloride oversee extracellular fluid. The electrolyte composition of the water inside and outside a cell's membrane is not the same. Intracellular fluid contains large concentrations of positively charged potassium particles and small amounts of similarly charged sodium particles; in extracellular fluid, the proportions are reversed. Potassium, sodium, and chloride also regulate the equilibrium between the *acidity* and *alkalinity* of body fluids. A shift in either balance—water and electrolytes; *acids* and *bases*—can disrupt the normal functioning of the cells.

Someone who is dehydrated typically has elevated levels of sodium and chloride and deficiencies of potassium, calcium, and magnesium. If not rectified, a low concentration of any of the latter three electrolytes can trigger a number of potentially serious complications, including an abnormal heartbeat.

HOW DEHYDRATION IS MANAGED

Intravenous Fluids—If you become dehydrated and simply cannot drink enough to replace the lost fluids, your doctor will order an infusion of water and sugar *(dextrose)*, plus any minerals that need to be replenished. This may be done in a medical facility or at home by a home-care nurse.

HOW YOU CAN HELP YOURSELF

The simple answer—drink the equivalent of eight to ten eight-ounce glasses of cool liquids per day—is not so simple. Downing a glass of water is a feat surprisingly few of us seem able to manage when we're healthy, much less when we're not feeling well. Instead, keep a glass of water at your side throughout the day, sipping and replenishing it. Feeling thirsty tells you that your body is two cups (sixteen ounces) of water short.

There are many other ways to meet your daily fluid quota:

- Suck on ice chips, Popsicles, electrolyte freezer pops, and ice pops made from your favorite beverages.

- Eat sherbet, sorbet, and Jell-O.

- For variety, try alternatives to water such as Hi-C, Kool-Aid, broth, soup, liquid Jell-O, milk, and juices, nectars, and sports drinks diluted in water. Go easy on citrus juices (orange, grapefruit, lime, lemon), which can irritate the urinary tract.

- Cold beverages, including water, are often more palatable when served over ice. Avoid coffee, tea, chocolate milk, sodas, and other caffeinated beverages. Caffeine, a *diuretic,* increases urination.

Indigestion, Nausea, Vomiting

COMMON CAUSES

- Chemotherapy • Radiation to the abdomen, pelvis, or brain
- Total-body irradiation in preparation for bone-marrow transplantation • Narcotic pain medications, immunosuppressant agents, and other drugs • Gastrointestinal graft-versus-host disease following bone-marrow transplantation • Mucus draining from the mouth and sinuses • A tumor of the gastrointestinal tract, liver, or central nervous system • Dehydration • Infection • "Dumping syndrome" following surgery to remove a large portion of the stomach (see "Dumping Syndrome" under "Cancer of the Stomach" in Chapter Six, "State of the Art: Your Treatment Options").

"Of all the possible symptoms and side effects," observes nurse Maureen Sawchuk, "patients are most fixated on nausea and vomiting." A sick stomach isn't an inevitable consequence of having cancer, even during chemotherapy, the form of treatment most likely to bring about nausea. How your body will react is partly unpredictable, but also partly dependent on the regimen. Chemo drugs are grouped according to their potential for inducing nausea and vomiting: severe, high, moderate, low, very low. At the "severe" end of the spectrum are cisplatin (Platinol), dacarbazine (DTIC-Dome), streptozocin (Zanosar), mechlorethamine (Mustargen), and high-dose cytarabine (Cytosar-U), which produce these side effects in more than 90 percent of patients. However, nausea and vomiting will affect less than 10 percent of patients taking a drug belonging to the "very low" category: busulfan (Myleran), thioguanine (Tabloid), vincristine (Oncovin), and hormonal agents. The dose, schedule, and method of delivery also influence the incidence and severity of chemo-related stomach sickness.

PREVENTIVE MEASURES

Many patients find that maintaining a clear-liquid diet (see page 736) one to twelve hours prior to chemo treatments helps them to avert nausea. Fasting for several hours before and after radiation treatments may eliminate queasiness. Another strategy is for your oncologist to prescribe antinausea drugs prophylactically. The American College of Physicians recommends taking the antiemetic at bedtime the night before chemotherapy, again the morning of treatment, and then repeating the dose every four to six hours (or as directed) for a minimum of twelve to twenty-four hours or as long as your nausea and vomiting continue. In order for the antinauseant to be effective, it must maintain a consistent presence in the bloodstream. Taking the medicine half an hour before meals will help you to feel more like eating and help to keep your food down.

HOW INDIGESTION, NAUSEA, AND VOMITING ARE MANAGED

Antinausea Medications—Today's antiemetic drugs are extremely effective at curbing nausea, although you and your doctor may have to experiment with different types of medications or a combination of agents before you find relief. Probably the most widely prescribed antinauseant is prochlorperazine (Compazine), which works by interfering with the action of a brain chemical called dopamine. Ondansetron (Zofran) and granisetron (Kytril) block a different neurotransmitter, serotonin. Marinol, the dual antinausea drug and appetite stimulant, is rarely a first choice. But that may be largely due to some doctors' and patients' discomfort with the fact that it is derived from the marijuana plant, *Cannabis sativa.*

The corticosteroids dexamethasone (Decadron) and methylprednisolone (Medrol) are usually administered in conjunction with antiemetics but may be used alone to alleviate mild or moderate nausea. Since physicians have come to recognize that anxiety exacerbates nausea, a mild tranquilizer is frequently prescribed too.

Antacids and Antiflatulents—Two symptoms of indigestion are heartburn and gas pains. Heartburn occurs when the stomach regurgitates its acidic contents up into the esophagus, often as a result of our eating too quickly. Over-the-counter *antacids* such as Mylanta and Tums relieve simple acid indigestion by neutralizing gastric acid, while Tagamet, Pepsid AC, and Zantac reduce the amount of acid secreted. If you suffer from recurrent heartburn, though, notify your doctor. Not only might this signal a more serious underlying problem, but the repeated backflow of acid can damage the esophagus.

Burping or flatulence, often accompanied by abdominal swelling and pain, announces the presence of gas or air in the stomach or bowels. As virtually every grade-schooler can tell you, beans and other foods produce intestinal gas, while chewing with the mouth open can cause a person to swallow too much air. The antacid Mylanta doubles as an *antiflatulent*, dispersing gas in the GI tract.

Gas pain is also a common aftereffect of surgery and endoscopic procedures like colonoscopy and laparoscopy, during which air or gas is often introduced into the bowel and abdominal cavity, respectively, to give the physician a clearer view.

HOW YOU CAN HELP YOURSELF

- Set aside sufficient time for meals. Eating when you're tense, upset, or in a hurry can bring on heartburn. Chew your food thoroughly for easier digestion and try not to talk while eating so that you don't gulp air.

- Sipping liquids slowly decreases the amount of air you ingest.

- Chemotherapy can heighten your sensitivity to smell, so even the aroma of your favorite foods may make you sick to your stomach. Poultry, fish, dairy products, and eggs usually have a milder aroma than beef, lamb, and other red meats, and foods in general emit less of an aroma when served cold or at room temperature.

  Heating frozen dinners or reheating leftovers in the oven or microwave cuts down on cooking odors and liberates you from the kitchen. Better yet, ask someone else to do the cooking. When a particular smell is making you queasy, try breathing through your mouth instead of your nose.

- During hospital stays, ask the nurse to deliver your food tray without a cover on the plate so that the smell doesn't overwhelm you.

- Other odors, such as tobacco smoke, perfumes, cosmetics, and colognes, may unsettle your stomach while you're on chemotherapy. Don't hesitate to request that friends, family, and coworkers refrain from smoking (a good idea anyway) and wearing body fragrances around you. If you patiently explain why, most folks will be understanding.

- Sit up or walk around after eating. This helps to empty the stomach and dissipate gas.

- If you must lie down, do so on your left side, which allows air to escape through your mouth.

- If you find that even small servings of food leave you feeling full, drink liquids at least an hour before or after eating instead of with meals.

- Fresh air helps to calm the stomach and ease nausea. Don't let your home or workplace get too warm or too stuffy. Open a window and take slow, deep breaths.

- Wear comfortable, loose-fitting clothes. Constrictive garments put pressure on the stomach and throat, which adds to stomach upset.

- *Don't* eat your favorite foods when you're nauseous. The reason? Because you may come to permanently associate them with feeling sick.

- Distract yourself. Phone a friend, watch TV, read a book—anything to take your mind off your nausea. Learning relaxation and visualization techniques can be helpful in this regard, as can other alternative measures that are also used to relieve pain and anxiety, including acupuncture, biofeedback, and hypnotherapy.

See "Relieving Pain Without Medicine," page 793.

Dietary Do's and Don'ts When You're Feeling Nauseous

- Think bland: crackers, melba toast, dry toast, dry cereal, yogurt, sherbet, fruit ice, angel food cake, vanilla wafers, oatmeal, pretzels, baked or broiled skinless chicken, soft fruits such as canned peaches, clear liquids.

- Avoid fatty, greasy, or fried foods, which linger in the digestive tract. Also cross the following off your menu until you're feeling better:

  Candy, cookies, cakes, and other sweets

  Spicy or hot foods

  Foods and beverages that produce gas, including beans, onions, cabbage, broccoli, cauliflower, turnips, cucumbers, corn, green peppers, brussels sprouts, sauerkraut, milk, and chewing gum

  Acidic foods and beverages such as fruit juices and vinegary salad dressing

What to Do After an Episode of Vomiting

- Wait an hour or two before reintroducing food or drink.

- Start with clear liquids, an ounce or two at a time. If you're able to keep these down, graduate to full liquids, then work your way back to solid food. Don't stay on the clear-liquid diet for more than three to five days; it is intended primarily to keep you hydrated and does not supply all the nutrients you need. The *full-liquid diet*, when planned by a doctor or dietitian, can be followed indefinitely. (See table 8.6.)

- To restore fluids and minerals, sip fruit juices and sports drinks such as Gatorade.

- Carbonated sodas, waters, and juices can unsettle your stomach and produce gas. Remove the fizz by opening bottles or cans and letting the beverages go flat.

  ♦ Contact your doctor if your vomiting is severe, contains blood, or lasts more than a few days.

Diarrhea

COMMON CAUSES

- Radiation to the abdomen or pelvis ▪ Chemotherapy
- Some antibiotics, antinauseants, and other drugs ▪ Intestinal infections ▪ Gastrointestinal graft-versus-host disease following bone-marrow transplantation ▪ Lactose intolerance ▪ Blockage of the intestinal tract due to a tumor, hard stools, or scarring

---

TABLE 8.6 CLEAR-LIQUID AND FULL-LIQUID DIETS

Clear-Liquid Diet	Full-Liquid Diet *Same items as clear-liquid diet, plus:*
Beverages: water; carbonated beverages; cereal beverages such as Postum; decaffeinated coffee or tea; fruit-flavored drinks and fruit punches; apple, grape, and cranberry juice, and strained lemonade and other citrus juices if they agree with you	*Beverages:* all juices and nectars; thin fruit purees; tomato and vegetable juices; milk, chocolate milk, buttermilk, skim milk, milk shakes
Soups: bouillon, consommé, clear fat-free broth, strained vegetable broth	*Soups:* clear cream soups, cheese soup, any strained or blenderized soup, pureed tomato or potato soup
Sweets: small amounts of honey, jelly, syrup, plain gelatin, or plain sugar candy; ice pops, frozen fruit juice	*Sweets:* junket, soft or baked custard; sherbet; plain cornstarch pudding; fresh or frozen yogurt, ice milk, smooth ice cream; pasteurized eggnog
	Meats: small amounts of strained meat in broth or gelatin
	Fats: butter, cream, oils, margarine

---

from surgery or radiation ▪ Surgery to remove part of the stomach, small intestine, or colon ▪ Intestinal surgery requiring an ileostomy or colostomy ▪ Deficiencies in pancreatic enzymes following pancreatic surgery or during pancreatic radiation therapy ▪ Malabsorption ▪ Emotional upset

Patients don't always appreciate how quickly diarrhea can leave them dangerously dehydrated and depleted of electrolytes. During diarrhea, semidigested food speeds through the bowel before the body can draw off enough vitamins, minerals, and liquid, which is why the stools are watery and more frequent than the average one bowel movement a day.

Malabsorption

Diarrhea may be a sign of *malabsorption,* a condition in which the bowel is unable to take in nutrients. This sometimes happens following surgery, particularly operations involving the intestines. Malabsorption usually lasts a short time and goes away on its own. If it should persist, your doctor may recommend taking vitamin and mineral supplements and cutting out fatty foods.

HOW DIARRHEA IS MANAGED

Antidiarrheal Medications—Loperamide (Imodium), diphenoxylate (Lomotil), paregoric, and similar drugs slow down peristalsis, the undulating motion that propels food through the gut. With normal motility restored, the intestinal walls have sufficient time to absorb the nutrients and digestive juices. Follow the directions exactly; if you take too much of an antidiarrheal, you could wind up constipated. An *anticholinergic/antispasmodic* agent such as Donnatal may be prescribed to alleviate intestinal cramping. For severe abdominal pain, a narcotic analgesic is commonly added.

HOW YOU CAN HELP YOURSELF

- Drink those eight to ten glasses of fluid a day. Clear liquids are preferable: They don't overexert or irritate the bowel and are easily absorbed into the bloodstream. Smart choices include apple, cranberry, or grape juice; Jell-O; chicken broth; ice pops; plain gelatin; weak decaffeinated tea; peach nectar; flat ginger ale; and Gatorade. Pedialyte, available in almost any pharmacy, is specially formulated to quickly restore lost fluid, minerals, and electrolytes following bouts of diarrhea or vomiting.

- Diarrhea is acidic and can irritate the skin around the anus. Instead of using toilet paper after each bowel movement, gently wash yourself with warm water or take a tub bath or sitz bath. To prevent chapping, moisturize the rectal area or wipe it with a Tucks astringent pad. If the skin becomes red and sore, smooth on an over-the-counter diaper-rash ointment, which promotes healing, relieves chafing, and protects the skin. Popular brands include Desitin, Diaparene, and A&D.

- To ease cramps, wrap a warm-water bottle in a towel and hold it against your abdomen. Because radiation and chemotherapy can cause the skin to become overly sensitive to heat, don't fill the bottle with hot water or use a heating pad.

Dietary Do's and Don'ts When You Have Diarrhea
- Avoid foods that intensify the churning action of the intestines, leading to more discomfort—and diarrhea. Among the culprits: foods that produce gas; overly spicy foods; greasy, fatty, or fried foods; acidic foods; caffeinated foods and beverages; and high-

fiber foods such as bran, whole-grain bread and cereal, popcorn, nuts and seeds, and raw vegetables and fruit. Broccoli, corn, cabbage, cauliflower, peas, and beans—already off-limits because of their tendency to cause gas—are especially difficult to digest.

- Allow food and drinks to cool off before consuming. Hot solids and liquids activate the intestines.

- Anytime you have a severe bout of diarrhea, switch to a clear-liquid diet for the first twelve to fourteen hours. This gives your bowel a rest while you stock up on fluids. Once your symptoms have improved, follow the BRAT diet. The acronym stands for Bananas, Rice, Applesauce, and decaffeinated Tea, all of which are binding and low in fiber.

- Low-fiber foods are ideal, because they are less dehydrating than high-fiber fare. Each item below is gentle on the bowel:

White rice	**Applesauce**
Noodles	**Eggs**
Creamed cereals	**Cottage cheese**
Dry toast	**Cream cheese**
Ripe bananas	**Pureed vegetables**
Smooth peanut butter	**Yogurt**
Canned or cooked fruit without the skins	**Skinless mashed or baked potatoes**
Lean beef	
Skinless chicken or turkey	
Fish	
White bread	
Crackers	

Meat, poultry, and fish should be baked, not fried.

- Diarrhea is often a side effect of antibiotics. The antibacterial drugs also destroy the "good" bacteria in your intestines. Eating yogurt replaces the intestinal *flora*, but only if the product contains *live and active cultures*. These microorganisms also help to reduce diarrhea. Look for containers bearing the National Yogurt Association's "LAC" seal and stay away from any yogurt that doesn't require refrigeration: The high temperatures used in processing to prolong the product's shelf life destroy live cultures.

- Lean toward foods and drinks that are rich in potassium, a vital mineral frequently lost during diarrhea. Good sources include meat; fish; bananas (I probably ate a jungleful when I was suffering from severe mucositis); boiled or mashed potatoes; orange or tomato juice; peach, pear, or apricot nectar; colas; and tea.

- If you are lactose intolerant, like millions of Americans, take *lactase supplements* before drinking milk or eating dairy products such as ice cream or cheese. Lactase, manufactured in the small intestine, is an enzyme that breaks down *lactose,* the principal sugar in milk. Some people find that as they become older, drinking milk gives them diarrhea, gas, and bloating. This is because it is normal for our bodies to produce less lactase as we age. Chemotherapy and radiation therapy can deactivate the enzymes, thereby inducing temporary lactose intolerance.

Lactase caplets or drops make dairy foods more digestible. Lactaid, a popular brand, also markets several varieties of natural-tasting lactose-free milk. A number of men and women unable to assimilate lactose find that they can eat yogurt and hard cheeses without experiencing adverse GI symptoms.

Dairy products are by far the best source of calcium, but they're not the only ones. You can shore up this important mineral by eating canned sardines, salmon and mackerel (with bones), smelts, collard greens, broccoli, tofu, almonds, and filberts.

♦ Contact your doctor if your diarrhea contains blood, lasts more than a few days, or if you have more than three bowel movements a day. To help her pinpoint the exact cause, your doctor will want to know how much diarrhea you've had, its consistency, and whether or not there's been any change in color.

Constipation

COMMON CAUSES

  - A low-fiber diet ▪ Dehydration ▪ Narcotic pain medications, antidepressants, antihistamines, and other drugs ▪ Chemotherapy ▪ Blockage of the bowel due to a tumor or scarring from surgery or radiation ▪ Inactivity ▪ Hypercalcemia, an abnormal buildup of calcium in the blood ▪ Uremia, an abnormal buildup of toxins in the blood due to the kidneys' inability to filter them out of the circulation and excrete them in the urine ▪ Compression of the spinal cord that interferes with normal bowel movements ▪ Overuse of laxatives

"Constipation" describes either of two conditions: (1) A person's bowel movements occur far less frequently than normal and produce discomfort or pain, or (2) the fecal matter passes through the large intestine so slowly that too much fluid is absorbed, resulting in dry, hard stools. As with diarrhea, many people underestimate the potential seriousness that constipation poses. A *fecal impaction,* where the feces collect in the lower colon or the rectum, can be fatal if not treated promptly.

PREVENTIVE MEASURES

The same steps used to relieve constipation can be taken to prevent it. Ask your doctor if you might benefit from a daily *bowel routine,* which simply consists of physical activity, changes in diet, and laxatives. The National Cancer Institute recommends that any patient taking a narcotic analgesic should follow a bowel routine for as long as he's on the pain reliever.

- Exercise every day. A daily walk helps to keep your bowel moving. If you're confined to bed, ask your doctor or nurse to show you abdominal exercises that can be performed lying down.

- Try to avoid straining while on the toilet, which can contribute to hemorrhoids.

Dietary Do's and Don'ts for Preventing and Managing Constipation

- Gradually increase the fiber in your diet to about five to ten grams a day. Fiber-abundant foods include whole-grain bread, cereal, pasta, brown rice, and barley; dried peas and beans; dried fruit; fresh fruit and vegetables, with the skins left on; and nuts, popcorn, and seeds.

- Sprinkle unprocessed wheat bran on cereal, homemade bread, casseroles, and other foods. Bran stimulates colon activity. But don't add too much too quickly. The American College of Physicians suggests starting with two teaspoons a day and eventually progressing to two tablespoons a day.

- For softer stools, consume your eight to ten glasses of fluids a day, including a hot beverage about half an hour before you normally go to the bathroom. Coffee, tea, hot lemon water, and warm prune juice all help to activate the bowels. Prune juice works just as well cold.

- If your doctor has prescribed narcotic analgesics or the chemotherapy drug vincristine (Oncovin), he may want you to take a nonprescription *stool softener* once or twice a day. Leading brands include Colace, Dialose, and Fleet Sof-Lax.

HOW CONSTIPATION IS MANAGED

Laxatives—It's important to keep a record of your bowel movements so that your physician can recommend a suitable intervention. Going three days without defecating may warrant using a stool softener, a *stimulant* laxative, or a combination stool softener/laxative such as Senokot-S. Stimulant laxatives like Dulcolax and Senokot tablets promote bowel movements by acting on the smooth muscle of the colon wall. When taken at bedtime, they often achieve the desired effect the next morning. *Bulk-forming* laxatives jump-start peristalsis and soften the stool. They must be mixed with water, and can take anywhere from twelve hours to three days to work. Metamucil is probably the best-known brand.

     ◆ Bulk laxatives should not be used to counteract constipation brought on by narcotic painkillers.

If you're still not able to move your bowels, your physician will most likely increase the daily dosage. Or he may advise you to switch to a *rectal suppository* or an *enema* solution. Both methods can usually evacuate the contents of the bowel within about thirty minutes.

     ◆ Do not use either one if your platelet count or white-cell count is below normal. Inserting the suppository or the plastic tip of the enema bottle in the rectum could puncture a tiny blood vessel, causing bleeding; or it could tear rectal tissue, heightening the risk of infection.

Because excessive doses can actually impair the intestine's natural muscle tone, all patients should exercise caution with any type of laxative. Ironically, laxatives contribute to fecal impaction more than any other drug.

Fecal Impaction

The symptoms of a fecal impaction may resemble those of constipation, or they may seem completely unrelated. For instance, if the mass of hardened stool is compressing the nerves at the base of the spine, the person will experience back pain. If it presses against the urinary tract, he will have to relieve himself frequently or, conversely, find it difficult to empty his bladder. A distended abdomen can infringe on the lungs, making it hard to breathe.

Sometimes an impaction goes undetected because a patient appears to have the very opposite problem: diarrhea. In fact, what looks like watery stool is really backed-up fecal matter that's been forced around the blockage in the intestine. The diarrhea may be explosive or dribble out, particularly after a cough or some other stress on the abdomen.

HOW FECAL IMPACTION IS MANAGED

Enemas—Impactions are typically treated with one or more enemas, to soften the stool and lubricate the intestine. Do not administer yourself an enema unless your physician has instructed you to. Instilling enema solution one too many times may cause the already-irritated bowel to become perforated, a life-threatening situation. Often, if the fecal matter is sitting low enough in the rectum, a doctor or nurse will insert a gloved finger and manually break up the mass. *Disimpaction* should never be attempted by anyone who isn't a health-care professional.

Bowel Obstruction

Constipation may also indicate that the intestines have become partially or completely blocked. Four in five bowel obstructions occur in the small intestine. The most frequent cause is a primary tumor of the colon, stomach, or ovary, while malignancies of the breast and lung and melanoma can metastasize to the abdomen and narrow the path of liquefied food in the small bowel or feces in the large bowel. Along with constipation, patients typically experience severe vomiting (including throwing up fecal matter when the blockage is in the lower portion of the small intestine). They also become extremely dehydrated.

Other conditions can give rise to an intestinal obstruction: bowel inflammation or trauma; compression from outside the bowels; or, as happened to me—twice, no less—a twisted loop of colon. *Volvulus,* the medical term for this, can literally strangle the bowel, cutting off its blood supply. If the situation is not reversed, the oxygen-starved tissue will die.

HOW BOWEL OBSTRUCTION IS MANAGED

Decompression/Surgery—By placing a nasogastric tube down my throat and into my stomach, the doctors at Lombardi spared me from having to undergo what would have been my third abdominal surgery in three months. Fluid and gas were drained from the swollen colon, which finally unkinked itself. This nonoperative approach can also be achieved via a flexible endoscope inserted into the rectum and snaked up the bowel. Four in five episodes of large-intestine volvulus occur in the lowermost segment of the colon.

An operation may still be necessary following decompression. Without a surgical solution, more than half of all patients will suffer recurrences. Total bowel obstruction calls for prompt surgery. Additionally, patients are given medications to control nausea, constipation, and abdominal pain.

♦ Contact your doctor if you normally move your bowels once a day but haven't done so in three or four days; or if you've gone for four or five days without a bowel movement when your normal routine is every other day. Also report constipation accompanied by any of the following: severe abdominal pain, bloody stool, nausea and vomiting, or an abdomen that feels full and hard to the touch.

Weight Gain/Fluid Retention

COMMON CAUSES

- Hormonal therapy ▪ Immunotherapy

Hormonal agents such as estrogens and prednisone (Deltasone) and the immunologic interleukin-2 (Proleukin) can cause the body to retain water. Despite the weight gain, this doesn't mean that you are overeating.

HOW FLUID RETENTION IS MANAGED

Diuretic Medications—There are several different types of diuretics, drugs that rid the body of excess water by increasing the frequency of urination. *Thiazide diuretics,* the most commonly prescribed kind, typically begin working within a few hours and produce few side effects.

HOW YOU CAN HELP YOURSELF

- If your legs have become swollen with fluid, try not to cross them, and keep them elevated when resting.

Dietary Do's and Don'ts When You're Retaining Fluid

- Eat less salt. Sodium retains water. Don't add salt to foods, and avoid items that are high in sodium, such as:

Bologna, ham, and other cold cuts	Hot dogs
Bacon	Corned beef
Sausage	Salt pork
Canned and salted meats	Chipped beef
Canned or frozen soups	Bouillon
Olives	Pickles
Frozen dinners	Pizza
Potato chips, pretzels, corn chips, and other salty snacks	Ketchup and mustard
	Chili sauce
Soy sauce, steak sauce	Monosodium glutamate (MSG)
Beans cooked with salt pork	Sauerkraut

Oral Complications

The oral cavity and the throat are frequent sites of complications from radiation to the head and neck region and drug therapy. While a metallic taste or a dry mouth may seem like a minor nuisance compared to some of the harsher side effects associated with cancer treatment, any oral complication has the potential to interfere with eating to the point where patients can become malnourished.

During therapy, it's essential to practice meticulous dental hygiene. Saliva, secreted by the salivary glands, acts as a protective buffer against tooth decay. These glands are extremely sensitive to radiation and chemotherapy. Radiation damage can cause saliva production to dry up, predisposing patients to cavities and gum disease. The ionizing rays also alter the composition of the saliva, as can chemotherapy. The thin, watery fluid turns acidic, thick, and ropy.

The National Cancer Institute recommends scheduling a dental checkup two to four weeks before starting chemo or radiation so that you'll have ample time to heal from any dental work that may be necessary. For instance, a person with bleeding gums (gingivitis) should be treated now, since chemotherapy can impair the blood's ability to clot. Don't forget to inform your dentist that you'll be undergoing cancer treatment. If your blood counts are too low, a dental procedure may have to be postponed until the levels are acceptable.

Your dentist will undoubtedly encourage you to follow a daily program of oral hygiene like the one below.

- Clean your teeth with a soft-bristle brush and a mild, nonabrasive toothpaste after every meal and at least once in between—no less than every four hours. Spongy-tipped toothbrushes should be used only when absolutely necessary.

- Change brushes and apply a topical fluoride gel, foam, or rinse. Be forewarned that fluoride can irritate the inside of the mouth and sometimes make you nauseous. You can also place these fluoride products in a soft-plastic device that you wear over your teeth like the mouth guard used by boxers and football players.

- Rinse the toothbrush thoroughly and store it in a dry place.

- After each brushing, mix half a teaspoon of baking soda and half a teaspoon of salt in an eight-ounce glass of warm water and vigorously swish the solution around in your mouth.

- Floss gently every night before bedtime. When your blood counts are below normal, make sure not to let the floss come into contact with the gums.

- If you wear dentures, brush and rinse them after meals and clean them regularly. Take them out at night; false teeth can scrape the gums, leading to an infection.

- Unless you need the calories because you've been losing weight, cut down on sugar and other foods and beverages that contribute to tooth decay. If you crave the taste, use sugar substitutes such as aspartame, saccharin, xylitol, sorbitol, and lycasin.

- Avoid chewy candy bars, caramels, gummy-style candies, taffies, processed dried-fruit candies, raisins, and other foods that stick to the teeth.

- If you develop cavities, see your dentist every three to four months.

Dry Mouth (Xerostomia)

Saliva, in addition to fending off cavities, moistens the mouth and aids digestion by lubricating food for the ride down the throat. It also contains an enzyme that begins the process of breaking down food. Normally, the salivary glands discharge about three pints of the fluid a day. A lack of saliva flow or a change in the makeup of the secretion can affect the abilities to chew, speak, swallow, and taste flavors.

There are three major pairs of salivary glands. The *parotids,* the largest, are located on either side of the face, below and in front of each ear. The *subinguinal* glands lie beneath the tongue, and the *submaxillary* glands are inside the lower jaw. Smaller glands are distributed within the tongue and the cheeks. Once injured by radiotherapy, salivary-gland tissue does not recover. Depending on the total radiation dose and the number of glands affected, the dryness may be permanent.

COMMON CAUSES

- Radiation to the head and neck ▪ Chemotherapy
- Antihypertensives, antidepressants, antinauseants, antihistamines, antidiarrheals, antianxiety agents, narcotic painkillers, and many other commonly prescribed medications
- Chronic oral graft-versus-host disease following bone-marrow transplantation

HOW DRY MOUTH IS MANAGED

Drug Therapy—Pilocarpine (Salegen), an oral prescription medication taken three times a day, stimulates saliva production from the glands unharmed by radiation. It may be three months before patients notice a significant improvement. Salegen is typically reserved to treat severe xerostomia. Amifostine (Ethyol) is an injectable drug that protects the salivary glands from postsurgical radiotherapy to the head and neck. In the study that ultimately won it expanded approval from the FDA, amifostine reduced the incidence of moderate to severe xerostomia by 35 percent.

Artificial Saliva—Saliva substitutes, available without a prescription, temporarily moisten the mouth and simulate some of the effects of saliva. Brands to look for include Glandosane, Moi-Stir, Mouthkote, Optimoist, Salivart, and Xerolube.

HOW YOU CAN HELP YOURSELF

- Rinse your mouth before eating and throughout the day. Avoid products containing alcohol, which will only dry out your mouth more.

- Keep a glass of water handy and sip frequently, especially when eating. This will help you to speak and swallow more easily. You can also moisten your mouth by sucking on ice chips, ice pops, and frozen fruit-juice pops.

- If your lips are dry, apply lip balm, petroleum jelly, cocoa butter, or another moisturizer to your lips frequently, particularly before eating.

- Use a humidifier at night, and if you can, during the day.

- Don't suck on lemon or glycerine mouth swabs, which often exacerbate dryness.

Dietary Do's and Don'ts When Your Mouth Is Dry

- Chewing low-calorie, sugarless gum stimulates saliva flow. Other foods known to increase salivation are carrots and celery; tart sugar-free sucking candies and lozenges; and citric acid, found in lemons and oranges. Lemons also help to thin thick saliva.

- Moisten foods by adding low-fat gravies, sauces, melted butter or margarine, salad dressings, mayonnaise, and yogurt.

- Don't eat dry foods. Marinate meats, and dunk bakery products and crackers in soup, milk, coffee, and other liquids.

- Serve food and beverages warm, but never hot.

- Avoid tobacco and alcohol. Both dry out the mouth.

- If viscous saliva is a problem, don't eat thick, creamy soup or drink fruit nectar.

- Stick to soft foods and blenderize hard-to-chew foods. For examples of soft foods, see the dietary do's and don'ts under "Difficulty in Swallowing (Dysphagia)," page 749.

Changes in Taste

Cancer therapies often dull the sense of taste or give foods a metallic, salty, or pungent flavor—one more reason not to feel like eating. Following radiation to the head and neck, taste acuity usually returns to normal after two to four months. Until then, the tips below should help to make food more appealing again.

COMMON CAUSES

- Radiation to the head and neck ▪ Chemotherapy
- Some narcotic painkillers and antibiotics ▪ Dry mouth
- Dental problems

HOW YOU CAN HELP YOURSELF

- To cover up disagreeable tastes, chew sugar-free gum, suck on peppermint or sour hard candies, drink peppermint tea and ginger ale, and remember to rinse your mouth frequently.

- Use plastic utensils if food has a metallic taste.

- After treatment, take zinc supplements, which help to revive the ability to taste.

Dietary Do's and Don'ts When You Have Changes in Taste

- Unless you have mouth sores, eat tart or spicy foods. Spice up recipes by liberally adding strong-flavored herbs such as oregano, curry, rosemary, mint, and basil.

- Enhance the flavor of meat, chicken, and fish by marinating them in sweet wine, fruit juices, sweet-and-sour sauce, salad dressings, soy sauce, or barbecue sauce. Or eat them with applesauce, cranberry sauce, or jelly.

- Serve food cold or at room temperature, which diminishes aromas and numbs the tongue to some unpleasant flavors.

- Don't go overboard on sweets. One common complaint during cancer treatment is that many foods taste excessively salty. To compensate, patients often eat more sugar. Some people on chemotherapy have the opposite problem: They become overly sensitive to sweet tastes.

Sore Mouth or Throat (Stomatitis/Oral Mucositis)
Difficulty in Swallowing (Dysphagia)

The rapidly dividing cells in the lining of the mouth and throat attract the attention of both anticancer drugs and radiation. Sores typically develop within a week of starting chemotherapy, and two to three weeks into radiotherapy. Irritation may give way to full-fledged inflammation, or what's referred to as either stomatitis or mucositis. In severe cases, the membranes become frayed or ulcerated.

A tender mouth or throat can make swallowing painful, if not impossible. Unless the tissue becomes infected, the sores typically clear within two to four weeks. In the meantime, there are many steps you and your doctor can take to ease discomfort and to keep eating.

COMMON CAUSES

- Radiation to the head and neck and to the chest
- Chemotherapy, especially drugs administered by continuous infusion, or over the course of several consecutive days
- Oral infections ▪ Oral graft-versus-host disease following bone-marrow transplantation ▪ Dry mouth

> Patients who've had part or all of their tongue or lower jaw removed, or who are experiencing a temporary narrowing of the esophagus, must adapt to new ways of eating.
>
> *See "Other Causes of Swallowing Problems," page 752.*

HOW MOUTH AND THROAT SORES ARE MANAGED

Drug Therapy—Different medical centers have their own recipes for a syrupy concoction dubbed "magic mouthwash." Among other effects, it numbs the mouth and tongue long enough so that patients can eat. The Lombardi Cancer Center's magic mouthwash consists of an anesthetic, to relieve pain; an antibiotic, to protect against infection; and an antacid, to help soothe the inflammation. "We recommend that patients take it twenty to thirty minutes before meals," explains nurse Maureen Sawchuk. Other hospitals' combinations may include other types of medicines. Patients swish the elixir around in their mouth, then swallow it, which coats the throat and the esophagus; or the preparation can be applied directly to ulcerated areas of the mouth.

When mouth pain is so intolerable that it's preventing a person with cancer from getting adequate nutrition, the doctor may prescribe a topical ointment or a systemic painkiller.

Mucosal Guard—For patients who have ulcers on the insides of their cheeks or the sides of their tongue, a soft-plastic mouth guard can be molded to fit over the lower teeth so they don't rub against the irritated tissue.

Tube Feedings—Severe stomatitis/oral mucositis may make it necessary for patients to be temporarily fed through a nasogastric tube or gastrostomy tube, or intravenously.

See "Tube Feedings" under "Appetite Loss (Anorexia)," page 726.

HOW YOU CAN HELP YOURSELF
- Every morning, inspect your mouth for any swelling, bleeding, or tissue deterioration, including under dentures.

- Rinse your mouth several times a day with one cup of warm water mixed with (1) one-quarter teaspoon of salt, or (2) half a teaspoon of baking soda, or (3) one-quarter teaspoon each of salt and baking soda. *Don't* use hydrogen peroxide, however, which dries out tissue.

- If your dentures no longer fit well because of swollen gums, ask your doctor whether or not you should keep them out until you're finished with treatment. A poor-fitting dental prosthesis could break the tissue, causing infection to set in.

- Don't use tobacco or alcohol (including commercial mouthwashes that contain alcohol). Both irritate the delicate mucosal lining.

- If a regular toothbrush is too harsh on your mouth, use a brush tipped with a sponge- or cotton-tipped applicator, or wrap some wet gauze around your finger and gently wipe the teeth and gums.

Dietary Do's and Don'ts When Your Mouth and/or Throat Is Irritated

- Serve foods at room temperature or cold. Warm or hot foods can irritate raw tissue.

- Cut food into small pieces, which are easier to swallow. Tilting back your head or dipping your chin also helps to overcome dysphagia.

- To soothe your mouth or throat, enjoy ice cream, sherbet, frozen yogurt, Popsicles, Jell-O, and soft, canned fruit.

- Spicy, salty, and acidic foods and drinks are temporarily off-limits. You'll never appreciate a bland diet more than during an episode of mucositis.

- Instead of citrus juices, drink fruit nectars, apple juice, and fruit-flavored beverages.

- Drink liquids through a straw so that they don't come into contact with sores in the mouth. Carbonated beverages, incidentally, may exacerbate sore gums.

- Protein-rich foods will expedite the healing process.

- Drink water and other thin liquids carefully. Contrary to what you might think, these can slip down the windpipe and into a lung more easily than thicker fluids.

- Drowning foods in butter, milk, cream, gravies, and sauces helps them slide down the throat more easily. This is also a good way to add calories.

- Rough, coarse, or dry foods are more painful to swallow. No popcorn, peanuts, fresh fruit and vegetables, nuts, dry toast, crackers, dry cereal, or granola until this passes.

- Ask your doctor if she thinks you should go on a *soft diet* until you're able to eat comfortably. The diet, which is made up of soft, relatively bland, low-fat foods, contains all the nutrients you need. As you can see from table 8.7, there's plenty of variety. If you have trouble swallowing any of the items on the "Enjoy!" list, consider blending or pureeing them. You can even tenderize and puree boneless steak and other meats without sacrificing their flavor.

Other Causes of Swallowing Problems

▪ Surgery to remove part or all of the tongue *(glossectomy)* or one side of the jawbone *(hemimandibulectomy)* ▪ Narrowing *(stricture)* of the esophagus, an occasional temporary side effect of esophageal surgery or radiation therapy

HOW "MECHANICAL" DYSPHAGIA IS MANAGED

Palatal Prosthesis—People who lose part or all of the tongue or jawbone can be fitted with a custom-made *palatal drop,* a device not unlike the retainer worn by many teenagers. The prosthesis, molded to conform to the upper palate, gives the tongue a surface to mash food against during the act of chewing and swallowing. Total-glossectomy patients can use the palatal drop in a similar way, but with no tongue, they must rely on the muscles in the floor of the mouth. This frequently proves too tiring. Most people who've undergone a total glossectomy can consume only liquids and pureed foods through their mouth, and require a feeding tube. Jaw surgery leaves swallowing intact; the problem for these patients tends to be chewing. Once they learn techniques for effective swallowing, something also taught to glossectomy patients, they often manage to forgo a feeding tube.

> *See "Will Treatment Affect Your Speech, Voice, or Swallowing?" under "Cancers of the Lip and Oral Cavity" in Chapter Six, "State of the Art: Your Treatment Options," and "Tube Feedings" under "Appetite Loss (Anorexia)," page 726.*

Esophageal Dilation—A narrowing of the gullet makes it difficult for food to travel to the stomach. Dilation, undertaken to widen this passage, entails inserting a series of progressively larger rubber tubes down the esophagus and past the affected area, one at a time. If this technique fails, the doctor may recommend implanting a feeding tube until the stricture heals, or switching to a full-liquid diet.

HOW YOU CAN HELP YOURSELF

- Sit up straight while you're eating, and remain upright for about twenty minutes after meals.

- Take deep breaths before you swallow, then be sure to exhale or cough afterward.

TABLE 8.7 **Soft Diet**		
Type of Food	**Enjoy!**	**Avoid**
Beverages	No restrictions	
Bread	All soft breads and rolls, except for those made from whole grain, bran, or unrefined whole wheat; seedless rye bread *If you can tolerate them:* crackers; French toast; pancakes; waffles; biscuits; muffins	Whole-grain, bran, cracked-wheat, or buckwheat breads and bread products; crusty breads; breads containing seeds, nuts, coconut, or dried fruit; raisin bread; granola bars; tortillas
Cereal	All cooked or dry soft cereals	Whole-grain or bran cereals
Cheese	All except those on the "Avoid" list	Sharp or strongly flavored cheeses; cheeses containing whole seeds and spices
Desserts	Ice cream; ice milk; sherbet; sorbet; gelatins; custard; pudding; applesauce and other desserts containing any of the fruits on the "Enjoy!" list	Desserts made with nuts, coconut, or any of the fruits on the "Avoid" list
Eggs	All except raw or fried	Raw or fried eggs
Fats	Butter; cream and cream substitutes; vegetable shortening and oils; margarine; mayonnaise; sour cream; commercial French dressing	Other salad dressings; fried foods; salt pork
Fruit	Raw bananas and avocados; canned or cooked apples, apricots, cherries, peaches, pears, seedless grapes, tomatoes *If you can tolerate them:* watermelon and other soft melons	All raw fruit except bananas and avocados; dried fruit; berries; crab apples; coconut; figs; grapes; pineapples; plums; rhubarb; all citrus fruits
Fruit juices	All juices and nectars except citrus juices	Orange, grapefruit, and other citrus juices
Meat	*Tender* beef, lamb, veal; roasted or stewed pork; baked, broiled, roasted, stewed, or creamed liver	Fried, salted, and smoked meats; corned beef; cold cuts; sausage; chitterlings

Poultry	Chicken; Cornish game hen; turkey; chicken liver	Duck; goose; fried poultry
Fish	Cooked, fresh, or frozen fish without bones; tuna; salmon	Fried fish; shellfish; anchovies; caviar; herring; sardines; snails; skate
Legumes and nuts (peas, beans, etc.)	Creamy peanut butter	All other legumes, nuts, and seed kernels
Milk and milk products	No restrictions	
Pasta	Spaghetti; noodles; dumplings	Chow mein noodles
Potatoes	Baked, boiled, creamed, mashed, or au gratin; mashed sweet potatoes	French fries; hash browns; potato salad; whole sweet potatoes or yams
Rice	White or brown rice	Wild rice; barley
Soup	Bouillon; broth; consommé; strained cream and vegetable soups	Bean, split-pea, and onion soups; unstrained clam chowder; bisques; gumbos
Sweets	Apple butter; butterscotch candy; caramels; chocolate; fondant; plain fudge; lollipops; marshmallows; mints; honey; jelly; syrups; sugars in small amounts	Candied fruit; nut brittle; jam; preserves; marmalade; marzipan; fruit sauces containing any of the fruits on the "Avoid" list
Vegetables	Canned or cooked asparagus; carrots; beets; eggplant; mushrooms; parsley; pumpkin; spinach; squash; vegetable-juice cocktail *If you can tolerate it:* raw lettuce	All raw vegetables except lettuce; all canned or cooked vegetables not on the "Enjoy!" list
Miscellaneous	Ketchup; gravy; pretzels; soy sauce; tomato sauce; cream sauce; brown sauce; cheese sauce; white sauce; vinegar; all finely chopped or ground leaf herbs and spices; aspic; liquid nutritional supplements	Garlic; horseradish; olives; pickles; popcorn; potato chips; relishes; chili sauce; à la king sauce; Creole sauce; barbecue sauce; cocktail sauce; sweet-and-sour sauce; Newburg sauce; Worcestershire sauce; whole and seed herbs and spices

Source: National Cancer Institute.

- Keep your chin down while swallowing; tilting the head back increases the risk of inhaling food into the lungs.

- Drinking fluids from a glass is often easier than trying to suck them through a straw.

- If your tongue movement is limited, you may have to spoon food deep into your mouth. You can also do this by using your fingers.

- Ask the speech and language pathologist to show you range-of-motion exercises for the tongue and jaw, and practice them every day.

Dietary Do's and Don'ts When You Have Mechanical Difficulty in Swallowing

- Liquids and mashed foods should be soupy in texture, not too thin and not too thick.

- You may find it easier to eat gelatin as a liquid.

- The American Institute for Cancer Research recommends avoiding milk products if they seem to increase your mucus production, which further complicates swallowing.

Oral Infections

Oral mucositis and infection often go hand in hand. Not only can the mouth become infected, but the damage to its protective lining allows microorganisms a clear path directly into the bloodstream. Patients whose white-cell counts are battered down are especially susceptible to systemic oral infections.

The most common oral infection in people with cancer is *candidiasis* (also known as *thrush),* followed by the *herpes simplex virus* (HSV). Candidiasis, an overgrowth of a yeastlike fungus, presents as raised white patches on the tongue or inner cheeks; oral herpes, as blisters. Both are usually painful. The oral cavity may also attract bacterial infections.

COMMON CAUSES

- Chemotherapy ▪ Antibiotics ▪ Long-term use of steroid medications ▪ Bone-marrow transplantation
- Stomatitis/mucositis • Emotional stress

PREVENTIVE MEASURES

If you are receiving treatment that could compromise your defenses against infection, your doctor may prescribe clotrimazole (Mycelex) lozenges or a mouthwash containing nystatin (Mycostatin). Both are *antifungal* agents.

HOW ORAL INFECTIONS ARE MANAGED

Drug Therapy—Another antifungal, fluconazole (Diflucan), is the drug of choice for treating oral candidiasis, although topical nystatin cream or ointment may be sufficient to clear superficial infections. HSV calls for acyclovir (Zovirax), an antiviral medication that comes in oral and intravenous forms, while antibiotics are used to fight bacterial infections. Thrush and herpes sufferers may be put on antibiotics as a precaution against secondary bacterial infections.

HOW YOU CAN HELP YOURSELF

Oral Thrush

- Before taking antifungal drugs, clean your mouth; denture wearers should remove all appliances when applying a topical medication.

- Use a new toothbrush each time you brush and throw away the old one. You can brush off the white patches, but do so gently. The tissue under the lesion will be red and tender and may bleed slightly.

- To soothe your mouth and throat, rinse frequently with a mixture of one cup of warm water and half a teaspoon of salt.

Oral Herpes Simplex Virus

- Avoid spicy, acidic, or abrasive foods, which can irritate the sores.

- When brushing, take care not to jab your cheek, tongue, or gums.

- Herpes blisters, unlike canker sores, are contagious. Until the sores have healed, you'll have to give up kissing. Also avoid touching the inside of your mouth so that you don't spread the virus to your eyes or genitals or infect someone else.

Urinary Disorders

Bladder Inflammation (Cystitis)

Bladder irritation is a relatively common side effect of radiation to the pelvic area as well as some anticancer drugs, among them ifosfamide (IFEX), mitomycin (Mutamycin), and paclitaxel (Taxol). Infections, too, can inflame the bladder. Normally, the organ is free of bacteria. Either the germs slip inside the thin urethra tube and make their way up to the bladder, or the ureters deliver them from the kidneys.

Symptoms of cystitis to watch for include pain or burning when urinating *(dysuria)*, frequent urination, and a sudden urge to relieve your bladder. Fever and chills often signal that the rest of the urinary tract is also involved. Occasionally, patients will pass bloody urine *(hematuria)*. If you ever notice blood in the toilet, alert your doctor right away.

However, be aware that chemotherapy drugs such as daunorubicin (Cerubidine), doxorubicin (Adriamycin), and idarubicin (Idamycin) frequently turn the urine red for a day or two after each dose. Needless to say, this can be disconcerting, especially the first time it happens. But there's nothing to be worried about. Other antineoplastics and noncancer medications can temporarily tinge urine yellow, orange—even blue or green.

◆ The pigment melanin, found in melanoma tumors, is sometimes excreted in the urine, giving it a brown or black color.

COMMON CAUSES

- Chemotherapy ▪ Radiation therapy to the bladder, prostate, uterus, cervix ▪ Bacteria ▪ Bladder irritation resulting from a catheter tube or cystoscope being inserted into the urinary tract

HOW CYSTITIS IS MANAGED

Drug Therapy—Ifosfamide and other anticancer drugs are often given in conjunction with mesna (Mesnex), an injectable detoxifying agent that lessens the chances of developing chemotherapy-induced cystitis. Bacterial infections are controlled with antibiotics.

Other drugs may be ordered to make you feel better. Phenazopyridine (Pyridium), a urinary analgesic, is effective in relieving the pain, burning, and other urinary symptoms. If the inflammation causes the bladder walls to contract involuntarily, an antispasmodic such as hyoscyamine (Urised) might be prescribed. Both medications, incidentally, are known to produce discolored urine.

HOW YOU CAN HELP YOURSELF

- *Intake! Outtake! Intake! Outtake!* Because fluids flush out germs and noninfectious irritants, the keys to avoiding cystitis are to drink plenty of liquids and to empty your bladder regularly.

See "Dehydration," page 729.

- Conscientious hygiene helps. Keeping the genital area clean reduces your risk of contracting an infection. After a bowel movement, always wipe from front to back, so as not to introduce bacteria from the rectum into the urethra.

Metabolic Disorders

Hypercalcemia

Hypercalcemia, an abnormal buildup of calcium in the blood, affects between one in ten and one in five cancer patients, usually when the disease is advanced. Although it can occur as a complication of many illnesses, a physician would probably want to rule out a malignancy and a hormonal disorder called hyperparathyroidism before considering less common causes. Tumor-induced hypercalcemia is life-threatening but treatable, especially if recognized early.

Elevated blood calcium can interfere with the central nervous system, kidney function, and digestion. Most patients come to their doctor complaining of weakness and listlessness, impaired reflexes, and dulled mental abilities. These nerve and muscle symptoms are less common in young patients than in the elderly.

Other effects can include personality changes, appetite loss, extreme thirst and frequent urination, constipation, nausea and/or vomiting, and abnormal heart rhythms. Bear in mind that few people experience all of these symptoms. In fact, mild hypercalcemia may produce none at all.

COMMON CAUSES

- Secondary cancers of the bone ▪ Substances released into the bloodstream by malignant cells ▪ Impaired kidney function, a common complication of multiple myeloma ▪ Hormonal therapy incorporating androgens, estrogens, antiestrogens, or progestins

Though we tend to think of the bones as solid and unchanging, they are constantly undergoing renovation. The hard, dense material of the skeleton is composed of calcium and phosphorus. Normally, special cells called *osteoclasts* attach themselves to a microscopic section of bone and, over a period of about ten days, eat away enough tissue to create a small cavity. This is called *resorption.* Then a work crew of *osteoblasts* enters the site to lay down new bone. The bloodstream carries off the resorbed calcium to the kidneys, which are charged with filtering out excess quantities of the mineral and eliminating it from the body as part of urine.

In hypercalcemia, the osteoclasts dissolve bone faster than the osteoblasts can replace it. The imbalance results in weakened bones and can predispose patients to fractures, skeletal deformities, and pain. At the same time, the kidneys are unable to process the influx of calcium in the blood. The mineral accumulates in the blood, further impairing renal function. If the condition is allowed to persist for a long time, enough calcium can amass in the kidneys to cause permanent damage.

Cancers Most Likely to Cause Hypercalcemia

Cancer Type	Percentage of Patients to Develop Hypercalcemia
Multiple myeloma	More than 33 percent
Lung	25 to 35 percent
Breast	20 to 40 percent
Head and neck	3 to 25 percent
	(depending on the site)

Other Cancers Associated with Hypercalcemia

- T-cell lymphomas ▪ Parathyroid cancer ▪ Kidney cancer
- Gastrointestinal cancers

There are two ways that cancer can accelerate bone resorption. Metastatic bone disease—most often originating in the breast or the myeloma cells in marrow—may ravage tissue directly. These lesions are said to be *osteolytic,* which loosely translated means bone ("osteo") destruction ("lysis"). But many tumors can trigger what's called *humoral* hypercalcemia without spreading to the bone. Primary cancers of the head and neck, breast, lung, kidney, and other sites secrete substances into the bloodstream that step up osteoclastic activity while at the same time diminishing the kidneys' ability to remove surplus calcium from the body.

HOW HYPERCALCEMIA IS MANAGED

IV Hydration/Diuretic Drug Therapy—Definitive therapy for hypercalcemia consists of treating the underlying cancer. But the immediate concern is to keep the patient out of danger. First, you're given intravenous hydration and administered a *loop diuretic* such as furosemide (Lasix) to increase urine output and speed the excretion of calcium. *Thiazides,* the most frequently prescribed type of diuretic, should be avoided in this situation because they have the opposite effect.

Hypocalcemic Drug Therapy—If the symptoms subside and cancer therapy is to begin shortly, no further treatment may be necessary. But when symptoms persist or the doctor expects the tumor to respond slowly, the next step is to start the patient on one or more *bone-resorption inhibitors* to normalize the concentration of calcium in the blood. Probably the most potent and safest is pamidronate (Aredia), which belongs to the drug category known as *bisphosphonates.* It requires only a single IV infusion, whereas etidronate (Didronel), the other bisphosphonate approved for use in the United States, must be given over the course of three to seven days. Pamidronate also delays the progression of secondary bone tumors.

Bisphosphonates take a few days to begin working. The naturally occurring hormone calcitonin (Calcimar, Miacalcin) is the fastest acting of all hypocalcemics. It usually begins to decrease the rate of bone resorption within hours. Plicamycin (Mithracin) also corrects hypercalcemia rapidly, but given its toxicity to the kidneys, liver, and blood platelets, this anticancer agent isn't called on as frequently as it was before the arrival of pamidronate.

Patients with lymphoma, myeloma, or one of the other tumors

that respond to steroid medications may be prescribed a *glucocorticoid* such as dexamethasone (Decadron). Like plicamycin, the potential side effects associated with glucocorticoids make them a less appealing option; another downside is that a week or two may pass before a reduction in calcium is evident.

◆ Changes in intellectual function and behavior due to hypercalcemia may linger for a while after the calcium level has returned to normal.

Kidney Dialysis—The overload of calcium can impair the kidneys to the point of renal failure. When this complication occurs, patients may need to go on *dialysis* until the calcium level is brought under control.

Both types of dialysis carry out the blood-purifying function of healthy kidneys. *Hemodialysis,* performed three times a week on an outpatient basis, routes the patient's blood through a machine that contains a dialyzer—essentially, an artificial kidney—then returns the filtered blood to the patient. Each treatment lasts approximately four hours.

In *peritoneal dialysis,* patients infuse a plastic pouch of cleansing solution through a tube that's been surgically placed in their abdomen. The *dialysate* fluid fills the space between the two layers of the *peritoneal membrane* that lines the abdominal and pelvic cavities. Calcium and other waste products from the blood flow through the membrane and into the solution. After about thirty minutes, the dialysate is drained back into the bag and discarded. This method of internal dialysis allows patients to go about their day without having to report to a dialysis facility; however, it must be done three to five times a day, every day.

HOW YOU CAN HELP YOURSELF

• *Don't* eliminate calcium from your diet, even if you're hypercalcemic, because your body is absorbing less calcium than normal.

Suggestions for Preventing Hypercalcemia

• Drink the equivalent of four quarts of liquid a day. This helps the kidneys to clear the excess calcium from the blood. You should also look for signs of fever, nausea and vomiting, and other medical conditions that can dehydrate you so that you and your doctor can treat them promptly.

- Stay as physically active as you can. Not getting up and around tends to increase the bones' resorption of calcium, heightening the risk of hypercalcemia.

Lymphedema

Lymphedema is the medical term for swelling *(edema)* brought on by a damaged or overloaded portion of the lymphatic system. This network contains vessels that drain off excess *lymph* fluid from the spaces between body tissues and return it to the circulation as *plasma,* the liquid portion of the blood. The lymphatic system joins the bloodstream at the neck, where two large ducts empty into a pair of veins.

Any cancer surgery that calls for a regional lymph-node dissection has the potential to cause lymphedema, although the clusters most frequently affected are those in the armpit *(axillary* nodes), the groin *(inguinal* nodes), and the pelvis *(pelvic* nodes). Without the vessels and nodes that normally serve a particular body site, the lymph collects in the *interstitial* spaces between tissue cells. The swelling may come on either suddenly or gradually.

An estimated 2 to 3 million men and women in the United States have *secondary lymphedema,* the type that develops as a complication of cancer. (In *primary lymphedema,* a rare hereditary condition, lymphatic vessels are either missing or impaired.) Swelling that subsides within six months is said to be *acute.* It may occur days, weeks, or years after surgery. The condition can be painful but usually isn't. Patients develop *pitting edema,* in which pressing the fingers against the skin leaves an indentation. Typically, acute lymphedema can be alleviated simply by keeping the affected limb elevated and exercising the muscles in the area. Sometimes the physician may prescribe an anti-inflammatory drug.

Chronic lymphedema is far more serious and is difficult to manage. It can arise as a complication of radiotherapy as well as surgery: Radiation damage to nodes and vessels may cause scar tissue to form, obstructing the flow of lymphatic fluid. Among women with breast cancer, those who undergo radiation following axillary-node dissection face double the incidence of lymphedema as those treated surgically but without radiation: approximately one in two versus one in four.

The chronic form is staged as mild, moderate, or severe. Mild lymphedema produces little more than pitting and a feeling of heaviness or fullness in the extremity. In moderate lymphedema, the skin takes on a spongy consistency; when pressure is applied, you see no indentation.

If the condition isn't arrested, it will progressively involve more and more of the limb. Following an axillary-node dissection, a breast-cancer patient might develop lymphedema in the hand and forearm initially. From there it might eventually spread to the shoulder and the upper trunk on the same side of the body. Once lymphedema is classified as severe, it is not unusual for the limb to swell to twice its normal size. The skin becomes hard and stiff and unresponsive to touch. At this point, patients become susceptible to infections of the lymph channels *(lymphangitis)* and the tissue beneath the skin *(cellulitis)*. Besides inducing fever, chills, and other flulike symptoms, the bacteria inflame the infected area. As with any infection, there is always the risk that the microorganisms will contaminate the bloodstream.

In extremely rare instances, untreated chronic lymphedema can progress to *lymphangiosarcoma,* a malignant tumor of the lymphatic vessels in the arm or leg. Other serious complications are skin ulcers and impaired function of the affected limb.

Cancers and Treatments That Heighten the Risk of Lymphedema

Cancer	Treatment
Breast	• Dissection of nodes under the arm
	• Subsequent radiation to the area increases the odds of developing lymphedema.
Melanoma of the arms or legs	• Dissection of nodes under the arm or in the groin
	• Radiation to either area, alone or following surgery
Prostate	• Radiation to the pelvis
	• Prostate surgery
Advanced endometrial, ovarian, cervical	• Dissection of pelvic lymph nodes
	• Radiation to the pelvis

A tumor that has metastasized to the abdomen—often from the ovary, testicle, colon, rectum, pancreas, or liver—can block the lymphatic vessels from draining.

COMMON CAUSES

Acute Lymphedema
▪ Surgery to remove lymph nodes ▪ Immobility of the affected leg or arm • Inflamed lymphatic vessels ▪ Fluid leakage from a surgical drain ▪ Temporary malfunctioning or loss of function of the lymphatic system in an area of the body

Chronic Lymphedema
▪ Surgery to remove lymph nodes ▪ Radiation therapy ▪ Immobility of the affected leg or arm ▪ Infection and/or injury of the lymphatic vessels ▪ Other medical conditions,

such as congestive heart failure, liver disease, kidney disease, diabetes, hypertension, metabolic disorders ▪ Obesity ▪ Advanced age

◆ A sudden, considerable increase in swelling may be indicative of a new or recurrent tumor that is blocking the flow of lymph fluid; call your doctor immediately.

HOW LYMPHEDEMA IS MANAGED

Once lymphedema gains a foothold, it cannot be cured. But proper treatment can prevent the typical progression and return the deformed part of the body to its normal size and shape. Early diagnosis improves the prospects for recovery. Therefore, it is important to familiarize yourself with the warning signs of the condition so that you can report any symptoms to the physician:

- Pain, aching, fullness, or heaviness in a limb or another part of the body
- Rings, bracelets, watches, shoes, or clothing that suddenly do not fit
- A "tightness" of the skin
- Less flexibility and strength in the hand, wrist, or ankle
- Persistent swelling
- Redness, warmth, itching, discoloration, and other symptoms of an infection

Drug Therapy—If the swelling can be traced to an infection, antibiotics will be prescribed. Other medications that may be ordered include analgesics, to control pain; anti-inflammatories, to reduce inflammation; and antipyretics, to bring down fever. Diuretics have no place in lymphedema; although these agents are able to rid the body of excess fluid, over time they actually exacerbate swelling and the hardening of skin tissue.

Mechanical Measures—Mild swelling can often be controlled by practicing light hand-and-arm or leg-and-foot exercises and by wearing *compression garments*. These adjustable sleeves and stockings, available at many medical supplies dealers, exert pressure on the limb. Important: Make sure that the product covers the *entire* problem area; otherwise, it may further constrict circulation.

A *pneumatic pump* can also help reverse early lymphedema. The device alternately inflates and deflates a cuff that you slip around your leg or arm, improving lymph drainage. An oncologist might recommend against using it, however, when cancer treatment has been unable to eradicate a malignancy, and when there is concern that the pump might cause part of the tumor to break off and enter the blood or lymph vessels.

Advanced lymphedema may call for *Complete Decongestive Physiotherapy* (CDP). The program incorporates (1) a specialized massage technique called *manual lymph drainage;* (2) *low-compression bandaging,* which reduces swelling and softens tissue; followed by (3) a series of mild exercises.

The first phase of therapy typically consists of intensive daily outpatient treatments. Each session, conducted at the treatment facility, lasts approximately an hour and a half. You may need five, ten, or twenty-one days

---

Finding a Lymphedema Treatment Center

The National Lymphedema Network (NLN), a support organization founded by a registered nurse, can refer you to treatment facilities and to individual health-care professionals experienced in Complete Decongestive Physiotherapy.

Although there are currently no standards in the United States for certifying CDP therapists, the NLN suggests using practitioners who have been certified by either of two training programs: the Lerner Lymphedema Academy of Lymphatic Studies, located in Sunrise, Florida; or the Dr. Vodder School of North America, in Victoria, British Columbia, Canada.

National Lymphedema Network
2211 Post Street, Suite 404
San Francisco, CA 94115-3427
800-541-3259 or 415-921-1306
http://www.lymphnet.org

---

of CDP, possibly more. Phase two takes place at home. The physical therapist will teach you exercises and skin care and demonstrate how to properly wear compression garments and bandages. Through Complete Decongestive Physiotherapy, most patients will see a significant reduction in their lymphedema.

HOW YOU CAN HELP YOURSELF

Whether you are at risk for lymphedema or are experiencing symptoms, observing these precautions from the National Cancer Institute can help to keep the disorder at bay or halt its progression.

Upper and Lower Extremities

- When resting, keep your arm or leg elevated above heart level as much as possible.

- Conscientiously inspect the limb every day. Measure the circumference of the arm or leg at least once a day or as per your doctor's recommendation. Wrap the tape measure around the same *two* points (e.g., upper arm, lower arm) and write down both measurements.

  ◆ Tell your doctor about any abrupt increase in size.

- Take good care of your skin. Not only are people with lymphedema vulnerable to infection, but any wounds or other breaks in the skin heal slowly. Be sure to keep the swollen limb clean and follow these safety measures for avoiding cuts, cracks, and punctures:

  Generously apply a lanolin-based skin moisturizer at least twice a day and always after bathing.

  Shave your underarms and legs with an electric razor only.

  Don't use strong, abrasive detergents or other harsh chemicals on your skin.

  Maintain good nail care and don't trim cuticles or hangnails.

  When gardening, wear heavy gloves and long pants.

  Avoid getting sunburned. Use sunscreens and stay out of intense sunlight.

  Don't subject the skin to extreme heat or cold when bathing and washing dishes. No-no's include heating pads, ice packs, saunas, and Jacuzzis.

  Take whatever preventive steps you can to avoid sports injuries, burns, insect bites, and animal bites and scratches.

- Don't wear clothing with constrictive elastic cuffs, such as stockings.

- Wear a compression sleeve or stocking when flying on an airplane, even if you don't have lymphedema. The lower cabin pressure may contribute to the onset of lymphedema after cancer surgery.

- Don't overexert the affected limb through prolonged, strenuous work or exercise. If your arm or leg starts to ache, lie down and keep it elevated.

- Because you may have limited sensation in the swollen extremity, use your other arm or leg to test the temperature of bathwater and so on.

- Eat a nutritious diet high in protein and low in salt. Although the stagnant lymph contains an overabundance of protein collected from the body tissues, cutting down on protein-rich foods does nothing to reduce the protein in the fluid. In fact, it only makes the lymphedema worse. Two good sources of protein are chicken and fish.

- If you cut yourself, wash the wound thoroughly with soap and running water, apply an antibacterial ointment, then cover it with a sterile bandage. Check frequently for redness, warmth, soreness, and other signs of infection.

  - Report any evidence of infection to your physician at once.

- Simple exercises such as those in table 8.8 can help you to regain strength and maintain muscle tone in your arm and shoulder. Exercise number one can even be done in bed. *Important: Consult with your surgeon before beginning any exercise program.* Barring any postoperative complications, you should receive the go-ahead within just a day or two of surgery.

The Arms and Hands

- Don't wear tight-fitting jewelry; wear your watch on the other wrist.

- When washing the dishes, wear loose-fitting rubber gloves.

- When cooking, wear heavy-duty oven mitts.

- When sewing, use a thimble.

- Carry handbags and other heavy objects with your healthy arm. Don't use over-the-shoulder straps on luggage and briefcases. They restrict circulation.

- Avoid rapidly circling your arm, which can cause fluid to pool in the lower part of the limb. You should also stay away from any exercise, activity, or chore that requires vigorous repetitive motions, such as scrubbing, pushing, or pulling.

- Don't hold a cigarette in the affected hand. Better yet, don't smoke at all.

- Remind medical personnel to use the other arm for injections, intravenous blood drawings and fluid administration, finger sticks, and taking blood pressure.

TABLE 8.8   Strengthening Exercises, Step by Step

The Flat-on-Your-Back Range-of-Motion Bed Workout

---

1. Lie on a bed, with your arms at your sides. Raise the affected arm straight up in the air, then reach back and try to touch the headboard or wall.

2. To stretch the muscles in your shoulders, chest, and upper back, hunch up your shoulders, then rotate them forward, down, and back in a circular motion.

3. Clasp your hands behind your head and push your elbows into the mattress.

4. With your elbow bent and your arm at a ninety-degree angle to your body, rotate your shoulder until the forearm is down, and then back the other way until it is up.

5. Raise your arm, then clench and unclench your fists.

6. Take a deep breath.

7. Turn your chin to the left, and now to the right. Turn your head sideways.

Wall Walking

---

1. Stand facing a wall—feet apart and toes up against the wall.

2. Place your palms against the wall at shoulder level, keeping your elbows slightly bent.

3. Flexing your fingers, move your hands up the wall until your arms are fully extended. Then "walk" your way back down.

♦ Until the lymphedema subsides, it's a good idea to invest in a Medic Alert bracelet engraved with the inscription "Caution: Lymphedema Arm. No Tests or Injections." For more information, call Medic Alert: 800-432-5378.

The Legs and Feet

- Don't sit in the same position for more than thirty minutes.

- Don't cross your legs while sitting.

- Keep your feet dry and clean and wear cotton socks.

- Wear something on your feet when at the beach, even when you're in the water.

Skin Disorders

Itching (Pruritus)

Pruritus, a common complaint among people with cancer, might not rank among the more serious symptoms and side effects of the disease and its treatment, but a nagging itch that keeps you awake at night can be maddening. The condition does pose a possible health hazard too, in that a patient's incessant scratching can break the skin, setting the stage for an infection. Pruritus associated with various types of tumors tends to ease or disappear once the cancer is in remission.

COMMON CAUSES

- Many malignancies, including Hodgkin's disease, non-Hodgkin's lymphomas, leukemia, and solid tumors of the stomach, pancreas, lung, colon, brain, breast, and prostate
- A number of chemotherapy drugs, hormonal agents, and immunotherapies ▪ External-beam radiation ▪ Combination chemotherapy and radiation ▪ Certain painkillers, antibiotics, tranquilizers, anti-inflammatories, and numerous other medications ▪ Infections, caused by the tumor, a fungus or parasite, or discharge or drainage from a surgical incision
- Graft-versus-host disease (GVHD), a frequent complication of allogeneic bone-marrow transplantation ▪ Noncancerous diseases of the kidney, liver, gallbladder, and thyroid
- Dry skin ▪ Emotional stress

HOW ITCHING IS MANAGED

Systemic Drug Therapy—When pruritus is a feature of infection, the doctor will prescribe an antimicrobial agent. Other systemic medications that may be used to quell itching are antihistamines such as the ubiquitous Benadryl (known generically as diphenhydramine). There are several classes of antihistamines. If none proves effective, the physician may prescribe an antidepressant—which may have powerful antihistamine and anti-itching effects—a sedative, or a tranquilizer. To help patients sleep, the doses are frequently increased at bedtime. Itching that stems from kidney disease or liver disease may be brought under control by a *sequestrant* drug like cholestyramine (Questran Light). It binds pruritus-inducing substances in the intestine so that they are excreted instead of reabsorbed into the bloodstream.

Topical Drug Therapy—Applying a mild corticosteroid cream or ointment to the skin may relieve pruritus known to respond to steroid medications. However, they should never be used to treat itching caused by radiotherapy or if the underlying condition isn't known. One drawback to topical steroids is that they reduce blood flow to the skin, causing it to become thinner and more prone to injury.

Nonmedical Measures—Scratching a persistent itch may feel heavenly, but it can actually aggravate pruritus, setting off an "itch-scratch-itch" cycle. Impulses of itching and pain both travel the same circuits of the central nervous system. Scratching an itch to the point of pain can disrupt the cycle—substituting one sensation for the other. If you're immunosuppressed, though, you don't want to damage the skin, which is your main barrier against infection. Instead, try placing a cool washcloth or ice over the area or pressing the palm of your hand against it. Another trick is to distract yourself from the itching by watching TV, listening to music, or practicing relaxation and visualization exercises.

See "Relieving Pain Without Medicine," page 793.

HOW YOU CAN HELP YOURSELF

The fundamentals of tender, loving skin care—clean, moisturize, nourish, protect—go a long way toward alleviating itching. Here are do's and don'ts for pruritus sufferers:

- Hydrate your skin, inside and out. Itching is often due to dry skin, a recurrent problem for many older men and women. Because the skin derives most of its moisture from blood vessels in the tissues below, it's essential to keep yourself adequately hydrated by drinking four quarts of fluid a day.

  A well-balanced diet is also important. Be sure you get the recommended daily value of vitamins A and C, preferably through natural sources like fruit and vegetables rather than supplements. Deficiencies of vitamin A can leave the skin dry and rough, while a lack of vitamin C slows healing.

- Generously apply a fragrance-free, preservative-free *emollient* moisturizer at least twice a day and immediately after bathing—preferably while your skin is still slightly wet. (Instead of toweling yourself dry, just shake off the water.) Besides keeping skin supple, these lotions seal in moisture. Popular brands include Aquanil, Moisturel, and Eucerin.

Emollients containing either lactic acid or urea are even better because the added ingredient enables the lotion to better penetrate the skin's outer layers. Look for brands such as LactiCare, Lac-Hydrin, and Eucerin Plus. However, the acid content can actually irritate the skin. Any of these products, in fact, may induce allergic reactions in some people. Ask your physician or nurse for advice on choosing a moisturizer.

- When it comes to bathing, less is sometimes more. Tiny glands in the skin's inner layer secrete a film of oil that insulates the skin from the drying effects of the elements. As we grow older, the glands usually produce less oil, so it's a good idea to change bathing habits that strip away the skin's oily coating and lead to dryness:

    Buy mild soaps such as Dove, Neutrogena, and Basis, instead of harsh brands containing detergents. Use less of it too: Lather up only your armpits, your privates, and your backside, then rinse off.

    Bathe every other day instead of daily; limit baths and showers to no more than half an hour.

    Wash with lukewarm water instead of hot water.

    Just before you get out of the tub, add some bath oil to the water.

    Soak in a tubful of warm water and a soothing *colloidal* bath treatment containing powdered oatmeal, bran, or starch. Bubble baths, however, dry out the skin and should be avoided.

- In cold, windy weather, wear gloves and a scarf or ski mask outdoors to protect your hands and face from chafing. When indoors, don't overheat your home. Heat is believed to exacerbate itching. It also reduces the humidity, which further contributes to pruritus. Although the skin drinks up water mainly from within, in humid conditions it can absorb moisture in the air. A humidifier, therefore, is a wise investment.

- In hot, dry weather, stay indoors as much as possible. If you must go out in the sun, slather on a sunscreen with a sun protection factor (SPF) of at least 15.

- Wash your clothes and bed linens in mild, unscented detergents and run them through an extra rinse cycle. The residue from scented detergents, bleaches, fabric softeners, antistatic products, and other additives can aggravate itching. One trick for neutralizing this residue, recommended by the National Cancer Institute, is to add vinegar during the rinse cycle: one teaspoon per each quart of water.

◆ Always wash new clothing, sheets, and towels before you use them.

• Wear loose-fitting, lightweight clothing made of cotton or other soft fabrics. Synthetics and abrasive materials such as wool can irritate your skin, as can wrinkle-free and permanent-press apparel containing formaldehyde and other chemicals. Similarly, cover your bed with cotton sheets and cotton flannel blankets. Sleeping under heavy comforters can raise your body temperature.

• Don't consume hot foods, hot beverages, or alcohol. All cause blood vessels to enlarge, thereby inflaming pruritus.

• Use only hypoallergenic cosmetics and avoid all perfumes, colognes, aftershaves, and soaps containing alcohol.

• If you use cornstarch, a helpful remedy for dry skin caused by radiation therapy, be sure not to pat it on areas that tend to become clammy: under the arms, skin folds, and wherever you sweat the most. Also keep the powder away from the anus and the vagina. Moist cornstarch can promote the growth of fungal infections.

See "Potential Side Effects of Radiation Therapy" in Chapter Seven, "What You Can Expect During Treatment."

Respiratory Complications

Shortness of Breath (Dyspnea)

COMMON CAUSES

▪ A tumor in the respiratory tract ▪ Radiation therapy to the lung, chest, esophagus ▪ Chemotherapy ▪ Anemia ▪ Anxiety and stress ▪ Pneumonia ▪ Pleural effusion, a buildup of malignant or nonmalignant fluid between the membranes surrounding the lungs ▪ Pericardial effusion, a buildup of malignant or nonmalignant fluid in the pericardial sac that encloses the heart

TABLE 8.9 Other Effects on Skin and Nails

Side Effect	Can Be Caused by	How It Is Managed
Acne	Chemotherapy	• Keep your face clean. • Use nonprescription acne creams and medicated soaps.
Dark, brittle, or cracked nails	Chemotherapy	• Wear protective gloves when washing dishes, gardening, and performing other chores around the house. • Try nail-strengthening products, but check your nails daily for signs of irritation.
Darkening of the skin along the vein used to deliver chemotherapy	Chemotherapy	• You can use makeup to camouflage the area. However, this may not work so well if more than one vein is affected. The discoloration typically fades several months after chemotherapy ends.
Heightened skin sensitivity to the sun's rays	Chemotherapy, radiation therapy	• Ask your doctor or nurse which sunscreen or sunblock to use when you're out in the sun, or whether you should try to avoid direct sunlight altogether. • Wear wide-brimmed hats, long-sleeved shirts and pants, and other protective clothing. • Never use a tanning bed.
"Radiation recall," a reaction to chemotherapy following radiation treatments. Shortly after chemo is administered, the skin in the radiation field turns red and may itch and burn for hours or days.	Chemotherapy that follows radiation therapy	• Place a cool, wet washcloth over the affected area. • Notify your doctor or nurse.

Also alert your physician or nurse to any of the following:

- Severe itching that persists for more than three days

- A red, open wound from scratching an itch

- Pus oozing from a wound or cut, which typically indicates an infection

- A rash; hives; rough, red, painful areas of the skin. All are possible symptoms of an allergic reaction to a medication.

As many as half of all cancer patients experience shortness of breath *(dyspnea)* at some point, for one or more of the reasons above. It is often a symptom of advanced disease, although approximately three in five people with lung cancer complain of breathing difficulties at the time of diagnosis.

Fifty percent of *pleural effusions* in cancer patients are benign. The incidence of malignant pleural effusions is highest for tumors of the lung, breast, gastrointestinal tract, urinary tract, and ovary, and for lymphomas and leukemias. *Pericardial effusions,* while less common, can develop as a complication of some of the same cancers.

HOW SHORTNESS OF BREATH IS MANAGED

If the cause is an obstructed air passage, successful definitive therapy to eradicate the tumor will relieve the symptom. Anemia, a common side effect of chemotherapy, depletes the body of the red blood cells that deliver oxygen to all tissues. A patient may receive a blood transfusion or a drug that stimulates the production of new red cells. For mild anemia, the doctor may elect to do nothing, since normally the red count will rebound in time for the next drug cycle. When primary cancer treatment cannot improve dyspnea, measures such as the following may be used.

See "Anemia (Erythropenia)," page 714.

Drug Therapy—To feel like you're starving for air is a frightening experience. Breathing distress also exhausts patients and interferes with sleep. Unfortunately, when a person's muscles tense up from anxiety, the act of breathing becomes even more difficult. Antianxiety medications may help to return respirations to the normal sixteen to twenty breaths per minute.

Narcotic analgesics, or opioids, may also help to improve breathing by relaxing the muscles. If you're already taking morphine or another narcotic to ease pain, your physician may increase the dose. For patients who are not on opioid painkillers, a low dose may be prescribed strictly to aid respiration.

Other drugs used to alleviate dyspnea include diuretics, to unload excess fluid from the body; *bronchodilators,* which open up the airways; and *mucolytics,* for dissolving mucus plugging up the respiratory system.

Oxygen Therapy—These days, portable oxygen tanks are routinely delivered for use at home. Someone from a medical equipment company or a home-care nurse will teach you and your loved ones how to operate it. Most people get the hang of it pretty quickly.

Patients requiring supplemental oxygen must usually wear a *nasal cannula:* a pair of soft-rubber prongs, one for each nostril. These lead to a tube that connects to the oxygen source. For severe breathing problems, the oxygen may be administered through a disposable face mask that is frequently attached to a humidifier. The snug-fitting devices can be hot and uncomfortable, so be sure to take good care of the skin around your mouth, nose, and chin.

Thoracentesis/Pericardiocentesis—In both these procedures, performed under local anesthesia, the doctor inserts a needle through the skin and muscle and into the membrane surrounding the lung (in thoracentesis) or the heart (in pericardiocentesis). The excess fluid is then aspirated through the syringe. Another method is to place a catheter in the *pleural space* or the *pericardial space* and drain the fluid over the course of one to three days. Medicine to prevent a recurrence is then instilled through the chest tube.

> **Safety Tips When Using Supplemental Oxygen**
>
> Think of supplemental O_2 as you would medication and don't deviate from the prescribed dosage—or in this case, the *concentration* (percentage of oxygen) and *flow rate* (the number of liters per minute). An overdose can lull your brain into thinking that you don't need as much oxygen and can actually impair your breathing.
>
> Never allow anyone to smoke near an oxygen tank, even when it's not in use.

HOW YOU CAN HELP YOURSELF

- Put gravity to work by propping yourself up in bed with pillows or with a soft-foam wedge, available at most medical supplies stores. Sitting partially upright, at about a forty-five-degree angle, allows the lungs to expand more. It's also easier to cough up phlegm this way than when lying flat on your back. You may want to sleep in this position as well, either in bed or in a reclining chair.

> **MONEY MATTERS**
>
> Some chapters of the American Cancer Society lend reclining chairs to patients who need them. Call 800-227-2345 to be put in touch with your local ACS chapter.

- Practice relaxation exercises such as those described in this chapter's section on alternative methods of pain control. A gentle massage can also help to calm patients, making it easier for them to catch their breath.

- Know your physical limits and plan your day accordingly. If you become winded after exerting yourself, schedule periods of rest between activities. Even the act of eating or talking can leave some patients short of breath at times. In that case, it's wise to relax after meals and to keep visits from well-wishers shorter than usual.

- Practice controlled breathing, in which you take a lingering breath through your nose, then purse your lips and exhale twice as slowly out your mouth.

- Drink the recommended eight to ten eight-ounce glasses of cool liquids per day. Water thins out secretions that might otherwise become lodged in the respiratory tract.

- Sit in front of a fan or an air conditioner. Cool air on your face will help you to breathe more easily.

- Keep a humidifier on day and night during the winter months. When you can't catch your breath, it's natural to inhale more through your mouth, which dries out the tissue. Breathing moistened air helps prevent dryness and loosens thick mucus too.

  See "Dry Mouth (Xerostomia)," page 746.

- Stop smoking! As if smokers needed another reason to give up the habit, tobacco use interferes with the effectiveness of chemotherapy and radiotherapy and increases the likelihood of side effects. Smokers do not heal from surgery as quickly as nonsmokers; they also tend to experience more postoperative complications, such as pneumonia and other infections.

In addition to these immediate benefits, giving up cigarettes lowers the future risk of developing a second tobacco-related cancer or *chronic obstructive pulmonary disease* (COPD), the fourth leading cause of death in the United States. Most compelling of all: Cancer patients who stop smoking live longer.

Finding the Right Smoking-Cessation Strategy for You

There are three approaches to overcoming nicotine addiction, which for some people is no less enslaving than heroin or cocaine. One is to stop abruptly—go "cold turkey"—and contend with the subsequent withdrawal symptoms until they subside. Longtime, heavy smokers are more likely to experience anxiety, irritability, insomnia, coughing, dry mouth, lack of concentration, and an increased craving for food.

Nicotine-replacement therapy supplies the body with a small, steady dose of the drug; enough to make withdrawal more bearable. These products come in four forms: skin patch, gum, nasal spray, and inhaler. The success rates from using the patch and gum together are significantly higher than from using the gum alone. Both are available over-the-counter in different strengths. A doctor must write you a prescription for the nasal spray and the inhaler.

> **The Agency for Health Care Policy and Research, part of the U.S. Department of Health and Human Services, publishes a highly informative, readable booklet on smoking-cessation techniques, titled "You Can Quit Smoking." For a free copy, call the AHCPR Publications Clearinghouse at 800-358-9295 or visit its Web site: *http://www.ahcpr.gov.***

The oral antidepressant bupropion (Zyban) became the first non-nicotine prescription medication for treating tobacco dependency. It reduces withdrawal symptoms and the urge to smoke, although just how is not known.

Smoking-Cessation Programs

Studies show that nicotine withdrawal is most effective when undertaken in conjunction with some form of behavioral modification: short-term counseling by a doctor or nurse, or participation in a *smoking-cessation program*. Relapses are extremely common. The long-term success rate for stop-smoking groups is about 25 percent, which is far higher than for people who try to quit without the encouragement and support of other smokers.

The typical program consists of four to eight sessions led by a trained ex-smoker. For instance, smokers who enroll in the American Cancer Society's Fresh Start program attend four one-hour sessions over the course of two weeks, while the American Lung Association's Freedom from Smoking clinics run for eight sessions. Many hospitals sponsor their own groups.

See "Smoking-Cessation Programs" in Appendix B to learn how to find a program near you.

◆ Summon emergency medical service should you ever be unable to catch your breath while resting or if you experience chest pains.

Fatigue

COMMON CAUSES

- Extreme physical or emotional stress ▪ Anxiety ▪ Depression
- Sleeplessness ▪ Anemia ▪ Radiation therapy
- Chemotherapy ▪ Immunotherapy ▪ Other medications,
including those used to treat pain, depression, seizures, and
nausea ▪ Surgery ▪ Sleep interruptions while in the hospital
- Chronic pain ▪ Nausea and vomiting ▪ Infections
- Appetite loss ▪ Dehydration ▪ Electrolyte imbalance
- Weight loss ▪ Difficulty in breathing

Roughly three in four cancer patients complain of feeling physically and mentally fatigued throughout treatment. In some cases, the exhaustion persists for a considerable time afterward as well.

This tiredness is different from just wanting to take a nap. Cancer-related fatigue can impact upon every aspect of daily life. The Fatigue Coalition, part of the National Coalition for Cancer Survivorship support organization, surveyed more than four hundred patients who were then in treatment. About three in five said that chronic exhaustion interfered with their sense of physical well-being, their ability to work, and their enjoyment of life. In another Fatigue Coalition poll, the same percentage of patients cited fatigue as the most debilitating side effect of therapy. Yet fatigue tends to get overlooked by physicians, family members—and even patients, who may assume that they have to put up with this kind of exhaustion. Only about one in ten of those surveyed received appropriate treatment for their fatigue.

HOW FATIGUE IS MANAGED

Emotional stress and the disease process itself can also wear down the body. One way to alleviate fatigue is to treat the underlying cause(s). This could entail surgically removing a patient's tumor; using drugs or blood transfusions to reverse chemotherapy-induced anemia; or prescribing medication to relieve depression.

Otherwise, there is relatively little the doctor can do to treat fatigue specifically. The best way to restore your energy is to eat a balanced diet, regularly engage in mild to moderate exercise, and get lots of rest. The National Cancer Institute recommends discontinuing any medications that act on the brain, unless they're essential to treatment. This is a point to take up with your doctor.

HOW YOU CAN HELP YOURSELF

- Stay active, but don't overdo it. "When you get out for a little bit of physical activity, you tend to feel better and you can be more productive during the time that you're awake," says Dr. Christine Berg. "Plus, you'll sleep better at night." A short walk or light exercise regimen is ideal, but if you're not up to that level of physical exertion, just make sure to keep your body moving at least once a day, even if it's only to get dressed.

- Get extra sleep at night and nap as needed. Dr. Berg, a radiation oncologist, typically advises her patients to go to bed "half an hour earlier than normal and get a good, long night's sleep." If you're feeling fatigued during the day, don't fight the urge to doze. But napping too much can throw off your body clock and prevent you from sleeping through the night.

- Keep a diary of how you feel during the day. When do you seem to have the most energy? When do you tucker out? Let your body's natural rhythm guide you in planning your day. Build extra time into your schedule to allow for periods of rest, and don't be discouraged if you can't accomplish everything on your list.

- Now is a good time to call in favors from family and friends; ask them to pitch in around the home, run errands for you, and so on.

   See Chapter Ten, "Getting Help When You Need It."

- When sitting or lying down, get up slowly. This will help to prevent dizziness and falls.

Dietary Do's and Don'ts When You're Feeling Fatigued

Include liver, red meat, and green, leafy vegetables in your diet in order to replace iron. You also want to eat chicken, fish, and other foods rich in protein. But the most important food group for you is complex carbohydrates, which pack the most energy. Excellent sources include pasta, bread, fruit, and potatoes.

Can't Sleep? Join the Club

Nearly half of all cancer patients suffer from some form of sleep disorder, largely *insomnia* and disruptions of the *sleep-wake cycle*. That's about double the rate of sleep disturbances among the general population. One possible solution is for your physician to prescribe a sleeping aid. However, be aware that continued use of such drugs can alter your natural sleep pattern and lead to physical and psychological dependence after as little as one to two weeks.

Before going that route, try the following tips. Start by assessing your bedroom. Is it conducive to sleep? Perhaps you need room-darkening shades to keep out the morning sunlight and let you catch that extra hour of shut-eye.

At bedtime, adjust the thermostat, fan, or air conditioner to a comfortable temperature and make sure that you have the right amount of bedcovers. Change the bed linens frequently. Fresh, clean, unwrinkled sheets, blankets, and pillowcases are far more inviting than clammy, rumpled bedding. Bedclothes should be soft and loose-fitting, never constricting. Put on some soothing music if that works for you.

Other ways to help lure Mr. Sandman:

- Don't go to bed when you're hot and sticky. If a bath or shower is impractical, lather up a warm, wet washcloth and clean one section of your skin at a time. Use a fresh washcloth to wash off all the soap. Then dry the area and move on to the next. Clean as much of your body as you can; whatever's in reach.

- Have someone give you a gentle back rub.

- Relieve your bladder and bowel before going to sleep so that you're not getting up in the middle of the night to use the toilet. This is especially important for older men with enlarged prostates.

- Along similar lines, don't drink before you go to bed; try to consume your recommended four quarts of fluids earlier in the day. And avoid beverages containing caffeine, which acts as a diuretic.

- Exercise is wonderful, but finish at least two hours before retiring for the night.

- To help you fall asleep, eat a small snack high in carbohydrates and low in protein two hours before bedtime. This increases the level of a natural brain chemical called *tryptophan,* which has been called nature's sleeping pill. Try munching on popcorn, toast with jam, a bagel, an apple, or a banana. As an added bonus, tryptophan triggers the release of another substance in the brain, *serotonin,* which can ease mild depression.

If you're still tossing and turning at night and bleary-eyed during the day, tell your oncologist. Sleep deprivation diminishes pain tolerance, deepens depression, and impairs immunity against infection. As a temporary measure, the doctor might suggest a sleeping aid.

The most popular *hypnotic* agents are the *benzodiazepines,* which induce a natural sleep: diazepam (Valium), temazepam (Restoril), triazolam (Halcion), flurazepam (Dalmane), and clonazepam (Klonopin). In the event that a patient cannot tolerate benzodiazepines, the physician may choose an antihistamine, an antidepressant, an antipsychotic, or a nonbenzodiazepine hypnotic called zolpidem (Ambien). Barbiturates, however, are generally discouraged because they can become habit-forming and because of their narrow margin of safety.

Cancer Pain

COMMON CAUSES

- A tumor pressing against organs, nerves, or bone, or blocking an organ, blood vessel, or lymph vessel ▪ Incisional pain from surgery ▪ Infection ▪ Inflammation ▪ Chemotherapy
- Radiation therapy ▪ Constipation ▪ Indigestion ▪ Immobility

The 1990s brought such significant advances in pain management that by middecade the American College of Physicians could claim: "Most cancer pain can be eliminated, and all cancer pain can be controlled."

In theory, yes. In practice, far too many men and women with cancer still experience pain. According to a 1998 poll conducted by the pain-research group at Houston's M. D. Anderson Cancer Center, four in five oncologists surveyed conceded that cancer pain was undertreated. It seems that attitudes, on the parts of both the medical profession and the public, have not kept pace with the strides in pain medications and nonpharmacologic techniques.

Two major obstacles stand in the way of patients receiving adequate pain relief: One is the unfounded fear that prescription painkillers lead to addiction. The other is a long-standing cultural bias that encourages stoicism in the face of suffering and regards the use of pain medication as a sign of moral weakness. *Half* the oncologists in the M. D. Anderson study considered it acceptable for patients to have to

---

TABLE 8.10 **Cancer-Related Pain**

· Back pain	· Jaw pain
· Bone pain	· Joint or muscle pain
· Breast pain/tenderness	· Nerve pain
· Chest pain	· Phantom-limb pain
· Ear pain	· Rectal pain
· Genitourinary pain	· Testicular pain
· Headaches	· Visceral (abdominal) pain
· Incisional pain	

---

bear mild pain as well as to endure intervals of "distressing" pain between doses.

When cancer pain is managed well, you're better able to battle the disease and go on living. Chronic pain disrupts sleep, which can impair the body's defenses against potentially deadly infections. It curbs appetite, which can prevent you from getting the nutrients needed for healing. It can make you anxious, depressed, and irritable, which in turn can exacerbate pain, setting up a vicious cycle.

Medical Terms You're Likely to Hear

Phantom-limb pain: Many people who have lost an arm or a leg to amputation experience a curious phenomenon called *phantom-limb pain.* They feel—not imagine, *feel*—a burning or shooting sensation arising from the missing part of the body or the stump. Doctors aren't certain why this happens, although the suspicion is that changes in the spinal cord cause the brain to misinterpret new signals sent from the area as pain. Women who have undergone a mastectomy may also perceive phantom pain in their chest.

Types of Cancer Pain

Simply put, the word "pain" means any sensation that hurts. Pain is said to be acute or chronic. "Acute" describes the severe but relatively short-lived pain you feel when you cut yourself. Once the injury heals, the pain usually subsides. Chronic pain is longer lasting and ranges from severe to mild.

Just as cancer isn't a single entity, there are different types of pain associated with the disease and its treatment, as shown in table 8.10.

One important point to bear in mind: "A significant number of cancer patients don't have pain at all," notes Dr. Jane Ingham, director of palliative care at the Lombardi Cancer Center. Only one in four men and women with early-stage cancer experience pain, and they are not in pain all the time. "Pain is more common in advanced disease," she continues. "Whatever the stage, there are many effective treatments."

HOW CANCER PAIN IS MANAGED

When a tumor is the source of pain, the primary treatment to eradicate it or reduce it in size should bring relief. But if the cancer is beyond therapy, or the origin of the pain can't be identified, the oncologist looks to treat the symptom. Ninety percent of the time, this involves oral pain medications alone, although any of a number of alternate routes or nonpharmacologic techniques may be implemented.

The guiding principle of pain management is to start with the least invasive method first. With this in mind, cancer doctors cautiously follow a three-step ladder for prescribing analgesic medicines.

Types of Pain Medications

For mild pain, the first step is to try an over-the-counter remedy such as acetaminophen or a *nonsteroidal anti-inflammatory drug (NSAID)*. (Some NSAIDs require a prescription.) Studies show that these products are often as effective as many of the prescription painkillers, while producing fewer side effects and saving you money. They reduce postoperative pain and the pain from metastatic bone tumors. In addition, nonsteroidals reduce inflammation in swollen joints and other inflamed areas of the body; acetaminophen does not.

When a medication doesn't ease the discomfort sufficiently, the dosage may be increased, or the physician may substitute another nonopioid drug. If the pain still fails to respond, she moves one rung up the ladder and introduces a weak prescription *opioid,* often in conjunction with one of the nonopioids mentioned above. Step-two medications are for moderate pain.

> **Medical Terms You're Likely to Hear**
>
> Referred pain: Pain originating in the heart and many abdominal organs is sometimes felt elsewhere in the body. For instance, a pain in the right shoulder or the back can actually be "referred" pain from the liver. Referred pain is often felt in the skin, probably because pain impulses from the skin and the abdominal organs share the same nerves.

Opioids, the mainstay therapy for cancer pain, are chemically related to natural opium from the opium poppy flower. Doctors regard these potent painkillers as the first choice for managing moderate to severe cancer pain. They work by scrambling pain messages before they reach the brain.

Seventy to 90 percent of patients will see their pain controlled with oral opioids, but should the drug not perform as expected, a patient may be instructed to take more or switch to another weak opioid, such as propoxyphene (Darvon) or oxycodone (Percodan). Severe pain, step three, calls for a strong opioid analgesic. The most commonly ordered agent is morphine, which goes under several brand names.

The Informed Patient
What You Need to Know About Taking Pain Medications

Nonopioid Analgesics
- acetaminophen (Excedrin, Tylenol)
- nonsteroidal anti-inflammatory drugs

   aspirin (Bufferin, Ecotrin)

   choline magnesium

   trisalicylate (Trilisate)

   fenoprofen (Nalfon)
- ibuprofen (Advil, Motrin, Nuprin)
- naproxen (Aleve, Naprosyn)
- tramadol (Ultram)

NSAIDs impair the function of the platelet cells that enable blood to clot. What's more, they can irritate the stomach and cause internal bleeding. Avoid these pain relievers under the following conditions: if you are

---

The World Health Organization Three-Step Analgesic Ladder

1: Mild Pain	2: Moderate Pain	3: Severe Pain
A nonopioid pain reliever	A mild opioid painkiller	A strong opioid painkiller
alone or with	*with or without*	*with or without*
a nonanalgesic drug	a nonopioid medication	a nonopioid medication
	with or without	*with or without*
	a nonanalgesic drug	a nonanalgesic drug

scheduled for surgery within seven days; if you have stomach ulcers; or if you have a history of ulcers, gout, hemorrhoids, or other bleeding disorders.

Patients taking any of the following drugs should also not use NSAIDs: chemotherapy agents known to cause bleeding; steroid medications; prescription arthritis medications; oral hypoglycemic agents used to manage adult-onset diabetes; and anticoagulants.

Over-the-counter pain relievers may contain additives such as buffers, to help protect the stomach; the stimulant caffeine; and antihistamines. Since the additives can alter the action of other drugs you may be taking, check with your doctor or nurse before using one of these combination products.

Aspirin's Aliases

Aspirin is present in many different kinds of medicines, including the over-the-counter pain reliever Excedrin and the prescription opioid Percodan. Get into the habit of scrutinizing labels for aspirin, which may be listed under its chemical name, *acetylsalicylic acid,* or another alias, *salicylate.* Or ask your pharmacist for assistance.

Opioid Analgesics
- Weak opioids

  codeine (present in many products)

  hydrocodone (Hydrocet, Lorcet, Lortab, Vicodin)

  oxycodone (Percocet, Percodan, Roxicet, Tylox)

  propoxyphene (Darvocet-N, Darvon, Wygesic)

- Strong opioids

  fentanyl (Actiq lozenge on a stick, Duragesic transdermal patch)

  hydromorphone (Dilaudid)

  levorphanol (Levo-Dromoran)

  merperidene (Demerol)

  methadone (Dolophine, Methadose)

  morphine (Astramorph, Duramorph, MS Contin, Oramorph, Rescuedose, Roxanol)

  oxymorphone (Numorphan)

When Dr. Jane Ingham broaches the subject of taking opioid pain medications, her first words to leery patients are, "Many people are fearful of these drugs; let me explain to you what the situation really

Common Side Effects of Opioid Pain Medications

Notify your doctor or nurse if you experience any of the following:

- Constipation ▪ Nausea and vomiting ▪ Sleepiness

Less Common

- Dry mouth ▪ Itching
- Moderately slower and shallower breathing
- Difficulty in urinating
- Nightmares, confusion, hallucinations, sleep disturbances ▪ Depression and anxiety ▪ Convulsions

is." One concern that she hears expressed again and again is, "What if I become addicted?"

Less than 1 percent of patients who rely on opioids to relieve pain acquire an addiction, which the dictionary defines as a "compulsion or overpowering drive to take a drug in order to experience its psychological effects." With some drugs, though, you may find that over time you need a higher dose to achieve the same analgesic effect as before. This is not addiction. Perhaps your pain has intensified. Or it could be that your body has developed a *tolerance* for the medication.

Yet patients can often remain on opioid painkillers for years if necessary. Morphine, fentanyl, methadone, oxycodone, and several other narcotics classified as *full agonists,* have no "ceiling" to their effectiveness. Unlike the NSAIDs and drugs such as Tylenol, the dosage can be increased until the pain is relieved or until side effects occur.

Doctors with little experience in using opioids may be averse to prescribing the heavy doses that may be necessary to control pain because they're afraid of overdosing the patient into respiratory failure. This rarely happens. Most people who take opioid pain medications for an extended amount of time eventually develop tolerance to the effects on breathing.

The first sign of an overdose is typically extreme drowsiness or difficulty in waking up. Your family should be aware of this and know to contact your physician or nurse immediately. However, some degree of sleepiness is normal for the first two to three days that you take an opioid analgesic. The dosage may need to be adjusted. Or it could be that you're sleeping more than usual because the nagging pain that had been keeping you awake is diminished or gone altogether.

It goes without saying that you never get behind the wheel of a car or operate heavy machinery when you're feeling lethargic. Even cooking and walking up and down stairs should be postponed until you're more alert. Discuss with your doctor the possibility of his ordering a stimulant to help offset the sedating effect of the pain medication.

♦ Never take more pain medication than your physician has prescribed without first consulting him or the nurse. By the same token, never stop pain medicine suddenly if you've been taking it for several weeks. "Just as giving up nicotine or caffeine can cause physical symptoms," says Dr. Ingham, "patients can develop flulike withdrawal symptoms when being gradually weaned off opioids. Some mistakenly believe this means they must be addicted to the medication. That is not so," she emphasizes.

Adjuvant Medications

One of the developments in pain management has been the heightened appreciation that pain is both a physiological and an emotional response, says Matthew Loscalzo, codirector of the Center for Cancer Pain Research at Johns Hopkins Oncology Center in Baltimore.

"We're learning that pain and emotions are all interwoven within the central nervous system," he explains. "Anxiety, stress, and depression don't cause pain, but they do increase pain." In addition to prescribing analgesics, a doctor may incorporate one or more adjuvant medications into treatment in order to improve pain control and/or to relieve other symptoms (see table 8.11).

The Principles of Pharmaceutical Pain Relief

The key to relieving cancer-related pain is to "stay on top of it," as doctors and nurses like to say. For instance, if a person is suffering from persistent pain, it's important that a constant level of painkiller in the bloodstream be maintained. Therefore, analgesics are usually dispensed at set intervals around the clock, including at night.

"It could be every four hours," explains Dr. Ingham, "or if it's a long-acting drug, perhaps once or twice a day." Sustained-release morphine tablets are metabolized by the body in such a way that they can provide pain relief for eight to twelve hours, whereas fentanyl comes in the form of a *transdermal* patch. When applied to the upper arm, back, chest, or side, they continuously release the medicine through the skin for forty-eight to seventy-two hours.

If you've been experiencing unremitting pain, your doctor will generally suggest that you never skip a dose, even during times when you're feeling fine. Once pain is allowed to peak, it can be more diffi-

TABLE 8.11 **Nonanalgesic Drugs Used in the Treatment of Cancer Pain**

Type	Generic Name	Brand Name	Possible Uses
Antianxiety drugs	alprazolam lorazepam	Xanax Ativan	May be used to manage *muscle spasms* that frequently accompany severe pain, as well as *anxiety.*
Anticonvulsants	clonazepam carbamazepine phenytoin	Klonopin Tegretol Dilantin	May be used to manage *nerve pain,* especially burning or sharp pain.
Antidepressants	amitriptyline doxepin imipramine	Elavil Sinequan Tofranil	May be used to manage *nerve pain.* Antidepressants have painkilling properties themselves and may enhance the analgesic effects of narcotic medications.
Antihistamines	hydroxyzine	Atarax Vistaril	May be used to ease *pain* and *anxiety,* help control *nausea* and *itching,* and act as a *sleep aid.*
Bone-resorption inhibitors	pamidronate	Aredia	Pamidronate, a bisphosphonate, controls pain while slowing down the progression of a type of bone tumor that "devours" bone. It is used to treat multiple myeloma and metastatic breast cancer. *See "Metastatic Cancer of the Bone" in Chapter Six, "State of the Art: Your Treatment Options."*
Corticosteroids	dexamethasone prednisone	Decadron Deltasone	May be used to manage a wide range of symptoms and side effects, including *bone pain* that does not respond to other therapies; *swelling of the brain and spinal cord;* and *spinal-cord compression.* Corticosteroids *stimulate appetite, alleviate nausea,* and *improve mood.* However, if used for a long time, these drugs can bring about depression, agitation,

			bleeding, diabetes, muscle loss, infection, and a hormonal disorder called Cushing's syndrome.
Neuroleptics (major tranquilizers)	methotrime- prazine	Levoprome	May be used to treat *chronic pain*. Less constipating than opioids. Neuroleptics also have *antianxiety* and *antinausea* effects.
Stimulants	dextroamphet- amine methylphenidate	Dexedrine Ritalin	May be used to offset the drowsiness that narcotics can induce. Dexedrine also enhances the pain-relieving action of opioids.

cult to bring it back under control and may require larger doses or stronger medicine. People who take analgesics only when they're hurting may actually use a higher total dose than those who take their medication on a regular, preventive basis.

Arriving at the optimal pain reliever and dose for you may involve some experimentation. "We also prescribe a 'rescue' or 'breakthrough' dose," Dr. Ingham continues, "to be taken in the event that the around-the-clock dose isn't sufficient." Supplemental medicine is taken on an as-needed basis. The medical abbreviation for this is *p.r.n.:* short for the Latin expression *pro re nata,* or "according to circumstances."

You may find that these flare-ups are related to a specific activity, such as driving a car. In that case, take the extra medicine before you leave. However, *breakthrough pain,* as this is called, may also be an indication that your timed doses are losing their effectiveness, or *duration of action,* before it's time for the next dose. It is important to know this as well as the rescue dose's *onset of action.* For instance, aspirin usually starts to work thirty to sixty minutes after being swallowed; but coated aspirin can take as long as *eight hours* before producing an effect.

When using drugs p.r.n., never exceed the dose frequency stated on the label. If you're constantly having to rely on the rescue dose, try to time your regularly scheduled doses as consistently as you can. If that doesn't work, clearly the amount needs to be adjusted or the intervals between doses shortened—possibly both. Over time, the doctor will typically increase a patient's pain medication by 25 to 50 percent.

HOW YOU CAN HELP YOURSELF

Pain is one symptom that can't be diagnosed on X ray or through a blood test. It is completely subjective: You are the only person who knows what you're feeling. The more accurately and vividly you convey this to the doctor, the quicker she'll be able to get to the root of the problem.

The beginning of this chapter offers suggestions for how to characterize symptoms: describing pain on a scale of 1 to 10, pinpointing the location, and using adjectives such as "burning," "throbbing," and so on. Recording details in a "pain diary" is certainly a good idea. According to Dr. Ingham, the information most useful to your doctor includes the following:

- Where is the pain located?
- Is the pain constant, or does it come and go?
- How long does the pain last?
- How many times per day and per week do you experience pain?
- What seems to make the pain worse?
- What seems to make it better?
- Is the pain preventing you from eating, sleeping, going to work, participating in a certain activity?
- What pain medication are you taking, and how much?
- When do you take your pain medication?
- How long does the pain medication work?
- Are you experiencing any side effects from the medication?
- Do you use any nonpharmacologic methods of pain management?

"It's also extremely helpful for us to know the history of what's gone on," she says, offering an example. "If a patient tells me that he's having a constant, stabbing pain in the middle of his abdomen, it's obviously relevant for me to know whether or not he had an operation last week or a history of ulcers!"

No Relief Yet? Don't Give Up

When you're in pain, tell your doctor or nurse right away. Finding the most effective combination of pain-relieving methods can take time. Don't be discouraged if the medical team doesn't come up with the optimal solution on the first try. We all feel pain differently, so what works for one person may not work for another. (It's a fact: Opioids tend to control pain more effectively and longer in the elderly and in women than in younger men.) At the same time, with a little tweaking of dosage or scheduling, what didn't work for you yesterday may work today.

Most pain from cancer *can* be substantially relieved or reduced, says Matthew Loscalzo of Johns Hopkins. "If a person in pain is told that nothing else can be done, he should insist on a second opinion or ask to be referred to a pain-care team for a consultation." The ideal team should have access to an internist, a neurologist, an anesthesiologist, a social worker, and a psychologist or a psychiatrist.

Outside of major cancer centers, though, few hospitals provide multidisciplinary pain management. It's worth the search. The American Pain Society, a professional organization made up of more than 3,200 pain-management professionals, can refer you to pain centers and clinics that specialize in cancer-related pain, as can the Commission on Accreditation of Rehabilitation Facilities and the Cancer Information Service of the National Cancer Institute. The American Society of Anesthesiology can refer you to individual pain specialists. We'd suggest also calling a hospice or the department of anesthesiology at a cancer center or university hospital.

American Pain Society
847-375-4715
http://www.ampainsoc.org (Web site)
info@ampainsoc.org (e-mail)

American Society of Anesthesiologists
847-825-5586
http://www.asahq.org (Web site)
mail@asahq.org (e-mail)

Cancer Information Service
800-422-6237
http://cancernet.nci.nih.gov (Web site)
cancernet@icicb.nci.nih.gov (e-mail)

Commission on Accreditation of Rehabilitation Facilities
4891 East Grant Road, Tucson, AZ 85712
520-325-1044
http:www.carf.org (Web site)

Write to CARF and enclose a self-addressed, stamped envelope for a listing of facilities with accredited pain programs.

Other Types of Pain Relief

ALTERNATE ROUTES OF ADMINISTERING PAIN MEDICATION

About half of all cancer patients receive medication via a route other than the mouth at some point during treatment, perhaps because they're encountering temporary difficulty in swallowing.

Rectal Suppositories—Dilaudid and Numorphan are two examples of opioids that come in suppository form. Once inserted in the rectum, they melt and the body absorbs the medicine.

Injections—Pain medications can be injected beneath the surface of the skin (subcutaneously) or directly into a vein (intravenously). The latter route offers the quickest relief but also the shortest duration of action. Intramuscular injections are not recommended. Absorption is unreliable this way; in addition, repeated shots into muscles become painful.

Intraspinal Injections—Injecting analgesics into the epidural space (the space between the lining of the spinal canal and the outermost layer of the three-ply membrane that surrounds the spinal cord) or into the subarachnoid space (the space between the two innermost layers, nearer the spinal cord) is usually reserved for intractable pain, particularly of the lower part of the body, or for patients who cannot tolerate other methods of delivering the drug.

Pump-Delivered Analgesia—In *continuous subcutaneous infusion,* a small needle inserted beneath the skin leads to a small computerized electronic pump that dispenses the drug automatically at regular intervals. The pump can also be used to infuse pain medication directly into either of the two spaces outside the spinal cord, as described under "Intraspinal Injections."

The premise behind *patient-controlled analgesia* (PCA) is that patients know best when they need pain medication. The battery-operated pump delivers a small continuous flow of analgesic into a vein, into the spine, or under the skin. But patients also have the option of pressing a button on the device to release preset rescue doses. You don't have to worry about giving yourself too much drug. Once the infuser has administered the maximum total amount of painkiller per hour, as predetermined by your doctor, it disables the button until the allotted time is up. Interestingly, studies have found that patients on PCA often use *less* medication, not more. The lightweight, portable pump attaches to an IV pole or a belt, allowing you to remain mobile.

RELIEVING PAIN WITHOUT MEDICINE

Noninvasive Mind-Body-Control Interventions

In response to growing public interest in so-called alternative medicine, many cancer centers now routinely offer a number of unconventional noninvasive pain-management techniques as complements to pain medications: acupuncture, hypnotherapy, relaxation, visualization, biofeedback, distraction.

"By themselves, probably none of these interventions would work," says Matthew Loscalzo, who specializes in the psychobehavioral aspects of cancer pain. "But when integrated with a patient's overall medical care, they can give him a sense of control and hope, and under some circumstances, they can definitely reduce pain."

Institutions like Houston's M. D. Anderson Cancer Center have gone so far as to establish wellness clinics, where complementary therapies are used to ease stress, alleviate side effects and symptoms, and enhance patients' well-being.

Nowadays, instruction in relaxation and visualization techniques is available in many treatment settings. Other specialities, though, may be delegated to outside practitioners. At the Lombardi Cancer Center, for instance, biofeedback is performed on the premises, but patients seeking acupuncture or massage therapy are referred out.

To locate specialists in these modalities on your own, call the department of social work or the department of psychiatry/psychology/psycho-oncology at a local hospital and ask if they could recommend anyone. According to Loscalzo, "Most professionals in this field do a number of interventions."

You can also contact the professional organizations in the box at right for the names,

---

Acupuncture
American Academy of Medical Acupuncture
800-521-2262
http://www.medicalacupuncture.org

National Certification Commission for Acupuncture and Oriental Medicine
703-548-9004
http://www.nccaom.org

Biofeedback
Association for Applied Psychophysiology and Biofeedback
http://www.aapb.org

For more information about these organizations, see Appendix B.

addresses, and telephone numbers of practitioners in your area. Apply the same criteria as you would when seeking an oncologist. The two crucial questions to ask are: "How many patients do you see a year?" and "Have you ever worked with anyone who had my specific complaint?"

◆ Many of these interventions are also useful for helping to control nausea and anxiety.

Relaxation—There are several techniques for relaxing the muscles, which can relieve minor pain. Relaxation doesn't come naturally to many of us, but keep practicing, and you should get the hang of it within a week or two at the most.

To begin, find a quiet spot and lie prone on the floor or sit in a cushioned chair. It doesn't matter which, as long as you're comfortable. Rest your arms at your sides and keep your legs slightly apart; crossing the limbs can cut off circulation. Now close your eyes.

Exercise 1. Rhythmic Breathing

1. Inhale s-l-o-w-l-y and deeply.
2. Now exhale slowly. Feel the tension drain from your body.
3. Continue breathing slowly and rhythmically for five to ten minutes at a rate of approximately ten breaths per minute. As you inhale, count silently, *In, one, two.* Then exhale: *Out, one, two.*
4. Take a final slow, deep breath. Then say to yourself, *I feel alert and relaxed.*

Exercise 2. Progressive Muscle Relaxation

1. Inhale s-l-o-w-l-y and deeply.
2. At the same time, tense the muscles in your feet and ankles for a count of four.
3. Now slowly let out your breath while you release the tension in the muscles. Let that part of your body go limp.
4. Repeat this with all of the body's major muscle groups: calves and knees, thighs, upper arms and shoulders, stomach, chest.

Some cancer patients study the Far Eastern discipline of *transcendental meditation* or *yoga* to help them learn to clear their minds and achieve a deeply relaxed, peaceful state.

Visualization—This technique, also known as *imagery,* combines rhythmic breathing with your imagination to create mental images or scenes for the purpose of relieving pain, anxiety, boredom, and sleeplessness. One patient might concentrate on a warm ball of healing energy radiating from inside her body, bringing comfort; another might envision the nerves that deliver pain signals being snipped one by one. A person suffering from a burning pain might picture cool water cascading over the painful area. The possibilities are endless.

Matthew Loscalzo of Johns Hopkins guides cancer patients in developing visualizations that have meaning for them. First he asks them to compare the painful sensation to a color, shape, size, taste—"anything," he says, "that gives them a sense of distance and control over it." He recalls the case of one twenty-five-year-old woman, an artist, with leukemia. "She was one of the 10 percent of cancer patients whose pain we couldn't adequately manage. We had her on doses of pain medication that made her too sleepy, and she didn't want that," says Loscalzo.

"I asked her, 'What is the pain like?' She said, 'It's achy, and it's hot.'

" 'Wonderful. Tell me what color most reminds you of something cool and comfortable.'

"She said purple. I had her imagine herself using a thick brush to paint her entire body purple. First each toenail, then each toe, then each foot. This took about twenty minutes. She went into a very deep, relaxed state, smiled, and said, 'This is the first time I've been comfortable and totally without pain in months.' "

Loscalzo tape-records patients' favorite visualizations and gives them audiocassettes to play at home, to help them call up the scene again. Many bookstores and record stores carry relaxation instruction tapes. Ask your physician or nurse if they can recommend any titles.

Distraction—Distraction is exactly what it sounds like: tricking the brain into focusing on something other than the pain. Immersing yourself in a good book, a video, or music can take your mind off mild pain for hours. It can even make you forget about intense pain, though generally for five minutes to forty-five minutes, maximum. Some patients learn to distract themselves by counting, praying, or repeating a positive statement, such as "I can cope."

Hypnotherapy—In hypnosis, a trained professional guides the subject into a trancelike state, during which he becomes highly receptive to the power of suggestion. The hypnotist might plant the idea that the pain

TABLE 8.12   **Methods of Skin Stimulation to Alleviate Pain**

Method	Effective for Relieving This Type of Pain	Precautions
Heat, using a heating pad, hydroculator, gel pack, hot-water bottle, hot towel, warm bath or shower	• Sore muscles • Bone pain • Weakness	• Always wrap the heat source in a towel; never place it against bare skin. • Don't set a heating pad on High. • Never fall asleep with the heating pad on. • Placing heat over a new injury can increase bleeding; wait a minimum of 24 hours. • Don't apply heat to an area with poor circulation or sensation. • Time limit for applying heat: 5 to 10 minutes.
Cold, using a gel pack, ice pack, ice cubes wrapped in a towel	• Chronic pain • Inflammation • Swelling	• Wrap the gel pack or ice pack in a towel. • If you start shivering, remove the cold source from the skin. • Don't apply cold to an area with poor circulation or sensation. • Time limit for applying cold: 5 to 10 minutes.
Menthol preparations such as BenGay, Heet, Mineral Ice, Icy Hot. They work by increasing blood flow to the area, which produces a warm or cool sensation.	• Muscle and joint pain • Backache	• Before you use one of these products, test your reaction to it by rubbing a small amount over an inch or so of skin. You may feel a burning sensation for the first several uses. If it's comfortable and doesn't irritate the skin, apply more. • Don't apply over open wounds or rashes, and avoid getting menthol preparations inside your mouth, around your rectum, or in your eyes. • If you've been instructed to avoid aspirin, ask your doctor whether or not it's safe for you to use a menthol preparation, many of which contain an aspirin-like ingredient. • To intensify the effect of the menthol, take a hot shower or go out in the sun. Heat opens the pores in the skin. ♦ Caution: Do not use a heating pad when using menthol preparations.
Massage, pressure, and vibration can bring temporary relief	• General aches and pains • Headache	*Massage:* • Try a massage using talcum powder, warm oil, or lotion.

by distracting patients from their pain or relaxing them. You can perform these techniques yourself or have a family member or friend do them.

Massage Techniques:
• To give a relaxing massage, use long, slow, fluid strokes.
• To increase circulation to an area, stroke rapidly, or squeeze and knead the tissue, or move your hands in a slow, steady, circular motion.

• Don't massage areas that are swollen, tender, red, or raw.
• Time limit: 3 to 10 minutes.

Pressure:
• Apply pressure to the pain site, or near it, using your whole hand, the heel of your palm, the tips of your fingers, two knuckles, or both hands.
• Don't press so hard that it hurts.
• Time limit: up to 1 minute.

Vibration:
• A handheld vibrator placed against the scalp is great for relieving headaches.
• A vibrator placed near the small of the back can reduce lower-back pain.
• Don't use vibration over areas that are swollen, tender, red, or raw.

will have vanished the moment the patient wakes up. Patients can be taught to induce a hypnotic state themselves whenever mild to moderate pain strikes.

Exactly how hypnotherapy eases pain remains a mystery, "but it can be very effective in certain patients," says Matthew Loscalzo. However, self-hypnosis does not work for everyone. "Although virtually all people can put themselves into a hypnotic trance," he points out, "they may not be skilled enough at it that they can block pain."

Biofeedback—Biofeedback uses special equipment to train people to regulate bodily processes that are normally involuntary. Among these is muscle tension, which exacerbates pain. Sensors applied to the skin monitor electrical signals from the muscles and convert it to a visual or auditory cue. Every time the patient tenses, the biofeedback machine beeps or activates a flashing light. From heeding the feedback, patients eventually learn how to use mind control to relax their muscles at will without having to be hooked up to the unit.

Another biofeedback technique helps subjects ward off anxiety. They place two fingers on a small sensor device. One of the symptoms of stress is restricted blood flow to the fingers, which makes them feel cool. The monitoring instrument perceives changes in the skin and emits a rising or falling tone. Adjusting one's response to stress lowers the pitch, until, if possible, it becomes ingrained. According to

Loscalzo, this technique has been especially helpful for relieving headache pain.

Noninvasive Physical Interventions

Mind-body-control interventions like visualization and distraction demand concentration and energy and are best reserved for those times when you're well rested and mentally alert. If you're feeling worn down, though, various techniques that stir the nerve endings in the skin can bring welcome relief with minimal effort.

Skin Stimulation—The principle behind skin stimulation is that pain impulses ride the same neural pathways to the brain as sensations of heat, cold, and pressure. Thus, stimulating the skin on or near the area that's hurting can block or at least reduce the perception of pain. Stimulating the skin on the opposite side of the body can also work.

Table 8.12 describes the various techniques. Many will be off-limits to cancer patients who are undergoing or recently completed radiation therapy. Extreme heat or cold should never be applied to or near the radiation site; nor should menthol gels, lotions, and other topical preparations.

♦ Check with your oncologist or nurse before trying any method of skin stimulation.

Transcutaneous Electrical Nerve Stimulation (TENS)—A small battery-operated power pack no larger than a pager generates a mild electric current through two or more small electrodes placed near the painful area. The tingling sensation produced by the electricity is believed to disrupt the pain signal to the brain.

TENS seems to be most effective at relieving migraine headaches, sciatica, and phantom-limb pain. The units, which require a doctor's prescription, cost anywhere from $130 to $350 and may be covered by insurance. You might want to consider renting the device first to make sure that it works for your type of pain. Your physician or a physical therapist will adjust the settings for you and show you where to place the disc-shaped sensors.

♦ Transcutaneous electrical nerve stimulation should not be used for anyone with a cardiac pacemaker, a metal plate, or pins, or anyone who has one of the following conditions: pregnancy, diabetes, or hypertension.

Acupuncture—The ancient Chinese healing art of acupuncture can be traced back to the year 500 B.C., if not earlier. In the United States, thousands of acupuncturists, physicians, dentists, and other health-care professionals have used acupuncture to treat a number of medical conditions, including postsurgical pain, headache, and lower-back pain.

Acupuncture is based on the premise that good health relies on certain patterns of energy flow, or *Qi,* along pathways called *meridians;* disease represents a disruption of this flow. Placing hair-thin metallic needles in the skin at specific *acupoints* on the body is believed to correct imbalances of flow. Western physicians have their own hypotheses about how acupuncture might work. One theory is that the needles stimulate the release of natural substances that exert opioid-like effects.

Although the mechanism by which acupuncture works remains unclear, there is little argument about its effectiveness. At a 1997 conference conducted by the National Institutes of Health, a panel of experts named more than a dozen conditions for which acupuncture appeared to be useful. They concluded: "There is sufficient evidence of acupuncture's value to expand its use into conventional medicine and to encourage further studies of its psychological and clinical value."

Before you make an appointment to see an acupuncturist, be sure to confirm that he or she is licensed to practice in your state—presuming that your state is among the majority that allows and sets standards for acupuncturists—and also that he or she uses *only* sterilized needles.

◆ Patients receiving chemotherapy cannot undergo acupuncture because of the danger of increased bleeding at the insertion site.

Invasive Interventions
In instances where noninvasive approaches have been ineffective or caused intolerable side effects, more-invasive measures may be necessary.

Palliative Radiation Therapy—External-beam radiation is highly effective in relieving skeletal pain from cancers that have metastasized to the bone. Whereas the standard dose for curative radiotherapy is approximately six weeks, a week or two of treatment is usually sufficient to manage bone pain.

A single injection of an intravenous radioactive substance such as strontium 89 (Metastron), samarium 153 (Quadramet), or sodium phosphate P-32 can alleviate pain from widespread bone metastases. Should the pain recur, half of those patients treated with radiopharmaceuticals will respond to a second injection.

Surgery—Palliative surgery to remove part of a tumor, while not curative, can alleviate the pain of a lesion that was pressing on an organ or a nerve or was obstructing one of the body's passageways.

Nerve Blocks—When nothing else is helping a patient's pain, a procedure to bar pain messages from entering the brain may need to be performed. In a nerve block, an agent that either anesthetizes or destroys nerve tissue is injected directly into or near a nerve. This can be done through the skin (percutaneously) or as open surgery. For example, people with pancreatic cancer often undergo a *celiac plexus block* at the same time as palliative surgery to bypass a tumor obstructing the abdomen.

The celiac plexus is a bundle of nerves that forwards pain information from the pancreas, liver, gallbladder, kidney, spleen, and small bowel. Injecting an anesthetic such as lidocaine into the celiac nerves silences the transmission of pain temporarily. Using alcohol or the toxic compound phenol can bring months of pain-free living. Fifty to 90 percent of people with pancreatic-cancer pain will achieve relief for anywhere from one month to as long as one year.

A celiac block may induce diarrhea and a feeling of light-headedness upon standing up quickly. Uncommon complications include a collapsed lung; partial paralysis; and a collection of blood, or hematoma, in the abdomen. The potential side effects from other types of nerve blocks depend upon the site affected, but they frequently cause a loss of all sensation in the area.

Rhizotomy/Cordotomy—Another method for shutting down neural pathways is to sever a nerve close to the spinal cord (rhizotomy) or to

---

Other Types of Nerve Blocks

- *Chemical cordotomy,* for treating pain in arms, trunk, or legs
- *Chemical rhizotomy,* for treating pain in the chest wall, arms, legs, pelvic region, and abdomen
- *Dorsal root blocks,* for treating localized bone lesions
- *Intercostal nerve blocks,* for treating chest-wall pain or pain from secondary tumors of the ribs
- *Lumbar sympathetic blocks,* for treating leg pain
- *Paravertebral blocks,* for treating localized bone pain or chest-wall pain
- *Stellate ganglion blocks,* for treating pain involving the face and arms

cut bundles of nerves in the lower end of the spinal cord itself (cor-dotomy). Whether a scalpel or chemical is used to destroy nerve tissue, the technique is referred to as *neuroablation.*

Rhizotomy can be performed percutaneously or through open surgery. Chemical rhizotomy is essentially the same as a lumbar punc-ture: While the patient curls up on his side, a small amount of alcohol is injected into the cerebrospinal fluid, which cushions the spinal cord. The block typically lasts three to six months. Head and neck pain that doesn't respond to other treatments may require incisional cranial rhi-zotomy.

Cordotomy is usually done through the skin, with the open pro-cedure reserved for men and women who are unable to lie on their back. The technique is highly effective for relieving pain on one side of the torso or one leg, as well as chest-wall pain. Nine in ten patients see significant, long-lasting improvement. After one year, half will experi-ence recurrent pain, at which point the treatment may be offered again.

Temporary complications of rhizotomy and cordotomy include partial paralysis, lack of coordination, and bladder dysfunction; in some cases, though, the effects may linger or become disabling.

The point where the nerves from a limb enter the spinal cord is called the *dorsal root entry zone*—DREZ, for short. Cutting the dorsal root entry zone in the neck relieves arm pain; to treat leg pain, the in-cision is made farther down the spinal cord, in the lower-chest area. The technique works for four in five patients and shows promise as a treatment for phantom-limb pain.

Electrical Stimulation—*Spinal-cord stimulation* (SCS) and *deep-brain stimulation* (DBS) are not typically employed to treat cancer-related pain. SCS is usually performed for back pain that has not responded to back surgery; DBS, for nerve disorders of the lower limbs and midback pain.

Both techniques call for surgically implanting a small wire elec-trode in the central nervous system: for SCS, in the spinal canal, near the section of the spinal cord that receives the pain information; for DBS, in the sensory pathways within the brain. The electrode attaches to a small electrical generator, much like a cardiac pacemaker. It, too, is placed in the body during an operation—either in the chest or near one of the hips.

A low-energy electric current emitted by the generator halts the transmission of pain fibers from a specific area of the body. Unlike neuroablation, SCS and DBS do not interfere with normal function or sensation. A major drawback to these two techniques is cost. Deepbrain stimulation, for example, costs approximately $30,000.

Hair Loss (Alopecia)

COMMON CAUSES

- Radiation therapy to the head - Some chemotherapy drugs

Losing your hair as a result of chemotherapy or radiotherapy to the head doesn't make you feel sick, nor is it a threat to your health. Yet it is the side effect that patients find most disturbing. In a Gallup survey, some fifteen hundred people with cancer were asked to rank side effects according to the emotional distress they caused. On a scale of 1 to 6—with 6 denoting "extremely upsetting"—hair loss placed first (4.6), followed by fatigue (4.4) and nausea and vomiting (4.2). Infection, which can be deadly for patients receiving chemotherapy, finished a distant fourth (3.5).

Eventually, most men and women who experience hair loss accept it as part of the ransom they're forced to pay for the chance to get their health back. But I can tell you from experience that it is a shock to discover clumps of hair on your pillow or clogging the shower drain. The transformation is often startlingly quick, with many patients going bald or near bald in a matter of days.

Now, we can easily cover up a hairless head—attractively too—with a variety of flattering wigs, scarves, caps, and so forth. The psychological impact of this side effect runs far deeper than concerns about changes in physical appearance, though cancer can certainly play havoc with one's body image. Seeing a different face in the mirror is a constant reminder of the disease and how your body has let you down.

It is also visible evidence that you are sick, which can rattle a person's self-image and how others perceive them. The Lombardi Cancer Center counts among its patient population a number of high-powered men and women, including politicians and captains of industry. "Although hair loss is usually more acceptable for men than for women," says nursing coordinator Maureen Sawchuk, "we have male patients who choose to wear wigs because they're extremely concerned about the impact an ill appearance could have on their business and how they are perceived."

Bear in mind that many patients do *not* lose their hair. External-beam radiotherapy causes hair to fall out solely in the area being treated, so unless you're undergoing radiation of the scalp, there's no need to worry. As for chemotherapy, only about one in five anticancer drugs, hormonal agents, and immunologics bring about alopecia frequently. The culprits include three widely used antineoplastics: doxorubicin (Adriamycin), paclitaxel (Taxol), and fluorouracil (5-FU), one of the two drugs that I was on. However, as with other side effects, every patient reacts differently. The fact that a person is receiving an agent known to often cause hair loss doesn't guarantee that it will happen.

Alopecia typically occurs one to three weeks into treatment. Chemotherapy and radiotherapy are designed to target rapidly dividing cells. Although they primarily go after cancer cells, both therapies are toxic to the cells that make up the hair roots, which are also prolific proliferators. Facial hair, arm and leg hair, underarm hair, and pubic hair may be affected as well.

Sure enough, I lost a considerable amount of hair during my first two cycles of 5-FU and leucovorin. I had so much hair to begin with, though, that it wasn't too noticeable. And once my oncologists lowered my dosage in December, the hair began growing back. Had I continued at the original dosage, undoubtedly all my hair would have fallen out.

Many times, a patient's hair does not begin growing back for six to twelve months after the completion of chemotherapy. Don't be surprised if at first it is very fine or is of a different texture or color altogether. These changes are usually temporary. Hair loss from radiation is usually permanent.

HOW HAIR LOSS IS MANAGED

According to the American Hair Loss Council, no hair-growth stimulants, shampoos, conditioners, or other cosmetic treatments can prevent or delay hair loss from cancer therapy. It has been theorized that applying cold to the scalp just before chemotherapy is administered can preserve the hair. Patients put on a "cold cap"—essentially an ice pack for the head. Supposedly, the blood vessels in the scalp constrict, preventing a high concentration of medicine from getting through to the hair follicles that surround each hair. "We've never found the cap to be effective," says Maureen Sawchuk, "but we'll use it if a patient wants to try it."

HOW YOU CAN HELP YOURSELF

Hair Today, Gone Tomorrow: Caring for Your Hair and Scalp During Treatment

Hair loss from cancer therapy doesn't necessarily leave patients totally bald. The hair may merely become thinner, as existing hair falls out faster than new hair grows in. Therefore, gentle but thorough hair and scalp care is essential during treatment.

- Brush and wash away hair that is falling out. If you're shedding a lot of hair, consider shaving off the rest of it. As Maureen Sawchuk notes, "It can become tremendously annoying to have hair in your mouth, all over your pillow, and on your clothes. Many of our patients choose to shave their heads."

- A short, easy-to-manage style will make your hair look fuller and require less brushing and combing.

- Gently wash your hair and scalp with a mild protein shampoo no more than three times a week. Excessive shampooing can dry the scalp. Be sure to massage the scalp thoroughly to prevent itching and scaling. Next, work in a protein conditioner and rinse thoroughly with lukewarm water. This will add body to fine or limp hair.

- Sleeping on a satin pillowcase helps to eliminate tangling.

- Wear a hairnet to bed. Hair that is contained by a net sheds more evenly.

- Style hair with a soft brush and a wide-toothed comb. If you encounter tangles, don't pull—fragile hair will break right off. Hold your hair above the tangle and gently work the comb through.

- Avoid hair-care products that contain harsh chemicals such as bleach, ammonia, peroxide, lacquer, or alcohol. Use sprays, mousses, and gels with light or medium holding power. Stronger styling preparations are harder to shampoo out and will build up on the hair shafts.

- Do not perm, straighten, color, or highlight your hair. The chemicals used in these processes damage hair and will cause it to fall out faster.

- Set your blow-dryer to low. Following chemotherapy, your scalp is likely to be tender and highly sensitive to heat. Similarly, retire all curling appliances and hot rollers for the time being.

- Protect newly exposed skin from the sun. Before going outside, apply a sunblock with a sun protection factor (SPF) of at least 15. Then wear a wide-brimmed hat and sunglasses to shield your eyelashes from the sun's rays.

- Heat escapes through the top of the head. Wearing a hat or wrapping a scarf around your head in cold, harsh weather not only retains body heat but keeps the scalp from drying out.

Head Coverings

It is up to each patient to decide whether or not to cover a hairless head with a wig, hairpiece, turban, scarf, or cap, or to go "au naturel." Many people switch back and forth among different head coverings, depending on the setting. At home or around family and friends, they might clap on a baseball cap or wear nothing on their head; before going to work, they don a wig. The bottom line is: Do whatever suits you.

If you do decide to wear a wig, get it prior to beginning chemotherapy or cranial irradiation. That way you can get used to wearing the hair prosthesis at home, then start to wear it in public while your hair is still full. Some patients do this and find that no one is the wiser when their natural hair is falling out. Once you commit to the wig, we suggest shaving your scalp. Not only will your new wig fit better, but the adhesives used to adhere wigs to the skin will work better.

Perhaps the drug regimen your oncologist has prescribed rarely causes hair loss. In that case, you may want to wait and see what happens before buying a wig. That's fine too. Just save a lock of your hair. If your hair does fall out, you'll then be able to match the color and texture exactly. On the other hand, maybe you want to adopt a radically different look. "Some women," observes Maureen Sawchuk, "will decide, 'I've always wanted to be a platinum blonde; now is my chance to do it.'"

MONEY MATTERS

Insurance Coverage for Hair Prostheses

Some insurance companies will cover all or part of the cost of a wig if it has been prescribed by a doctor. Medicare, however, does not pay for hair prostheses.

Save your receipt. Under these circumstances, a wig qualifies as a medical tax deduction.

Custom-made wigs are more expensive than off-the-shelf models, but they tend to be more comfortable. You should know in advance, however, that custom wigs can take anywhere from a month and a half to four months to be manufactured and delivered to you.

Your oncologist can probably recommend local wig and hairpiece salons that specialize in fitting and styling wigs for people undergoing cancer treatment. Or look in the Yellow Pages under "Wigs and Hair-pieces." If money is a problem, local chapters of the American Cancer Society (800-227-2345) and the patient-support organization Y-ME (800-221-2141) loan or donate wigs to patients who cannot afford them. Many hospitals run their own "wig banks."

When Your Hair Grows Back

Once cancer treatment is over, your hair needs tender loving care as it heals and rebuilds itself. The American Hair Loss Council recommends the following hair-care tips during this time:

- Wait until your hair is at least three inches long before having it chemically curled or permed. A mild body wave produces the best results, with the hair wrapped loosely around the largest size curler possible. Tight curls can damage the recovering hair shafts, causing them to break.

 ◆ Many patients' scalps remain extremely sensitive for up to one year following the completion of chemotherapy. They may not be able to withstand the application of the permanent-wave solution. Hair coloring, too, may irritate a sensitive scalp and should be postponed until the skin has healed.

- Semipermanent hair colorings that gradually wash away after four to six shampooings are less damaging to the hair than permanent hair-coloring products. In addition, do not attempt to dye your hair more than three shades from its present color. Drastic color changes may result in increased hair breakage.

- Do not bleach your hair at this time.

Sexual Problems

COMMON CAUSES

In Men and Women

Lack of Interest in Sex

▪ Hormonal Therapy ▪ Chemotherapy ▪ Depression, stress ▪ Distorted body image and/or sexual identity, perhaps as a result of hair loss, infertility, or decreased fertility; disfigurement from surgery (limb amputation, facial surgery, breast surgery, surgery to remove reproductive organs, surgery to create an artificial opening for breathing, feeding, speaking, or passing urine or stool) ▪ Feeling just plain *lousy*

In Women

Painful or Difficult Sexual Intercourse

▪ A tumor in the uterus, cervix, or another reproductive organ[4] ▪ Radiation to the uterus, cervix, or another reproductive organ ▪ Surgery that involves shortening the vagina, such as radical hysterectomy for early stage cervical cancer and, rarely, endometrial cancer; and pelvic exenteration for recurrent cervical cancer

Vaginal Dryness

▪ Radiation to the bladder, ovary, uterus, cervix, and other reproductive organs ▪ Chemotherapy

Inability to Achieve Orgasm

▪ Surgery to remove the vulva (vulvectomy), which includes excising the clitoris

Heightened Sexual Desire

▪ Hormonal therapy using estrogens

In Men

Male Erectile Dysfunction

▪ A tumor in the prostate or one of the other organs that make up the male reproductive tract[5] ▪ Surgery to remove the prostate

---

[4] Cancers of the vagina, vulva, fallopian tubes, and the female urethra are rare.
[5] Cancers of the male urethra and the penis are rare.

gland (radical prostatectomy), the bladder and the prostate (radical cystoprostatectomy), or only the cancerous portion of the prostate (transurethral resection) ▪ Cryosurgery of the prostate ▪ Radiation to the prostate or the bladder ▪ A tumor or treatment affecting the central nervous system ▪ Surgical castration (orchiectomy) to remove the testicles, the main production site of the male sex hormone testosterone ▪ Medical castration, using hormonal agents, to shut down testosterone production ▪ Other drugs, such as antidepressants, antihistamines, and blood-pressure medications ▪ Depression, stress

Heightened Sexual Desire and Frequent or Continuing Erections
▪ Hormonal therapy using androgens

Inability to Ejaculate
▪ Surgery to remove part or all of the prostate, or the bladder and the prostate

Most sexual problems related to cancer or its treatment are emotional in origin rather than physical. Probably the greatest obstacle to patients' love lives is a listless libido—a common response to a life-threatening illness. If you think back to other times when you've felt stressed or blue, you know how anxiety and depression generated by a crisis can diminish not just sexual feelings but enjoyment of life's pleasures in general.

Sexual side effects that stem from psychological causes can be more complicated to manage than physical, or *organic,* problems. Frequently both must be addressed together, as when the disease or therapy distorts body image and sense of self, making a patient feel less attractive, less "manly," less "feminine," less productive, less independent, and so forth. Self-confidence is the most powerful aphrodisiac of all, whereas self-doubt usually has the opposite effect. Consequently, a person with cancer may shy away from intimacy at a time when physical affection from a loved one would bring much-needed joy and comfort.

HOW SEXUAL PROBLEMS ARE MANAGED

In Women

Painful or Difficult Sexual Intercourse

Patients are often advised to forgo sexual intercourse during radiation therapy to the pelvic region. Because the treatment can cause the vagina to narrow, afterward a woman may find intercourse painful. If this happens, the doctor will most likely show her how to use a *dilator*, a smooth, rod-shaped instrument that is inserted in the vagina to gently stretch the tissue.

Vaginal Dryness

Surgery, chemotherapy, and pelvic radiation can dry out vaginal tissue. This, too, can make intercourse uncomfortable. To compensate for the lack of natural lubrication, apply K-Y jelly or another *water-soluble* lubricant inside the vagina and around the opening before having sex. Vaginal lubricating products also come in suppository form.

Don't use an *oil-soluble* lubricant like petroleum jelly. The tissue changes may predispose you to vaginal infections. Water-based products provide protection. Other ways to prevent gynecologic infections include wearing loose-fitting pants and shorts, and cotton panties and panty hose with ventilated cotton linings.

In Men

Erectile Dysfunction

Erectile dysfunction, or impotence, is the inability to attain and maintain an erection sufficient to permit sexual intercourse. By age sixty-five, one in four men experience some degree of erectile dysfunction, and the prevalence increases with age. Yet, contrary to what many people assume, impotence is not an inevitable consequence of growing old. Besides the numerous medical causes listed earlier, other factors can contribute to erectile dysfunction, among them alcohol and drug abuse, hypertension, high cholesterol, diabetes, and diseases of the blood vessels.

The form of cancer most associated with impotence is prostate cancer. Surgery to take out the gland frequently injures the nerves that control the penis's rise and fall, even when the nerve-sparring approach is used. Other operations in the abdomen may cause damage to the nerves or to the blood vessels that carry blood to the penis when the body and brain are in a state of sexual excitement. A low level of testosterone also interferes with the erection connection; more significantly, it douses sexual desire as thoroughly as emptying a bucket of water upon a campfire. Insufficient testosterone is rarely the guilty party, however, except in advanced prostate cancer, where the treatment calls for shutting off the testes' production of the male sex hormone. This is accomplished by surgically removing both testicles or through the use of hormonal drugs.

Organic erectile dysfunction tends to be compounded by psychological problems such as performance anxiety or a poor self-image. Therefore, therapy may consist of counseling, preferably with the man's spouse, and one or more of the measures described below. The Impotence Institute of America, which sponsors support groups for impotent men and their partners, can refer you to urologists and therapists who specialize in treating erectile dysfunction. Call the IIA at 800-669-1603 or 301-262-2400.

No Treatment—Given time, erections may return on their own. The usual recovery following therapy for prostate cancer is six to twelve months. If impotence persists beyond that, a man may want to consider treatments that can restore his potency.

Or not. Many couples are quite satisfied with a sex life that revolves around noncoital expressions of intimacy, like kissing, snuggling, caressing, mutual masturbation, and oral sex. The interventions to treat erectile dysfunction vary greatly in invasiveness and expense. Whichever method suits the pattern of lovemaking that you and your partner find fulfilling is the right one.

Penile Pump—a simple device consisting of a plastic cylinder attached to a hand-operated pump. You place the cylinder over the penis and begin squeezing the handle. The vacuum created inside the tube draws blood into the three chambers of the penis, causing it to expand. Once you are fully erect, you remove the cylinder and slip an elastic constrictive ring around the base of the penis. This traps the blood inside, preserving the erection. The ring should not stay on for more than thirty minutes.

Success Rate: 40 to 65 percent, with no major side effects.

Drawbacks: Some men find the device cumbersome.

Drug Therapy—The introduction of several prescription drugs during the second half of the 1990s revolutionized impotence treatment. They work somewhat differently, but the principal behind them is the same: to promote blood flow to the penis. Alprostadil(Caverject, Edex), the most popular, is self-administered by injection into the spongy tissue (the *corpus cavernosum*) on either side of the penis about five to ten minutes before sexual intercourse.

Medicated Urethral System for Erection, acronymed MUSE, is a synthetic version of alprostadil. It comes as a tiny suppository housed in a small, disposable plastic applicator, which is inserted about one inch into the urethra. A slight jiggle deposits the pellet, then you carefully withdraw the device. You will sense the response within minutes.

Sildenafil (Viagra), marketed amid much fanfare, is the first oral medication approved by the U.S. Food and Drug Administration for the treatment of erectile dysfunction. You take the tablet(s) one to four hours prior to lovemaking.

Success Rates: MUSE, 65 percent; Viagra, 70 percent; Caverject, 80 percent; Edex, 90 percent. All produce erections lasting roughly thirty to sixty minutes and have minimal side effects.

Drawbacks: Men who cannot abide the thought of inserting *anything* into their penis should consider Viagra.

Penile Implant Surgery—One in ten men suffering from impotence chooses to have a rod-shaped prosthesis surgically implanted in each of the two corpus cavernosum. They typically turn to this option, the most invasive and expensive approach, after nonsurgical measures have proved unsatisfactory.

There are three types of implants. With a *semirigid* prosthesis, the penis is elongated and stays partially erect all the time. The *malleable* type has been compared to a pipe cleaner, in that it can be bent into an upright position, then down. *Inflatable* prostheses replicate the natural hydraulic system of the penis. During the operation, the surgeon implants two hollow cylinders and a fluid-filled reservoir attached to a tiny bulblike pump. When the man wants an erection, he squeezes the pump, which sits either externally, behind the head of the penis, or internally, inside the scrotum. The fluid fills the cylinders and inflates the penis, much like a natural erection. Bending the penis or pressing the valve on the pump returns the liquid to the receptacle.

Success Rate: 95 percent.

Drawbacks: The noninflatable prostheses can be uncomfortable; imagine walking around with a permanent semierection. The more complicated pump models are more prone to malfunctioning, which requires corrective surgery.

Vascular Surgery—If the cause of impotence is found to be a leaky blood vessel in the penis, *venous ligation* to tie off the defective vein may be considered. The procedure has a low success rate, though, and is rarely performed. *Penile artery bypass graft surgery*, while effective, also has a limited role. In an operation similar to a coronary artery bypass graft, the surgeon uses a vessel from the abdomen to reroute blood around the blockage that is impeding circulation to the penile arteries.

Success Rates: Venous ligation, 15 percent; penile artery bypass graft surgery, 70 percent.

Drawbacks: With either procedure, it is difficult for physicians to predict which patients can expect to benefit from surgery.

Inability to Ejaculate

A man's inability to attain an erection does not preclude his reaching a climax. However, because the prostate produces seminal fluid, removing the whole organ results in so-called "dry" orgasms: the sensation of orgasm without ejaculation.

Transurethral resection, the other prostate-cancer operation, usually puts an end to ejaculation as well, but for a different reason. The procedure causes the reproductive system to misfire. Instead of the semen being discharged out of the penis, it is ejaculated in the opposite direction and lands in the bladder. The fluid leaves the body as part of the urine, which will appear abnormally cloudy. *Retrograde ejaculation* is not harmful, aside from leaving a man unable to father children. Drugs such as the decongestant pseudoephedrine or the antidepressant imipramine may be able to reverse this condition, but it is often permanent.

HOW YOU CAN HELP YOURSELF

Talk about your desires, your insecurities, your concerns. In any relationship, problems can often be traced to a lack of communication, especially where sex is concerned. Let's use as an example a woman who recently lost a breast to cancer. She's worried that her husband won't be as attracted to her.

He, in turn, has been less physically affectionate than usual since the mastectomy. It's not for lack of desire: He's keenly aware of her self-consciousness and doesn't want her to feel as if she's being pressured into intimacy before she's ready. Secretly, he may also be harboring some insecurities of his own. Will he still know how to please her sexually? She's just had a major operation; what if he accidentally hurts her?

Unfortunately, she misinterprets his consideration as aloofness, which confirms her fears that her body no longer turns him on. The situation unravels from there, with each partner feeling increasingly hurt, lonely, and frustrated—all the while waiting for a romantic cue from the other person. If only one of them would break the stalemate by expressing how he or she truly felt. Some couples get to that point on their own; others need a marital counselor or sex therapist to act as a catalyst to more open communication.

Be willing to work at redefining "sex." Perhaps treatment has left you or your spouse less sexually responsive than before or unable to have intercourse. Try not to focus so much on what is missing from your love life; think of all the fun that can be had exploring new ways of physically expressing your love.

Set aside plenty of time for each other, so that lovemaking is relaxed and unhurried. At first, one or both of you may seem tentative and less spontaneous. That's okay. Were you naturally attuned to each others' bodies and needs when you first met however many years ago? Probably not. It took time to achieve sexual harmony before; you can do so again. There are books and sex therapists to teach you sensual exercises that will help you to rediscover each other. If this is "work," it's the kind of work where you hope for lots of overtime.

Long-Term Effects of Cancer Treatment

Only in the last few decades have the long-term effects of cancer therapy emerged as a medical issue, simply because prior to the treatment breakthroughs of the 1960s and 1970s, not enough patients lived long enough for the subject of long-term effects to be much of an issue.

But between 1960 and 1994, the five-year survival rate for all cancer sites combined rose impressively from 39 percent to 62 percent for white Americans and from 27 percent to 47 percent for African Americans. As more and more men and women leave chemotherapy and radiation therapy farther and farther behind, patterns of delayed organ damage and a heightened risk of second primary cancers are surfacing. Here are a few for-instances:

- Roughly three in four patients to receive single-dose total-body irradiation in preparation for a bone-marrow transplant develop cataracts, a clouding of the lens of the eye, typically three to six years later.

- The antiestrogen drug tamoxifen (Nolvadex), used to treat and prevent breast cancer, doubles a woman's chance of one day developing endometrial cancer.

- Transplant recipients who were treated aggressively with immunosuppressant drugs are at least fifty times more likely to incur non-Hodgkin's lymphoma in the future.

Should these statistics deter anyone from pursuing cancer therapy? Only if the potential risks outweigh the potential benefits. Naturally, this is partly dependent on factors such as a patient's age, stage of disease, and general health. But all of the above-mentioned treatments are highly effective.

In testicular cancer, for example, chemotherapy regimens incorporating the antineoplastic etoposide (VePesid) have been associated with a slightly elevated risk of leukemia: less than 0.5 percent five years after diagnosis. The overall cure rate for cancer of the testes, though, is 95 percent, and higher still if the disease is detected early.

A cancer patient's first priority has to be getting well *now* and not worrying about what might happen years down the road, although researchers are looking for ways to lower the toxicity of the drugs without compromising their effectiveness. As Dr. Bruce Redman of the University of Michigan Comprehensive Cancer Center tells his patients with testicular cancer, "Yes, there's a risk from treatment. It's less than 1 percent. But if you don't take chemotherapy, there's a 100 percent chance that you will die."

Chapter Nine

Don't Neglect Your
Emotional Health

During the fall, when I was at my sickest, I read a book that someone had given me, *Head First: The Biology of Hope and the Healing Power of the Human Spirit*, by Norman Cousins. In 1964, the
author had been stricken with a painful and potentially crippling form
of rheumatoid arthritis that stiffens the joints and stabilizing ligaments
of the spine, making movement difficult. If the disease progresses to
the ribs, it can impair breathing as well.

Cousins asked his physician what his prospects were for a full recovery. Only one in five hundred, he was told.

Figuring he had little to lose, Cousins convinced his doctor to
allow him to incorporate elements of holistic medicine into his treatment. He wound up beating the odds, something he attributed largely
to megadoses of intravenous vitamin C and daily doses of laughter—
courtesy of old Marx Brothers movies and episodes of TV's *Candid
Camera.*

Cousins's account of his experience originally appeared in the
New England Journal of Medicine and was later turned into *Anatomy of
an Illness as Perceived by the Patient,* one of the first books to explore the
mind's power to heal the body. In *Head First,* published ten years later,

Cousins attempted to support that theory with scientific proof. Many doctors scoffed at his notion that laughter might indeed be the best medicine; they contended that the spinal arthritis would have subsided whether he spent his months of recuperation laughing or brooding. Other M.D.'s believed it wasn't far-fetched at all that a patient's will to recover might be powerful enough to help reverse the disease process.

How Much *Does* Attitude Count?

I found *Head First* inspiring. But did I believe that maintaining a positive attitude would cure my cancer? In all honesty, no.

Few cancer patients go through treatment without well-meaning loved ones and friends lecturing them about the importance of keeping up their spirits. "Attitude is *so* important," they'll say knowingly. I certainly heard that more than once.

If everyone who survives cancer is presumed to have courageously battled the disease, what does that imply about the nearly 50 percent who eventually die? That they didn't "try" hard enough to get better or were weak-willed? To possibly add feelings of guilt or inadequacy to the psychological burden of a life-threatening illness is, I believe, unconscionable. And irresponsible, because there is no evidence to conclusively prove the power of positive thinking as a weapon against cancer.

In an attempt to answer this question, British researchers followed 578 women with early-stage breast cancer, making this one of the largest studies of its kind. Twice during the first year, participants were given psychological tests designed to gauge their responses to having cancer. After five years, three-fourths of the women were still alive. The study, published in 1999, found that the patients who could be said to approach their disease with a fighting spirit fared no better or worse than those who did not share that outlook. Nor did an inability to express anger and other negative emotions have any impact on a woman's likelihood of suffering a relapse or dying.

Whether a patient's mental outlook can or cannot fight cancer directly is really beside the point. Who wouldn't prefer to face illness optimistically? In addition to improving one's quality of life, there *are* health benefits to be gained. Countless studies have documented the mind's considerable influence upon the body. How else are we to explain the *placebo effect,* in which inactive medications—dummy pills—are able to induce responses nearly equivalent to those achieved with the real drug. Until the 1950s, doctors routinely relied on this phenomenon to help patients feel better (as well as to appease known hypochondriacs), because for many medical conditions they had little else to offer.

Placebos work by essentially tricking the brain into believing the body is about to receive the same medication that had brought relief in the past. Based on what it expects to occur, the brain then sets in motion the necessary biochemical changes. In a study on the placebo effect and depression, conducted at Los Angeles's University of California Neuropsychiatric Institute, one group of volunteers was given the antidepressant Prozac; the other group received inert sugar pills. After eight weeks, the number of patients to report that their depression had lifted was nearly the same in the placebo group as it was in the Prozac group.

Both groups underwent electroencephalograms (EEGs), which record brain-wave activity in various parts of the brain. The participants given Prozac showed decreased activity in the front of the brain, as would be expected. However, those who ingested the bogus pills exhibited *increased* brain activity in the same area.

In other studies investigating the mind-body connection, placebos have been found to relieve pain, improve breathing in asthmatic children, treat the symptoms of bleeding ulcers—even stimulate hair growth in balding men who believed they were taking a remedy for hair loss. When the bubble bursts and the subjects discover they've been receiving fake pills all along, the salubrious effect inevitably subsides. On average, one in three patients given placebos as part of clinical trials benefit.

Mood is also known to impact on immunity. Anxiety, psychological stress, and depression are associated with reductions in the activity levels or numbers of various defenders against infection, such as natural-killer (NK) cells, which are thought to play a role in protecting the body from certain types of cancer, and helper T cells, the white cells decimated by the human immunodeficiency virus (HIV).

Conversely, staying upbeat may enhance your body's immune system. Another UCLA study examined the differences in immune function between two groups of law students. Half described themselves as optimists; the other half tended to respond negatively to stress. At the beginning of the school year and again at midsemester, the students were asked to fill out questionnaires and give blood samples. The optimists were found to have higher numbers of helper T cells and significantly more NK cells. In that regard, a positive outlook can be said to contribute to a positive outcome by reducing the risk of infection—always a potentially serious complication. But as for a direct link between immunity and cancer, scientists have yet to substantiate whether or not the immune system's response to, say, bacteria, a foreign agent, is the same as its response to a malignant tumor, which has hijacked the body's own cells and converted them into cancer.

If there is a link between emotions and cancer, it may be that people with a fighting spirit take better care of themselves and follow their oncologist's instructions more faithfully than do patients who are mired in depression, anxiety, and/or anger. Or perhaps a positive attitude promotes health simply by making patients more bearable to be around *and less likely to be murdered by the loved ones caring for them!*

Getting Through the Low Moments

Throughout the course of treatment, you will undoubtedly experience moments of discouragement and frustration. You're entitled. Maybe after a day of feeling sick from chemotherapy, you grumble, "I can't do this anymore," and threaten to give up therapy. Those around you will fearfully try to convince you that you don't really mean that. They're right, of course; you're just letting off steam. You don't have to apologize for your emotions, which are perfectly normal under the circumstances.

But continuing to feel blue or jittery day after day, while it may be understandable, should not be accepted as something you must endure. The problem is, the depressed person doesn't always recognize how despondent she is. Meanwhile, family members may assume this is a normal state of mind for someone with a serious illness. "Of *course* she's depressed and nervous," they reason. "She has cancer. Who wouldn't be?"

Depression and Anxiety

In reality, "the vast majority of cancer patients are not depressed," says Dr. Julia Rowland, director of psycho-oncology at the Lombardi Cancer Center. Transient periods of mild depression and anxiety are relatively common, but only one in four men and women suffer from major depression and/or severe anxiety, which often go hand in hand.

"What we usually see," she continues, "are people with adjustment disorder." Adjustment disorder is the inability to cope with cancer or another life-altering event. It is characterized by persistent moodiness, agitation, and anger. From the moment you're diagnosed with cancer, an undercurrent of anxiety runs through you each day. Most of the time you're able to suppress it; the level typically peaks during doctor's visits, at the start of new treatments, when you're awaiting the results of a test, and at other critical points.

COMMON CAUSES

Symptoms such as pain, fatigue, insomnia, and severe nausea and vomiting • Medications, including corticosteroids, opioids, some chemotherapy agents (asparaginase, vinblastine, vincristine, procarbazine), biologic therapies such as interferon and interleukin, antibiotics, neuroleptic drugs used to control vomiting, others • Abnormal metabolic states such as hypoglycemia, hypercalcemia, and electrolyte imbalances • Tumors that affect the central nervous system or secrete hormones • Whole-brain irradiation • A history of depression

People with cancer sometimes suffer needlessly from depression and anxiety because those around them dismiss their sadness or agitation as emotions they can control if only they'd try. Many times, though, the symptoms can be traced to one of the medical causes listed above, including hormonal imbalances, medications used to treat cancer or its side effects, and chronic pain. (Anxiety, in turn, can heighten the perception of pain, creating a vicious cycle.) Either disorder could be a sign of metastasis to the area of the brain that regulates mood. Therefore, it's important for loved ones to report these conditions to the patient's physician promptly.

> **Medical Terms You're Likely to Hear**
>
> Psycho-oncologist: a psychologist with a special interest in patients' psychological responses to cancer, as well as the psychological well-being of family members. Psycho-oncologists also study the influence that psychological, behavioral, and social factors have on the disease process.

How Depression and Anxiety Are Treated

Family members and friends aren't the only ones who may overlook a patient's obvious depression or anxiety. Patients themselves may choose

TABLE 9.1 Symptoms of Depression and Anxiety

Depression	Anxiety

Contact your doctor if two or more of these symptoms persist for at least two weeks.

Depression	Anxiety
• Chronic sadness, anxiety, complaints of feeling "empty"	• Feeling shaky, jittery, or nervous
• Loss of interest or pleasure in ordinary activities, including sex	• Feeling tense, fearful, or apprehensive
• Fatigue, lack of energy	• Avoiding certain places or activities because of fear
• Difficulty in falling asleep or getting back to sleep, or sleeping excessively	• Pounding chest or racing heartbeat
• Appetite loss or overeating	• Difficulty in catching breath when nervous
• Frequent crying	• Sweating or trembling for no apparent reason
• Poor concentration and memory; difficulty in making decisions	• Butterflies in stomach, accompanied by nausea and diarrhea
• Increased irritability	• Lump in throat
• Lack of interest in routine grooming or hygiene	• Tendency to pace
• Expressions of guilt, helplessness, worthlessness	• Fear of dying in sleep
• Uncharacteristic withdrawal from other people	• Worrying about the next diagnostic test, or the results of it, weeks in advance
• Increased alcohol consumption or drug use	• Fear of losing control or "going crazy"
• Sudden manic activity	• Sudden fear of dying
• Aches and pains	• Worrying about when pain will return and how bad it may be
• Headaches	• Worrying about getting next dose of pain medication on time
• Indigestion	• Staying in bed for fear that the pain will intensify if you stand up or move about
• Sexual dysfunction	• Feeling confused or disoriented
• Thoughts of suicide; a suicide attempt	• Worrying about becoming a burden to family and friends

to suffer in silence rather than admit to an emotional disorder, "which still carries a social stigma in our culture," says Dr. Rowland. According to the National Institute for Mental Health, only about one in five clinically depressed men and women receive medical treatment; among cancer patients, the ratio may be significantly lower.

"For people with cancer," she continues, "it can feel like a dual stigma. 'Not only are you telling me I have a life-threatening illness, but now you're telling me I'm crazy too.' Patients want to feel that they're coping well with their disease, and when we suggest that they would probably benefit from an antidepressant or an antianxiety medication, they may see this as a direct threat to their ability to get through treatment." Enlightenment has been slow in coming, she says, but both the public and the medical profession are beginning to accept that cancer therapy involves treating the whole patient. "Now when people are diagnosed, some will ask for a consultation with a mental-health professional. They'll say, 'I want to be sure I have the right attitude to survive this illness.' Ten or fifteen years ago, that didn't happen."

At a multidisciplinary cancer center like Lombardi, the psychiatry service is integrated into the team. Not every patient sees a mental-health specialist unless he or she requests a consultation, but the medical and nursing staffs regularly refer men and women believed to be at risk for developing a psychiatric problem.

Most institutions, however, do not place the same priority on psychological care, so you may be left to fend for yourself. The organizations listed in table 9.3 can refer you to a practitioner in your area. Or you can ask your primary oncologist or nurse for several recommendations. Less important than the person's degree is his or her experience in counseling people with a life-threatening illness. In that respect, a psycho-oncologist would be ideal. Medication is the mainstay of treatment for moderate to severe depression and anxiety, typically in combination with talk therapy. Since only M.D.'s can prescribe medicine, you may very well wind up with a psychiatrist *and* a psychologist or social worker. General physicians and oncologists can also write out prescriptions, but

Who Treats Depression and Anxiety
Mental-Health Specialists
• Psychiatrist
• Psychologist
• Social worker
• Psychiatric nurse specialist
General Practitioners
• Physician
• Physician's assistant
• Nurse practitioner

with an expanding arsenal of antidepressants and *anxiolytics,* you really want a specialist who understands the subtleties of each drug.

Psychotherapy—The general goals of short-term psychotherapy are twofold: to encourage patients to discuss and understand their fears about having cancer, as well as to learn coping skills and techniques for overriding despair, anxiety, or other self-defeating thoughts that are interfering with their quality of life. This can often be accomplished in three to ten sessions.

> *See Table 9.4, "National Organizations That Run Support Groups," page 826.*

Behavioral Approaches—Therapy may also incorporate one or more of the same behavioral interventions employed in pain management: hypnotherapy, meditation, distraction, biofeedback, progressive muscle relaxation, and guided imagery.

The latter method can be used both for relaxation and for helping patients to confront their fears. Matthew Loscalzo, director of patient and family services and codirector of the Center for Cancer Pain Research at Johns Hopkins Oncology Center in Baltimore, offers an example of each:

Exercise Your Way Out of Depression

Moderate exercise can relieve depression and anxiety. One theory is that physical activity builds up the body's response to stress.

"Let's say a patient tells me that she's nervous and can't sleep at night," he says. "I ask her to give me a sense of where she feels safest and most comfortable, and she replies, 'At home on my blue couch.' I then make her an audiotape on which I describe, through visual imagery, the comfort she feels: 'You're sinking into the blue couch and beginning to feel the special feel of the color blue. You're relaxing, and you drift into a deep, comfortable sleep . . .'

"Another patient says, 'Every time I begin to drift off to sleep, I get scared.' For him, I might say, 'I want you to imagine that you're sitting in a chair, and lo and behold, behind you is what you're fearing. I want you to turn around and look at it. And I want you to allow yourself to become afraid but not overwhelmed, and to tell me what you see.'

"So," Loscalzo explains, "guided imagery is a way of helping patients control their emotional responses to a situation and feel more in charge. It can be used for relaxation, or it can be used to enable a person to confront her fears."

Don't feel bad if you're unable to visualize. A lot of people can't, points out Dr. Rowland. They may be too easily distracted or too fa-tigued. "I might lead them in progressive muscle relaxation, deep breathing, yoga, tai chi," she says. "Something that's meditative as op-posed to visualization."

Some patients find it empowering to imagine their white blood cells gobbling up cancer cells or some other inner picture representing their battle against the disease. If that brings you comfort or a sense of control, wonderful. Remember, though: We have no proof that people can "think" their way free of cancer. As Dr. Rowland reminds patients who practice this type of visualization, "Should your cancer recur one day, it wouldn't be because you didn't think the 'right' way."

See "Noninvasive Mind-Body-Control Interventions" in Chapter Eight, "Take Control: Managing Symptoms, Side Effects, and Complications."

Drug Therapy—The same barriers to adequate pain control can stand in the way of patients getting proper relief from depression and anxi-ety: namely, their unfounded fears of becoming addicted to the med-ications and viewing the need for pharmacologic intervention as some sort of character flaw.

There are a number of different antidepressants and anxiolytics, which act upon the brain in different ways and produce different side effects. Both the drugs and their dosages must be carefully matched to each patient's psychological symptoms, overall health, and so on. For instance, if depression has you feeling fatigued, the psychiatrist might prescribe a *selective serotonin reuptake inhibitor* (SSRI). But if you're feeling agitated during the day and unable to fall asleep at night, a *tri-cyclic antidepressant* (TCA), known for its sedating effect, would prob-ably be the more suitable choice; or perhaps an antidepressant *and* a benzodiazepine anxiolytic.

It is not unusual for patients to have to try one, two, or more med-ications before finding the one that works best or the right combina-tion. Don't be discouraged. Relief will come. You should also be aware that antidepressants typically must build up in your body for anywhere from three to six weeks before you feel the effects, another reason to contact your doctor before the symptoms of an emotional disorder be-come unbearable.

A 1999 study from the federal Agency for Health Care Policy and

TABLE 9.2	Commonly Prescribed Antidepressants and Antianxiety Medications		
Antidepressants		**Anxiolytics**	
Generic Name	**Brand Name**	**Generic Name**	**Brand Name**
Tricyclic Antidepressants (TCAs)		**Benzodiazepines**	
amitriptyline	Elavil, Endep	alprazolam	Xanax
desipramine	Norpramin	chlordiazepoxide	
doxepin	Sinequan	clonazepam	Klonopin
imipramine	Tofranil	clorazepate	Tranxene
nortriptyline	Aventyl, Pamelor	diazepam	Valium
protriptyline	Surmontil	flurazepam	Dalmane
		lorazepam	Ativan
Selective Serotonin Reuptake Inhibitors (SSRIs)		oxazepam	Serax
		temazepam	Restoril
		triazolam	Halcion
fluoxetine	Prozac	***Non-Benzodiazepines***	
paroxetine	Paxil		
sertraline	Zoloft	buspirone	BuSpar
Monoamine Oxidase (MAO) Inhibitors		thioridazine	Mellaril
		haloperidol	Haldol
		hydroxyzine	Vistaril
phenelzine	Nardil		
tranylcypromine	Parnate		
Others			
bupropion	Wellbutrin		
mirtazapine	Remeron		
nefazodone	Serzone		
trazodone	Desyrel		
venlafaxine	Effexor		

Research reported that tricyclics, the older generation of antidepressants, were as effective as the relatively new selective serotonin reuptake inhibitors. SSRIs, which quickly surpassed TCAs in popularity, still have several advantages over their predecessor: more tolerable side effects, no need for periodic blood tests, and less chance of a patient overdosing. SSRIs would also be chosen over tricyclics for a cancer patient with a history of heart problems, sinceTCAs can cause abnormal heart rhythms.

Antidepressant therapy typically lasts one year. "It used to be six

TABLE 9.3 Organizations That Can Refer You to Mental-Health Specialists

American Psychiatric Association
1400 K Street, N.W., Washington, DC 20005
202-682-6000
http://www.psych.org

American Psychological Association
750 First Street, N.E., Washington, DC 20002-4242
202-336-5500 or 800-964-2000
http://www.apa.org

National Association of Social Workers
750 First Street, N.E., Suite 700, Washington, DC 20002-4241
800-638-8799 or 202-408-8600
http://www.naswdc.org

Also contact your state or county department of mental health; the American Cancer Society; your local Area Agency on Aging; Catholic Charities; United Way of America; a hospital's department of social work, psychiatry, or psychology; or local chapters of disease-related organizations. For more information, see "Mental-Health Services" in Appendix B.

months," explains Dr. Rowland, "but we discovered that patients who went off of it after only six months were more likely to become depressed again.

"Antianxiety medications, on the other hand, are usually taken on a short-term or as-needed basis." Benzodiazepines, the most popular anxiolytic, come in short-, intermediate-, and long-acting forms. They may be prescribed in conjunction with an antidepressant, then gradually be withdrawn once the antidepressant begins to take effect.

Six Essential Skills for Coping with Cancer

1. Talk! Don't suppress your feelings. The problem, though, can be finding others to talk to, people who don't become visibly uncomfortable when you remark that you've made out a living will, or who don't

---

TABLE 9.4 **National Organizations That Run Support Groups for People with Cancer and Cancer-Related Complications**

AboutFace (support groups, patient-to-patient support, phone pal and pen pal programs)

Alliance for Lung Cancer Advocacy, Support and Education (phone pal program)

AMC Cancer Research Center Cancer Information and Counseling Line (telephone counseling)

American Amputee Foundation (support groups)

American Brain Tumor Association (pen pal program)

Bloch Cancer Hot Line (telephone counseling)

Blood & Marrow Transplant Newsletter (patient-to-patient support)

Brain Tumor Society (phone pal program)

Cancer Care (support groups and on-line support groups)

Cancer Hope Network (phone pal program)

Cancervive (support groups and telephone counseling)

CanSurmount (American Cancer Society) (patient-to-patient support)

Cure for Lymphoma Foundation (patient-to-patient support and phone pal program)

Impotence Institute of America (support groups)

International Association of Laryngectomees (American Cancer Society) (support groups and patient-to-patient support)

International Myeloma Foundation (patient-to-patient support)

Leukemia Society of America (support groups and patient-to-patient support)

Lymphoma Foundation of America (patient-to-patient support)

Lymphoma Research Foundation of America (support groups and phone pal program)

Make Today Count (support groups)

Man to Man (American Cancer Society) (support groups, telephone counseling, and patient-to-patient support)

National Alliance of Breast Cancer Organizations (support groups)

National Bone Marrow Transplant Link (telephone counseling)

National Brain Tumor Foundation (support groups and phone pal program)

National Carcinoid Support Group (phone pal program)

National Kidney Cancer Association (on-line support groups)

National Lymphedema Network (support groups, pen pal and Net pal programs)

National Organization for Rare Disorders (support groups and patient-to-patient support)

National Ovarian Cancer Coalition (support groups)

National Transplant Assistance Fund (patient-to-patient support)

Reach to Recovery (American Cancer Society) (patient-to-patient support)

Simon Foundation for Continence (support groups and on-line support groups)

United Ostomy Association (support groups and patient-to-patient support)

US TOO International (support groups)

Y-ME National Breast Cancer Organization (support groups and telephone counseling)

See Appendix A for these organizations' addresses and telephone numbers.

---

feel compelled to try solving your medical problems for you ("You really should ask your oncologist about . . ."), when all you were seeking was a sympathetic ear.

It's true what they say: With a few exceptions, only other cancer patients truly understand what you're going through; hence the appeal of *peer support groups,* where people in similar circumstances meet to share experiences amid a supportive, nonjudgmental atmosphere. Most patients should be able to find a cancer support group in their area, through one of the national patient organizations listed in table 9.4, hospitals, medical clinics, and other health-related agencies.

Peer support can take other forms as well. For example, the American Cancer Society sponsors a program called CanSurmount, which matches a newly diagnosed cancer patient with a cancer survivor for one-to-one support; a similar ACS program, Reach to Recovery, is specifically for women recently diagnosed with breast cancer. Other organizations offer one-to-one pen pal programs, telephone-buddy programs, and on-line support groups.

Besides the obvious benefits of attending a support group—a comforting sense of community and the realization that others are going through trials similar to yours—you will come away with arcane knowledge not found in any book. Members share tricks they've discovered for managing side effects, compare notes on local physicians, inform one another of investigational studies that are in the process of accruing patients, and so on. *"I've* learned a lot from patients," says Dominica Roth, a clinical social worker who conducts support groups at the Lombardi Cancer Center.

So even if pouring out your emotions to a roomful of strangers isn't your style, consider sitting in on a few meetings just to soak up a few helpful tips. Attending a group may also help you to identify the unfamiliar feelings that can accompany a diagnosis of cancer. "Many times," says Roth, "patients express something that one individual is feeling but is unable to verbalize himself."

Finding the Right Group

A support group will be most valuable if it is made up of people whose situations mirror yours. While many issues are universal to all types of cancer, the concerns of an elderly man who's undergone surgery to remove a cancerous prostate are likely to be different from those of a young woman with Hodgkin's disease. If he is upset because the operation has left him impotent or incontinent, he may be too embarrassed to reveal intimate details to a mixed group of men and women, few or none of whom can relate to his experience. The ideal group for him would be Man to Man, sponsored by the American Cancer Society, or another support group exclusively for men with prostate cancer.

"In addition to disease-specific groups," says Roth, "there are age-specific groups and stage-specific groups." She recommends *closed* support groups, which meet for a prescribed period of time and do not accept new members. This way, everyone is at a reasonably similar point on the road to surviving cancer. When groups are *open-ended*, with no time limits, the dynamics can change from meeting to meeting, based on who attends. For a woman with early-stage breast cancer and an excellent prognosis, belonging to a group comprised mainly of patients whose breast cancer has metastasized or recurred could shatter her hard-won optimism.

We also advise staying away from groups not led by a health-care professional. The *facilitator,* usually an oncology nurse or social worker, acts as a vital interpreter of information and screens out misinformation. In addition, she redirects the discussion when members digress from the topic at hand and prevents sessions from degenerating into gripe-fests.

Dr. Rowland's advice for her patients is simple: "I tell them that support groups are not for everybody. Go to a group; if it makes you feel better, you enjoy being there, and it addresses problems for you, fine. If it makes you feel worse, get out, and don't beat up on yourself because it didn't work for you."

I thought about going to a support group. But to be honest, I felt that I had more than enough support from family and friends, and that my time would be better spent at home with Valerie and the girls. The disease consumes so much time and energy as it is, which makes phone-buddy programs and on-line chat groups appealing alternatives. Should you decide that a support group isn't for you, consider joining one of the national organizations listed in table 9.4., if only to receive its informative newsletter. Membership usually costs a nominal fee, which most groups will waive if you're unable to afford it.

2. *Indulge in a little denial. Go ahead!* "Denial has gotten a bum rap," says Christine Swift, a chaplain at Georgetown University Medical Center. Provided that it doesn't prevent patients from obtaining appropriate medical care, some level of denial can help them to surmount the various hurdles before them. They're not denying reality, merely suppressing it.

"A patient of mine who is three years into treatment for lung cancer expressed it very well," reflects Chaplain Swift. "He says he puts his cancer in a box and places it upon a shelf in his closet. When he needs to, he takes down the box, opens it, and looks inside. And then he closes it and returns it to the shelf. He's not in true denial, but he doesn't feel the need to confront it every day of his life, either."

That describes me throughout much of my illness. When mucositis landed me in the hospital following my second course of chemotherapy, I enjoyed the company of an elderly roommate named Callahan, a short-order cook from Charlottesville, Virginia. He'd already lost a lung to lung cancer; it had now spread to the other one. He knew his prognosis was bleak, and he accepted his impending death with remarkable serenity and dignity. I chose *not* to contemplate my mortality, despite odds of 50 to 70 percent that I would not survive. I worried that to dwell on it might undermine my progress. For better or worse, my attitude was that if I could survive pneumonia, I could beat this. That became my focus.

Whenever I felt pessimistic thoughts steal over me—usually late at night, if I was reading alone in the living room—or felt myself breaking down emotionally, I'd fight it off. This may sound silly, but I'm a die-hard Notre Dame football fan. (I have no explanation for why a son of Detroit by way of England would be drawn to the Fighting Irish, but they've always been my team.) I'd put down my book and think ahead to next Saturday's game or wax nostalgic over a couple of old articles, anything to force myself to think about something enjoyable.

That was *my* coping mechanism. Faced with similar odds, someone else might need to ponder every conceivable "what if?" Whatever brings you comfort and allows you to go on living with a sense of purpose is the right outlook for you. But if you haven't reached that peaceful refuge on your own, consult a mental-health professional, who perhaps can suggest different approaches to getting there.

3. *No time for negativity.* Apparently, not everyone shared my optimism that I would live. My friend Michael Kramer, then a columnist for *Time* magazine, visited me at home over the winter. About a month later, I needed a taxi to the cancer center. The same battered station wagon that had taken me there the first time lumbered up.

"How're you doin'?" asked the driver, who by this time felt like an old friend.

I told her I was doing quite well.

"Oh, I'm really happy to hear that," she said, as if not quite believing me.

"Why do you say that?"

"Well," she replied, "I picked up that friend of yours at this house a few weeks ago and drove him to the airport. And when I asked him how you were doing, he told me you were going to die." I thought to myself, *That son of a bitch!* I may not have looked terrific at the time, but I was feeling pretty good about my prospects for recovery. All these years later, I never miss an opportunity to kid Kramer about my imminent demise.

At least he managed to mask his feelings in my presence. Not everyone is capable of remaining so poker-faced. On several occasions, Valerie and I caught glimpses of pitying expressions. "It was painful to be with friends who looked at Peter as if he were dying," she recalls. "I don't fault them for it, because to many people, cancer equals death. I might have reacted the same way. But it hits you hard when you realize that's what others are thinking."

The few times it happened, it bothered me to have my positive attitude intruded upon. When you're undergoing cancer treatment, you don't have the reserves of mental energy it takes to fend off someone else's negativity. Nor should you have to. To the extent that you can, steer clear of people (and you know their names) who sap your energy, no matter how well intentioned they might be.

I'm going to tell you a story even though it's far from my proudest moment. But it's the truth.

A reporter whom I'd known casually from several campaigns developed a brain tumor around the same time that I was diagnosed with colon cancer. We used to talk on the phone now and then and trade stories about how our respective treatments were going. Every time I spoke to him, he seemed to have a complaint about this, that, and the other thing. In all fairness, he was in a far worse situation medically than I was.

But one night I hung up and said to Valerie, "I can't talk to him anymore; he's just too depressing."

Had I been healthy myself, of course I would have continued our conversations. But with your life at stake, you have a right to be that protective of your morale. You *need* to be that protective.

Putting the Brakes on Negative Thinking

When we're tired and depressed, our minds can become trapped in negativity like the tires of a car stuck in a snowbank. The self-defeating thoughts whir round and round, digging a rut so deep you feel like you'll never get out. The next time you find yourself sinking into pessimism, try these mental tricks suggested by the American College of Physicians. They'll help to put you in command of your thoughts instead of the other way around.

- Break the cycle of negativity: Yell "Stop!" silently or aloud; visualize a large stop sign; slap yourself on the wrist; splash cold water on your face; get up and move to another room.

- Allow yourself a time each day for negative thinking. If a pessimistic thought enters your mind any other time, tell yourself that you must save it for later or for tomorrow. Hopefully you'll have forgotten about it by then.

- Similarly, designate one area, and one area only, as your negative-thinking "workshop." But don't set up shop in the kitchen or your bedroom.

- Practice distraction (a personal suggestion: Notre Dame football), meditation, yoga, guided imagery, or other techniques to clear your mind or to transport your thoughts elsewhere.

- Debate yourself. Depression has a way of coloring our worldview. Find yourself bogged down in negative thinking? Take the opposing position. For example:

Point: *"I've just been diagnosed with cervical cancer. What if the tumor comes back?"*

Counterpoint: *"The doctor said I had stage I cervical cancer, which means the tumor was confined to the cervix. Nine in ten patients with stage I cervical cancer are cured. I've done my research, I've chosen an excellent gynecologic oncologist. I'm going to be one of those nine women."*

4. *Refuse to play the blame game.* Take responsibility for your recovery by getting the best medical care possible, but don't blame yourself for your disease. Contrary to what others may believe (and feel compelled to tell you):

- You didn't get cancer because you're the "nervous type" or "high-strung," two characteristics of the so-called type C personality. There is no evidence of any association between a person's personality and developing cancer.

- Too much stress did not cause your cancer. "If that were true," observes Dr. Rowland, "we'd *all* have cancer." However, get into the habit of practicing the stress-reduction techniques described in Chapter Eight and sidestepping stressful situations whenever possible. Getting a better handle on stress isn't going to save your life, but it will most definitely enhance it.

See "Noninvasive Mind-Body-Control Interventions" in Chapter Eight, "Take Control: Managing Symptoms, Side Effects, and Complications."

- Don't incriminate yourself for having indulged in smoking, unprotected sunbathing, and so on. For one thing, it's nonproductive. For another, nine in ten smokers never get cancer; other factors, such as genetic predisposition, play a part in determining who develops the disease.

- When you're feeling dispirited, don't compound your troubles by worrying that you're letting down those who care about you. No one can maintain a positive outlook twenty-four and seven, least of all someone with a serious illness. Depressive thoughts do not cause tumors to grow more rapidly.

5. *Seek comfort in spirituality and faith.* In times of crisis, many people draw strength from religious beliefs. Whether or not we attend a house of worship, observe religious practices, or pray privately to a higher power, each of us has a spiritual dimension. "We're not human beings trying to be spiritual," says Christine Swift, quoting a favorite saying, "we're spiritual beings trying to be human."

Although she was ordained in the Roman Catholic Church, Chaplain Swift counsels patients of all denominations—or no denomination. Her definition of spirituality changes with each visit to a hospital room, she says. "We all have our own belief systems. If a patient believes in his treatment, or his doctor, or his family, that's his spirituality."

A diagnosis of cancer often spurs a need to form a spiritual connection with God, with other members of a religious community, but ultimately with ourselves. For many patients, like me, cancer is a first brush with mortality. You're truly forced to reflect on the meaning and purpose of life and perhaps to reset your priorities and strive to become a better human being. *Please, God, let me*

Journal Writing

Consider starting a journal in which you record your thoughts about having cancer, as well as past events from your life and your hopes for the future. Journal writing may be therapeutic physically *and* psychologically. Several studies have found that men and women who wrote about their illness or other traumatic experiences felt a heightened sense of well-being. They also bolstered their immune function and made fewer visits to the doctor.

The Stony Brook School of Medicine, in Stony Brook, New York, studied patients with mild to moderately severe asthma or rheumatoid arthritis. On three consecutive days, the subjects were asked to write about past traumas for twenty minutes. Four months later, nearly 50 percent showed significant improvement in their health.

In each journal entry, describe recent happy times. *"Felt pretty good. Got out of the house for the first time since radiation ended. Took grandson Justin to the playground, then out to lunch."* Whenever you're feeling blue, flip through the pages to remind yourself of the wonderful days you've had and will enjoy again.

live, and I promise to . . . Making pacts with the Almighty, or bargaining, is one of the five stages of coping with a life-threatening medical condition. Contrary to popular myth, not every patient goes through all five stages, the others being denial, depression, anger, and acceptance. Nor do all ill people march sequentially from one stage to the other; circumstances could send you dancing across all five on any given day.

Every experience brings opportunities for growth. That includes having cancer. Unlike some survivors, you will never hear me say I'm grateful to have had cancer because of the lessons it taught me. Believe me, I'd have preferred to receive my education any other way. But it *was* enriching in that it made me more compassionate toward other people and more appreciative of all the good things in my life.

When Faith Is Put to the Test

A life-threatening illness can fortify a person's faith; it can also cause patients to question their beliefs. Sometimes the more devout they are, the greater the sense of betrayal. "How could God do this to me?"

Chaplain Swift has heard it all before. "It's okay for patients to be angry with God," she says. "He can take it better than anybody else!" For patients who have been religious most of their lives, this can give rise to seesawing emotions of anger and guilt. If you're feeling conflicted about your faith, or want to delve into it more deeply, talk to your cleric or to a hospital chaplain. Not all religious leaders are comfortable counseling the ill, however. Ask if he or she has had any training in ministering to people with serious illnesses like cancer.

6. *Reclaim yourself.* Having cancer can distort your self-image on many levels, from how you perceive yourself physically and sexually to how you see your place in your marriage and in the workplace. Literally overnight, you can be plunged into a world you don't recognize. A self-assured, highly competent CEO wakes up from surgery utterly dependent upon others, unable to take care of his most basic needs. Or a mother whose self-identity has been that of nurturer and caregiver has a difficult time accepting that for the first time in her adult life, her grown children must take care of her. These adjustments are often equally awkward for loved ones, because when one person in a family is incapacitated due to illness, everyone feels displaced.

Being informed that you have cancer is like being shoved out of an airplane at twelve thousand feet with no instructions on how to operate the parachute. No one ever informed you you were going skydiving in the *first* place. You're disoriented, you're free-falling, free-falling, the ground is coming up much too fast, you're free-falling, but then your hand finds the rip cord and *whoosh!* The chute billows open and you begin to get your bearings as you survey the ground below. Here are some suggestions to help you land on your feet once you've completed treatment:

- Return to old routines as much as possible. You may not have your usual stamina, though, so don't overdo it. Whereas normally you would attend your teenage grandson's high school football games, maybe he joins you for a Sunday afternoon of watching football together on TV instead. Or if you're renowned for throwing lavish dinner parties but you're not feeling up to it right now, invite a few friends over for dessert. Or order in. People will understand. The point is, have realistic expectations and don't be too hard on yourself.

- Prioritize. Do the things that are most important to you right now.

- Focus on short-term goals; consider activities and projects that will yield results and a sense of accomplishment reasonably quickly:
  Cook an elegant meal.
  Repair something around the house.
  Take up a new hobby.
  Complete a crossword puzzle or a jigsaw puzzle.
  Mow the lawn.
  Build a model for an appreciative child or grandchild.
  Paint.
  Write poetry.
  Knit a scarf for someone you love.

- Celebrate what you can do rather than lament what you can't do at the moment. Be patient; your body is healing.

- Make as many decisions for yourself as you can. Probably the most upsetting aspect of any illness is that it temporarily robs you of control—over your body, your day-to-day life, your destiny. Seize control wherever you can, even if it's merely by deciding what to wear or what to eat.

"A good health-care team will try to give patients as much control as possible over their treatment," says Maureen Sawchuk, nursing coordinator at the Lombardi Cancer Center. "With some chemotherapy regimens, you can be treated in the afternoon versus the morning. It's your choice. You want to work therapy around your lifestyle. This should not be your entire life."

- Few people feel attractive when they're sick. To feel better about yourself and to get reacquainted with your body, engage in mild to moderate physical activity: exercise, dance, sports, yoga, tai chi, and so on. Clear this with your physician first.

  And never forget: Cancer treatment has done nothing to change your intangible inner qualities, which are truly what makes us attractive to others.

- Get back into the social swim, but at your own pace. Companionship is so important to the ill, especially if they are stranded in the hospital or at home. Having visitors forces your mind off your situation. It also provides a fresh perspective that perhaps allows you to see things more clearly. The conversation brings the outside world to you, whether you're discussing news headlines or dishing the latest neighborhood gossip. Best of all, it reminds you of how much people care.

  Throughout the fall, when I was in and out of the hospital, in and out of the coma, and in general one hell of a mess, I was deeply touched by the outpouring of concern from my friends and colleagues in politics and the press. This may surprise you, given the low opinion many people seem to have of both professions nowadays, but there were hundreds of cards and letters and phone calls. Secretary of State Jim Baker would phone from Europe to see how I was doing, and the White House was checking in every day during my initial hospitalization.

  A few days after I'd pulled through from the pneumonia, the phone in my hospital room rang. Because I was still on a respirator, I couldn't talk. A nurse answered, and I watched as her eyes

---

Look Good, Feel Better

Look Good, Feel Better is a free program developed by the Cosmetic, Toiletry and Fragrance Association (CTFA) Foundation, the National Cosmetology Association, and the American Cancer Society. It teaches cancer patients undergoing chemotherapy or radiation how to use makeup, wigs, and other accessories to enhance their self-image and self-confidence. The single-session program is usually held at a hospital. For more information, contact the American Cancer Society (800-227-2345) or the CTFA Foundation (800-558-5005).

widened. "It's President Bush calling, wanting to know how Mr. Teeley's doing!"

She spun around and thrust the receiver at the head nurse. "*You* take it!"

"No, *you* take it!"

"You're the head nurse! It's your job to talk to him!"

"I can't talk to him," the woman spluttered. "I'm a *Democrat*!" In the end, she spoke to the president and nervously assured him that I was coming around.

I was fortunate not to have friends drop out of my life, as can happen in these situations. Other cultures take a rather matter-of-fact view of sickness, death, and dying. Broach the subject here, and someone is bound to snap uncomfortably, "Can't we change the conversation to something a little less morbid?" Consequently, a friend's or loved one's illness often blindsides many of us emotionally.

When people don't know how to react or what to say (or are too frightened or threatened, because they are reminded of their own mortality), they may avoid the patient, which compounds her mounting feelings of loss. It is better to say the wrong thing to someone who is sick than to desert her when she needs you most. Family members and friends shouldn't hesitate to use that line on anyone who is conspicuously absent from the bedside. Beyond that, there isn't much else you can do to compel them to pay a visit.

On a more heartening note, some of your sturdiest sources of support will be people who transcend all expectations. "I'll hear patients exclaim that a casual acquaintance from down the street has been bringing over cooked meals every night for weeks," says Dr. Rowland. "So that can offset somewhat those friends who take a walk."

Sometimes, though, patients cause their own isolation by withdrawing from others. If you're feeling abandoned by someone close to you, why not pick up the phone and call him? Please, let's not stand on ceremony.

"Hi, how's it goin'? I hadn't heard from you in a while and just wanted to say hello." The person is liable to be startled by the call, and probably chagrined as well. But he might be grateful too, for your generosity in offering him a second opportunity to step up to the plate and to mend a friendship.

- As your health improves, start planning for the future and getting on with life. One paragraph in particular from Norman Cousins really stayed with me. I'm paraphrasing loosely, but essentially he wrote that setting your sights on future goals—"the next mountain to climb"—can keep patients alive.

  I thought to myself: *I'm going to get through this and then do something else with my life.* Although I had a thriving corporate-relations business, to tell you the truth, I was growing bored with it. I was midway through chemotherapy, 1992 had just begun, I'd recently turned fifty-two, a birthday I wasn't sure I'd see; it seemed an appropriate time for a fresh challenge and to return to government work in some capacity.

  I visited Secretary of State Baker and told him of my intentions. "Fine," he said. "Whenever you're ready, just let me know." One of the positions we discussed was an ambassadorship. At my next medical checkup, I asked my oncologist, Dr. Woolley, "What would you think about me taking a post abroad?"

  I'm still indebted to him for his answer.

  "You're doing well," he said. "I want you to start making personal and professional decisions about your life as if you'd never been ill." I went ahead and accepted the ambassadorship to Canada, to commence as soon as I completed treatment. Having that to look forward to was a wonderful focus and extremely therapeutic for me.

A Word to Family and Friends:

Seven Things a Person with Cancer Wants You to Know but May Not Tell You

1. Let me do as much for myself as I can.
2. Don't force me to talk about my illness if I'm not ready to or simply not in the mood. Some days it's the *last* thing I want to talk about. What's going on in the news?

   On the other hand, please don't shrink away if I share my deepest fears with you—and at times, my tears. Please take your cues from me. And if you're not sure whether or not I feel like talking about my cancer, all you have to do is ask.
3. Don't feel compelled to "entertain" me all the time. I'm perfectly content to sit together in silence, watching TV together or reading separately. Your presence is entertainment enough.

4. If I'm feeling down, please don't act falsely cheerful around me. (Besides, you don't really think I'm buying your performance, do you?)

5. Likewise, please don't encourage me to "cheer up!" It makes me feel self-conscious, as if I can't be honest with you. And when you feel like hell, there's nothing worse than to have a healthy person lecture you about the importance of maintaining a positive attitude.

6. Please try not to take it personally if I snap at you or lash out at you on occasion. Sometimes the frustration and anxiety get the better of me. Or maybe I'm just having a bad day. This may be small consolation, but one reason you bear the brunt of my frustration is that I know you won't abandon me, which makes you a "safe" target.

    None of this excuses my behavior, but I hope you will try to be understanding, even if deep down inside you'd really like to throttle me.

7. You can never reassure me too many times, especially in my low moments, that I am still the same person I always was, that I am not a burden, and that you will be by my side forever.

Cancer Is a Family Disease

Your family may be wrestling with many of the same emotions as you are, though not always in sync with you or with one another. Half of all men and women caring for someone who is sick suffer from depression; that is higher than the rate among people with cancer.

The remedies for allaying the anger, fear, and helplessness that often grip loved ones are no different than for the patient: Become an active participant in helping him obtain the cancer care that he needs. Then, once the initial medical crisis is over, try to reestablish as normal a family life as possible, even though things will be anything but normal at first.

Family members can expect to assume new responsibilities while you're recuperating from surgery or under the weather from chemotherapy. Perhaps a husband with rusty domestic skills must cook for himself and do his own laundry during his wife's hospitalization. Or a wife finds herself the household's sole breadwinner because her husband has taken early retirement following treatment for a brain tumor. If there are children living at home, they'll be asked to handle more chores than usual. Eventually life will return to its familiar rhythms, but until then, those around you should try to:

- Relax household standards. Meals don't have to be elaborate, plasticware and paper plates will suffice, and unless *House Beautiful* is featuring your home on its next cover, does it really matter if the floors aren't immaculate right now?

- Be organized but flexible. Accept that unforeseeable complications will disrupt the best-laid plans from time to time.

- Pace themselves and know their own limitations. In most instances, our home care will fall mainly to one other person; usually a spouse, grown child, or other relative. Prolonged periods of stress and sleep deprivation can grind them down physically and emotionally. But because all attention is focused on us, their symptoms frequently go unnoticed.

  As Valerie discovered, when you're the primary caregiver, it's easy to tell yourself that only you can meet the patient's needs. You brush aside offers of help with an insistent "Thanks, but I really don't need anything. I'm fine." Maybe you are, but if you've gone days without a good night's sleep while wolfing down sandwiches from the hospital cafeteria, you may not be in the best position to judge.

  Valerie rarely left my side during the three weeks I spent in the community hospital in September and October. "I felt I had to be there," she says, "just to know what was going on and to raise hell whenever necessary." Two months later, the mucositis I developed after my second round of chemo was severe enough that I had to be admitted to Georgetown University Medical Center for eight days. Once again Valerie would stay virtually the entire day, every day.

  "It got to the point where I was running out of strength and falling into a deep pit of depression," she recalls. "And when you're exhausted and depressed, you're not very effective. I had to recognize that it wasn't as crucial for me to be around all the time at Georgetown as it was when he was in the other hospital."

  Valerie's father, a photographer and writer who'd roamed the world for *National Geographic* magazine, saw how tired and stressed she was. "He said to me, 'You don't have to be there all the time. Sit with Peter a couple of times a day, but not the entire day.' I welcomed his advice; it was the permission I needed. After that, I could deal with everything better. I was okay."

I would have told her the same thing, but she never brought it up for fear of hurting my feelings. I believe that patients have a responsibility to look after their caregivers' health, provided that we're alert and not incapacitated by illness. For one thing, *our* well-being depends on it. What happens if your caregiver throws out her back because she's been shortchanged on sleep and exercise? As much as you would love to have her at your bedside, if you see her becoming run-down, insist that she go home to rest. "I'll be fine here in the hospital, honest. *Now go relax!*"

- Most important of all: Family members need to keep talking to one another. When individuals retreat into themselves and stop communicating, simmering anxieties and resentments inevitably boil over. Does somebody in the family feel unfairly put upon? Maybe the responsibilities of caring for the person with cancer can be distributed more equitably. Somebody else is feeling unappreciated? "I'm sorry, I should have told you what a terrific job you're doing. Thanks for taking Grandma to the oncologist's office." Let's address these matters before they snowball.

Renewing Romantic Relationships

As with any protracted crisis, one partner's cancer can strain a marriage,* although the incidence of separation and divorce in the wake of a diagnosis "is about the same as it is for the general population," says Dr. Julia Rowland. The first step toward maintaining a healthy relationship when a husband or wife is sick is to acknowledge the stress you're under and to extend each other a little leeway. Exhaustion alone can fray tempers and patience. And when we're tired and distracted, we don't always have full command over our tone of voice or how we express ourselves.

Try to bear this in mind the next time your partner makes a re-

---

*For the sake of convenience, we use the word "marriage," but this refers to any romantic partnership between two people.

mark that you interpret as hurtful. Instead of reacting as you would normally, maybe you say to yourself, *He's been feeling lousy all day. I'm going to let this one slide.* Then do so. Here's a good rule: Any snapping or carping calls for an immediate apology. The two of you have too much important work to do than to walk around angry at each other.

In addition, you need to devote time and energy to nursing your relationship. Carve out time for just the two of you once a week if possible. Start "dating" again. Go to a favorite restaurant, a movie—anything fun—and try to steer the conversation away from cancer.

In addition, don't allow illness to become an excuse for avoiding physical intimacy. What sometimes happens is that patients feel self-conscious sexually, particularly if they've undergone disfiguring surgery or if treatment has rendered them sterile. Their partners, not wanting to appear insensitive or to pressure them, may hesitate to initiate physical affection. Cancer patients may misinterpret this as a lack of desire, which only reinforces their insecurity.

The way to avoid this cycle is for both partners to be open with their emotions. If you're feeling shut off from each other, consider going to a marriage counselor or a sex therapist. As always, inquire beforehand whether or not the practitioner has experience in counseling couples with similar problems.

> *See "Sexual Problems" in Chapter Eight, "Take Control: Managing Symptoms, Side Effects, and Complications."*

What About the Kids? (Or Grandkids?)

Naturally, Valerie and I were deeply concerned about the effect my illness might have on our two young daughters. Randall was four years old at the time; Adrienne, one and a half. Valerie chose to be up front with them about the situation, without needlessly frightening them.

One day she sat the girls down and calmly explained, "Daddy is sick. He had an operation on his tummy. Now he has to take a medicine that is probably going to make him feel sick and tired. He's going to be okay," she assured them, "but it's going to take some time." They seemed to accept her explanation.

In telling children, you want to effect a hopeful tone—neither overly optimistic nor pessimistic. *Never* withhold the truth from them, as parents sometimes do in an effort to spare them. Kids have remarkable radar for sensing crisis in the air. What's more, they may imagine scenarios that are far worse than the reality. Having to perpetuate the lie also adds unnecessary stress to the lives of the adults in the family.

The amount of detail you go into varies according to their intellectual development (see table 9.5). Respond to their questions simply but honestly and don't be afraid to admit that you don't know an answer. Your initial discussion should touch on these major points:

1. Cancer is not contagious.
2. You did nothing to cause this.
3. So-and-so will take care of you while I am in the hospital (or recuperating at home). Don't worry: You will not be alone.

Depending on their age, you may want to prepare them for possible treatment-related side effects that may change your appearance. "I may look a little different without my hair, but I'm still the same Mommy on the inside. And before you know it, my hair will grow back."

Discussions about death are appropriate when a patient is ex-

---

**TABLE 9.5 How Much Do They Understand?
Kids and a Parent's Cancer**

Infants do not understand the concept of illness and death, but they are aware of a parent's absence.

Ages two to three may feel anxious when someone in the family is sick; they often confuse death with sleep.

Ages three to six understand that people die, but do not comprehend the finality of death. Children in this age range may also believe that their thoughts can cause another person to become sick or die. So, for example, if they once entertained an angry thought about Mommy ("I wish Mommy would go away and never come back!"), they might feel guilty as well as scared.

Ages six to nine view death as final and frightening, but think of it as an entity separate from the ailing person. This is the age range during which most boys and girls first become curious about death.

Ages nine and older realize that illness and death can occur at any age, not just when people are old. By age twelve, most children have an adult's understanding of death.

tremely ill or when an older youngster has questions. Experts agree that no matter what age a child is, parents should avoid using euphemisms for death such as "Grandma is asleep forever." Younger boys and girls may equate sleep with death and be afraid to go to bed at night, terrified that they won't wake up in the morning.

HOW CHILDREN MAY REACT WHEN A PARENT HAS CANCER

Youngsters don't necessarily respond to grief the same way adults do. "Sometimes concerned parents will worry because their kid is acting as if nothing out of the ordinary is happening," says Dr. Rowland. "That's *appropriate* for children. They are programmed to act that way." Their cries for attention are likely to be expressed through behavior instead of words or tears, so you'll want to monitor them carefully. It's also recommended that you make your child's school aware of the situation. Ask to be contacted if his or her schoolwork begins to suffer or if teachers notice uncharacteristic behavior. Children sometimes wear halos at home but trade them in for a pair of horns and a pitchfork upon entering the school doors.

> **You Are Not Alone**
>
> Chapters of the American Cancer Society (800-227-2345) offer short-term crisis counseling, consisting of four to six sessions, for patients and family members who cannot afford professional therapy.

"Any overt changes in behavior are always a flag that a child is having problems," Dr. Rowland says. "Grades falling off sharply is a key marker. Or is this a child who's always gone on play dates or had friends over, and suddenly he isn't socializing with anyone? It may not be critical, but you'd want to talk to somebody about it." Individual counseling or family counseling might prove helpful. The hospital psychologist or social worker can guide you to a therapist skilled in this area.

See "Mental-Health Services" in Appendix B.

Teenagers, says Dr. Rowland, often have the most difficulty in coping with a parent's cancer. "It's the worst time for them to have an ill parent," she explains. "They're trying to become independent, and one way they do that is to rebel against Mom and Dad. But now they're being asked to toe the line because of the crisis at home, and they have nothing to rebel against because the home front has been destabilized."

Unfortunately, one parent's illness often robs children of the attention they need from the healthy parent, who is consumed with car-

---

TABLE 9.6 Common Physical/Behavioral Reactions to Grief, by Age

Children may exhibit one or more of the following:

Infants—Sluggishness ▪ Unresponsive to smiling, cooing ▪ Weight loss ▪ Difficulty in sleeping ▪ Drop in activity level

Ages two to three—Less talkative than normal ▪ Appear anxious, distressed

Ages three to six—Lack of appetite ▪ Difficulty in sleeping ▪ Regressive behavior such as thumb-sucking, bed-wetting

Ages six to nine—A decline in schoolwork ▪ Not wanting to go to school ▪ Concern about their own health ▪ Aggressive, defiant behavior ▪ Dependent, clingy behavior

Ages nine and older—A decline in schoolwork ▪ Not wanting to go to school ▪ Concern about their own health ▪ Aggressive, defiant behavior ▪ Dependent, clingy behavior ▪ Not wanting to bring friends home, out of embarrassment ▪ A need to act "perfect"

---

ing for the patient and tending to her own emotional pain. The following suggestions can help them to keep their heads above water during this turbulent time:

- Make homelife as normal as possible. Kids find comfort in routines such as family meals, a parent's reviewing their homework, and other family traditions.

- Spend time alone with each child. Even if you can squeeze this into the day only occasionally, opt for quality over quantity. Let each youngster know that he can come to you with his sadness, happiness, and fears, and that a jumble of emotions is normal when someone you love is sick.

- Let youngsters help care for the parent with cancer, but never force them. Running up to the corner drugstore to fill a prescription, fetching a glass of juice, and other tasks appropriate to age can make children feel less powerless. But don't overburden them with responsibilities.

- The best thing you can do for your family while you're undergoing treatment, says Dr. Rowland, is this: "Take care of yourself and do whatever you need to do to keep yourself on an even keel, because your family is going to pick up its cues from you. If you fall apart, the family falls apart."

- The best thing you can do for *yourself* is to use this enforced "downtime" to cherish your family. For me, one of the most meaningful moments came when my two older daughters flew in from Michigan following my release from the hospital. Susan was twenty-eight; Laura, twenty-one. For a father who'd nearly died, to be surrounded by them and my two young ones was so, so important.

Chapter Ten

Getting Help When You Need It

Cancer can be an isolating experience, both for patients and for those taking care of them. Most people rely on family and friends to help lighten their load. If that's sufficient to meet your needs, wonderful.

But you should know that if you dig deeper, you'll discover patient-support organizations and community programs that offer services such as home-delivered meals, transportation to and from medical appointments, and assistance in resolving insurance disputes.

Just how *much* help is available will depend on the size and proximity of your personal support network and where you live. Generally, large cities and their suburbs provide more services than you would find in a small town many miles from the nearest urban center. But one thing is for certain: You won't receive help from anyone unless you ask for it.

"Patients are usually reticent to reach out," says Maureen Sawchuk, nursing coordinator of the Lombardi Cancer Center. "So many people want to be of assistance. They can't take away your cancer or your symptoms. But it makes them feel good to take away some of your anxiety about the day-to-day details of life that need to be addressed."

Help from Family and Friends

When a relative, friend, or neighbor says to you, "If there's any-thing I can do, don't hesitate to call," they're looking for guidance. Because unless they've been through this situation before, they honestly aren't sure what they can do for you.

Don't hesitate to specify what you or the person caring for you needs. Usually, it's the small things, like running a chore or errand, or watching the kids for an afternoon. As Valerie can attest, when you're trying to run a household in between commuting back and forth to the hospital, even the simplest act of kindness is a godsend.

"Our friend Alixe used to come by the hospital quite a bit," she recalls. Alixe Glen was a tremendous inspiration to me. At sixteen, she'd been diagnosed with sarcoma of the leg muscles. According to her doctors, the disease was fatal. But radical surgery saved her life. Five years later I hired her to work on the 1980 presidential campaign, and ten years after that she was visiting me when I had cancer.

"One time," says Valerie, "I remarked to Alixe how I was always running out of quarters for phone calls. She disappeared and returned ten minutes later with a roll of quarters, which was exactly what I needed at that moment."

Usually, though, when you're asked what you need, you draw a blank. Ask someone to photocopy table 10.1. Make your own additions, then post it near the telephone so that the next time someone says, "If there's anything I can do," you or your caregiver can reply, "That's so considerate of you. Yes, there is . . ."

Resources in Your Community

Contacting some of the organizations and agencies listed in table 10.2 can lead you to support services right in your own community. You may find what you need at any of four levels:

1. Federal, state, or local government agencies, like the Social Security Administration
2. Private networks of social service organizations and charities, such as Catholic Charities USA
3. The American Cancer Society and other patient-support organizations

---

TABLE 10.1 **Ways for Family and Friends to Be Helpful**

General Help:

- Sit with the patient.
- Assist with feeding the patient, helping her get dressed, administering routine medications.
- Give the patient a shave, shampoo, haircut, manicure, pedicure, or massage.
- Drop in regularly on a patient who lives alone.
- Baby-sit the patient's or primary caregiver's children or elderly relatives, or invite them to dinner.
- Find cancer-related information requested by the patient or the caregiver.
- Offer to let one of the patient's relatives or friends from out of town stay with you as a temporary houseguest.
- Take the patient for a walk.
- Accompany the patient to religious services.

Errands:

- Go to the supermarket.
- Fill prescriptions and purchase medical supplies.
- Pick up the mail and accept hand deliveries.
- Drop off and pick up dry cleaning.
- Take out cash or make deposits for the person.
- Accompany the patient to appointments at the Social Security office.

Transportation:

- Chauffeur the patient to and from medical appointments, the store, the bank, the park, and so on.
- Drive children and elderly relatives to and from daily activities.
- Take the car to the auto-repair center for seasonal maintenance and annual inspections.
- Drive the car to the gas station and fill up the tank.
- Wash and vacuum the car.

Help Around the Home:

- Prepare freezable meals in advance. Ask the patient to name her favorite foods and how she likes them prepared.
- Do the laundry and put it away.
- Make sure the garbage is put out on trash-collection days.
- Do routine outdoor work, such as mowing the lawn, trimming the hedges, cleaning the gutters, shoveling snow.
- Clean the house.
- Clean out the garage.
- Wash and dry the dishes.

- Hire and supervise electricians, plumbers, and other repairmen for necessary jobs around the house.
- Feed pets and walk the dog.

Bills and Personal Affairs:

- Handle the patient's monthly bills and balance her bank accounts.
- File insurance claims and track down payments.
- File tax forms and other legal documents.
- Arrange for home services such as nursing care, home health aides, and so on.
- Offer to let concerned friends and relatives call you for information about the patient's condition, so her phone isn't ringing off the hook.
- Help the patient answer letters and make phone calls.

---

4. Local service clubs, civic organizations, and fraternal orders, including church and synagogue groups, Elks Club, YMCA/YWCA, Lions Club, Masons, American Legion, Rotary Club, Knights of Columbus, B'nai B'rith, Sons of Italy, Kiwanis International, Community Chest organizations, Veterans of Foreign Wars, Jaycees, Salvation Army

Although a resident of Dallas, Texas, will no doubt be offered a wider array of services than someone from tiny Dallas, North Carolina, availability is often a hit-or-miss proposition wherever you live. For instance, many chapters of the American Cancer Society provide trans-

---

TABLE 10.2 Resources Offering Services for People with Cancer

Organization/Agency (* = government agency)	Telephone Number
American Amputee Foundation	501-666-2523
American Cancer Society	800-227-2345
Area Agencies on Aging*	800-677-1116
Blood & Marrow Transplant Newsletter	888-597-7674
Cancer Care	800-813-4673
Cancervive	310-203-9232
Catholic Charities USA	703-549-1390
Civilian Health and Medical Program of the Department of Veterans Affairs(CHAMPUS)*	800-733-8387

Organization/Agency (* = government agency)	Telephone Number
Department of Social Services (state/local/city)*	Check the government listings section of the white pages.
Health Care Financing Administration*	800-638-6833 (Medicare) 410-786-3000 (Medicaid)
Hill-Burton Program*	800-638-0742
Human Rights Commission*	Check the government listings section of the white pages.
Leukemia Society of America	800-955-4572
Lymphoma Foundation of America	202-223-6181
National Association of Community Action Agencies	202-265-7546
National Association of Hospital Hospitality Houses	800-542-9730
National Association of Insurance Commissioners	816-842-3600
National Coalition for Cancer Survivorship	877-622-7937
National Foundation for Facial Reconstruction	212-263-6656
National Foundation for Transplants	800-489-3863
National Kidney Cancer Association	800-850-9132
National Leukemia Research Association	516-222-1944
National Marrow Donor Program*	888-999-6743
National Meals on Wheels Foundation	616-531-9909
National Organization for Rare Disorders	800-999-6673
National Transplant Assistance Fund	800-642-8399
Patient Advocate Foundation	800-532-5274
Social Security Administration*	800-772-1213
State Pharmaceutical Assistance Programs*	See "Prescription-Drug Patient-Assistance Programs" in Appendix B.
Tricare Management Activity*	303-676-3526
United Way of America	703-836-7100
U.S. Equal Employment Opportunity Commission*	800-669-4000
Veterans Health Administration Cancer Program*	800-827-1000
Y-ME National Breast Cancer Organization	800-221-2141

portation to and from treatment. But if no volunteer drivers happen to be free in the morning for the six weeks that you're scheduled to undergo daily radiation therapy at 10:00 A.M., you'll have to try your luck elsewhere.

Lining up community services is an ideal task to delegate to a loved one or friend; preferably someone with impeccable organizational skills, a pleasant phone manner, and inexhaustible patience. He or she should expect to be ping-ponged from one extension to another, receive conflicting information, and so on. We don't want to give the impression that you pick up the phone an hour before an appointment and "order" a driver the way you would call for a taxicab. This is a frustrating assignment. But don't give up. If you're able to land, say, *respite care* (a trained volunteer, home health aide, or nursing assistant who can watch the patient for a few hours, giving the caregiver a chance to get out of the house) for the weeks you figure to be recuperating at home from cancer surgery, you'll be thankful you were so persistent.

Whoever mans the phones, equipped with a pen and writing pad, be sure to inquire: (1) how to apply for the service; (2) whether or not there are any eligibility requirements, such as age, income level, and assets; and (3) how long the application process takes. Also ask the person at the other end (always take names and extension numbers) if he or she could recommend other organizations or agencies that might prove helpful.

Your New Best Friend: The Hospital Social Worker

Hospital social workers are invaluable sources of information about services to which you may be entitled and where to find them. Counseling cancer patients and their families is just one facet of their job. In the hospital environment, the social worker's main function is to guide you through the process of applying for government-funded programs such as Medicare and Medicaid, financial assistance, and practical services.

"We perform a lot of roles," says *oncology social worker* Dominica Roth of the Lombardi Cancer Center. Oncology social workers specialize in the issues unique to people with cancer. "We link patients with resources and coordinate care plans for once they leave the hospital," she explains. "We'll even advocate for them with insurance companies." You may hear the social worker referred to as a *discharge*

Six Essential Resources for Cancer Patients

American Cancer Society—the largest and best-known support organization for patients and their families. Services may include financial aid, medical equipment loans, transportation services, free lodging, and legal advice/referrals.

Area Agencies on Aging—an excellent resource for Americans aged sixty and older. There are more than 660 AAAs in the United States. As federally mandated by the Older Americans Act, all AAAs arrange services such as transportation, home health care, homemaker and chore-maintenance services, and legal assistance, to name but a few.

Catholic Charities USA—the largest private network of social service organizations in the United States. May be able to help you access free or low-cost transportation, family counseling, home health care, and respite care, among other services.

Social Security Administration—the government agency that oversees Social Security, Supplemental Security Income, and Medicare.

State, County, or City Department of Social Services—coordinates Medicaid and other programs, such as Temporary Assistance for Needy Families (formerly known as welfare), food stamps, and state-funded financial aid.

United Way of America—a national network of local charity organizations. Services of interest to people with cancer may include home health care, adult day care, child care, family counseling, and transportation.

---

planner. At Lombardi, men and women receiving outpatient chemotherapy or radiotherapy may see the social worker; other medical centers, however, restrict this service to hospitalized patients only.

Types of Services

Home Health Care

Since private health-insurance protection varies from one policy to the next, we can't definitively state what insurers will and won't cover. In general, many policies follow the lead of *Medicare*, the government health-insurance program for people aged sixty-five or older, and for people of any age who have received disability payments for twenty-four months. If anything, private plans often pay for more services than Medicare does. Similarly, benefits under *Medicaid*, the government health-insurance program for low-income families, are determined by each state. The only way to know for sure what services you're entitled to is to thoroughly read your private policy or the "Medicare Handbook," or, if you're on Medicaid, to contact your local department of social services or human services.

SKILLED NURSING CARE

Medicare covers part-time *skilled nursing care* performed by a registered nurse (R.N.), provided that you are confined to your home and your physician approves a home-care plan. Skilled nursing care includes administering oxygen and medications, giving injections and setting up IVs, and tending to wounds, catheters, and ostomies. Many state Medicaid programs provide for home care.

The Informed Patient
Medicare and Medication at Home

Although many insurance companies will pay for home chemotherapy, Medicare does not. Nor does it cover the considerable expense of oral medications prescribed to alleviate treatment-related side effects. At Lombardi, says Maureen Sawchuk, "our Medicare patients receive their nausea medication intravenously before they leave here.

"Most of those medications," she adds, "last twelve hours, twenty-four hours, or longer." This way the drug, administered on an inpatient basis, is paid for. If you're on Medicare, ask your oncologist about the possibility of making similar arrangements.

HOME HEALTH-AIDE SERVICE

Home health aides can assist you with the activities of daily living: bathing, cooking, household chores, and so on. They are not nurses. Under Medicare, the same eligibility requirements for skilled nursing care apply to home health aides, physical therapists, occupational therapists, and speech and language pathologists. Some state Medicaid programs will pay for home health aides, so long as they are supervised by a nurse. As for private insurers and managed-care plans, benefits rarely include home health-aide service unless you also need a registered nurse.

◆ Your local Area Agency on Aging or United Way of America may be able to provide a home health aide.

FINDING HOME HEALTH CARE ON YOUR OWN

Of course, there's nothing to stop you from privately hiring a nurse or health aide, perhaps to temporarily ease the burden on your family or other loved ones. Your oncologist, nurse, or social worker may know of reputable, home health-care agencies in your area. If not, contact the National Association for Home Care for a list of state-licensed agencies near you. More than four hundred Visiting Nurse Associations around the country provide skilled nursing care, home

> **National Association for Home Care**
> 228 7th Street, S.E.
> Washington, DC 20003
> 202-547-7424
> *http://www.nahc.org*
>
> **Visiting Nurse Associations of America**
> 11 Beacon Street, Suite 910
> Boston, MA 02108
> 888-866-8773
> *http://www.vnaa.org*

health aides, social work and counseling, and other in-home health services. The national organization's toll-free referral line will direct you to the closest VNA. When you call, inquire whether or not the fees are based on income, or *sliding scale.*

Don't hire any agency without first checking to see if it is accredited by one of three professional associations: Community Health Accreditation Program, the Foundation for Hospice and Home Care, or the Joint Commission on Accreditation of Healthcare Organizations. Accreditation, while not a guarantee of satisfaction, at least affords you an additional avenue for lodging any complaints.

> See *"Home Health Care" and "Health-Care Accreditation Organizations" in Appendix B.*

◆ The American Cancer Society and the National Transplant Assistance Fund offer modest financial assistance to offset the cost of a home health aide.

RESPITE CARE, ADULT DAY CARE, CHILD CARE, HOMEMAKER SERVICES AND CHORE-MAINTENANCE SERVICES

What if your next cycle of chemotherapy is scheduled for the same week as school vacation, and you have no one to look after a young child or an elderly relative? Child care and adult day-care services may be available through the Area Agency on Aging, Catholic Charities USA, or the United Way of America. These organizations may also be able to provide respite care, to give the loved one caring for you a much-needed break; or services to help with household chores during those times when you're too fatigued to tidy up yourself.

◆ The American Cancer Society provides limited financial assistance for child care.

Assistance with Insurance Disputes

During the time that I was being treated for cancer, I was fortunate to have excellent insurance coverage through my company's private plan. In 1991, the year I was diagnosed, 47 percent of employees in firms of two hundred or more were enrolled in *managed-care* plans. As of 1997, that figure had shot up to 85 percent, and American workers with traditional *indemnity* policies like mine were all but a vanishing breed.

There are different types of managed-care plans (see table 10.3), but in general, policyholders are restricted to a network of physicians and hospitals. The goal of managed care is to contain medical costs by seeing to it that tests aren't prescribed indiscriminately and that patients aren't referred to expensive specialists when a medical condition could be managed adequately by their primary-care doctor (usually an internist or family practitioner, often referred to as a gatekeeper). Emphasis is also placed on preventive measures and on performing procedures on an outpatient basis whenever possible instead of admitting patients to the hospital. Members of managed-care plans pay lower premiums, and so long as they see health-care practitioners within the network, they are charged nominal *copayments* at the time of medical visits and don't have to file claim forms. Who could argue with that?

One of the downsides is that in the managed-care companies' effort to curb wasteful spending, people with life-threatening diseases such as cancer may be denied access to services that are essential to their survival. In a 1997 survey by the Association of Community Cancer Centers, approximately three in ten oncologists said that primary-care physicians regularly or frequently delayed routing their patients to a cancer specialist. The same percentage noted that patients regularly or frequently had to switch oncologists, either because of changes in their managed-care contract or because they changed insurers. Patients don't always realize that by switching plans in midtreatment, they may no longer be able to see their original oncologist; there may even be a question as to whether or not the therapy they're currently on will be approved by the new policy. Continuity of care isn't essential, but it certainly is the preferable course.

In addition, one in three oncologists who participated in the study reported that their patients regularly or frequently had to travel long distances or to several locations for medical care instead of receiving those services locally and under one roof.

Another survey, this one conducted by pollster Louis Harris for the organization the Commonwealth Fund, looked at the advantages and disadvantages of managed care from the perspective of some seventeen hundred primary-care physicians who worked for *health-maintenance organizations,* or HMOs. The drawbacks were most glaring for *capitated* plans, which pay their doctors a flat fee for each patient regardless of how many services he or she requires.

Disturbingly, one in ten of the doctors polled acknowledged that they had a financial incentive *not* to refer a patient to a specialist or subspecialist in cases where they, as gatekeeper, had some doubt about the necessity of such services. The vast majority of physicians put their patients' interests first, but not all, unfortunately.

Dr. Larry White, president of the Association of Community Cancer Centers, offers a graphic example: "A radiation-oncologist friend of mine was working with a urologist who was very popular in his community and saw a lot of patients. Apparently, this urologist would operate on every case of prostate cancer that he could. The only time he'd refer a patient to radiation therapy was if the tumor was inoperable or the patient flatly refused to have surgery.

"When the urologist decided that he couldn't survive in private practice anymore, he joined an HMO and went on a capitated system. His practice changed 180 degrees. From then on he referred every man with prostate cancer for definitive radiation treatment and operated only on those who refused radiation.

"It's very sad to see," he says, "because that's a poor reflection on medicine. But the public needs to realize that the economic system can have a tremendous impact on a doctor's incentives to take care of patients and what he does in terms of treatment."

WILL YOUR INSURANCE COVER EXPERIMENTAL THERAPIES? WHAT ABOUT DRUGS USED OFF LABEL?

The fiercest battles between those who care for cancer patients and those who insure them have been waged over two issues: coverage of

---

TABLE 10.3   Types of Medical Insurance

Private Insurance—an insurance plan purchased by an individual or by a group, typically an employer. Patients pay a monthly premium and are free to see any doctor they wish. Medical charges are covered on a *fee-for-service* basis, with the patient usually responsible for 20 to 30 percent of all costs except for emergency care, which is fully covered. Once the patient has paid a certain amount of money in a calendar year, the insurer assumes 100 percent of all claims for the remainder of the year. This is called a *stop-loss* feature.

    Some private policies are *self-funded*. An employer or group creates its own plan. Although an insurance company may be retained to process the claims and pay the health-care providers, the money comes from the employer or group.

HMO (Health Maintenance Organization)—A member may receive services only from health-care practitioners and hospitals under contract with the HMO. A primary-care physician coordinates his care and refers him to specialists within the network as seen fit.

Preferred Provider Organization (PPO)—PPOs, the most popular form of managed care, are more flexible than HMOs. Enrollees may see any health-care provider from the plan's roster (which is usually considerably larger than an HMO's), sometimes without written referrals from their primary physician. If they go outside the network, they pay a deductible. Once that is met, the insurer pays a percentage of the bills.

Point-of-Service Plan (POS)—This hybrid of HMO and traditional indemnity plans allows members to receive full benefits for seeing practitioners belonging to the network. Coverage for fees charged by nonnetwork providers ranges from 60 to 80 percent.

Medicare/Medicaid—Both of these federally subsidized programs were established by Congress in 1965. Medicare is administered by the Social Security Administration; Medicaid is overseen by the Health Care Financing Administration (HCFA).

    Medicare has two parts: Part A, which pays 80 percent of inpatient hospital care and various follow-up services, is free. Part B pays 80 percent of doctors' services, outpatient hospital care, and other medical expenses. Patients who enroll in part B pay a monthly premium. Some additionally choose to purchase *Medigap* insurance, to cover the remaining 20 percent of medical costs.

    Men and women aged sixty-five or older qualify for Medicare, as do people with permanent kidney failure and those who have been receiving Social Security Disability Income (SSDI) payments for twenty-four months. Less well known is the fact that cancer patients diagnosed with metastatic disease are usually considered permanently disabled and therefore eligible for Medicare. "Most people don't know this," says social worker Dominica Roth. "But, generally, if the cancer is in a major organ such as the lung, liver, or brain, they will be approved."

    The Medicaid program is for people under age sixty-five who cannot afford health insurance. Their income and assets must be below a certain level in order to qualify. Both Medicaid and Medicare were originally conceived as fee-for-service plans. But now many beneficiaries are enrolled in managed-care plans. In the 1990s, the number of Medicaid recipients belonging to Medicaid Managed Care quadrupled to more than 10 million participants.

Military Health Services System—Any veteran who served in the active military, naval, or air service and was discharged or released under honorable conditions has basic eligibility for Veterans Administration (VA) care. For medical services to be covered, vets must be treated in VA facilities, unless VA authorities determine that certain services are unavailable or cannot be provided economically. Under those circumstances, care will be authorized at a private facility at VA expense.

The Civilian Health and Medical Program of the Department of Veterans Affairs (CHAMPVA) is the health-benefits program for dependents of veterans who became ill or permanently disabled while on active military duty.

Tricare Management Activity, administered by the Department of Defense, insures military retirees and their dependents, as well as families of deceased servicemen or those on active military duty. It used to be known as the Civilian Health and Medical Program of the Department of the Uniformed Services (CHAMPUS).

investigational therapies and coverage of drugs used "off label"—that is, used for a purpose other than the "indications" specified on the package insert that comes with the drug (and is reprinted in the reference book *Physicians' Desk Reference).*

In the 1980s, insurance companies began questioning the off-label use of anticancer drugs, complaining that it amounted to experimental treatment. The U.S. Food and Drug Administration, which approves medications for commercial use, essentially disagrees. Off-label usage is a common practice, with more than half of all cancer patients receiving at least one chemotherapy drug off label. Once the FDA greenlights a medication, doctors can prescribe it for any medical condition, not just the ones indicated on the label. This is how new, improved applications are discovered. As a report from the U.S. General Accounting Office noted, "It is even possible that for a specific form of cancer, a drug given off-label may have been proven to be more beneficial than any drug labeled for that cancer."

In that report, "Off-Label Drugs: Reimbursement Policies Constrain Physicians in Their Choice of Cancer Therapies," more than half of the oncologists surveyed said that they had encountered resistance in getting reimbursed for anticancer drugs prescribed off label. Three in five said they had admitted their patients to the hospital for chemotherapy treatments, since insurers' drug-reimbursement policies tend to be stricter for outpatient care. One in four oncologists acknowledged having switched patients' treatment protocols from the preferred drug regimen to one with no off-label agents because they anticipated that the insurer would refuse payment.

The GAO report was made public in September 1991, the same

month that I was diagnosed with colon cancer. At the time, only two states, Michigan and New York, had enacted legislation requiring insurers to cover off-label uses of FDA-approved chemotherapy drugs. As of 1999, thirty-one other states had followed suit.

Getting Medicare to pay for cancer clinical trials is the next battleground. It has been the government health-insurance program's long-standing policy not to cover any service that could be considered experimental. Bear in mind that more than half of all cancers are diagnosed in men and women who are aged sixty-five or older and thus eligible for Medicare. In 1997, two bipartisan bills were introduced in the U.S. House of Representatives and in the U.S. Senate to change that. Both measures were reintroduced two years later as the Medicare Cancer Clinical Trial Coverage Act(s) of 1999. The House bill was sponsored by Representatives Nancy Johnson (R-CT) and Benjamin L. Cardin (D-MD), and the Senate bill by Senators Jay Rockefeller (D-WV) and Connie Mack (R-FL). Senator Mack, incidentally, lost a brother to melanoma.

No action has been taken on either bill as of yet, but one hopes that Medicare will join the U.S. Department of Defense and the Department of Veterans Affairs in offering their beneficiaries opportunities to join investigational studies of promising cancer treatments. In 1996 and 1997, the two departments entered into separate agreements with the National Cancer Institute to allow their members to participate in NCI-funded clinical trials. Veterans who receive medical care at VA facilities or who are authorized to receive care privately do not have to pay for medications.

Private policies vary in their coverage of investigational therapies, while most managed-care contracts routinely exclude experimental care from any coverage at all. Patients have the option of bringing a lawsuit against their insurers, to force them to pay for experimental treatments. But as Dr. David Tubergen, medical director of managed care at M. D. Anderson Cancer Center in Houston, observes, "Unfortunately, the process often takes longer than the patient has to live without that treatment."

WHAT TO DO IF YOUR INSURER DENIES A CLAIM:
A STEP-BY-STEP GAME PLAN

With more than eight in ten patients enrolled in managed-care plans, most people with cancer will need to receive *preauthorization* (also called *precertification)* before certain medical services or hospitalizations are approved. Maureen Sawchuk of the Lombardi Cancer Center recommends that Medicare beneficiaries and those with private policies also notify their insurer in advance of any therapy that could conceivably be deemed experimental, "because what you don't want," she explains, "is to start a therapy, then find out three months later that it's been denied."

Should precertification or a claim be turned down, you or your doctor will receive a letter advising you that the insurer has reviewed your case and is not going to authorize payment for the proposed treatment. Time is of the essence, so if you plan on appealing the decision, get the process rolling right away. Some policies impose time limits on how long a patient has to challenge a denial.

1. If you don't already have a copy of your plan's descriptions of the appeals process (it is usually explained in writing as part of your policy), call the insurer and obtain one.

2. Ask your physician or nurse to write to your insurer and justify why the doctor believes the treatment in question is necessary. The physician should rebut the reasons given for rejecting the claim and submit any materials that could bolster your case, such as medical studies and articles supporting the use of the therapy for your diagnosis, or second opinions from other physicians.

> **Situations That May Warrant an Appeal**
>
> *Your health insurer has stated that it will not pay for:*
>
> - A referral to a specialist
> - A cancer therapy under investigation
> - Chemotherapy used off label
> - A hospital stay
> - A diagnostic procedure

♦ Most of the major pharmaceutical manufacturers operate reimbursement hotlines staffed by trained specialists whose sole job is to assist physicians and their office staffs persuade insurers to pay for the contested treatment. Among other services, they will dig up pertinent studies and other medical literature, recommend strategies for appealing denied claims, and search for alternative medical coverage for the patient. When appropriate, they may even negotiate directly with the third-party payer on your behalf—all of this free of charge.

Along with the doctor's letter, enclose your own cover letter outlining the problem. Be sure to photocopy all letters, articles, and other papers that you send. Either follow up with a phone call to ensure that the package found its way to the person(s) who issued the denial, or send it certified mail, return receipt requested.

Keep a log in which you jot down notes of all telephone conversations with representatives of your insurer. Date the entries and remember to ask for the name, title, and phone number of each person to whom you speak.

The combined clout of your physician's input and supporting documentation is often enough to persuade an insurance company that a medical service warrants coverage.

3. If your claim is turned down a second time, the next step, if you wish to pursue it, is a *hearing appeal.* You, your physician, and anyone else able to offer evidence supporting your case would appear before an appeal panel from the insurer. Ask beforehand who may accompany you. In a *third-party appeal,* your information is turned over to an independent review organization, which renders a written decision as to the merit of the prescribed treatment.

4. While you await a hearing, it is advisable to file a written complaint with your state regulatory agency. All plans except for self-funded policies fall under the jurisdiction of the *Commissioner of Insurance.* In your state, it may be called the Department of Insurance or the Division of Insurance. To find its address and telephone number, call the National Association of Insurance Commissioners or tap into its Web site:

120 West 12th Street, Suite 1100
Kansas City, MO 64105-1925
816-842-3600
http://www.naic.org

You can also contact your state's Department of Health and the Attorney General's Office. Complaints should include copies of all correspondence with the insurer and copies of relevant medical studies. The agency may be able to help mediate a resolution, or it may intervene directly on your behalf if it determines that the insurer is violating either the terms of your policy or state law. How much authority these agencies have over managed-care plans varies from state to state.

Self-funded plans are monitored by the federal Department of Labor, which generally does not involve itself in complaints stemming from the denial of an experimental cancer therapy. Members of these plans can try appealing to the insurance company that administers the policy or go directly to the employer or group that established it. If that fails, they should consult an attorney experienced in representing consumers against self-insured plans.

5. As a last resort, or at any step along the way, you may consider suing an insurer who refuses to pay for a particular treatment. This is an expensive option, naturally, with no guarantee that the court will rule in your favor.

6. Another costly strategy is to pay for the proposed treatment out of pocket while you pursue the appeal process or wait for your day in court. Maureen Sawchuk recalls one breast-cancer patient whose insurer denied her permission to enter a clinical trial being conducted at the Lombardi Cancer Center. The protocol con-

---

Important Resources for People on Medicare or Medicaid

To learn how to appeal payment denials

MEDICARE
State Health Insurance Assistance Program
To get the phone number for your state's program, contact:
Health Care Financing Administration
800-638-6833
http://www.medicare.gov/contacts

MEDICAID
State Medicaid Office
To get the phone number for the office serving your state, contact:
Health Care Financing Administration
410-786-3000
http://www.hcfa.gov/medicaid

Insurance-Related Terms You Should Know

Deductible: the amount of medical expenses the policyholder must pay out of pocket (not including premiums) before coverage begins. Generally, the higher the premiums, the lower the deductible.

Lifetime cap: the maximum benefits to be paid out over the course of the plan's lifetime. Your policy may also spell out the maximum amounts it will pay for specific health-care services.

Major medical insurance: covers doctors' fees and other expenses excluding the hospital fee.

Usual, reasonable, and customary (URC): Instead of paying a stipulated amount for a service or procedure, the insurer pays a benefit based on what it considers average charges for specific services in a particular region of the country.

sisted of a standard two-drug regimen for breast cancer: cyclophosphamide (brand name: Cytoxan) and doxorubicin (Adriamycin). To this, Lombardi researchers added the immunologic agent interleukin-11, which is not approved for commercial use. At least not yet. On that basis, her insurer rejected the claim.

"The research nurse spent a lot of time on the phone with the payer, going back and forth," Nurse Sawchuk says. "We provided literature. We did a lot of maneuvering to make it less expensive. But it was to no avail.

"We offered the patient routine Cytoxan-Adriamycin," which is one of the most frequently used drug combinations. "But she was determined to join the clinical trial." So determined, in fact, that she took out a second mortgage on her home in order to pay for the three-drug regimen: approximately $1,800 per cycle for six cycles. Not everyone would have made the same choice, but that was the choice that was right for her.

Who Else Can Help
From your health-care team:
- The hospital social worker

- Your physician or nurse

Social service agencies and patient-support organizations:
- American Amputee Foundation (for information)

- American Cancer Society (may intervene on behalf of patients)

- Area Agencies on Aging (assistance in resolving insurance disputes)

- Blood & Marrow Transplant Newsletter (for referrals to attorneys specializing in insurance cases)

- Cancer Care (for information)

- Cancervive (for referrals to attorneys specializing in insurance cases)

- National Coalition for Cancer Survivorship (for information)

- National Kidney Cancer Association (may intervene on behalf of patients)

- National Marrow Donor Program (for information)

- Patient Advocate Foundation (for free legal counseling)

See "Keeping Your Insurance If You Become Unemployed,"
page 869.

Assistance for Victims of Job Discrimination

From a medical standpoint, our knowledge about cancer is light-years ahead of where it was just twenty years ago. Public attitudes about the disease, however, haven't always kept pace. Old myths still abound, such as the assumption that a cancer diagnosis is synonymous with death or that cancer is contagious.

These and other misconceptions have little impact on a patient's life unless the setting happens to be your place of employment. If you worked before you developed cancer, staying on the job is vital to your emotional equilibrium. The biotechnology company that I work for, Amgen, Inc., sponsored a survey about job discrimination faced by cancer survivors. Five hundred patients were polled, along with one hundred supervisors and one hundred coworkers of people with cancer.

The survey found that cancer survivors were five times more likely than other workers to be fired or laid off. Judging by some of the opinions held by the supervisors and coworkers, that should come as little surprise. One-third of the supervisors said that they felt employees with cancer could not handle the workload and needed to be replaced. The truth is that most adult patients work while they're undergoing treatment and maintain a level of productivity comparable to other workers. Once my dose of chemotherapy was lowered, starting with my third cycle in January, I hardly ever missed a day at the office.

Fortunately, laws are in place to protect many people with cancer from job discrimination. The *Americans with Disabilities Act of 1990* (ADA) prohibits private employers with fifteen or more employees from treating qualified cancer patients or cancer survivors differently from other workers in job-related activities. Also covered under the law are employees of state and local governments, employment agencies, and labor unions. The federal *Rehabilitation Act of 1973* and various state and local laws provide additional protection.

You probably don't think of yourself as disabled. According to the ADA, a person is considered to have a disability "if he/she has a physical or mental impairment that substantially limits one or more major life activities, has a record of such an impairment, or is regarded as having such an impairment." In other words, you are also shielded from being discriminated against because you have a history of cancer.

RIGHTS AND WRONGS

An employer is guilty of discrimination for committing any of the following acts on the basis of an employee's disability, including having cancer or having survived cancer:

- Not hiring an applicant for a job or training program
- Firing a worker
- Providing unequal pay, working conditions, and benefits, such as health insurance, pension, and vacation time
- Punishing an employee for having filed a discrimination complaint
- Screening out disabled employees

WHAT IS "REASONABLE ACCOMMODATION"?

By law, employers are required to modify the work hours or responsibilities—within reason—to help a person with cancer do her job while she's undergoing treatment and afterward. For instance, if you have to come in a few hours late during the month and a half you're receiving radiation therapy, your employer may accommodate you by letting you work flexible hours until you're finished with therapy. Perhaps you stay after hours, take work home, or telecommute. Reasonable accommodation might also include acquiring or modifying equipment or providing qualified readers or interpreters.

The accommodation does not have to ensure equal results or provide exactly the same benefits as before, but employers are not obligated to find positions for unqualified applicants or to lower quality standards. Nor must they institute changes that would create an "undue hardship" for the business because they're either too costly or too disruptive. What constitutes an appropriate accommodation is judged on a case-by-case basis by the Equal Employment Opportunity Commission (EEOC), the federal regulatory agency that enforces federal statutes prohibiting job discrimination.

◆ Suggest to your employer that he or she contact the Job Accommodation Network, 800-232-9675, a free service of the President's Committee on Employment of People with Disabilities. The network helps companies tailor accommodations for disabled workers.

TAKING TIME OFF FROM WORK

Under the 1993 *Family and Medical Leave Act* (FMLA), employees with a serious health condition that prevents them from working are entitled to a total of twelve weeks of *unpaid* protected leave per year without risking their position. However, the law pertains only to businesses with fifty or more employees, and companies are allowed to exempt their highest-paid employees. In order to be covered, the person with cancer must have worked at least twenty-five hours per week for one year. Only about one in twenty of all U.S. businesses are affected by the FMLA, so realistically, it benefits relatively few workers.

To learn more about the law, call your local Department of Labor, Employment Standards Administration, Wage and Hour Division. You'll find its number under "U.S. Offices" in the government listings section of the white pages. Or visit the Wage and Hour Division Web site at: *http://www.dol.gov/dol/esa/public/whd_org.htm*

FILING A DISCRIMINATION COMPLAINT AGAINST AN EMPLOYER

You have 180 days from the date of the action taken against you to lodge a complaint with the U.S. Equal Employment Opportunity Commission; 45 days if you're employed by the federal government. Most state laws also give workers 180 days in which to file.

The EEOC investigates the charges (pretty remarkable, when you consider that 75,000 to 80,000 complaints are filed each year). If the agency determines that there is "reasonable cause" to believe that the employer has broken the law, it will attempt to resolve the dispute without a trial. Perhaps the employee gets his job back, or reasonable accommodation is made, or the worker receives a written apology from his employer.

At all stages of the process, the commission tries to broker an informal settlement, because *nobody* wants to go to court. In fiscal year 1998, the agency obtained $169.2 million in monetary benefits for charging parties through settlement and conciliation, and millions more through its *Alternative Dispute Resolution* (ADR) program, in which a trained, neutral mediator works with the two sides to reconcile their differences. Mediation takes place before the charges are investigated, and the process is confidential and free. Most mediations are completed in one session lasting one to five hours.

But if the two parties cannot be brought together, the EEOC may bring suit in federal court. In fiscal year 1998, the EEOC's litigation program recovered nearly $90 million for victims of discrimination. Whenever it finishes processing a case, the agency gives the complainant the go-ahead to pursue individual legal action. Be forewarned that these cases can drag on for years, eating up time, energy, and money—with no guarantee of victory. And don't overlook the fact that even if you were to win a large cash award, much of any money collected would go to your lawyer. We suggest traveling this route only if you and an attorney experienced in job-discrimination lawsuits both believe that you have an airtight case.

At the state-government or local-government level, about ninety *Fair Employment Practice Agencies* (FEPA) process more than 48,000 discrimination charges annually. These include complaints concerning alleged violations of state and local laws prohibiting employment discrimination and federal laws enforced by the EEOC.

> **U.S. Equal Employment Opportunity Commission**
>
> 1801 L Street, N.W.
> Washington, DC 20507
> 800-669-4000 or
> 202-663-4900
> *http://www.eeoc.gov*

The National Coalition for Cancer Survivorship recommends that if you sense a pattern of discriminatory behavior on the part of your employer, start keeping meticulous records of all job actions. For example: Following a mastectomy, a woman whose position has always included interaction with the public is suddenly moved to a position where she no longer comes into contact with customers. Also write down summaries of conversations, phone calls, and so forth that could become significant down the line should you decide to file a complaint.

♦ In your area, the Fair Employment Practice Agency may be known as the Commission on Human Rights, the Fair Housing and Employment Agency, or the State Human Relations Commission. You'll find the number in the government listings section of the white pages.

Who Else Can Help
From your health-care team:
- The hospital social worker

Social service agencies and patient-support organizations:
- Cancervive (for referrals to attorneys experienced in employment-discrimination cases)

- Lymphoma Foundation of America (for referrals to attorneys experienced in employment-discrimination cases)
- National Coalition for Cancer Survivorship (for information)
- Patient Advocate Foundation (for free legal counseling)

Keeping Your Insurance If You Become Unemployed

What would you do if you were too ill to work or were laid off, and lost your group health-insurance benefits? The federal *Consolidated Omnibus Budget Reconciliation Act* (COBRA), signed into law in 1986, allows ex-employees of companies with twenty or more workers to purchase group coverage for themselves and their families for eighteen months, and, under certain circumstances, up to thirty-six months. If you were covered by a group health policy on the day before you left a company, either voluntarily or involuntarily, you qualify for COBRA benefits. You have sixty days to accept coverage, or you lose all rights to benefits. Spouses and dependent children are also covered. Group health coverage under COBRA usually costs more than what you paid in the past, because when you were an active employee, your employer paid a part of the premium. Still, it is less expensive than individual health coverage.

MORE GOOD NEWS FOR PEOPLE WITH CANCER: THE HEALTH INSURANCE PORTABILITY AND ACCOUNTABILITY ACT (HIPAA)

In 1989, the COBRA law was expanded so that beneficiaries could maintain their coverage for the full eighteen months in the event that they found a new insurer but would not be covered immediately for preexisting conditions, such as cancer. Many plans will accept people with cancer and other preexisting medical conditions, but they typically impose a waiting period before paying expenses related to that malady. The *Health Insurance Portability and Accountability Act* limits these restrictions to twelve months in most cases, and a maximum of eighteen for late enrollees. (Many insurers do not exclude coverage for preexisting conditions.)

Another provision of HIPAA can whittle down those twelve months or eliminate them altogether. Employees receive credit for the length of time that they had continuous health coverage prior to joining the new plan. The law defines "continuous health coverage" as not

TABLE 10.4 Eligibility for COBRA

You are eligible for continued coverage by your group health-insurance plan if:	Months Covered	Your spouse is eligible for continued coverage by your group health-insurance plan if:	Months Covered	Your dependent children are eligible for continued coverage by your group health-insurance plan if:	Months Covered
You left your job or were terminated for any reason other than "gross misconduct"	18	You left your job or were terminated for any reason other than "gross misconduct"	18	You left your job or were terminated for any reason other than "gross misconduct"	18
Your hours of employment were reduced	18	Your hours of employment were reduced	18	Your hours of employment were reduced	18
		You are now entitled to Medicare, but your spouse is not	36	You are now entitled to Medicare, but they are not	36
		The two of you legally separate or divorce	36	You and their mother/father legally separate or divorce	36
		You predecease him/her	36	You predecease them	36
• Federal employees are covered by a law similar to COBRA. They should contact the personnel office serving their agency for more information on temporary extensions of health benefits.				Your child is no longer considered "dependent" under the rules of the plan	36

going without coverage for sixty-three days or more. So if you were at your old job for one year or longer, and fewer than sixty-three days passed between the time your previous insurance expired and your current policy began, you would not be subject to an exclusion for any preexisting conditions.

One exception might be if you received medical advice, a diagnosis, or treatment *six months or less* prior to the day you enrolled in your new insurance plan. Thus, a person who is several years away from a cancer diagnosis and who sees his oncologist for checkups only once a year is considered to have no preexisting condition. Some states impose even

stricter obligations on health issuers; they may shorten the six-month period that defines a preexisting condition or increase the sixty-three-day
gap in coverage that determines whether or not a patient receives credit
for the length of time that he had continuous health coverage.

If you have questions about COBRA and HIPAA, contact:

U.S. Department of Labor
Pension and Welfare Benefits Administration
Division of Technical Assistance and Inquiries
200 Constitution Ave., N.W., Room N-5619, Washington, DC 20210
202-219-8776
800-998-7542 (for publications)
http://www.dol.gov/dol/pwba

Finding a New Insurer When You've Had Cancer

The U.S. Agency for Health Care Policy and Research estimates that 2
million men and women have been denied health insurance due to a
medical condition. Many states offer their uninsurable residents protection through programs called *Comprehensive Health Insurance Plans*
or *high-risk pools.*

Be forewarned: The policy premiums are 25 to 50 percent higher
than comparable plans available to a healthy person. (In Montana,
some people pay as much as four times the standard premium.) The
reason the rates are so astronomical is that the risk pools are funded primarily by the beneficiaries themselves.

Fortunately, few people stay in risk pools for long. Perhaps they
turn sixty-five and become eligible for Medicare, or they change jobs
and get accepted into their new employer's plan, and so on. In the best
of all outcomes, their medical condition subsides or is cured.

To learn if your state has a risk-pool insurance program, contact
the Department of Insurance. The staff there can also tell you about
additional plans that may be available covering only specific health-
care costs. Some of these restricted policies go by names such as
Medicare Supplement Plans, Specified Disease Policies, and Catastrophic (Excess Major Medical) Policies.

Who Else Can Help
From your health-care team:
- The hospital social worker

Assistance with Financial Matters

Even if you are comfortably insured, having cancer can drain family finances. Besides the portion of medical expenses for which you may be liable, many policies do not cover the expense of prescription drugs. In addition, there are the hidden costs that often take patients and their families by surprise, says Maureen Sawchuk, who offers several examples.

"Many people have to pay for additional day care that they didn't plan on, or they may have to pay for a housekeeper to help with the day-to-day chores because they're so tired. They may be buying more frozen meals because it's too fatiguing to cook. Maybe they used to walk to work, and during treatment they have to take a cab."

Little exists in the way of monetary aid unless you qualify for one of the government entitlement programs described at right. However, with the help of the hospital social worker you should be able to take advantage of several free or low-cost services in your community: transportation, lodging for your family if you have to undergo treatment away from home, loans of medical equipment, and more. These can help to pare down expenses, but they're probably more useful in terms of preserving two of your most valuable assets: time and energy.

MONEY MATTERS

Tips for $tretching Those Dollars

- Speak to a financial counselor in the hospital's business office about developing a monthly plan to pay off hospital expenses.
- Save your receipts! Medical costs not covered by insurance may be tax-deductible, including gas and car mileage for trips to and from medical visits, prescription and over-the-counter drugs, medical equipment, meals eaten out during all-day medical appointments, and modifications made to your home, such as installing a grab bar in the shower.
- If funds are tight, make arrangements with creditors to pay them back over time. Many utility companies have instituted special payment programs for the sick and elderly.
- It's not uncommon for people with cancer to drop $200, $300, $400, for a single prescription. When your doctor prescribes a medication, ask if there's a less expensive but equally effective alternative you could take. If it's a drug you've never used before, request that she start you off with a trial supply instead of the usual amount, because what if you find that you need a stronger medication or you can't tolerate the side effects?

GOVERNMENT-FUNDED FINANCIAL AID PROGRAMS

Social Security Retirement Benefits—monthly-income program for men and women aged sixty-five or older (sixty-two, for early benefits), administered by the Social Security Administration (SSA).

Supplemental Security Disability Income (SSDI)—monthly payments from the SSA made to people under age sixty-five who are disabled as a result of illness or injury. If you're going to be receiving treatment for twelve months or more, you may qualify for SSDI.

Supplemental Security Income (SSI)—monthly assistance, also from the Social Security Administration, to the blind, disabled, or those over age sixty-five, with limited income and assets. Qualifying for SSI automatically makes you eligible for state-run programs such as food stamps and Medicaid.

Temporary Assistance for Needy Families (TANF)—the successor to what used to be called welfare. This federal program for impoverished families with children under the age of eighteen is administered by each state's Department of Health and Human Services; therefore, regulations, restrictions, and benefits vary widely. In exchange for monthly financial aid, TANF recipients must work a minimum of thirty hours per week annually. Some states, however, pay benefits for up to two years before requiring recipients to put in their hours at a subsidized or unsubsidized job; in other states, benefits are contingent upon immediate employment.

Food Stamp Programs—The U.S. Department of Agriculture administers the food-stamp program through state agencies such as the Department of Public Health and Human Services.

General Assistance Programs—administered by the state or county Department of Social Services. These programs typically provide food, housing, prescription drugs, and other medical expenses for those who do not qualify for other programs. Funds are often limited.

Community Action Agency (CAA)—Nearly one thousand CAAs across the country help people in need through a variety of programs, including financial aid.

Hill-Burton Program—The approximately eighteen hundred hospitals that receive Hill-Burton funds from the federal government are required by law to provide some free or low-cost medical services to people who cannot afford to pay for hospitalization.

State Pharmaceutical Assistance Programs—As of 1999, eleven states provide financial assistance to residents who are ill and need help in paying for medications: Connecticut, Delaware, Illinois, Maine, Maryland, Michigan, New Jersey, New York, Pennsylvania, Rhode Island, and Vermont.

See Appendix B for addresses and telephone numbers.

PRIVATELY FUNDED FINANCIAL AID PROGRAMS AND SERVICES

Financial Assistance—A few patient-support organizations offer modest monetary aid to cancer patients: American Cancer Society, National Foundation for Transplants, National Transplant Assistance Fund, Leukemia Society of America, and National Leukemia Research Association. The National Foundation for Facial Reconstruction provides state-of-the-art facial reconstructive treatment, regardless of the patient's ability to pay, at its Institute of Reconstructive Plastic Surgery at New York University Medical Center. The American Amputee Foundation can advise callers on how to obtain financial aid for artificial limbs and home modifications.

Prescription-Drug Patient-Assistance Programs—Many drug manufacturers offer medications at reduced cost to patients who meet certain income requirements. A few allow annual incomes as high as $35,000 to $40,000. Your doctor may know if any of the drugs he's prescribed for you are being offered through one of these programs. Or you can call the manufacturer yourself.

The Pharmaceutical Research and Manufacturers of America publishes an annual directory of prescription-drug patient-assistance programs, with all the pertinent phone numbers, the names of the drugs covered, and the eligibility requirements. You can also access publication on the organization's Web site.

Prescription-Drug Buyers' Clubs—Buyers' clubs can save you 30 to 50 percent on the cost of prescriptions. Like any cooperative, these clubs purchase products in large volume, which enables them to pay wholesale prices to the pharmaceutical companies. The American Association of Retired Persons (AARP) Pharmacy Service, for men and women over age fifty, has more than 33 million members nationwide. This and other buyers' clubs are listed below.

- American Association of Retired Persons (AARP) Pharmacy Service: 800-456-2277
- American Preferred Prescription: 800-227-1195
- Medi-Mail, Inc.: 800-793-3548
- Preferred Rx: 800-843-7038
- Stadtlanders Pharmacy: 800-238-7828

Medical Equipment Loans—The American Cancer Society loans wigs and breast prostheses free of charge to women who cannot afford them. Y-ME National Breast Cancer Organization also runs a wig and prosthesis bank.

Transportation Services—Your social worker or nurse may be able to find you a volunteer to drive you to and from medical appointments through the American Cancer Society, your Area Agency on Aging, Catholic Charities USA, your Community Action Agency, or the United Way of America. If the American Cancer Society has no drivers available, it will reimburse your expenses for public transportation. The National Transplant Assistance Fund and the Leukemia Society of America's patient-aid programs are intended partly to help patients afford transportation costs.

Also check with the medical facility itself. Some centers offer free van service to and from radiation and chemotherapy appointments. Your county's Department of Social Services may have its own low-cost van service for people who cannot use public transportation. Other possibilities include local service clubs, civic organizations, and fraternal orders.

Home Meal Delivery Services—Men and women homebound by illness can be delivered a hot lunch five days a week. There are more than twenty thousand federally funded and privately funded meal programs in the United States. Most are free; some request a small donation.

Your local Area Agency on Aging, Catholic Charities USA, Community Action Agency, or United Way of America should be able to direct you to a home meal delivery service in your area. Or contact the National Meals on Wheels Foundation.

Free Lodging or Housing—It is possible that at some point you might require the services of a specialized treatment center in another town. The American Cancer Society, Westin Hotels, and the National Association of Hospital Hospitality Houses offer patients and/or their families free accommodations.

Fund-Raising Drives—Some patients partially finance costly procedures such as bone-marrow transplantations by organizing a fund-raising campaign. Several organizations may be able to help you. The National Marrow Donor Program can assist you in finding alternative sources of funding. The National Foundation for Transplants and the National Transplant Assistance Fund provide assistance with raising funds and setting up a tax-exempt organization—called a 501 (C) (3) organization by the Internal Revenue Service—so that donations are tax-deductible and tax-exempt. One important rule of thumb when organizing your own fund-raising drive: The donated money should never be mixed with personal or family funds.

Who Else Can Help
From your health-care team:
- The hospital social worker

Social service agencies and patient-support organizations:
- American Amputee Foundation (for information on obtaining funds)
- American Cancer Society (for financial aid, drug assistance, loans of medical equipment, and transportation services)
- American Cancer Society Hope Lodges (for housing/lodging assistance)
- Area Agencies on Aging (for meal and transportation services)
- Catholic Charities (for meal and transportation services)
- Leukemia Society of America (for financial aid and drug assistance)
- National Association of Hospital Hospitality Houses (for housing/lodging assistance)
- National Association of Community Action Agencies (for financial aid, drug assistance, and meal and transportation services)

- National Foundation for Facial Reconstruction (for low-cost or free medical care)

- National Foundation for Transplants (for financial aid and information on obtaining funds)

- National Marrow Donor Program (for information on obtaining funds)

- National Leukemia Research Association (for financial aid)

- National Organization for Rare Disorders (for drug assistance and loans of medical equipment)

- National Transplant Assistance Fund (for financial aid and information on obtaining funds)

- Pharmaceutical Research and Manufacturers of America (for information on drug assistance)

- State Pharmaceutical Assistance Programs (for drug assistance)

- United Way of America (for meal and transportation services)

- Y-ME National Breast Cancer Organization (for loans of medical equipment)

See appendices for addresses and telephone numbers.

Chapter Eleven

When Treatment Ends

I completed my last cycle of chemotherapy on a Friday in April 1992. I felt tired but good, and was looking forward to assuming the ambassadorship to Canada. Dr. Woolley, who was about to leave Georgetown to direct the cancer program for a group of hospitals in and around Johnstown, Pennsylvania, compared me at the end to "a marathon runner in the twenty-fourth mile. When you get eight or nine months into treatment," he said, "it can be pretty tough."

The exhilaration over finishing is often tempered by uncertainty and fear, even for patients who have coped well throughout. As much as you're thankful to put doctors' appointments and blood tests and needles more or less behind you, the chemo drugs or the radioactive rays have been your lifeline. Now that therapy is being withdrawn, it is natural to worry, *What if the tumor comes back?* This has been called Damocles syndrome: feeling as if the sword of Damocles hangs over your head, suspended by a thin thread. It's an apt description of this next stage of surviving cancer.

You'll probably be surprised, though, by how you manage to banish such thoughts from your mind most of the time. The feelings of dread typically resurface around medical checkups or whenever you get a cold. Is it just a cold, or . . . ? If you find that depression and anxiety are dominating your life, call the hospital psychology department and ask for a referral to an experienced counselor.

It's also normal to feel somewhat out of place on your return to the healthy world. Family and friends may expect you to bounce right back to being your old self. But having cancer changes your perspective on life somewhat. For one thing, it shatters any illusions you may have held that illness and possible mortality were far off in the future. On the other hand, you do learn to treat most days as precious gifts to be enjoyed.

A support group could prove helpful during this time, to give you a forum for discussing these feelings. The hospital and the staff have provided steadfast support all these months. That won't immediately fade away, but the reassuring pats on the hand and the encouraging words will be less frequent. Some progressive cancer centers have begun programs for patients who have completed therapy. For instance, the Post-Treatment Resource Program at New York's Memorial Sloan-Kettering offers individual, family, and group counseling, and seminars and workshops addressing emotional and practical problems such as stress management and the balance between career and cancer.

Bear in mind that for a time you may not feel like your old self physically, either, as the effects of chemotherapy or the fatigue from radiation may continue for a while. Many people experience no side effects once therapy ends, but others may be bothered by symptoms for months and possibly years. Your oncologist will tell you which effects warrant his immediate attention.

The Next Phase of Treatment: Long-Term Follow-Up

Follow-up plans vary, depending on cancer type and the philosophy of your doctor, but a typical schedule includes examinations every three or four months for the first one to three years, then every six months through five years, and annually after that. Imaging procedures and/or endoscopic exams are usually conducted once a year, with physical exams and blood tests taken in between. I used to have a yearly X ray, CT scan, and colonoscopy. Once I reached the five-year mark, the colonoscopies were reduced to once every two to three years.

Since early detection saves lives, wouldn't it be beneficial to perform these procedures at shorter intervals? Why not four mammograms a year? It's a logical question. As Dr. Mitchell Morris of Houston's M. D. Anderson Cancer Center explains, "With a lot of cancers, if a patient has no symptoms, X rays and examinations rarely make a difference in the long run. In other words, detecting a recurrence a few months earlier doesn't necessarily improve the outcome. All it does is force patients to undergo a lot of expensive tests every few months.

"We and a lot of other cancer centers are in the process of cutting back our testing for many kinds of cancers." One exception is cervical cancer, Dr. Morris's specialty. "In cervical cancer, we are finding that a pelvic examination can detect an asymptomatic recurrence that is potentially curable; and a chest X ray can detect a potentially curable recurrence in the lung, also before symptoms occur. By the time these patients would be symptomatic a few months later, the tumor would usually be too big to cure. So there we have sound evidence that having these folks come in for examinations is a good thing."

How You Can Help Yourself

Besides following the surveillance plan outlined by your doctor, you can help to lower your risk of developing a second cancer by making improvements in your diet and level of physical activity and doing away with any unhealthful habits. In the process, you'll be protecting yourself against heart disease, stroke, diabetes, and other illnesses. There's nothing too drastic here. What we call the Cancer Prevention Program is really just a commonsense plan for healthful living. In fact, you probably incorporate many if not most of these steps in your daily life already.

The Cancer Prevention Program

YOUR DIET

- Limit the amount of dietary fat you eat to no more than 20 to 30 percent of your total daily calories.
- Eat at least 25 grams of dietary fiber per day.
- Eat five to nine servings of vegetables and fruit every day.

- Watch those calories! Stay at the weight recommended for your height and body type.

- Eat foods rich in vitamins A, C, and E—the *antioxidants.* These vitamins are believed to counter the effect of molecules known as *free radicals,* which can cause cancer by damaging the DNA in cells and by converting substances in the body into carcinogens.

YOUR DAY-TO-DAY HABITS

- If you smoke or chew tobacco, stop!
- Drink alcohol in moderation only: four drinks a week, maximum.
- Stay physically active.
- Avoid direct exposure to the sun.
- Do what you can to reduce the stress in your life, not because stress causes cancer, but because it can send you reaching for a cigarette, a pint of ice cream, and so forth.

Chemoprevention

A cancer center committed to research may be able to offer you another potential defense against your form of cancer: clinical trials testing natural and synthetic *chemopreventive* substances that show promise in possibly preventing or delaying a recurrence or the development of a second cancer. Some are over-the-counter medications that may be sitting in your medicine cabinet right now, like aspirin and nonsteroidal anti-inflammatory drugs (NSAIDs).

Since the National Cancer Institute established its chemoprevention program in the early 1980s, hundreds of compounds have been studied for their cancer-staving properties, and dozens have been evaluated in patient trials. Nineteen ninety-eight brought the first confirmed success in this area, when the synthetic hormone tamoxifen (brand name: Nolvadex) won approval from the U.S. Food and Drug Administration for use as a preventive agent against breast cancer in women considered at high risk. It has been a mainstay of breast-cancer treatment for many years. In clinical trials, tamoxifen's effectiveness was so convincing that the large study was halted more than a year early, and the drug was offered to all participants. Tamoxifen halves the risk of a recurrence as well as the formation of a second malignant tumor in the other breast. The preventive effect lasts for the five years a woman takes the oral anti-estrogen agent and for another five years after that. Clinical studies found no additional benefit to taking tamoxifen for more than five years; in fact, beyond that point, the drug loses its effectiveness and may even begin to fuel breast-cancer growth.

Tamoxifen belongs to the class of chemopreventive substances known as *blocking agents,* which includes flavonoids, oltipraz, indoles, and isothiocyanates. The other class is *suppressing agents:* vitamin D and related compounds, vitamin A and retinoids, NSAIDs, difluoromethylorithine (DFMO), monoterpenes, calcium. Table 11.1 lists just some of the chemopreventive substances that have advanced to human trials or are currently being studied.

What If the Cancer Comes Back?

When cancer comes out of remission, it is not a new cancer, but a new tumor formed by renegade cells from the original cancer. These cells resisted treatment and have eluded the body's natural defenses for anywhere from a few months to many years. Now they have become reactivated and begun to proliferate. A recurrence may arise in the same location as before or in nearby lymph nodes or tissue. Most relapses, however, are metastatic, growing in distant parts of the body.

Cancer's reappearance poses new challenges for you and your medical team. Your oncologist may have fewer chemotherapy agents to choose from (presuming drug therapy was used before and is warranted again), because the new tumor grew from the cells that withstood the agents' first offensive. Cancer cells, unlike normal cells, constantly reshuffle their DNA. That's how they evade the effects of chemotherapy. Then the survivors spin off new aberrant cells that are also resistant to the drugs.

When tumor tissue is sampled, 50 to 80 percent of relapsed patients will test positive for abnormally high levels of *P-glycoprotein (P-gp).* A product of the *multiple drug resistance (mdr1) gene,* this substance acts like a molecular pump, expelling certain types of cancer-killing drugs from malignant cells before they can inflict damage. In contrast, only 10 to 30 percent of people with cancer are P-gp positive at the time of their initial diagnosis. Some cancers, like tumors of the colon and the kidney, inherently overexpress P-glycoprotein; they tend to resist most cytotoxic drugs. Breast cancer, ovarian cancer, and

TABLE 11.1 **Chemopreventive Agents**

Agent	Description	Has Been or Is Being Tested for Effectiveness Against the Following Cancers
aspirin	Pain reliever and fever reducer	Colorectal
beta-carotene	Precursor of vitamin A	Bladder, cervical, colorectal, lung
calcium compounds	Most abundant mineral in the body	Colorectal
difluoromethylorithine (DFMO)	Synthetic enzyme inhibitor	Bladder, breast, cervical, colorectal, prostate, skin
finasteride (Proscar)	Enzyme inhibitor approved for use in treatment of benign prostatic hyperplasia	Prostate
oltipraz	Dual antiparasitic/anticarcinogenic agent	Bladder
piroxicam (Feldene)	Nonsteroidal anti-inflammatory drug used to treat arthritis	Colorectal
raloxifene (Evista)	Estrogen receptor modulator, used to help prevent thinning of the bones (osteoporosis). May exert the same effect as tamoxifen, but without some of tamoxifen's side effects, such as an increased risk of endometrial cancer.	Breast
retinoids 　fenretinide (4-HPR) 　retinols 　9-*cis*-retinoic acid 　13-*cis*-retinoic acid	Synthetic form of vitamin A	Bladder, breast, head and neck, lung, prostate, skin
sulindac (Clinoril)	Nonsteroidal anti-inflammatory drug used to treat arthritis	Colorectal
vitamin C	Vitamin C	Cervical
vitamin E	Vitamin E	Cervical, prostate

leukemias, on the other hand, do respond. But over time, they may become impervious.

A recurrence is certainly a time to consider all options. We would suggest asking your oncologist if he knows of any open investigational studies testing agents intended to circumvent multidrug resistance and whether or not you might be a candidate. Several old and new drugs under investigation appear able to reverse the mechanism that makes cancer cells invulnerable.

As for radiotherapy, generally it cannot be administered to the same area twice. If a tumor recurs outside of the original radiation "field," the new site can be irradiated safely. A local relapse within the field, however, rules out further use of the treatment. "The tumor may still be somewhat responsive to the radiation," explains Dr. Barnett Kramer of the National Cancer Institute, "but the surrounding healthy tissue can no longer tolerate another exposure."

While a recurrence may eliminate some treatment possibilities, new options often become available. "That is something very seldom discussed," Dr. Larry Norton of Memorial Sloan-Kettering Cancer Center says intently. "One of the big failings of books on cancer is that people with advanced or recurrent disease look for information that is relevant to them, and they rarely find it. Everything is geared toward early-stage cancers. They think, *God, they've given me up for lost!*" With most forms of the disease, your oncologist will have something to offer you.

Starting Over Again

To learn that your cancer has come back is devastating, naturally. You're liable to feel the same jumble of emotions as you did the first time the doctor delivered the dreadful news. If anything, the anger may be more palpable. After everything you've been through, now you're going to have to face treatment—and the prospect of possibly dying—all over again?

The fact that you have weathered this once before should also be a source of strength. Compared to when you were first diagnosed, you know what to expect, and you know where to find help if you need it. Perhaps a cure is no longer realistic, and the intent of treatment is to buy you a lengthy remission. For most patients, that in itself would be worth fighting for.

But never lose sight of this: No matter how dire the prognosis, *somebody makes it.* It might as well be you. The five-year survival rate may be a discouraging 1 percent, but that means one in one hundred people live. Five percent? One in twenty. We human beings think nothing of braving far higher odds every day.

Alternative Therapies: Buyer, Be Wary

Anytime there's a setback—a recurrence, a progression of the cancer, a failed attempt at symptom control—it's natural to wonder what answers therapies outside the therapies mainstream might hold. These are referred to variously as unconventional therapies, alternative therapies, and complementary therapies. Public interest in such interventions has soared in recent years, so much so that annual visits to practitioners of alternative medicine now eclipse the number of times Americans see their primary-care physicians.

According to a 1998 random survey of fifteen hundred adults across the country, the most popular alternative therapies were herbal therapy, chiropractic, massage therapy, and vitamin therapy, followed by homeopathy, yoga, acupressure, acupuncture, biofeedback, hypnotherapy, and naturopathy. The most common application, by far, is to ease chronic pain, although about one in five users turn to alternative care to alleviate anxiety or depression.

Without trying to discourage you, this is a path to be traveled cautiously, particularly if you are seeking not just symptom relief but treatment of the cancer itself. Many of the interventions mentioned above *have* proved valuable in reducing pain, nausea, and other symptoms. Maybe the pharmacologic 714-X and chelation therapy to rid the body of toxic chemicals are indeed the panaceas that cancer doctors and patients alike have been hoping for. But until they are subjected to carefully designed, tightly controlled patient studies, we have no way of substantiating whether they are of benefit or not.

Over the years, proponents of alternative medicine have repeatedly spurned overtures from the National Cancer Institute to submit their discoveries to the same research standards as conventional medicines. In 1990, an estimated 60 million Americans used alternative medical treatments, most of

Center for Alternative Medicine Research in Cancer

University of Texas, Health Science Center
P.O. Box 20186, No. 34
Houston, TX 77225
800-392-1611
http://www.sph.uth.tmc.edu/ utcam

National Center for Complementary and Alternative Medicine Clearinghouse

Call this number to speak to an information specialist and/or to receive print information about alternative medicine:
888-644-6226

which had never been evaluated for their effectiveness. The growing public demand led Congress to mandate the formation of the Office of Alternative Medicine (OAM), since renamed the National Center for Complementary and Alternative Medicine (NCCAM).

Ten research centers were opened in 1995, among them the University of Texas Center for Alternative Medicine at the M. D. Anderson Cancer Center in Houston. "There's no such thing as alternative medicine," says Dr. Mary Ann Richardson. That may sound peculiar coming from the program's director and coprincipal investigator, until she adds, "There are only alternative practitioners who aren't willing to present their therapy for rigorous evaluations."

The center is analyzing and conducting clinical trials of dozens of alternative cancer therapies. Two that have attracted a great deal of attention in recent years are shark cartilage and antineoplastons.

Scientists believe that the cartilage of sharks may contain a substance that inhibits angiogenesis—a tumor's ability to develop new blood vessels so that it can feast on nutrients and continue to grow. "We're testing it because people are taking it," Dr. Richardson says. The National Institutes of Health estimates that more than fifty thousand people in the United States use shark cartilage at a yearly cost of about $7,000 each. This therapy, like the vast majority of other unconventional techniques, is not covered by insurance. It is sold in health-food stores in pill and suppository forms. According to the American Cancer Society, however, shark cartilage can be effective only if injected intravenously.

Antineoplastons, naturally occurring substances that are believed to control tumor growth, were discovered by Dr. Stanislaw R. Burzynski of the Burzynski Research Institute in Houston. "His theory claims that the human body has a 'biochemical defense system,' which is like a parallel immune system," explains Dr. Richardson, "and antineoplastons are a part of this." By giving cancer patients antineoplastons, the biochemical defense system is restored. "Supposedly, antineoplastons change abnormal cells into normal cells, so that they begin to die." Once all the deviant cells have been eliminated, the patient can be pronounced cured.

In 1991, Dr. Burzynski allowed the National Cancer Institute to review the medical records of seven brain-tumor patients who'd been treated at his clinic. He selected the patients. When the NCI reviewers determined that there did appear to be evidence of antitumor activity, the institute proposed conducting a formal phase II investigational study, to further evaluate the therapy. Dr. Burzynski consented.

With his input, two experimental protocols were begun at the Mayo Clinic, Memorial Sloan-Kettering Cancer Center, and the National Institutes of Health Clinical Center. However, only nine patients enrolled in the clinical trial, which was aborted after less than two years, a rarity. Apparently, the NCI and Dr. Burzynski could not agree on how to modify the protocol to accrue more volunteers.

Never has there been a phase III randomized, controlled clinical trial of antineoplastons, in which one group of patients would receive the investigational therapy, and the other group would be given the current standard therapy for a particular cancer. Then at the end of a certain number of years, the investigators would tally up the results and see which group did better. This is the litmus test for all drugs approved by the U.S. Food and Drug Administration.

So for now, all we have is the anecdotal research of Dr. Burzynski and his colleagues. The University of Texas Center for Alternative Medicine reviewed eighteen clinical series, three of which studied patients with brain cancer and one of which studied patients with prostate cancer. The remainder studied patients with various other types of cancer. Thirteen of the studies contained fewer than twenty-five patients each. Most had advanced disease, although the stage wasn't always specified.

Sixteen of the studies assessed the cancer's response to the treatment. In all but three, more than half the patients achieved some degree of positive response: complete remission, partial remission, objective remission, or the disease remained stable. Of course, none of this tells us what percentage of the patients were still alive two, five, and ten years later, or whether or not any of the participants had undergone conventional treatment prior to antineoplaston therapy.

Dr. Barnett Kramer of the National Cancer Institute provides some perspective: "You can treat one thousand people or several thousand people with an unproven therapy, but if you don't have careful record-keeping and it doesn't measure up to the same scientific standards that other therapies do, it doesn't matter how many patients there were.

"I like to keep an open mind, because it may very well be that some of the treatments that are labeled 'alternative' work, and I wouldn't want to ignore them if they do," he emphasizes. "It's just a

---

TABLE 11.2 The Seven Categories of Alternative Therapies

Mind-Body Interventions—therapies that promote the mind's ability to influence our immune, hormonal, and neurological systems: psychotherapy, support groups, meditation and imagery, hypnosis and hypnotic suggestion, biofeedback, yoga, dance/movement therapy, music therapy, art therapy, prayer, and mental healing. The most dramatic example of the mind-body interaction at work is the placebo response, in which a patient's belief that a medication (in reality a dummy pill) will produce a physiologic effect brings about that very result.

Bioelectromagnetic Applications in Medicine (BEM)—an emerging science that studies the interaction between living things and electromagnetic fields. Major new applications of BEM in alternative medicine include nerve stimulation, bone repair, wound healing, treatment of osteoarthritis, electroacupuncture, tissue regeneration, and immune-system stimulation.

Traditional and Folk Remedies—encompass the following:

- Traditional oriental medicine (acupuncture, acupressure, herbal medicine, gigong, oriental massage)

- Ayurveda, India's traditional natural system of medicine (meditation, yoga, natural therapies, herbal preparations)

- Homeopathic medicine (remedies made from naturally occurring plant, animal, or mineral substances that are recognized and regulated by the FDA)

- Naturopathic medicine integrates traditional natural therapies (botanical medicine, clinical nutrition, homeopathy, acupuncture, oriental medicine, hydrotherapy, and naturopathic manipulative therapy) with modern medical diagnostic techniques and standards of care. There are more than one thousand licensed naturopathic doctors in the United States.

- Environmental medicine recognizes that illness can be caused by food and chemicals found at home, in the workplace, and in the air, water, and food.

Manual Healing—based on the theory that a dysfunction in one part of the body affects the function of another.

- Chiropractic therapy attributes most diseases to a misalignment of the bones, particularly the backbone, which applies pressure on the nerves. Doctors of chiropractic use their hands to manipulate various parts of the spine. They do not perform surgery and cannot prescribe medications.

- Massage therapy similarly manipulates soft body tissues.

- Laying hands on or near a patient's body; also referred to as healing touch, therapeutic touch, *shen* therapy, biofield therapeutics.

Pharmacological and Biological Treatments—the use of an assortment of drugs and vaccines not yet accepted by mainstream medicine or the FDA, including antineoplastons, cartilage products, ethylenediaminetetraacetic acid (EDTA), immunoaugmentive therapy, Coley toxins, neural therapy, apitherapy, iscador, and biologically guided chemotherapy.

Herbal Medicine—uses plants and plant products to treat illness. According to the World Health Organization, an estimated 4 billion people—or four-fifths of the global population—use herbal medicine for some aspect of primary health care. Green tea contains epigallocatechin-3-gallate (EGCG, for short), which in animal studies has been found to prevent tumor blood-vessel growth. Several studies have demonstrated an association between consumption of green tea and a reduced incidence of cancer. In 1999, researchers at California's Stanford University School of Medicine discovered that the Chinese herb triptolide can kill cancer cells.

Diet and Nutrition—an alterative philosophy that advocates supplementing one's diet with vitamins or nutrients beyond the recommended daily allowances. Orthomolecular medicine treats chronic disease with high doses of vitamins.

Source: National Center for Complementary and Alternative Medicine (NCCAM).

matter of subjecting them to the same level of statistically reliable evidence as we do with other treatments."

Is this sufficient proof on which to base a decision? If you had just been told by your oncologist that there was nothing else traditional medicine could offer you, it might be. Obviously, this is up to the individual to decide. In the end, the deciding factor for many of us would undoubtedly be the cost: on average, $32,000 for eight months of treatment, nonreimbursable by insurance.

If It Walks Like a Duck and Quacks Like a Duck: The Ten Warning Signs of Medical Quackery

1. *The treatment has never been evaluated in clinical trials.* Whatever "proof" is offered of the therapy's effectiveness is strictly anecdotal, if not outright false. As one advertisement that promises a cancer cure in ninety days boasts: "Our formulas have cured many people with cancer worldwide."

2. *The practitioner is unable to produce any articles about the treatment from reputable medical journals,* such as the *Journal of the American Medical Association,* the *New England Journal of Medicine,* the *Journal of Clinical Oncology,* and *Cancer.*

3. *Claims of persecution by the medical establishment. (And while we're at it, by the government and political organizations too.)* Remember laetrile, once hailed by proponents as the answer to cancer? As of 1980, seventy thousand Americans had tried the drug, despite a federal law that prohibited it from being shipped across state lines.

There was such a clamor for the law to be changed that a U.S. Senate subcommittee held hearings on laetrile, which is derived from the pits of apricots and other fruits. One of the "experts" to give testimony in praise of laetrile was Dr. John Richardson, a general practitioner from California who'd increased his net income seventeenfold once he began doling out the drug and promoting himself as a cancer expert. In 1972, he had been arrested for violating California's Cancer Law and eventually had his medical license revoked, at which time he went to Mexico to practice in a cancer clinic there. In his testimony, Dr. Richardson claimed that the Food and Drug Administration, the American Medical Association, the National Cancer Institute, the American Cancer Society, the Rockefeller family, *and* major drug and oil companies were banded together in a conspiracy against laetrile.

Bowing to public pressure, the National Cancer Institute conducted its own study. One hundred seventy-eight patients with different types of cancers were treated with laetrile at the Mayo Clinic and three other prestigious cancer centers. The results could not have been more definitive: Not one patient was cured or saw his tumor growth slowed. Most of the participants lived less than five months, as if they had received no therapy at all. What's more, several suffered symptoms of cyanide poisoning. An editorial in the *New England Journal of Medicine* concluded that laetrile had received its "day in court" and that the evidence, "beyond reasonable doubt," showed it to be utterly ineffective. Predictably, proponents of laetrile, including the Mexican company that manufactured it, denounced the study and filed three lawsuits against the NCI. All three were eventually dismissed.

As someone who works for a major biotechnology company, one of my favorite conspiracy theories put forth by practitioners of alternative medicine is that the medical community is trying to keep their cures from the public. Dr. Kramer of the NCI punctures such paranoid notions by pointing out that "a major pharmaceutical company can usually buy up any small company it wants." He notes drily that alternative manufacturers and practitioners don't exactly offer their products and services pro bono; unconventional therapies bring in close to $14 billion a year. The theorists also overlook the fact that "many doctors and many corporate executives from pharmaceutical houses die of cancer! For them to be at the base of a conspiracy to suppress a cure when they themselves die of the disease is a little hard to accept."

4. *Claims that the treatment causes no adverse side effects.* A 1991 study by Dr. Barrie R. Cassileth, then of the University of Pennsylvania Cancer Center, and now of Memorial Sloan-Kettering, found that terminal cancer patients treated with alternative means such as coffee enemas were more "miserable" than those who underwent chemotherapy and radiation.

5. *The practitioner discourages you from discussing the alternative therapy with your oncologist.* About three in four patients who use unconventional treatments continue with their traditional care but never inform their physician. It is *essential* that your doctor knows what you are putting into your body, particularly if you are receiving chemotherapy or radiation. Herbs, supplements, or high-dose vitamins taken before or after treatment can cause a drug interaction that could potentially inhibit or intensify the activity of the anticancer agent or the high-energy X rays. Dr. David M. Eisenberg, principal investigator at Boston's Center for Alternative Medicine Research, recommends that patients ask their physician to release information about the prescription medications they are taking, along with any other relevant medical details, to the person providing the alternative treatment.

6. *The practitioner boasts multiple, little-known degrees from obscure institutions or titles you've never heard of.* Examples: doctor of naturopathy, doctor of metaphysics, herbologist. Anyone can affix some impressive-sounding initials to his name or acquire phony certificates to hang on the wall.

7. *The treatment focuses primarily on diet.* Diet alone cannot rid the body of cancer. And certain diets, such as the *macrobiotic* diet, can be extremely harmful. Macrobiotics is a holistic way of life that includes adhering to a menu of organically grown whole grains, vegetables, beans, and nominal amounts of seafood and fruit. For a person going through chemotherapy, it may not supply enough protein, which is necessary to rebuild damaged tissue and blood cells.

"The macrobiotic diet takes away many nourishing foods," explains Susan Sloan, clinical dietitian at the Lombardi Cancer Center. "And although maybe cancer cells won't grow, your organs won't function properly and you'll be sacrificing your own body tissue. If someone is on a macrobiotic diet, and their blood counts aren't coming back up, they may not be able to get their next treatment."

8. *The treatment calls for heavy doses of "natural" herbs, minerals, and vitamin supplements.* You tend to hear the word "natural" a lot in alternative-medicine circles, usually spoken in a reverent tone of voice. But "natural" isn't necessarily "safe." Snake poison is natural. So are poison ivy, poison oak, and arsenic.

Many men with prostate cancer have been ingesting a mixture of herbs called PCP-SPES, under the assumption that the remedy is a nonhormonal alternative to the female hormone estrogen. Presumably, they hope to avoid some of the side effects of estrogen, such as breast tenderness and swelling, and a loss of libido.

When researchers at the Cancer Institute of New Jersey, in New Brunswick, tested the product, they discovered that the PCP-SPES was highly toxic and packed potent estrogenic activity. It caused the same side effects as estrogen therapy. Prostate-cancer patients have also taken the herb saw palmetto to relieve their urinary symptoms. Saw palmetto *contains* estrogen. Not only can it throw off the results of the prostate specific antigen test used to diagnose prostate cancer, it can cause the tumor to become "androgen independent." And incurable.

If someone walked up to you on the street, placed a bottle in your hand, and whispered, "Take a few of these," you'd toss it into the nearest trash can. Since the U.S. Congress deregulated dietary supplements in 1994, that is essentially what happens every time a consumer purchases a bottle of vitamins, herbal remedies, or minerals from the shelf of the local health-food store.

It often comes as a surprise to learn that, unlike drugs, supplements can enter the market without there being any proof that they are safe and effective. Nor are the manufacturers required to make consumers aware of potential side effects or drug interactions, or even to accurately list their substances on the label. One study of ginseng products, for instance, found that the active ingredient in each pill varied— in some instances, substantially—even though according to the label, all the pills contained the same amount. Some contained none at all.

Asian herbal remedies may contain lead and other heavy metals not listed on the label, while chaparral, germander, sassafras, and other herbs may cause liver damage. Congress's passage of the Dietary Supplement Health and Education Act has in effect tied the hands of the

FDA, which must prove that a product is dangerous before it can take it off the market.

9. *A refusal to divulge the "secret" behind their treatment.* Researchers who believe that they have developed an effective new therapy are typically eager to publish the results of their studies in respected medical journals so that other scientists with no vested interest in the outcome can review their work and attempt to duplicate their findings. "If a form of therapy is helpful," says Dr. Lamar McGinnis, medical director of the cancer center at DeKalb Medical Center in Atlanta, "it should be able to be reproduced by other doctors."

10. *Testimonials from movie stars, sports figures, and other celebrities.* However sincere they may be, these people are not trained or experienced in oncology.

The Informed Patient
Seeking Alternative Care—the Smart Way

Research as much as you can, then present the information to your primary oncologist. No matter how outlandish a practitioner's claims might seem, doctors should treat their patients' interest in an unproved therapy seriously and not dismiss it out of hand. An appropriate response would be, "Let me look through the material you've given me, then we can discuss it." Enough unconventional therapies have been integrated into traditional medicine that your request certainly won't be the first your physician has fielded. (In fact, Dr. Mary Ann Richardson notes that when the medical community learned of the opening of the University of Texas Center for Alternative Medicine, before the news was made public, "some of the first calls we received were from physicians who wanted to know if there were any promising alternative cancer treatments for family members who had run out of conventional options.")

All doctors should be as open-minded as my oncologist, Dr. John Marshall. "I'd say that at least one-third of my patients are taking shark cartilage, and several are using acupuncture and biofeedback," he says. "I'm supportive of them. If I had the answer and knew for certain that I could cure them, then I could be more critical of it. But I don't, and so I tend to say, 'I don't think it will hurt you, although I wouldn't waste a whole lot of money on it. If the treatment is making you feel better, for whatever reason, continue it.' "

Exercise healthy skepticism. When you call an alternative-medicine practitioner, ask as many questions as you need to.

Questions to Ask . . . About Unconventional Therapies

- Have you treated patients with my medical condition before?
- What benefits can I expect from this treatment?
- Is there any scientific evidence that this treatment may help me?
- How long will it be before we see if the treatment is effective?
- What are the known or possible risks and side effects?
- What is the anticipated cost per appointment?
- What is the anticipated cost of any medications I might need?
- Will my insurance cover this treatment?
- Will I have to travel to get the treatment? If so, how frequently?
- Could I speak to a few of your patients?
- Would you be willing to send my primary oncologist copies of your notes or reports of any diagnostic findings, your plans for my therapy, and any medications I might be taking?

- Do not start alternative cancer therapy before being diagnosed by a traditional doctor, and don't end conventional treatment without first consulting the physician who prescribed it.
- Reject any therapy that claims that patients create their own health. Because the flip side of that philosophy is that the patient conveniently bears the blame if treatment fails. You didn't "try" hard enough. You must not have wanted to get better. Getting cancer was your "choice." Et cetera, et cetera, et cetera.

 Cancer is *not* a choice, and no one doesn't go through hell to get better.
- Visit the Web sites of two consumer-advocacy organizations, the National Council for Reliable Health Information (NCRHI) and Quackwatch, or contact them for information. Both of these groups look to investigate and expose fraudulent claims made for

health products and services. They may seem overly skeptical and biased at times, but what else would you expect from a pair of consumer watchdog groups? The information they've uncovered may help you to decide whether or not an alternative therapy is right for you.

Psychiatrist Dr. Stephen Barrett, now retired, founded Quackwatch under a different name in 1969. NCRHI was established in 1977 and now has members in all fifty states. Its executive director, Dr. William Jarvis, is a consumer health education specialist and a professor at Loma Linda University in California. Combined, the two organizations' Web sites contain information about dozens of questionable alternative-medicine products, services, practitioners, and theories.

The two groups overlap in that Dr. Barrett heads the NCRHI's Task Force on Victim Redress. If you or someone you know has been seriously harmed by medical quackery, you can receive a free consultation. Attorneys seeking referrals or advice can also contact the Task Force.

You'll also find summaries of patients' experiences with alternative therapies, like the fifty-five-year-old woman with breast cancer who underwent surgery but refused to have follow-up chemotherapy. Instead, she sought treatment from a naturopath. She was given "Pesticide Removal Tinctures," among other dubious preparations. When the lymph nodes under one arm began to swell, the naturopath assured her that this was nothing more than a side effect of the herbal remedies he'd prescribed.

By the time she returned to her oncologist, the cancer had not only spread to the nodes but metastasized throughout her body. Once again she turned down conventional treatment. In her travels from one healer to another, she encountered one practitioner who claimed to have diagnosed her by using a pendulum. Another naturopath gave her a preparation that was to be painted on the skin in order to "draw" the cancer out of her. It merely succeeded in opening up an ugly abscess on her breast.

Shortly before the woman died, the second naturopath blamed her for her deteriorating condition, accusing her of "giving up."

Another woman with breast cancer, aged fifty-one, also chose to forgo conventional treatment. Instead, she flew to a Mexican cancer clinic run by a chiropractor. According to the account posted by her husband and a friend, the doctor would launch into daily tirades against the American Medical Association, the U.S. government, and the Rockefeller Foundation, which he claimed was importing guillotines from France to behead free spirits like himself in POW camps throughout the country.

Among the alternative treatments used were a mysterious black box with a probe that was run along the patient's finger to determine if she had the disease or if the medications given were working. A small box with blinking red lights was placed on her hip to relieve pain. The doctor asked the woman to lie on a padded examination table. He took a tiny vial of clear liquid ("for the tumor in the liver") and inserted it in the top of the patient's sock. Next he placed a "bone-cancer" vial under her sock. The doctor claimed to have just cured her of the metastases in her liver and hip.

As her condition worsened, the doctor tried injecting blood mixed with ozone; ordered regular colonics; painfully massaged her buttocks "to release the toxins" while she cried in pain; had her taken to a local dentist for the removal of four teeth, because the metal fillings, he insisted, were leaching mercury into the breast. *That* was what was causing her cancer.

All told, the woman was bilked out of $40,000. Three weeks before her treatments were to end, she informed the doctor that she couldn't pay him immediately but would somehow get the money to pay for the final three weeks of her stay. Her therapy ended abruptly the next day. She flew home, where a local hospital was able to relieve her excruciating bone pain with radiation before she died.

National Council for Reliable Health Information
P.O. Box 1276, Loma Linda, CA 92354
909-824-4690
http://www.ncrhi.org

Quackwatch
P.O. Box 1747, Allentown, PA 18105
610-437-1795
http://www.quackwatch.com

- ◆ The American Cancer Society and the National Cancer Institute both publish position papers on dozens of alternative treatments, which you can receive for free just by calling.

- If you decide to incorporate alternative medicine into your care plan, choose a practitioner who is certified and/or licensed. Certification from a professional organization or licensure from a state board provides some quality assurance that the health-care provider has met certain standards for education and clinical experience and has passed an examination. All of the organizations in table 11.3 can refer you to members near you. Of these five therapies, chiropractic is the only one that is licensed in every state. Acupuncture and massage therapy are licensed in about half the states; neuropathy, in thirteen; and homeopathy, in four.

Surfing the World Wide Web for Cancer Information? Better Wear Water Wings

Did you know that cancer is caused by a parasite? And not just cancer, but allergies, Alzheimer's disease, diabetes, human immunodeficiency virus (HIV), and many other health problems too. Fortunately, the worms slithering around inside of us can be killed by drinking a mixture of black walnut hulls, cloves, and wormwood.

So contends the Web site for the same herb and dietary-supplement company we quoted earlier in this chapter, the one that promised to make brain cancer vanish in ninety days. All you have to do is order a "cure package" containing a medley of nineteen different tinctures, herbs, and formulations for a shade under $1,000, plus shipping and handling. It's a small price to pay to be cured of brain cancer in three months—although, the company concedes, a repeat purchase may be necessary if you have had brain cancer for a long time.

Another Web site that peddles similar products quotes a doctor of naturopathy but has the good sense to add the following disclaimer in microscopic letters: "These products are not intended to diagnose, treat, cure, or prevent any disease." What exactly *is* their purpose, then? You can probably guess the answer.

Exploring the Internet is like rowing out into the middle of a vast ocean of medical information and misinformation, especially where alternative cancer treatments are concerned. It's easy to become lost at

TABLE 11.3   Finding an Alternative-Medicine Practitioner: Certification and Professional Organizations

Acupuncture

American Academy of Medical Acupuncture
5820 Wilshire Boulevard, Suite 500, Los Angeles, CA 90036
800-521-2262
http://www.medicalacupuncture.org

American Association of Oriental Medicine
433 Front St., Catasauqua, PA 18032
888-500-7999
http://www.aaom.org

National Certification Commission for Acupuncture and Oriental Medicine
11 Canal Center Plaza, Suite 300, Alexandria, VA 22314
703-548-9004
http://www.nccaom.org

Chiropractic

Federation of Chiropractic Licensing Boards
901 54th Avenue, Suite 101, Greeley, CO 80634
970-356-3500
http://www.fclb.org

Homeopathy

National Center for Homeopathy
801 North Fairfax Street, Suite 306, Alexandria, VA 22314
703-548-7790
http://www.homeopathic.org

Massage Therapy

National Certification Board for Therapeutic Massage and Bodywork
8201 Greensboro Drive, Suite 300, McLean, VA 22102
800-296-0664 or 703-610-9015
http://www.ncbtmb.com

Naturopathy

American Association of Naturopathic Physicians (AANP)
601 Valley Street, Suite 105, Seattle, WA 98109
206-298-0126
http://www.naturopathic.org

---

sea, as modern equivalents of snake-oil pitchmen vie for your attention alongside legitimate sites from highly regarded cancer institutions.

Advice on how to conduct research on the Web: The National Cancer Institute's CancerNet site *(http://www.cancernet.nci.nih.gov)* contains the broadest, most accurate, and up-to-date information on cancer and its treatment than anywhere else in cyberspace. Another excellent on-line resource is OncoLink *(http://www.oncolink.upenn.edu),* which is affiliated with the University of Pennsylvania Cancer Center. If you're interested in learning about unconventional therapies, we suggest visiting the University of Texas Center for Alternative Medicine homepage *(http://www.sph.uth.tmc.edu/utcam).*

You can supplement these with the Internet addresses for any or all of the major cancer centers (see table 5.1, The "A" List: Top Cancer Centers in the United States) and any patient-support organizations specific to your type of cancer (see Appendix A). In general, stick to sites supported by medical schools and universities, or organizations you're familiar with, like the American Cancer Society. A good rule of thumb is to see if the sponsoring organization exists outside of cyberspace. Is there a telephone number or street address?

Wander too far away from these reputable sites where the information is reviewed by cancer experts before it's put on-line for public consumption, and the accuracy becomes more and more tenuous. A 1999 study from the University of Michigan Medical School in Ann Arbor evaluated the medical information on 165 cancer-related Web sites. According to the researchers, one in every sixteen pages contained erroneous information, and a good deal more were misleading. Only three in five pages had been peer reviewed or listed the sources for their facts.

Furthermore, sites that appear to offer friendly medical advice and info often turn out to be marketing tools for pharmaceutical manufacturers, vitamin companies, herbalists, and so on. The fact that they're hoping to pique your interest in their products isn't an encouraging sign that their presentation of the facts will be free of bias.

In 1997 and again in 1998, the Federal Trade Commission had its investigators spend a day scanning the Internet for false health claims. They found hundreds. It would have been impossible to take legal action against all of them, so the agency went after the four most egregious culprits and e-mailed warnings to the rest. Only about three in ten ceased making their fraudulent on-line claims; the rest continued to hawk phony cures for dozens of diseases, including cancer.

Fight for Your (Quality of) Life

There may come a time when a person with cancer chooses to stop fighting. I hope that you never have to make that decision and that you join me as one of the millions of cancer survivors. But even once the goal of treatment has changed from cure to comfort, patients and the people who care about them need to remain involved in medical decisions, perhaps now more than ever. Your main concerns are that your symptoms are well managed, that your care takes place in the setting of your choice, and that your instructions regarding future medical interventions be honored.

When a patient accepts that his condition is terminal and begins to talk of hospice care, living wills, and such, family and friends may misinterpret this to mean that he has given up hope. No, his priorities have changed. Perhaps he hopes to spend more time with his loved ones and to be spared pain and suffering. He's still fighting, but for quality of life.

While you'll undoubtedly want to discuss these matters with your family and with your oncologist, the decision whether or not to pursue aggressive treatment is yours alone to make and should be supported by those around you.

Advance Directives

To ensure that your wishes are carried out in the event that you are unconscious or too ill to express them, you'll want to fill out an *advance directive,* if you haven't done so already. There are two types: a *living will* and a *medical power of attorney.* We recommend that you execute both, with the help of a lawyer experienced in end-of-life issues.

A living will stipulates which interventions a patient does or does not want used at the end of her life. A medical power of attorney (also called a *health-care proxy*) is a legal document in which she names someone to make medical decisions on her behalf. Your advance directives will not be put into effect until such time that you cannot make your preferences known.

The admissions office may have given you these forms the first time you checked into the hospital. You can also obtain them from an organization called Choice in Dying, either by mail or by downloading them for free over the Internet. In filling out the documents, be as specific as possible. Artificial life support encompasses a broad range of interventions intended to carry out vital functions that are temporarily or permanently impaired:

Cardiopulmonary Resuscitation (CPR)—giving mouth-to-mouth resuscitation and pressing on the chest to maintain breathing and circulation in the event that the heart and/or respiration ceases.

Defibrillation—an electrical charge applied through two paddles placed on the chest to correct an abnormal heartbeat or to restart a heart that has stopped pumping.

Intubation—the insertion of a flexible *endotracheal tube* down the mouth or nose and into the windpipe (trachea). The tube may be hooked up to a mechanical respirator if the patient cannot breathe independently.

> **Choice in Dying**
>
> 1035 30th Street
> Washington, D.C. 20007
> 800-989-9455 or
> 202-338-9790
> *http://www.choices.org*
>
> **If ordering advance-directive forms by mail, Choice in Dying requests that you enclose a $5 donation.**

Mechanical Respiration—a machine that forces air in and out of the lungs; attached to either an endotracheal tube or a surgically created opening through the neck and into the windpipe *(tracheostomy).*

Kidney Dialysis—a machine that filters the blood when the kidneys cannot do this on their own.

Drug Therapy—Powerful medications can be administered to stabilize the heart rhythm, break up blood clots causing a heart attack, reduce a potentially deadly swelling of the brain, or fight infection, among other uses. Patients have the right to refuse any type of drug.

Transfusions—both of whole blood or specific blood cells.

Artificial Feeding/Hydration—If a patient cannot eat or drink on his own, fluids and nutrients can be infused directly into the bloodstream.

Parenteral nutrition, as this is called, is usually a short-term measure. Liquid nourishment can also be poured into a feeding tube. A *nasogastric* (NG) *tube* is inserted through a nostril and into the stomach. A tube can also be surgically implanted into the stomach *(gastrostomy)* or the small intestine *(jejunostomy)*.

Emergency Surgeries/Invasive Tests—If you are unconscious, your loved ones may find themselves in the position of having to decide quickly whether or not to give their consent for a potentially lifesaving operative procedure.

The reason we recommend appointing a family member or friend your health-care proxy or *attorney-in-fact* is that the definition of "extraordinary measures" can fluctuate in conjunction with your condition. Is it an extraordinary measure for a doctor to place a patient with acute renal failure on dialysis if she could be expected to recover and perhaps enjoy another few productive months of life? If death were imminent, and your heart stopped beating, would you want to have a Do Not Resuscitate order in place, or would you want every attempt made to revive you? How you feel about this today may not be how you'll feel about it next year, next month, next week.

Again, these are your decisions to make. We suggest that patients specify what they would want done under the following circumstances: (1) if they fell into an irreversible coma or persistent vegetative state; (2) if implementing life support would merely be postponing the moment of death; (3) any situation in which the discomfort and/or emotional suffering that might be caused by an intervention outweighs its anticipated benefit.

Once your advice directives are completed, give copies to your attending physician (and include phone numbers for contacting the medical proxy). Equally important: Discuss your instructions with the person you have designated, more than once. You can never assume that other people know what you would want done medically in an emergency.

Choose the Setting for Your Care

The hospice-care movement has been quietly but steadily growing in the United States, where the first hospice opened in Connecticut in

1974. There are approximately 3,200 hospice programs across the country, serving half a million patients—seven in ten of whom are people with cancer. In the 1990s, the number of new hospices that opened and the number of patients that used hospice care rose roughly 15 percent every year.

Hospice's philosophy of humane, compassionate care delivered primarily at home holds a great deal of appeal. According to a nationwide 1996 Gallup poll, nine in ten adults said that if they were terminally ill and had six months or less to live, they would prefer to be cared for at home. Yet four in five of us spend the end of our lives in a hospital or nursing home. Among hospice patients, however, only about one in four do not die at home, as per their wishes.

A nurse coordinates the care plan for each patient. The nurses are particularly skilled at symptom control, an important feature of hospice care. Other members of the hospice team visit the patient at home as needed: physicians, home health aides, social workers, occupational therapists, counselors, and clergy. In addition, hospices provide medications, supplies, equipment, and hospital services related to the terminal illness. Volunteers are available to spell loved ones, who are also entitled to counseling. Although someone from the hospice will not be at your home all the time, staff members are on call twenty-four hours a day, seven days a week.

Hospice services are available to people who have been declared terminal by their doctor, with an estimated life expectancy of six months or less. Most types of health insurance cover hospice care, which wasn't the case just a short time ago. From 1984 to 1997, the total number of hospices participating in Medicare soared from 31 to 2,274. Currently, nearly 80 percent of hospices are Medicare-certified. The same percentage of managed-care plans and plans for employees in medium and large businesses also include hospice benefits. As for Medicaid, more than forty states plus the District of Columbia now pay for hospice care. Insurers have found that hospice care is highly cost-effective; because 90 percent of the hours of caring for an ill person take place in the home, it is about one-fifth as expensive per day than an average hospital stay.

Medicare hospice coverage pays for physicians' services; intermittent nursing care; medical appliances and supplies related to the terminal illness; outpatient drugs for symptom management and pain relief;

short-term acute inpatient care, including respite care; home health-aide and homemaker services; physical therapy, occupational therapy, and speech/language pathology; medical social services counseling, including dietary and spiritual counseling. The hospice benefit is divided into the following benefit periods:

- An initial ninety-day period
- A subsequent ninety-day period
- An unlimited number of subsequent sixty-day benefit periods as long as the patient continues to meet program eligibility requirements

If you should recover and your cancer goes into remission, you can be discharged from hospice care without forfeiting your coverage at a later date. In fact, Medicare and most private insurers will allow additional coverage for this purpose.

Hospice care is not for everyone, however. Some patients prefer the security of the hospital, particularly if there is no one at home capable of looking after them. It is important to discuss this option carefully with your family members and to ask the doctor, nurse, or hospital social worker for guidance.

The doctor or social worker can refer you for hospice care. Or, to find local programs on your own, contact either of the two organizations below. Both maintain on-line databases of hospice programs throughout the country.

National Association for Home Care
228 7th Street, S.E., Washington, DC 20003
202-547-7424
http://www.nahc.org

National Hospice Organization
1700 Diagonal Road, Suite 300, Alexandria, VA 22314
800-658-8898 (Hospice Information Line) or 703-243-5900
http://www.nho.org

I'm Cured! (Aren't I?)

In June 1992, Secretary of State Jim Baker swore me in as ambassador to Canada. Four hundred or so people attended the ceremony at the State Department, including my family, my elderly parents, and First Lady Barbara Bush.

It was certainly a time for reflection, not only upon the events of the past year but on my life. As I gazed at my mother and father from the stage, I thought of how we had been bombed out of two homes during the German air raids of World War II, and how I was the first person in the Teeley family to have graduated from college. My mother, who died later that year, had never been able to continue her education past grade school because the Depression was on in England too, and she'd had to go work in the weaving mills.

Our time spent in Ottawa, Canada, was marvelous. Adrienne and Randall especially loved it there, with all the snow and a terrific school. To this day, they still say wistfully, "I wish I was back in Ottawa." Unfortunately for us, that November the Democratic candidate for the White House, Arkansas Governor Bill Clinton, edged out George Bush for the presidency, and by early 1993 we were back in Washington. I accepted a position with Amgen, Inc., as vice-president of government and public relations.

I truly felt my cancer was behind me, though several more years would have to pass before I could be considered fully cured. Some forms of the disease, such as breast cancer and melanoma, can recur as long as thirty years later. With colon cancer, survival beyond two years is considered significant. As Dr. Marshall likes to tell patients, at two years past diagnosis they can throw a small party, and at five years, a big party.

The further away you get from your cancer diagnosis, the more it recedes into the past. But the passage of time never totally erases from the back of your mind the nagging fear of a recurrence or of a new cancer surfacing elsewhere.

Just a few months before I reached the five-year mark, I returned to the Lombardi Cancer Center for my annual CT scan. Everything seemed routine. The next day I came back to my office from lunch to find a message from Dr. Marshall waiting for me. *Uh-oh, something's wrong.* An earlier scan had revealed a mysterious spot on my liver, the most frequent site of metastasis from colon cancer. What if it had changed in size or shape?

We played phone tag for several hours, and as the day crawled by, I grew increasingly anxious. Finally, late in the afternoon, Dr. Marshall reached me. "Oh, by the way," he said, almost as an afterthought. "I just got your CT scan, and it looks great."

Right, I thought. *I knew that.*

Cancer Organizations Offering Information and Support for Patients and Families

Info on the Internet: Most organizations' educational materials, including their newsletters, are also available on their Web sites.

General Cancer Organizations and Hot Lines

AMC Cancer Research Center Cancer Information and Counseling Line
1600 Pierce Street, Lakewood, CO 80214
(800) 525-3777 or (303) 239-3424

Patient Services: The AMC's Cancer Information and Counseling Line, launched in 1981, handles ten thousand calls a year. Its professional counselors can give you information relating to treatment, obtaining a second opinion, and coping emotionally with the disease.

- Phone support/counseling
- Medical-care info/referrals
- Help in locating community services

Educational Publications: Yes.

American Cancer Society
1599 Clifton Road, N.E., Atlanta, GA 30329

(800) 227-2345 or (404) 320-3333
http://www.cancer.org (Web site)

Patient Services:

Calling the toll-free number above puts you directly in touch with your local division of the American Cancer Society. Either a nurse or the medical-affairs director can answer questions and make referrals regarding diagnosis, treatment, second opinions, clinical trials, and community resources. The ACS also offers a number of services and programs for people with cancer:

- Help in locating community services
- Financial aid
- Medical-equipment loans
- Patient advocacy
- Medical-care info/referrals
- Transportation services
- Lodging
- Legal advice/referrals
- Insurance info

Look Good . . . Feel Better, a free single-session program that is usually conducted in hospitals, shows patients undergoing chemotherapy or radiation how to use makeup, wigs, and other accessories to enhance their self-image and self-confidence.

The American Cancer Society also publishes *TLC,* a catalog of special products for breast-cancer patients and any woman experiencing treatment-related hair loss. Among the products described: hats, turbans, kerchiefs, hairpieces, mastectomy bras, and breast forms.

Transportation to and from cancer-treatment appointments. If no volunteer driver is available, the ACS will reimburse your expenses for public transportation.

Short-term crisis counseling, consisting of four to six sessions, for patients and/or family members who cannot afford professional therapy.

Interceding on behalf of patients involved in medical-insurance disputes. If, for instance, you are denied future health coverage after being treated successfully for cancer, the ACS might bring the case before the state insurance commissioner.

Free loans of wigs to patients experiencing hair loss from treatment and partial reimbursement to those who purchase their own wigs. If you've undergone or are about to undergo a mastectomy, and are considering wearing an artificial breast, you can make an appointment to visit your local ACS office, where a volunteer will show you the different types of external prostheses available. The American Cancer Society provides breast prostheses free of charge to women who cannot afford them.

Limited financial assistance for home health care, medical equipment, child care, and pain medication for patients with no medical insurance or with limited coverage.

> *Also see American Cancer Society Hope Lodges under "Housing/Lodging Assistance" in Appendix B.*

Support Groups:

CanSurmount, available upon request, links a newly diagnosed cancer patient with a cancer survivor for one-to-one support. Family members, too, can be put in touch with someone who has gone through a loved one's battle with cancer.

I Can Cope is a cancer-education program consisting of eight weekly two-hour classes, typically held at a local hospital. Physicians, nurses, social workers, and other health-care professionals explain the nature of the disease and its treatment, offer practical advice, and answer questions.

The ACS also sponsors several groups tailored to the needs of specific cancer-patient populations, such as those with breast cancer and prostate cancer and those who have had laryngectomies. *In this appendix, see Reach to Recovery under "Breast Cancer"; Man to Man under "Prostate Cancer"; and International Association of Laryngectomees under "Laryngectomy."*

Educational Publications: Yes.

Newsletter: Local divisions publish their own newsletters.

Bloch Cancer Hot Line
4400 Main Street, Kansas City, MO 64111
(800) 433-0464 or (816) 932-8453
http://www.blochcancer.org (Web site)

Patient Services: All the volunteers who staff the Bloch Cancer Hot Line are cancer survivors like Richard Bloch, founder of

- Phone support/counseling
- Medical-care info/referrals

the R. A. Bloch Cancer Foundation and the "R" in the venerable tax firm H&R Block. Call for information on obtaining a second opinion

---

National services:

- **Phone support/counseling**
- **Medical-care info/referrals**
- **Help in locating community services**
- **Legal advice/referrals**
- **Insurance info**

---

or if you simply need a sympathetic ear or a pep talk.

Cancer Care
275 Seventh Avenue, 22nd Floor, New York, NY 10001
(800) 813-4673 or (212) 221-3300
http://www.cancercare.org (Web site)
info@cancercare.org (e-mail)

Patient Services: Cancer Care, the largest agency dedicated exclusively to serving cancer patients and their families, provides a number of local services in the New York–New Jersey–Connecticut area, including support groups, professional counseling, and financial assistance. On the national level, the organization helps cancer patients and family members over the phone and on-line. No matter where you live, an oncology social worker can direct you to agencies that offer transportation to and from treatment, child care, and so on. Throughout the year, Cancer Care arranges free educational teleconferences—seminars that you can "attend" via telephone. Among the practical concerns that are addressed: how to cope with side effects of treatment, learning relaxation exercises, and legal advice.

Support Groups: In addition to the more than one hundred cancer support groups that meet at Cancer Care's offices, the agency conducts groups on the Internet, each led by an oncology social worker.

Educational Publications: Yes.

Newsletter: *CancerCare News.*

Cancer Hope Network
2 North Road, Suite A, Chester, NJ 07930-2308
(877) 467-3638 or (908) 879-4039
http://www.cancerhopenetwork.org (Web site)
info@cancerhopenetwork.org (e-mail)

Patient Services: Cancer Hope Network matches patients undergoing cancer treatment with trained cancer survivors who went through the same form of therapy, for one-to-one telephone counseling. Volunteers who have shared the cancer experience with a loved one are also available to provide hope and support to family members.

> • **Phone support/counseling**

Cancer Information Service
(800) 422-6237
Fax: (301) 402-5874
http://cancernet.nci.nih.gov (Web site)
cancernet@icicb.nci.nih.gov (e-mail)

Patient Services: The Cancer Information Service, a program of the National Cancer Institute, is a national telephone service for both the public and health professionals. Dialing the toll-free number connects you to one of nineteen regional offices. The CIS's trained information specialists can research the

> • **Medical-care info/referrals**
> • **Help in locating community services**

NCI's comprehensive PDQ (Physician Data Query) database and send you selected summaries of treatment options for more than seventy-five forms of cancer, printouts of open clinical trials in your geographical region, and a great deal more. Or you can access PDQ yourself by fax or by visiting the CancerNet Web site, which includes a listing of more than sixteen hundred clinical trials.

Educational Publications: Yes.

Cancervive
6500 Wilshire Boulevard, Suite 500, Los Angeles, CA 90048
(310) 203-9232
http://www.cancervive.org (Web site)

Patient Services: If no support groups exist in your area, Cancervive's head of patient services, a social worker, can offer counseling over the phone. The organization, founded in 1985 by a survivor of childhood cancer, provides referrals to attorneys around the country who specialize in representing victims of job discrimination or health-insurance discrimination.

> • **Phone support/counseling**
> • **Legal advice/referrals**
> • **Insurance info**

Support Groups: In California, Illinois, Texas, New York.

Educational Publications: In addition to publishing books on cancer-related issues, Cancervive has produced several educational videos, which it will send you free of charge. Topics include the impact of cancer on women survivors and on patients' spouses and children.

Newsletter: *Cancervive.*

Make Today Count
1235 East Cherokee, Springfield, MO 65804-2263
(800) 432-2273 (ask for Make Today Count)

Patient Services: A social worker is available to advise callers of services in their community, indigent-patient prescription-drug programs, and so on.

> • **Help in locating community services**

Support Groups: There are approximately two hundred Make Today Count support groups around the country for people with cancer and other life-threatening illnesses, as well as family members and friends.

Educational Publications: Yes.

Newsletter: *The Messenger.*

National Coalition for Cancer Survivorship
1010 Wayne Avenue, Suite 505, Silver Spring, MD 20910-5600
(877) 622-7937
http://www.cansearch.org (Web site)
info@cansearch.org (e-mail)

Patient Services: The NCCS, founded in 1986 by a group of cancer survivors, serves as a clearinghouse of information on issues such as job discrimination and health insurance. The organization can also refer you to cancer-patient support groups or help you start one. Its Web site includes CanSearch, an extensive guide to cancer-related information on the Internet.

> • **Legal advice/referrals**
> • **Insurance info**

Educational Publications: Yes.

Newsletter: *Networker.*

National Organization for Rare Disorders
P.O. Box 8923, New Fairfield, CT 06812-8923
(800) 999-6673 or (203) 746-6518
http://www.nord-rdb.com/~orphan (Web site)
orphan@nord-rdb.com (e-mail)

Patient Services: Many cancers meet the definition of a rare disease: one that affects fewer than 200,000 people in the United States. The National Organization for Rare Disorders is a federation of more than 140 voluntary health organizations serving people with rare medical conditions. You can order information from NORD's Rare Disease Database or access it yourself through the organization's Web site. Other services of interest include:

- Medical-care info/referrals
- Financial aid

NORD administers medication-assistance programs for approximately ten pharmaceutical companies. Different drugs, including those in clinical trials, are awarded to patients who cannot otherwise afford them.

The Medical Equipment Exchange program enables patients to buy and sell preowned medical equipment.

Support Groups: NORD runs several support groups throughout the United States and can refer you to others. It also maintains a confidential patient-networking program.

Educational Publications: Yes.

Newsletter: *Orphan Disease Update.*

Patient Advocate Foundation
780 Pilot House Drive, Suite 100-C, Newport News, VA 23606
(800) 532-5274 or (757) 873-6668
http://www.patientadvocate.org/ (Web site)
patient@pinn.net (e-mail)

Patient Services: PAF runs two programs designed to help cancer patients who need legal advice or representation.

National Legal Resource Network provides free legal counseling to patients who are experiencing problems such as employment dis-

• **Legal advice/referrals**
• **Insurance info**

crimination and are being denied insurance coverage. The foundation's attorney-consultants can intervene on your behalf with creditors to negotiate a reduction or deferment of outstanding payments while you are receiving treatment. They can also help you to obtain any federal or state aid to which you may be entitled. All reviews of patients' cases are *pro bono,* meaning donated free of charge. Should a patient choose to go forward with litigation, it is up to him and the lawyer to agree upon a fee. Attorneys often work on a contingency basis: If the suit is successful, they receive a predetermined percentage of the settlement or damages awarded.

National Managed Care Resource Network links you with an oncology case manager, who can answer questions you may have about your managed-care medical coverage. The case manager can also negotiate directly with your HMO to resolve disputes concerning coverage and benefits. This service, too, is free.

Educational Publications: Yes.

Organizations and Hot Lines for Patients with a Specific Form of Cancer or Cancer-Related Condition

Amputation

American Amputee Foundation
P.O. Box 250218, Little Rock, AR 72225
(501) 666-2523 or (501) 666-9540

Patient Services: The American Amputee Foundation can help patients with insurance disputes and explain how to obtain financial aid for artificial limbs and home modifications. Every two years the

• **Insurance info**

AAF publishes a *National Resource Directory* of services and products for amputees.

Support Groups: Over 120 support groups in thirty-six states and the District of Columbia.

Educational Publications: Yes.

Newsletter: *Life Care Planning.*

Bone-Marrow Transplant Recipients or Prospective Recipients

Blood & Marrow Transplant Newsletter
2900 Skokie Valley Road, Highland Park, IL 60035
(888) 597-7674 or (847) 433-3313
http://www.bmtnews.org (Web site)
help@bmtnews.org (e-mail)

Patient Services: If you're being denied insurance coverage for a bone-marrow transplant, the Blood & Marrow Transplant Newsletter, a nonprofit organization, can refer you to at-torneys who have successfully persuaded medical insurers to pay for transplant-related

- Legal advice/referrals
- Insurance info

expenses—usually without resorting to litigation. Most of the lawyers on its referral list do not charge for an initial consultation. Fees there-after vary and should be discussed directly with the attorney.

Support Groups: The Patient-to-Survivor Link matches patients about to undergo a bone-marrow, stem-cell, or cord-blood transplant with transplant survivors, for emotional support.

Educational Publications: Yes.

Newsletter: *Blood & Marrow Transplant Newsletter.*

Caitlin Raymond International Registry
University of Massachusetts Medical Center
55 Lake Avenue North, Worcester, MA 01655
(800) 726-2824 or (508) 792-8969
http://www.crir.org (Web site)
info@CRIR.org (e-mail)

Patient Services: The Caitlin Raymond International Registry conducts searches for unrelated marrow donors from all available donor registries and umbilical-cord blood banks around the world (except for

- **Medical-care info/referrals**
- **Help in locating community services**

the National Marrow Donor Program), giving it access to more than 2.2 million volunteer donors. The organization's patient-services staff can answer your questions about marrow transplantation, direct you to the nearest transplant center, and advise you on finding financial aid and services in your community.

National Marrow Donor Program
3433 Broadway Street, N.E., Suite 500, Minneapolis, MN 55413
(888) 999-6743 or (612) 627-5800
http://www.marrow.org (Web site)
webmaster@nmdp.org (e-mail)

Patient Services: The National Marrow Donor Program maintains an international registry of more than 3 million volunteer unrelated bone-marrow donors. Federally funded, it matches donors and recipients, coordinates the tissue-typing blood tests necessary for determining genetic compatibility, and helps to facilitate transplantation arrangements. The office of patient advocacy can advise you about choosing a transplant center, intervene on your behalf with insurance companies to win coverage, assist you in finding alternative sources of funding, and conduct personalized searches of current medical literature.

- **Patient advocacy**
- **Medical-care info/referrals**
- **Insurance info**
- **Help in locating community services**

Support Groups: The NMDP can refer you to support groups.

Educational Publications: Yes.

National Foundation for Transplants
1102 Brookfield, Suite 200, Memphis, TN 38119
(800) 489-3863 or (901) 684-1697
http://www.transplants.org (Web site)
nftpr@aol.com (e-mail)

Patient Services: The National Foundation for Transplants, formerly known as the Organ Transplant Fund, assists patients who are looking to raise money for a bone-marrow transplant or organ transplant. It also issues small financial grants to cover the cost of the immunosuppressive drugs that transplant recipients must take following the expensive procedure.

> • **Financial aid**
> • **Patient advocacy**

The Patient Fund-Raising Program assigns a staff person to each fund-raising drive. He or she meets with the family to help them launch the campaign, then stays in contact by phone after that. The foundation handles the account for the patient, paying the hospital and doctor bills and reimbursing the family for its expenses. Because it is a nonprofit organization, all fund-raising campaigns receive the tax benefits of nonprofit status.

The foundation, started in 1983, also serves as a patient advocate. For instance, a transplant center may refuse to add a patient to its list of prospective transplant recipients until a certain amount of money has been paid. If a patient is not yet at that threshold but funds are coming in regularly, the organization will intervene and try to influence the institution to list the person now.

National Transplant Assistance Fund

6 Bryn Mawr Avenue, P.O. Box 258, Bryn Mawr, PA 19010
(800) 642-8399 or (610) 527-5056
http://www.transplantfund.org (Web site)
NTAF@transplantfund.org (e-mail)

Patient Services: The National Transplant Assistance Fund serves patients and families seeking bone-marrow or organ transplants. Call the NTAF to find out the location of transplant centers, the cost of transplants,

> • **Financial aid**

and possible sources of financial assistance. The organization offers modest medical-assistance grants to eligible patients to help offset immediate transplant-related costs, such as relocations, medications, home care, and transportation. The NTAF can also assist you in establishing a tax-deductible account for raising funds, which it distributes for you. Four percent of all money is retained by the organization.

Support Groups: A transplant recipient who has raised funds through the NTAF can offer support and advice to patients just beginning the process.

Educational Publications: Yes

Newsletter: *The New Start News.*

Brain Cancer

American Brain Tumor Association
2720 River Road, Des Plaines, IL 60018
(800) 886-2282 (patient line) or (847) 827-9910
http://www.abta.org (Web site)
info@abta.org (e-mail)

> **Patient Services:** The ABTA's patient line can refer you to community services and aid for people with brain cancer.

> • **Help in locating community services**

> **Support Groups:** Connections, a pen-pal program.

> **Educational Publications:** Yes.

> **Newsletter:** *Message Line.*

Brain Tumor Society
124 Watertown Street, Suite 3-H, Watertown, MA 02472
(800) 770-8287 or (617) 924-9997
http://www.tbts.org (Web site)
info@tbts.org (e-mail)

> **Patient Services:** The Brain Tumor Society, primarily a research and education organization, publishes a useful resource booklet for patients titled *Color Me Hope.* Its telephone volunteers can give you up-to-date information on treatment options.

> • **Medical-care info/referrals**

> **Support Groups:** The BTS can refer you to brain-tumor support groups; the society also sponsors a telephone network program for patients and family members.

> **Educational Publications:** Yes.

> **Newsletter:** *Heads Up.*

National Brain Tumor Foundation
414 Thirteenth Street, Suite 700, Oakland, CA 94612-2603
(800) 934-2873 or (510) 839-9777
http://www.braintumor.org (Web site)
nbtf@braintumor.org (e-mail)

Patient Services: The National Brain Tumor Foundation, launched in 1981 by a group of brain-tumor survivors and their families, can apprise you of clinical trials for brain cancer and refer you to medical centers that specialize in treating the disease. Its Medical Advisor Helpline offers a free consultation with a neuroscience nurse.

> • **Phone support/counseling**
> • **Medical-care info/referrals**

Support Groups: The NBTF can refer you to more than 120 support groups nationwide or help you to start one. You can also be put in touch with other patients and family members through its Support Line Network.

Educational Publications: Yes.

Newsletter: Search.

Breast Cancer

National Alliance of Breast Cancer Organizations
9 East 37th Street, 10th Floor, New York, NY 10016
(800) 889-0606 or (212) 719-9154
http://www.nabco.org (Web site)
NABCOinfo@aol.com (e-mail)

Patient Services: NABCO represents more than 375 breast-cancer-related organizations. Its Web site lists all clinical trials for breast cancer contained in the National Cancer Institute's Physician Data Query (PDQ) database.

> • **Medical-care info/referrals**

Support Groups: The alliance can refer you to local support groups for women with breast cancer.

Educational Publications: Yes.

Newsletter: NABCO News.

Reach to Recovery
American Cancer Society
1599 Clifton Road, N.E., Atlanta, GA 30329

(800) 227-2345 or (404) 320-3333
http://www.cancer.org (Web site)

This program from the American Cancer Society pairs a newly diagnosed breast-cancer patient with a trained breast-cancer survivor,
who can provide emotional support and practical advice. She will visit
you at the hospital, your home, the local American Cancer Society office, or another location of your choosing.

Y-ME National Breast Cancer Organization
212 West Van Buren Street, 5th Floor, Chicago, IL 60607-3908
(800) 221-2141 or (312) 986-8338
http://www.y-me.org (Web site)
help@yme.org (e-mail)

Patient Services: Y-ME was founded in 1978 by two breast-
cancer patients. The organization can refer you to comprehensive
breast centers, breast-cancer specialists, and
treatment and research hospitals. It also runs
a wig and prosthesis bank.

- Phone support/counseling
- Medical-care info/referrals

Support Groups: Y-ME sponsors a network of chapters and support groups. Call its national hot line to speak to women who have had
breast cancer; men volunteers are also available to speak to the male
partners of women with breast cancer.

Educational Publications: Yes.

Newsletter: *Y-ME Hotline.*

Carcinoid Cancers

National Carcinoid Support Group
P.O. Box 44233, Madison, WI 53744-4233
http://members.aol.com/thencsg (Web site)
jean@mick.com (e-mail)

Patient Services: The National Carcinoid Support Group can
steer you to specialists with experience in treating these rare cancers.

- Phone support/counseling
- Medical care info/referrals

Support Groups: The NCSG sponsors
monthly conference calls, where men and

women with carcinoid cancer can swap tips, experiences, and emotions. E-mail the organization for the long-distance telephone number to call. You need a touch-tone phone.

Educational Publications: Yes.

Newsletter: *Rays of Hope.*

Head and Neck Cancers

AboutFace
123 Edward Street, Suite 1003, Toronto, Ontario, Canada M5G1E2
(800) 225-3223
In Canada: (800) 665-3223
http://www.interlog.com/~abtface (Web site)
abtface@interlog.com (e-mail)

Patient Services: AboutFace is an international support and information network for people with facial differences—mainly from birth defects and injuries, but also as a result of disfiguring surgery for head and neck cancers. It has approximately twenty-five chapters in the United States.

> • **Phone support/counseling**

Support Groups: Many AboutFace chapters run support groups. In addition, the organization can put you in touch with other members, either by mail or by phone. Trained volunteers can visit patients in the hospital, to provide support.

Educational Publications: Yes.

Newsletter: *AboutFace.*

Support for People with Oral and Head and Neck Cancer
P.O. Box 53, Locust Valley, NY 11560-0053
(516) 759-5333
http://www.spohnc.org (Web site)
info@spohnc.org (e-mail)

Newsletter: *News from SPOHNC,* published nine times a year, contains information on clinical trials, conventional and alternative therapies, employment issues, oral care, and personal stories from patients.

See National Foundation for Facial Reconstruction under "Financial Assistance" in Appendix B.

Impotence

Impotence Institute of America
Impotence World Association
P.O. Box 410, Bowie, MD 20718-0410
(800) 669-1603 or (301) 262-2400
http://www.impotenceworld.org (Web site)
info@impotenceworld.org (e-mail)

Patient Services: Surgery and radiation therapy to treat prostate cancer can result in impotence. To receive a list of physicians who specialize in diagnosing and treating the condition, and psychotherapists,

> • **Medical-care info/referrals**

send a self-addressed stamped envelope to the Impotence Institute of America.

Support Groups: The IIA can refer you to two related groups: Impotents Anonymous (IA), for men and their partners, and I-Anon for the partners of impotent men.

Educational Publications: Yes.

Newsletter: *Impotence Worldwide.*

Incontinence

National Association for Continence
P.O. Box 8310, Spartanburg, SC 29305-8310
(800) 252-3337 or (864) 579-7900
http://www.nafc.org (Web site)
llouden@nafc.org (e-mail)

Patient Services: Incontinence is a potential complication of prostate surgery and radiation. NAFC members can take advantage of

its Continence Resource Service: Send a self-addressed stamped envelope to receive a list of urologists who specialize in treating incontinence caused by cancer treatment. The | • **Medical-care info/referrals** |
association publishes *The Resource Guide,* a
directory of incontinence-related products and services. It also produces instructional videos and audiotapes such as *Pelvic Muscle Exercises,* which may be helpful for men experiencing urine leakage following prostate-cancer therapy.

Educational Publications: Yes.

Newsletter: *Quality Care.*

Simon Foundation for Continence
P.O. Box 835, Wilmette, IL 60091
(800) 237-4666 or (847) 864-3913
http://www.simonfoundation.org (Web site)
simoninfo@simonfoundation.org (e-mail)

Patient Services: Absorbent products for incontinence are expensive and not covered by insurance. Local chapters of the Simon Foundation's National Continence Cooperative can help to reduce the cost by purchasing products in bulk and making them available to members at substantial discounts. | • **Patient advocacy** |

Support Groups: The Simon Foundation sponsors support groups as well as on-line discussion groups.

Educational Publications: Yes.

Newsletter: *The Informer.*

Kidney Cancer

National Kidney Cancer Association
1234 Sherman Avenue, Suite 203, Evanston, IL 60202-1375
(800) 850-9132 or (847) 332-1051
http://www.nkca.org (Web site)
office@nkca.org (e-mail)

Patient Services: The NKCA, founded by a small group of patients and physicians, can refer you to kidney-cancer specialists. It has also assisted members in getting their insurance companies to pay for experimental treatments. Check the association's Web site for information about clinical trials, some of which may not be listed in the National Cancer Institute's database.

- Patient advocacy
- Medical-care info/referrals
- Insurance info

Support Groups: NKCA members host two on-line chat groups. Contact the organization for more information.

Educational Publications: Yes.

Newsletter: *Kidney Cancer News.*

Laryngectomy

International Association of Laryngectomees
American Cancer Society
1599 Clifton Road, N.E., Atlanta, GA 30329
(800) 227-2345 or (404) 320-3333
http://www.cancer.org (Web site)

Patient Services: The American Cancer Society helps sponsor most of the approximately three hundred IAL clubs in the United States. These clubs, known as "Lost Chord" or "New Voice" clubs, consist of anywhere from ten to three hundred members each, all of them laryngectomees. The association can refer you to a speech instructor.

- Medical-care info/referrals

Support Groups: Most IAL clubs conduct a visitors' program. At a doctor's request, members who are rehabilitated from their laryngectomies call on patients in the hospital, to show them that a return to normal life is possible.

Educational Publications: Yes.

Newsletter: *IAL News.*

Leukemia, Lymphomas, Multiple Myeloma

Cure for Lymphoma Foundation
215 Lexington Avenue, New York, NY 10016
(800) 235-6848 or (212) 213-9595
http://www.cfl.org (Web site)
infocfl@cfl.org (e-mail)

Support Groups: The Cure for Lymphoma Foundation, primarily a fund-raising organization that underwrites cancer research, can refer you to a support group. Its Patient-to-Patient Telephone Network matches newly diagnosed lymphoma patients with others who have been through treatment.

Educational Publications: Yes.

Newsletter: Together.

Leukemia Society of America
600 Third Avenue, New York, NY 10016
(800) 955-4572 or (212) 573-8484
http://www.leukemia.org (Web site)

Patient Services: The Leukemia Society of America offers supplementary financial assistance and support programs for people with leukemia, Hodgkin's disease, non-Hodgkin's lymphoma, and multiple myeloma. Its Patient Aid Program reimburses patients up to $750 a year for various treatment-related expenses, including specific drugs, therapies, and transportation to and from a doctor's office, hospital, treatment center, or one of the LSA's family support groups. To apply, call the toll-free number for a referral to one of the LSA's approximately 60 local chapters. You can also fill out an application on-line through the society's Web site.

> • Financial aid

Support Groups: The Family Support Group Program is provided free of charge to patients and family members. Each group is led by two credentialed health/mental-health professionals experienced in issues of importance to people with cancer. Another program, First Connection, matches a newly diagnosed patient with a volunteer who is in remission for a onetime visit or phone call.

Educational Publications: Yes.

Newsletter: *Newsline.*

Lymphoma Foundation of America
P.O. Box 15335, Chevy Chase, MD 20825
(202) 223-6181

Patient Services: The Lymphoma Foundation of America, founded in 1986 by people with lymphoma, can refer you to special-

> • **Medical-care info/referrals**
> • **Legal advice/referrals**

ists in the disease. If you've been a victim of job discrimination, it can direct you to legal experts who can advise you of your rights.

Support Groups: The foundation's buddy program can put you in touch with someone who has recovered from lymphoma.

Educational Publications: Yes.

Lymphoma Research Foundation of America
8800 Venice Boulevard, Suite 207, Los Angeles, CA 90034
(310) 204-7040
http://www.lymphoma.org (Web site)
LRFA@aol.com (e-mail)

Patient Services: In addition to funding research, the Lymphoma Research Foundation of America maintains a patient help line.

> • **Medical-care info/referrals**

Call for information on treatment options, including clinical trials.

Support Groups: Cell-Mates is a nationwide buddy program that links newly diagnosed callers with other lymphoma patients. The LRFA also sponsors support groups in Los Angeles.

Educational Publications: Yes.

Newsletter: *Lymphoma Update.*

International Myeloma Foundation
2129 Stanley Hills Drive, Los Angeles, CA 90046
(800) 452-2873

http://www.myeloma.org (Web site)
TheIMF@myeloma.org (e-mail)

Support Groups: The International Myeloma Foundation publishes a patient-to-patient directory that enables myeloma patients and/or their family members to meet, speak with, or e-mail other people with the disease.

Educational Publications: Yes.

Newsletter: *Myeloma Today.*

National Leukemia Research Association
585 Stewart Avenue, Suite 536, Garden City, NY 11530
(516) 222-1944

Patient Services: The National Leukemia Research Association, founded in 1965, raises funds to support leukemia research and to provide financial assistance to families whose insurance does not cover various medical expenses. Call or write for an application.

> • **Financial aid**

Lung Cancer

Alliance for Lung Cancer Advocacy, Support and Education
1601 Lincoln Avenue, Vancouver, WA 98660
(800) 298-2436 or (360) 696-2436
http://www.alcase.org (Web site)
info@alcase.org (e-mail)

Patient Services: ALCASE publishes *The Lung Cancer Resource Guide,* containing information and services for people with lung cancer and their families. The organization can conduct customized information searches of medical databases for patients.

Support Groups: The alliance sponsors Phone Buddies, a peer counseling program that matches lung-cancer survivors.

Educational Publications: Yes.

> • **Medical-care info/referrals**

Newsletter: *Spirit and Breath.*

Lymphedema

National Lymphedema Network
2211 Post Street, Suite 404, San Francisco, CA 94115-3427
(800) 541-3259 or (415) 921-1306
http://www.lymphnet.org (Web site)
lymphnet@hooked.net (e-mail)

Patient Services: The National Lymphedema Network, founded in 1988 by a registered nurse, can direct you to lymphedema treatment centers and health-care professionals. Its Web site is one of the most informative on the Internet.

- Phone support/counseling
- Patient advocacy
- Medical-care info/referrals

Support Groups: The NLN can refer you to a support group for people with lymphedema. It also sponsors a pen pals/Net pals network.

Educational Publications: Yes.

Newsletter: *NLN Newsletter.*

Oral Cancer

See "Head and Neck Cancers," page 921.

Ostomies

United Ostomy Association
19772 MacArthur Boulevard, Suite 200, Irvine, CA 92612-2405
(800) 826-0826 or (714) 660-8624
http://www.uoa.org (Web site)
uoa@deltanet.com (e-mail)

Patient Services: The United Ostomy Association can refer you to enterostomal nurses, as well as to distributors of ostomy equipment.

- Medical-care info/referrals

Support Groups: There are more than four hundred UOA chapters, each of which runs support groups for men and women with ostomies. The organization also sponsors a preoperative and postoperative patient-visitation program.

Educational Publications: Yes.

Newsletter: *Ostomy Quarterly.*

Ovarian Cancer

National Ovarian Cancer Coalition
P.O. Box 4472, Boca Raton, FL 33429-4472
(888) 682-7426 or (561) 393-0005
http://www.ovarian.org (Web site)
NOCC@ovarian.org (e-mail)

Patient Services: Contact the National Ovarian Cancer Coalition for referrals to gynecologic oncologists. Visitors to its extensive Web site can search a database containing thousands of books, audiotapes, and self-help resources for cancer survivors, chat with other patients, and have questions answered by the organization's medical advisory board.

> • **Medical-care info/referrals**

Support Groups: The NOCC has support groups in approximately two dozen states and can refer you to other support groups for women with ovarian cancer.

Educational Publications: Yes.

Newsletter: *NOCC Newsletter.*

Prostate Cancer

Man to Man
American Cancer Society
1599 Clifton Road, N.E., Atlanta, GA 30329
(800) 227-2345 or (404) 320-3333
http://www.cancer.org (Web site)

Patient Services: Man to Man's support-group meetings generally include an educational presentation by a health-care professional on a topic of interest to men with prostate cancer.

> • **Medical-care info/referrals**

Support Groups: In addition to its monthly support-group meetings, which are led by a trained facilitator, Man to Man provides one-to-one visitation and telephone support from specially trained prostate-cancer survivors.

Educational Publications: Yes.

Newsletter: *Man to Man News.*

US TOO International
930 North York Road, Suite 50, Hinsdale, IL 60521-2993
(800) 808-7866 or (630) 323-1002
http://www.ustoo.com (Web site)
ustoo@ustoo.com (e-mail)

Patient Services: US TOO's Web site lists clinical trials for prostate cancer, and its *Hot Sheet* publication features treatment-related news.

> • **Medical-care info/referrals**

Support Groups: US TOO support groups are located throughout the United States and Canada. Some sponsor Side by Side, a group for women partners of men with prostate cancer.

Educational Publications: Yes.

Newsletter: *US TOO Prostate Cancer Communicator.*

Thyroid Cancer

American Thyroid Association
Montefiore Medical Center, 111 East 210th Street, Bronx, NY 10467
(718) 920-4321
http://www.thyroid.org (Web site)
info@thyroid.org (e-mail)

Educational Publications: Yes.

Thyroid Foundation of America
350 Ruth Sleeper Hall, RSL 350, 40 Parkman Street,
Boston, MA 02114-2698

(800) 832-8321 or (617) 726-8500
http://www.tsh.org (Web site)
info@tsh.org (e-mail)

Educational Publications: Yes.

Newsletter: *The Bridge.*

Miscellaneous Resources for

People with Cancer

Acupuncturists
for Relieving Pain, Nausea, Anxiety

American Academy of Medical Acupuncture
5820 Wilshire Boulevard, Suite 500, Los Angeles, CA 90036
(800) 521-2262
http://www.medicalacupuncture.org (Web site)
JDOWDEN@prodigy.net (e-mail)

The academy will mail you, free of charge, a list of members in your state who have completed at least two hundred hours of training in medical acupuncture.

American Association of Oriental Medicine
433 Front St., Catasauqua, PA 18032
(888) 500-7999 or (610) 266-1433
http://www.aaom.org (Web site)
AAOM1@aol.com (e-mail)

To find AAOM-member acupuncturists in your state, visit the association's Web site and click on "Referrals."

National Certification Commission for Acupuncture and Oriental Medicine
11 Canal Center Plaza, Suite 300, Alexandria, VA 22314
(703) 548-9004
http://www.nccaom.org (Web site)
info@nccaom.org (e-mail)

For a list of certified acupuncturists in your state, send a $3 check or money order and a self-addressed stamped envelope.

Assistive Technology and Rehabilitation Equipment

Abledata
8401 Colesville Road, Suite 200, Silver Spring, MD 20910
(800) 227-0216
http://www.abledata.com (Web site)
belknap@macroint.com (e-mail)

Abledata, a free service of the National Institute on Disability and Rehabilitation Research, is an extensive database that contains detailed descriptions of more than 25,000 products for patients, from ostomy supplies and special bras for holding breast prostheses, to portable commodes and shower grab bars. Tell an Abledata information specialist the item you're looking for, and she can give you the manufacturer's phone number. You may also access this information twenty-four hours a day via the Internet.

Biofeedback Specialists
For Relieving Pain, Nausea, Anxiety

Association for Applied Psychophysiology and Biofeedback
10200 West 44th Avenue, Suite 304, Wheat Ridge, CO 80033-2840
http://www.aapb.org (Web site)
AAPB@resourcenter.com (e-mail)

Send a self-addressed stamped envelope to the AAPB to receive referrals to certified biofeedback therapists.

Clinical Trials Information

Centerwatch Clinical Trials Listing Service
22 Thomson Place, Boston MA 02210-1212
617-856-5900
http://www.centerwatch.com (Web site)
cntrwatch@aol.com(e-mail)

Centerwatch, a multimedia publishing company, hosts a Web site that provides all pertinent information about more than one thousand government- and industry-funded oncology clinical trials that are actively recruiting patients. You can search for investigational studies by geographic region. A related free feature is the Patient Notification Service. Type in your e-mail address and the type of cancer you have, and Centerwatch will automatically notify you by e-mail anytime a cancer drug receives FDA approval.

> *Also contact local cancer centers or the department of oncology at large teaching hospitals; local chapters of the cancer-patient support organizations listed in Appendix A; and call pharmaceutical manufacturers directly.*

> *Also see Cancer Information Service under "General Cancer Organizations and Hot Lines" in Appendix A.*

Community Assistance

Area Agencies on Aging
Eldercare Locator
(800) 677-1116
http://www.aoa.dhhs.gov/elderpage/locator.html (Web site)

Call Eldercare Locator for a referral to your Area Agency on Aging, of which there are more than 660 in the United States. AAAs arrange a variety of helpful services for elderly patients and family members, either directly or through contractors. Many are free; others are based on your ability to pay. You may find these and other programs:

- Transportation to and from medical visits
- Home health care
- Assistance with medical billing, filing claims and appeals, and resolving problems with Medicare, Medicaid, and Social Security supplemental insurance programs
- Homemaker and chore-maintenance services
- Adult day care
- Respite care
- Home meal delivery
- Telephone reassurance: regularly scheduled phone calls from volunteer seniors to homebound elderly persons living alone
- Legal assistance
- Mental-health services
- Case management

Catholic Charities USA
1731 King Street, Suite 200, Alexandria, VA 22314
(703) 549-1390
http://www.catholiccharitiesusa.org (Web site)
gwhite@catholiccharitiesusa.org (e-mail)

Catholic Charities USA is the country's largest private social service network, with more than fourteen hundred local agencies and institutions. Some of the organization's programs are free; others offer sliding-scale fees, based on your ability to pay. Among the services that may be offered:

- Transportation
- Family counseling
- Adult day care
- Child day care and after-school care
- Respite care
- Hospice care

National Association of Community Action Agencies
1100 17th Street, N.W., Washington, DC 20036
(202) 265-7546
http://www.nacaa.org (Web site)
info@nacaa.org (e-mail)

There are nearly one thousand Community Action Agencies across the United States, serving more than 34 million of the country's poorest people. Each nonprofit CAA receives government grants and private funds to help those in need through a variety of programs, including:

- Financial assistance
- Emergency food
- Child care
- Legal services
- Transportation to health-care facilities and appointments
- Low-cost pharmaceutical programs and health insurance
- Home meal delivery

United Way of America
701 North Fairfax Street, Alexandria, VA 22314-2045
(703) 836-7100 or (800) 411-8929
http://www.unitedway.org (Web site)

There are more than fourteen hundred local United Way organizations throughout the United States. Each funds an array of programs in its community. Services of interest to people with cancer may include home health care, adult day care, child care, family counseling, and transportation. Consult the white pages for your local United Way or call the organization's national headquarters. A toll-free number, listed above, can refer callers to many, though not all, United Ways.

Dietitians

American Dietetic Association's Consumer Nutrition Hotline
216 West Jackson Boulevard, Chicago, IL 60606-6995
(800) 366-1655
http://www.eatright.org (Web site)

The ADA can refer you to a registered dietitian, or you can conduct your own search on the association's Web site.

Financial Assistance

Government-Funded Programs

Social Security Administration
(800) 772-1213
http://www.ssa.gov (Web site)

Calling the toll-free number will direct you to one of the Social Security Administration's thirteen hundred local offices, where staff members can answer your questions about government-funded financial-assistance programs, eligibility requirements, and how to file for benefits. The SSA Web site contains information about Social Security Disability Income (SSDI), Supplemental Security Income (SSI), and Temporary Assistance for Needy Families (TANF).

Hill-Burton Program
5600 Fishers Lane, Room 7-47, Rockville, MD 20857
(800) 638-0742 or (301) 443-5656
In Maryland: (800) 492-0359
http://www.hrsa.dhhs.gov/osp/dfcr/about/aboutdiv.htm (Web site)

Approximately eighteen hundred hospitals in the United States receive federal funds in return for providing free or low-cost medical care to impoverished patients. Call the toll-free hot line for information on eligibility and a list of Hill-Burton programs in your area.

Privately Funded Programs

National Foundation for Facial Reconstruction
317 East 34th Street, Suite 901, New York, NY 10016
(212) 263-6656
http://www.nffr.org (Web site)
info@nffr.org (e-mail)

The NFFR, established in 1951, provides state-of-the-art facial re-constructive treatment, regardless of the patient's ability to pay, at its Institute of Reconstructive Plastic Surgery at New York University Medical Center. The foundation's primary focus is children with craniofacial abnormalities, but it has financed surgeries for men and women who were disfigured as a result of cancer.

Also see (in Appendix A):
American Amputee Foundation
   (for information on raising or obtaining funds)
American Cancer Society
   (for financial aid and low-cost or free medical care)
Leukemia Society of America
   (for financial aid)
National Foundation for Transplants
   (for financial aid and information on raising or obtaining funds)
National Marrow Donor Program
   (for information on raising or obtaining funds)
National Leukemia Research Association
   (for financial aid)
National Transplant Assistance Fund
   (for financial aid and information on raising or obtaining funds)
Y-Me
   (for loans of medical equipment or supplies)
Also see (in Appendix B):
National Association of Community Action Agencies
   (for financial aid)

Also see "Prescription-Drug Patient-Assistance Programs," page 947.

Health-Care Accreditation Organizations

Commission on Accreditation of Rehabilitation Facilities
4891 East Grant Road, Tucson, AZ 85712
(520) 325-1044
http://www.carf.org (Web site)
webmaster@carf.org (e-mail)

Send a self-addressed stamped envelope to CARF and receive a free list of accredited rehabilitation services near you.

Community Health Accreditation Program
61 Broadway, New York, NY 10006
(800) 669-1656 or (212) 363-5555
http://www.chapinc.org (Web site)
dfeinst@nln.org (e-mail)

CHAP, a subsidiary of the National League for Nursing, reviews and accredits several hundred home health-care agencies.

Foundation for Hospice and Home Care
228 7th Street S.E., Washington, DC 20003
(202) 547-7424
http://www.nahc.org (Web site)

Contact the foundation for help in locating an accredited home-care aide.

Joint Commission on Accreditation of Healthcare Organizations
One Renaissance Blvd., Oakbrook Terrace, IL 60181
(630) 792-5000
Department of Home Care Accreditation Services: (630) 792-3004
Complaint Office: (800) 994-6610 or (630) 792-5642
http://www.jcaho.org (Web site)

The JCAHO, the largest health-care accreditation organization of its kind, can refer you to home-care agencies and home medical-equipment companies.

Home Health Care

National Association for Home Care
228 7th Street, S.E., Washington, DC 20003
(202) 547-7424
http://www.nahc.org (Web site)

The NAHC can send you a list of state-licensed home-care agencies near you. Or tap into the association's Home Care/Hospice Agency Locator Web site, which contains information on more than 28,000 home-care and hospice agencies.

National Hospice Organization
1700 Diagonal Road, Suite 300, Alexandria, VA 22314
(800) 658-8898 (Hospice Information Line) or (703) 243-5900
http://www.nho.org (Web site)
webmaster@nho.org (e-mail)

The NHO can refer you to hospices in your area. Or use its "Find a Hospice" on-line database.

Visiting Nurse Associations of America
11 Beacon Street, Suite 910, Boston, MA 02108
(888) 866-8773 or (617) 227-4843
http://www.vnaa.org (Web site)
vnaa@vnaa.org (e-mail)

More than four hundred Visiting Nurse Associations around the country provide skilled nursing care, home health aides, social work and counseling, hospice care, and other in-home health services. The toll-free national referral line listed above will direct you to the nearest VNA.

Home Meal Delivery Services

National Meals on Wheels Foundation
2675 44th Street S.W., Suite 305, Grand Rapids, MI 49509
(616) 531-9909

If you're homebound, without anyone to cook for you, contact the National Meals on Wheels Foundation, which can direct you to the meals program serving your community. Approximately twenty thousand Meals on Wheels services nationwide deliver prepared lunches and sometimes dinners five days a week. The meals may be free, or a nominal donation is requested.

> *Also see:* Area Agencies on Aging (page 934)
> Catholic Charities USA (page 935)
> National Association of Community Action Agencies (page 936)
> United Way of America (page 936)

Housing/Lodging Assistance

American Cancer Society Hope Lodges
American Cancer Society
1599 Clifton Road, N.E., Atlanta, GA 30329
(800) 227-2345 or (404) 320-3333
http://www.cancer.org (Web site)

Cancer patients who are undergoing treatment can spend several nights along with their families at an American Cancer Society Hope Lodge free of charge. There are thirteen of these facilities in eleven states. More than two dozen Westin Hotels offer up to six weeks of free accommodations for cancer patients who have to travel considerable distances to receive outpatient care. To learn about eligibility requirements, call the American Cancer Society, which sponsors the program in cooperation with the hotel chain.

National Association of Hospital Hospitality Houses
4915 Auburn Avenue, Suite 303, Bethesda, MD 20814
(800) 542-9730 or (301) 961-3094
http://www.nahhh.org (Web site)
helpinghomes@nahhh.org (e-mail)

More than ninety Hospital Hospitality Houses are located in thirty-three states and the District of Columbia. They offer lodging for families of hospital patients as well as for hospital outpatients.

Job Discrimination

U.S. Equal Employment Opportunity Commission
1801 L Street, N.W., Washington, DC 20507
(800) 669-4000 or (202) 663-4900
http://www.eeoc.gov (Web site)

Calling the toll-free number automatically connects you to your nearest EEOC field office, which can advise you of your rights under the Americans with Disabilities Act and explain how to file a complaint against an employer.

Also contact your local human rights commission. You'll find the number in the government listings section of the white pages.

Also see (in Appendix A):
Cancervive
   (for referrals to attorneys experienced in employment-discrimination cases)
Lymphoma Foundation of America
   (for referrals to attorneys experienced in employment-discrimination cases)
National Coalition for Cancer Survivorship
   (for information)
Patient Advocate Foundation
   (for free legal counseling)

Medical Insurance

Medicare and Medicaid
Health Care Financing Administration
7500 Security Boulevard, Baltimore, MD 21244-1850
(800) 638-6833 (Medicare)
(410) 786-3000 (Medicaid)
http://www.hcfa.gov (Web site)
Question@hcfa.gov (e-mail)

You can call the HCFA, better known as "Hick-Fah," with general questions about Medicare or Medicaid. Request a free copy of the

Medicare Handbook or the *Medicaid Overview,* which explain the programs. These and many other publications are available on-line.

Veterans' Health Benefits
Department of Veterans Affairs Division of Veterans' Benefits and Services
Veterans Health Administration Cancer Program
(800) 827-1000
http://www.va.gov (Web site)
g.vhacss@forum.va.gov (e-mail)

Military veterans can call the Department of Veterans Affairs with questions regarding eligibility for medical care. The toll-free number above routes you directly to your regional VA office.

Civilian Health and Medical Program of the Department of Veterans Affairs
P.O. Box 65024, Denver, CO 80206-9024
(800) 733-8387 or (303) 331-7670
http://www.va.govhac/champva/champva.html (Web site)

CHAMPVA is the health-benefits program for dependents of veterans who became ill or permanently disabled while on active military duty.

Tricare Management Activity
16401 East Centretech Parkway, Aurora, CO 80011-9043
(303) 676-3526
http://www.tricare.osd.mil (Web site)
HelpDesk@tma.osd.mil (e-mail)

TMA, administered by the Department of Defense, insures military retirees and their dependents, as well as families of deceased servicemen or those on active military duty. (Formerly CHAMPUS: Civilian Health and Medical Program of the Department of the Uniformed Services.)

National Association of Insurance Commissioners
120 West 12th Street, Suite 1100, Kansas City, MO 64105-1925
(816) 842-3600
http://www.naic.org (Web site)

If you're unable to resolve a dispute with your medical insurer, contact your state insurance regulator. For the address and telephone number, call the National Association of Insurance Commissioners or tap into its Web site.

U.S. Department of Labor
Pension and Welfare Benefits Administration Division of Technical
Assistance and Inquiries
200 Constitution Ave., N.W., Room N-5619, Washington, D.C. 20210
(202) 219-8776 or (800) 998-7542 (toll-free publications hotline)
http://www.dol.gov/dol/pwba (Web site)

Contact the U.S. Department of Labor for information about the Consolidated Omnibus Budget Reconciliation Act (COBRA) and the Health Insurance Portability and Accountability Act (HIPAA), which allow ex-employees of companies with twenty or more workers to purchase group coverage for themselves and their families for up to eighteen months, and sometimes longer.

Also see: American Amputee Foundation (page 914)
  (for information)
American Cancer Society (page 907)
  (may intervene on behalf of patients)
Area Agencies on Aging (page 934)
  (assistance resolving insurance disputes)
Blood & Marrow Transplant Newsletter (page 915)
  (for referrals to attorneys specializing in insurance cases)
Cancer Care (page 910)
  (for information)
Cancervive (page 911)
  (for referrals to attorneys specializing in insurance cases)
National Coalition for Cancer Survivorship (page 912)
  (for information)
National Kidney Cancer Association (page 923)
  (may intervene on behalf of patients)
National Marrow Donor Program (page 916)
  (for information)
Patient Advocate Foundation (page 913)
  (for free legal counseling)

Mental-Health Services

American Psychiatric Association

1400 K Street, N.W., Washington, DC 20005

(202) 682-6000

http://www.psych.org (Web site)

apa@psych.org (e-mail)

The American Psychiatric Association's referral line will put you in touch with your local APA chapter, which can refer you to an appropriate psychiatrist.

American Psychological Association

750 First Street, N.E., Washington, DC 20002-4242

(202) 336-5500 or (800) 964-2000

http://www.apa.org/ (Web site)

publiccom@apa.org (e-mail)

The national office will refer you to your state's American Psychological Association affiliate, which can help you find a suitable psychologist. Or call the toll-free number above; the operator will connect you with the referral system in your area.

National Association of Social Workers

750 First Street, N.E., Suite 700, Washington, DC 20002-4241

(800) 638-8799 or (202) 408-8600

http://www.naswdc.org (Web site)

Call the NASW's referral service for the names of three social workers who specialize in counseling people with a serious illness.

Also contact your state or county department of mental health. You'll find the number in the government listings section of the white pages.

Also see: American Cancer Society (page 907)

Area Agencies on Aging (page 934)

Catholic Charities USA (page 935)

United Way of America (page 936)

Occupational Therapists/Physical Therapists

American Occupational Therapy Association
4720 Montgomery Lane, Bethesda, MD 20824-1220
(301) 652-2682
http://www.aota.org (Web site)
praoto@aota.org (e-mail)

For the names of certified occupational therapists, contact the AOTA and ask for Direct Mail Service.

American Physical Therapy Association
1111 North Fairfax Street, Alexandria, VA 22314
(703) 684-2782
http://www.apta.org (Web site)

Contact the APTA for the names of licensed physical therapists.

Pain-Management Specialists

American Pain Society
4700 West Lake Avenue, Glenview, IL 60025
(847) 375-4715
http://wwwampainsoc.org (Web site)
info@ampainsoc.org (e-mail)

The American Pain Society, comprised of more than 3,200 pain-management professionals, can refer you to pain centers and clinics near you, including those that specialize in cancer-related pain.

American Society of Anesthesiologists
520 North Northwest Highway, Park Ridge, IL 60068-2573
847-825-5586
http://www.asahq.org (Web site)
mail@asahq.org (e-mail)

This professional organization can refer you to individual pain specialists.

Cancer Information Service
(800) 422-6237
Fax: (301) 402-5874

http://cancernet.nci.nih.gov (Web site)
cancernet@icicb.nci.nih.gov (e-mail)

Among its many referrals, the Cancer Information Service of the National Cancer Institute can direct you to pain-management centers and pain specialists at hospitals.

Commission on Accreditation of Rehabilitation Facilities
4891 East Grant Road, Tucson, AZ 85712
(520) 325-1044
http://www.carf.org (Web site)

Write to CARF and enclose a self-addressed, stamped envelope for a listing of facilities with accredited pain programs.

Physical Therapists

See "Occupational Therapists/Physical Therapists,"
page 946.

Prescription-Drug Patient-Assistance Programs

Pharmaceutical Research and Manufacturers of America
1100 15th Street, N.W., Washington, DC 20005
(202) 835-3400
http://www.phrma.org (Web site)

PhRMA publishes an annual directory of prescription-drug patient-assistance programs sponsored by about fifty pharmaceutical companies. The free booklet lists the name, address, and telephone number of each manufacturer, the name of its program, the drug(s) covered, and eligibility requirements. You can also view this directory on PhRMA's Web site.

State Pharmaceutical Assistance Programs
Eleven states currently support prescription-drug programs for people who cannot otherwise afford necessary medications.

Connecticut	(860) 832-9265 or (800) 423-5026
Delaware	(302) 651-4400 or (800) 763-9326

Illinois	(217) 524-0435 or (800) 624-2459
Maine	(207) 626-8475
Maryland	(410) 767-5394 or (800) 492-1974
Michigan	(517) 373-8230
New Jersey	(609) 588-7049 or (800) 792-9745
New York	(518) 452-3773 or (800) 332-3742
Pennsylvania	(800) 225-7223
Rhode Island	(401) 277-3330 or (800) 322-2880
Vermont	(802) 241-2880 or (800) 987-2839

Also see (in Appendix A):
American Cancer Society
Leukemia Society of America
National Foundation for Transplants
National Organization for Rare Disorders

Also see (in Appendix B):
National Association of Community Action Agencies

Also see the "Manufacturers' Index" in the Physicians' Desk
Reference, *a medical reference book available in most libraries,
for the names of pharmaceutical companies not included in the
PhRMA directory.*

Pulmonary-Rehabilitation Therapists

American Association of Cardiovascular and Pulmonary Rehabilitation
7611 Elmwood Avenue, Suite 201, Middleton, WI 53562
(608) 831-6989
http://www.aacvpr.org (Web site)
aacvpr@tmahq.com (e-mail)

Contact the AACVPR via telephone or its Web site for referrals to
pulmonary-rehabilitation programs.

Sex Therapists and Counselors

American Association of Sex Educators, Counselors and Therapists
P.O. Box 238, Mt. Vernon, IA 52314-0238
Fax: (319) 895-6203
http://www.aasect.org (Web site)
AASECT@worldnet.att.net (e-mail)

Sending AASECT a self-addressed stamped envelope brings you a list of certified sex therapists and counselors in your area.

Smoking-Cessation Programs

Most local chapters of both the American Cancer Society and the American Lung Association sponsor low-cost smoking-cessation programs. For referrals to other programs, contact the Cancer Information Service of the National Cancer Institute.

Cancer Information Service
(800) 422-6237
Fax: (301) 402-5874
http://cancernet.nci.nih.gov (Web site)
cancernet@icicb.nci.nih.gov (e-mail)

Fresh Start
American Cancer Society
1599 Clifton Road, N.E., Atlanta, GA 30329
(800) 227-2345 or (404) 320-3333
http://www.cancer.org (Web site)

Freedom from Smoking
American Lung Association
1740 Broadway, New York, NY 10019-4374
(800) 586-4872 or (212) 315-8700
http://www.lungusa.org (Web site)

Speech-Language Pathologists

American Speech-Language-Hearing Association Action
10801 Rockville Pike, Rockville, MD 20852-3279

(800) 321-2742 or (301) 897-5700
http://www.asha.org (Web site)
actioncenter@asha.org (e-mail)

Call ASHA for referrals to certified speech-language pathologists.

Transportation to Medical Appointments

The following organizations may be able to arrange transportation to medical appointments; others reimburse patients for transportation expenses.

> American Cancer Society (page 907)
> Area Agencies on Aging (page 934)
> Catholic Charities USA (page 935)
> Leukemia Society of America (page 925)
> National Association of Community Action Agencies (page 936)
> United Way of America (page 936)

Index